Modified Glasgow Coma Scale for Infants and Children

	Child	Infant	Score
Eye opening	Spontaneous	Spontaneous	4
	To verbal stimuli	To verbal stimuli	3
	To pain only	To pain only	2
	No response	No response	1
Verbal response	Oriented, appropriate	Coos and babbles	5
	Confused	Irritable cries	4
	Inappropriate words	Cries to pain	3
	Incomprehensible words or nonspecific sounds	Moans to pain	2
	No response	No response	1
Motor response	Obeys commands	Moves spontaneously and purposefully	6
	Localizes painful stimulus	Withdraws to touch	5
	Withdraws in response to pain	Withdraws in response to pain	4
	Flexion in response to pain	Decorticate posturing (abnormal flexion) in response to pain	3
	Extension in response to pain	Decerebrate posturing (abnormal extension) in response to pain	2
	No response	No response	1

From Hazinski MF: *Nursing care of the critically ill child,* ed 2, St Louis, 1992, Mosby; modified from Davis RJ et al: Head and spinal cord injury. In Rogers MC, editor: *Textbook of pediatric intensive care,* Baltimore, 1987, Williams & Wilkins; James H, Anas N, Perkin RM: *Brain insults in infants and children,* New York, 1985, Grune & Stratton; and Morray JP et al: Coma scale for use in brain-injured children, *Critical Care Med* 12:1018, 1984.

Signs of Poor Systemic Perfusion

Tachycardia
Mottled color, pallor
Cool skin, prolonged capillary refill
Oliguria (urine volume <1-2 ml/kg/hour)
Diminished intensity of peripheral pulses
Metabolic acidosis
Change in responsiveness
Late: Hypotension, bradycardia

From Hazinski MF: *Nursing care of the critically ill child,* ed 2, St Louis, 1992, Mosby.

Signs of Respiratory Distress and Potential Respiratory Failure

Tachypnea, tachycardia
Retractions
Nasal flaring
Grunting
Stridor or wheezing
Mottled color
Change in responsiveness
Hypoxemia, hypercarbia, decreased Hgb saturations
LATE: Poor air entry, weak cry
        Apnea or gasping
        Deterioration in systemic perfusion
        Bradycardia

From Hazinski MF: *Nursing care of the critically ill child,* ed 2, St Louis, 1992, Mosby.

Manual of
Pediatric
Critical Care

Mary Fran Hazinski, MSN, RN

Division of Trauma
Departments of Surgery and Pediatrics
Vanderbilt Children's Hospital
Vanderbilt University Medical School
Nashville, Tennessee

With 200 illustrations

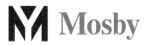 Mosby

St. Louis   Baltimore   Boston   Carlsbad   Naples   New York   Philadelphia   Portland
London   Madrid   Mexico City   Singapore   Sydney   Tokyo   Toronto   Wiesbaden

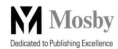
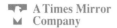

Mosby

Dedicated to Publishing Excellence

A Times Mirror
Company

Publisher: Nancy L. Coon
Editor: Barry J. Bowlus
Developmental Editor: Cynthia A. Anderson
Project Manager: Deborah Vogel
Project Specialist: Mary E. Drone
Designer: Bill Drone
Manufacturing Manager: Debbie Larocca
Cover Photo: Dan Grogan, Uniphoto

Composition by Clarinda Company
Lithography/color film by Clarinda Company
Printing/binding by R. R. Donnelley & Sons Company

Mosby, Inc.
11830 Westline Industrial Drive
St. Louis, Missouri 63146

International Standard Book Number 0-8151-4230-7

98 99 00 01 02 / 9 8 7 6 5 4 3 2 1

"Teachers affect eternity; they can never tell where their influence stops."
From: Henry Brooks Adams

To the outstanding teachers who have enriched my life, and the lives of many, including:
Farouk Idriss, MD *(In Memorium)*
William H. Tooley, MD *(In Memorium)*
Michele Ilbawi, MD
Sister Noreen McGowan, FSM, MSN, RN, PNP
Irene Riddle, RN, MSN, PhD

Also to the critical care nurses and physicians who teach, learn, and strive to heal children and families every day.

Finally, to Tom and Michael

Contributors and Reviewers

William Banner, Jr., MD

Pediatric Intensivist
Associate Medical Director
Children's Hospital at Saint Francis
Clinical Associate Professor of Pediatrics
University of Oklahoma College of Medicine
Tulsa, Oklahoma

John A. Barnard, MD

Associate Professor of Pediatrics
Director, Division of Pediatric Gastroenterology
Vanderbilt University Medical Center
Nashville, Tennessee

Derek Bruce, MD

Director, Pediatric Neurosurgery
Pediatric Neurosurgical Institute
North Texas Children's Hospital
Medical City Dallas Hospital
Clinical Associate Professor
Department of Neurosurgery
University of Texas Southwestern Medical Center
Dallas, Texas

Thomas Coates, MD

Associate Professor of Pediatrics and Pathology
Division of Hematology/Oncology
Children's Hospital of Los Angeles
Los Angeles, California

Jayant K. Deshpande, MD

Associate Professor of Pediatrics and
    Anesthesiology
Director, Pediatric Critical Care and Anesthesia
Vanderbilt Children's Hospital
Vanderbilt University Medical Center
Nashville, Tennessee

Joann Eland, RN, PhD, NAP, FAAN

Associate Professor
College of Nursing
University of Iowa
Iowa City, Iowa

Jade Floridas, RN, MSN

Clinical Specialist, Pediatric Critical Care
Vanderbilt University Children's Hospital
Nashville, Tennessee

Thomas A. Hazinski, MD

Professor, Department of Pediatrics
Vandervilt University Medical Center
Nashville, Tennessee

Cathy L. Headrick, RN, MS

Advanced Practice Nurse
Department of Neurosurgery
Children's Medical Center of Dallas
Dallas, Texas

John B. Pietsch, MD

Associate Professor
Department of Pediatric Surgery
Vanderbilt University Medical Center
Nashville, Tennessee

Joshua B. Pietsch, RN, BSN

Medical Intensive Care Unit
Vanderbilt University Medical Center
Nashville, Tennessee

Deborah Whitlock, RN, BSN

Pediatric Critical Care Unit
Vanderbilt Children's Hospital
Nashville, Tennessee

James Whitlock, MD

Chief, Division of Pediatric
    Hematology/Oncology
Associate Professor of Pediatrics
Vanderbilt University Medical Center
Nashville, Tennessee

Please also refer to the Acknowledgments in the Preface for a listing of contributors and reviewers to *Nursing Care of the Critically Ill Child,* edition 2, St. Louis, 1992, Mosby. That book provided the basis for the development of the *Manual.*

Preface

The care of seriously ill or injured children and their families becomes more challenging every day. Complex illnesses, multi-system injury, advanced technology, and children and families with special needs ensure that bedside nurses will have plenty to do and limited time in which to do it. In addition, the entire health care system continues to wrestle with the issues of cost and quality. Ideals can be sorely tested in situations in which time and resources are limited. This book is designed to enable the bedside nurse to keep essential information about patient care at his or her fingertips.

The emphasis in this text is *concise* presentation of core information, with many visual and memory aids, including boxes, tables, and illustrations. These visual aids should ensure that important facts can be gleaned in a few minutes.

Each chapter begins with a list of "Pearls"—points that the nurse should keep in mind whenever dealing with the problems discussed in that chapter. The "organ" or "system" chapters are divided into the same five sections as the large text *(Nursing Care of the Critically Ill Child, edition 2, St. Louis, 1992, Mosby):* Essential Anatomy and Physiology, Common Clinical Problems, Postoperative or Postprocedure Care, Specific Diagnoses, and Diagnostic Studies.

This book is *not* designed to provide a comprehensive reference of anatomy, physiology, and pathophysiology. It does not provide reference citations for every point made. There was a conscious decision to present facts rather than references. For more detailed information, the reader is referred to the publications listed as Suggested Readings at the end of each chapter and to the larger text.

I am constantly impressed by the enthusiasm and commitment that nurses bring to the care of critically ill or injured children and their families. I hope that the information contained in this book will be helpful at the bedside. However, the best thing the nurse brings to the bedside is not a book—it is the determination to optimize the care and comfort he or she provides for every child and family.

Acknowledgments

This manual developed as a condensed revision of the second edition of *Nursing Care of the Critically Ill Child.* Although a significant amount of new information is included in this text, the second edition provides the foundation. Therefore I would again like to express my appreciation for the work of the contributors to that book: William Banner, Jr., MD; John A. Barnard, MD; Kathy Byington, RN, MSN; Thomas D. Coates, MD; Joann Eland, RN, PhD, NAP, FAAN; Jeanette E. Kennedy, RN, BS; Linda Lewandowski, RN, PhD; Margaret Shandor Miles, RN, PhD, FAAN; Pam Pieper, RNC, MSN; Cathy H. Rosenthal, RN, MN, CCRN; Denise A. Sadowski, RN, MSN; Treesa Soud, RN, BSN; Gregory M. Susla, Pharm D; Julie Kay Wall, RN, MSN; Joan B. Warner, RN, MSN; Holly Weeks Webster, RN, MS; Deborah W. Whitlock, RN, BSN; James A. Whitlock, MD; and Jean Homrighausen Zander, RN, MSN.

Reviewers for the second edition of *Nursing Care of the Critically Ill Child* also added substantially to the focus and clarity of that book and provided the basis for many of the changes in the *Manual.* These reviewers include William Berman, Jr.; Cecily Lynn Betz, RN, PhD; Vicki Brinsko, RN, CIC; Ellen Cram, RN, MA, CCRN; Barbara Gill, RN, MN; Thomas A. Hazinski, MD; Michel N. Ilbawi, MD; Anthony Kilroy, MD; Eric Marsh, RN, MSN, CCRN, CEN; John B. Pietsch, MD; and Arno Zaritsky, MD.

Contents

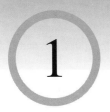

Children Are Different

Pearls

- Children are physically, physiologically, and emotionally immature and differ from adults in several important ways.
- Clinicians must be able to determine at a glance if child *"looks good"* or *"looks bad"* based on color, systemic perfusion, level of activity and responsiveness, position of comfort, and (in infants) feeding behavior.
- *Normal* vital signs aren't always *appropriate* vital signs for the seriously ill or injured child—tachycardia and tachypnea are usually more appropriate than "normal" rates.
- Signs of deterioration may be subtle in children, and decompensation may occur rapidly—be prepared to support ventilation and perfusion.
- Children are very dependent on heart rate to maintain cardiac output; bradycardia is often associated with inadequate cardiac output.
- Hypotension may be only a late sign of (decompensated) shock.
- Small compromises in airway radius caused by tongue obstruction, edema, mucus, or airway constriction can critically increase resistance to airflow and work of breathing.
- Fluid intake must be controlled and totaled, and the child's fluid balance must be monitored at all times.

Introduction

Many clinical signs and symptoms of disease or organ system failure are the same in children and adults, but some manifestations and complications are unique to children. The child's cardiovascular, pulmonary, and neurologic systems often operate with little reserve; and the child's condition is likely to deteriorate when injury, disease, or distress is present. Decompensation must be anticipated whenever the child is severely ill or injured.

Psychosocial Development

Children are emotionally and cognitively immature. Their immaturity will affect their comprehension of and response to illness or injury. The nurse must be able to approach and support the child in a manner appropriate for the child's development (see Chapter 2). The child may have difficulty localizing or quantifying pain; thus thorough assessment is required to identify, quantify and treat the child's pain (see Chapter 3).

General Assessment

Initial Impression: "Looks Good" vs. "Looks Bad"

Evaluate both qualitative and quantitative information to determine if the child *looks good or looks bad.*

1. *Color:* Color should be consistent over trunk and extremities. Mucous membranes, nailbeds, palms of hands, and soles of feet should be pink. Cardiorespiratory distress can produce mottling, pallor, or duskiness. Central cyanosis may be only a late or inconsistent sign of hypoxemia.

2. *Systemic perfusion:* Extremities should be warm with strong peripheral pulses. If the environment is warm, capillary refill should be brisk (≤2 sec). Cool extremities with weak peripheral pulses and prolonged capillary refill (despite warm environment) may indicate cardiorespiratory distress.

3. *Level of activity and responsiveness:* Evaluate child's responsiveness in light of age and clinical condition—look for unusual *irritability* or *lethargy* as a sign of cardiorespiratory distress or neurologic deterioration. *A decreased response to painful stimulus is abnormal* and, if it is a new clinical response, requires immediate investigation. Evaluate responsiveness in light of psychosocial development.

   a. Infants should make eye contact with and be comforted by parents/primary caretakers; older infants should protest when separated from parents/primary caretakers and should resist examination by strangers.

   b. Toddlers should protest when separated from parents/primary caretakers; should resist placement in supine position ("NO!"); and should speak in words, short phrases.

   c. Preschoolers should be able to point to painful areas of the body, should be comforted by parents, should speak in short sentences, and should know own name and name of all family members.

   d. School-age children should have good concept of time intervals and body parts and functions and should be able to converse in sentences. They can be comforted by health care providers. They are typically uncomfortable with focus on body.

   e. Adolescents are typically intensely private. They should be able to discuss their clinical condition and plan of care and to demonstrate short- and long-term memory.

4. *Position of comfort:* The child in respiratory distress often prefers to sit upright, and even the infant may protest when placed supine.

5. *Feeding behavior:* Failure to suck and swallow vigorously (infants) or intolerance of tube feeding may indicate cardiorespiratory or neurologic deterioration.

Evaluation of Vital Signs

Vital signs must always be interpreted in light of the child's clinical condition. *Normal vital signs aren't always appropriate vital signs for the ill or injured child.* Tachycardia and tachypnea are appropriate in the presence of serious illness or injury; thus normal vital signs under these conditions may well indicate deterioration—respiratory or cardiac arrest may be imminent. Small quantitative changes in vital signs may be significant.

The heart and respiratory rates of the child are more rapid than those of the adult and *should* be rapid in the presence of distress (Tables 1-1 and 1-2). The blood pressure is normally lower in children than in adults (Table 1-3) and may be normal, despite the presence of shock.

- Normal median (50th percentile for age) systolic blood pressure in the child >1 year can be estimated from the following formula:

  50th Percentile Systolic BP (mm Hg)
  $$= 90 \text{ mm Hg} + (2 \times \text{age in years})$$

Table 1-1
Normal Heart Rates in Children*

Age	Awake Heart Rate (per min)	Sleeping Heart Rate (per min)
Neonate	100-180	80-160
Infant (6 mo)	100-160	75-160
Toddler	80-110	60-90
Preschooler	70-110	60-90
School-age child	65-110	60-90
Adolescent	60-90	50-90

From Hazinski MF: *Nursing care of the critically ill child*, ed 2, St Louis, 1992, Mosby.
*Always consider patient's normal range and clinical condition. Heart rate will normally increase with fever or stress.

- A low systolic blood pressure (5th percentile) for age >1 year can be estimated from the following formula:

5th Percentile Systolic BP (mm Hg)
= 70 mmHg + (2 × age in years).

Table 1-2
Normal Respiratory Rates in Children*

Age	Rate (breaths per min)
Infants	30-60
Toddlers	24-40
Preschoolers	22-34
School-age children	18-30
Adolescents	12-16

From Hazinski MF: *Nursing care of the critically ill child,* ed 2, St Louis, 1992, Mosby.
*Your patient's normal range should always be considered. Also, the child's respiratory rate is expected to increase in the presence of fever or stress.

Table 1-3
Normal Blood Pressures in Children*

Age	Systolic Pressure (mm Hg)	Diastolic Pressure (mm Hg)
Birth (12 hr, <1000 g)	39-59	16-36
Birth (12 hours, 3 kg weight)	50-70	25-45
Neonate (96 hr)	60-90	20-60
Infant (6 mo)	87-105	53-66
Toddler (2 yr)	95-105	53-66
School age (7 yr)	97-112	57-71
Adolescent (15 yr)	112-128	66-80

From Hazinski MF: *Nursing care of the critically ill child,* ed 2, St. Louis, 1992, Mosby.
Estimated systolic blood pressure norms (for infants and children beyond 1 year of age):
- 50th percentile systolic blood pressure = 90 mm Hg + (2× age in years)
- 5th percentile systolic blood pressure = 70 mm Hg + (2× age in years)
*Blood pressure ranges taken from the following sources:
Neonate: Versmold H et al: Aortic blood pressure during the first 12 hours of life in infants with birth weight 610-4220 gms, *Pediatrics* 67:107, 1981. 10th-90th percentile ranges used.
Others: Horan MJ chairman: Task Force on Blood Pressure Control in Children, report of the second task force on blood pressure in children, *Pediatrics,* 79:1, 1987. 50th-90th percentile ranges indicated.

Noninvasive oscillometric blood pressure monitors may fail to reflect the development of hypotension in unstable children and may overestimate the blood pressure. A sphygmomanometer (mercury manometer) with cuff and stethoscope may underestimate blood pressure in the hypotensive child. An intraarterial catheter joined to an appropriately calibrated, zeroed, and leveled transducer and fluid-filled tubing provides the "gold standard" measurement of arterial blood pressure. This is the preferred method of arterial pressure monitoring when the child is unstable, particularly if vascular access for blood sampling is required.

Evaluation and Plan of Care

When encountering the seriously ill or injured child, the health care team should discuss the three most likely causes of deterioration in that child *each day* and discuss the plan for care if the deterioration occurs. This plan enables the team to function efficiently and effectively if the child deteriorates, and such discussion should be part of all morning and evening team rounds.

General Characteristics

Thermoregulation

Infants and young children have large surface area-to-volume ratios and lose a great deal of heat to the environment. Cold-stressed neonates can't shiver to generate heat; thus they must create heat in a process that consumes energy, increasing oxygen requirements. Cold stress may cause deterioration in unstable infants.

The following are important points to remember regarding thermoregulation:

- Monitor both skin and rectal temperatures in newborns and young infants and keep the child warm (use warming lights as needed). Evaluate skin temperature in light of rectal temperature.
- Hypothermia may be a sign of infection, cold stress, neurologic dysfunction, or a compromise in skin perfusion (including shock or sepsis). Poor perfusion may produce core body *fever* and cool skin temperature because intense peripheral vasoconstriction prevents dissemination of body heat.

- Warm blood products (using approved water bath) administered to unstable infants.

Fluid Requirements and Fluid Therapy

The absolute volume of fluids administered to children is very small and must be carefully regulated and totaled to prevent fluid overload. Fluid requirements can be estimated using a weight or body surface area-based formula (Table 1-4). However, the actual fluid administration rate must be *individualized* at a daily (or more frequent) interval based on the child's fluid balance and clinical condition.

Table 1-4
Maintenance Fluid and Caloric Requirements in Children

Weight	Formula
Body Weight Daily Maintenance Formula	
Neonate (<72 hr)	60-100 ml/kg
0-10 kg	100 ml/kg
11-20 kg	1000 ml for first 10 kg + 50 ml/kg for kg 11-20
21-30 kg	1500 ml for first 20 kg + 25 ml/kg for kg 21-30
Body Weight Hourly Maintenance Formula	
1-10 kg	4 ml/kg/hr
11-20 kg	40 ml/hr for first 10 kg + 2 ml/kg/hr for kg 11-20
21-30 kg	60 ml/hr for first 20 kg + 1 ml/kg/hr for kg 21-30
Body Surface Area Formula	
1500 ml/m² body surface area/day	
Insensible Water Losses	
300 ml/m² body surface area	
Daily Caloric Requirements by Age	
Infant	100-150 Calories/kg
1-2 yr Toddler/Preschooler	90-100 Calories/kg
School-age	70-80 Calories/kg
10-12 yr	50-60 Calories/kg

*Ill children (with disease, surgery, fever, or pain) may require additional calories above the maintenance value, and comatose children may require fewer calories (because of lack of movement).
From Hazinski MF: *Nursing care of the critically ill child*, ed 2, St Louis, 1992, Mosby.

1. Ensure that intravascular volume and systemic perfusion are adequate.
2. If intravascular volume is adequate, fluid administration may be limited to less than "maintenance" requirements in the presence of:
   a. Cardiac failure
   b. Respiratory failure
   c. Increased intracranial pressure (or head injury)
   d. Renal failure
3. Insensible water losses are calculated at 300 ml/m² body surface area/day.
4. Fever increases insensible water losses 0.42 ml/kg/hr/° C elevation in temperature above 37° C.
5. Measure child's weight daily and report significant weight gain or loss to a physician.

Fluids administered to replace excessive output should match that output in both volume and electrolyte content (e.g., gastric drainage is low in sodium and high in potassium, but ileostomy drainage is high in both sodium and potassium). Normal saline and lactated Ringer's solution are considered to be isotonic to serum, so these fluids should be used for bolus treatment of hypovolemia. Maintenance fluid requirements are generally administered in the form of a glucose/0.45% Na Cl solution. If intravenous fluids are used to provide maintenance fluids and nutrition, they must contain adequate calories, protein, and fat (see Nutrition).

Monitor child's fluid intake (include fluid used to flush monitoring lines and dilute medications) and output closely; evaluate fluid balance at least hourly. In a well-hydrated child urine output should average:

- 2 ml/kg/hour in neonate
- 1 ml/kg/hour in child
- 0.5 ml/kg/hour (or minimum of 25 ml/hr) in adolescent

Note: If incontinence or wound drainage is present, diapers and linens should be weighed to estimate fluid output (1 g weight gain equals approximately 1 ml fluid output).

Water constitutes a higher percentage of body weight in children than in adolescents or adults, and dehydration can rapidly develop in young children if fluid intake is inadequate or output is excessive. Signs of dehydration in the child are similar to those observed in adults. Peripheral circulatory compromise develops with 7% to 10% weight loss in an infant or child but with only 5% to 7% weight loss in an adolescent or adult because a smaller percentage of the adolescent's weight is water. Decompensated (hypotensive) shock may result from more than 10% weight loss in the infant or child with isotonic dehydration or 7% to 10% weight loss in the adolescent with isotonic dehydration.

Nutrition

Infants and children have a high metabolic rate and thus require more calories per kilogram for basal metabolism and cell growth than adults (see Table 1-4). During serious illness or injury, high caloric intake is usually required and can't be provided using 5% to 10% dextrose solutions. Therefore plans must be made during the initial days of the child's hospitalization to provide adequate nutrition (from glucose, protein, and fat) until oral intake is resumed.

Electrolyte Balance

Normal serum electrolyte concentrations are the same for adults and children. Common electrolyte imbalances in critically ill or injured children include the following:

Sodium Sodium is the major intravascular ion that affects extracellular osmolality.

Hyponatremia

Causes Causes are sodium (Na^+) loss (e.g., vomiting, diarrhea), or free water gain (including syndrome of inappropriate antidiuretic hormone secretion[SIADH]), adrenal cortical hyperplasia, or improper mixing of infant formula from powder. Severe hyperglycemia depresses serum Na^+ to under 135 mEq/L, *producing a fall of 1.6 mEq/L for every 100 mg/dl rise in glucose above 200 mg/dl;* as hyperglycemia is corrected, hyponatremia should also correct (serum Na^+ should rise 1.6 mEq/L for every 100 mg/dl fall in serum glucose concentration).

Complications (Rapid Fall in Serum Sodium Concentration) Extravascular fluid shift, cerebral edema, seizures, intracranial hemorrhage

Treatment Correct cause: eliminate free water (diuresis or fluid restriction if SIADH present). Ad-

minister 3% saline (3 to 5 ml/kg over 20 to 60 min) if neurologic symptoms develop.

Hypernatremia

Causes Dehydration, free water loss, sodium gain

Complications (Rapid Rise in Serum Sodium Concentration) Intravascular fluid shift develops as serum sodium rises. Note that rapid rehydration may produce extravascular fluid shift and cerebral edema, seizures, intracranial hemorrhage.

Treatment Administer fluid to restore intravascular volume and attempt to lower serum sodium slowly.

Potassium Potassium is the major intracellular cation. It affects cell resting membrane potential and affects excitability of muscle, including the heart (can affect the electrocardiogram [ECG]).

Hypokalemia

Causes Dilution, inadequate potassium (K^+) intake, excessive potassium loss (e.g., associated with administration of drugs such as furosemide or carbenicillin) or intracellular potassium shift (alkalosis or a rise in serum pH), hyperaldosteronism, and some renal tubular deficits

Complications Complications include arrhythmias, decreased myocardial contractility; ECG: low-voltage T wave, development of U-wave, then prolonged Q-T interval. Paralytic ileus may also develop.

Treatment Administer potassium supplement (usually 0.5 to 1 mEq/kg intravenously over 2 to 3 hours).

Hyperkalemia

Causes Reduced potassium excretion (e.g., renal failure), hemolysis, congenital adrenal hyperplasia, excessive potassium administration or intracellular potassium shift (acidosis or a fall in serum pH); may also develop as part of tumor lysis syndrome

Complications May produce arrhythmias; ECG: high-voltage T-wave, increased P-R interval, widened QRS, ventricular arrhythmias, heart block, or cardiac arrest

Treatment Stabilize myocardium (calcium gluconate: 60 to 100 mg/kg), shift potassium into cells (sodium bicarbonate, glucose, or glucose plus insulin), bind potassium in gut (kayexalate enema), exchange transfusion or dialysis.

Chloride   Chloride is the principle anion in both intravascular and gastric fluid. It moves passively with sodium.

Hypochloremia

Causes   Vomiting, diuretic therapy, cystic fibrosis

Complications   Aciduria can develop with hypochloremia associated with dehydration; hypochloremia can result in excretion of hydrogen and potassium ions in urine with resultant hypochloremic, hypokalemic alkalosis.

Treatment   Administration of sodium cloride (NaCl), ammonium chloride, or potassium chloride

Hyperchloremia   Not often observed in pediatric intensive care unit (PICU)

Calcium   Calcium affects the strength of muscle contraction. Calcium balance is closely regulated by parathyroid hormone (PTH), and the calcium concentration is inversely related to the serum phosphate concentration. The active part of the total calcium is the *ionized* calcium.

Hypocalcemia (Particularly Ionized Hypocalcemia)

Causes   Sepsis, alkalosis, hypomagnesemia, administration of citrate-phosphate-dextran-preserved blood; may also be observed with hyperphosphatemia (e.g., with tumor lysis syndrome), rickets, nephrosis, and in infants fed cow's milk

Complications   Reduced myocardial contractility, arrhythmias; ECG: increased Q-T interval

Treatment   Administer calcium (CaCl or Ca-Gluconate) supplement by slow intravenous (IV) push. If hypocalcemia is caused by hyperphosphatemia, the phosphate must be reduced.

Hypercalcemia

Causes   Excessive intake, hyperparathyroidism, hypophosphatemia, secretion of parathormone-like substance in some malignancies. Hypercalcemia is exacerbated in the presence of hypoalbuminemia.

Complications   Polyuria and dehydration, arrhythmias, nausea, anorexia, vomiting. Digitalis effects are amplified.

Treatment   Saline administration until diuresis occurs. If serum calcium is greater than 15 mg/dl, administer saline plus furosemide. IV phosphate (0.5 to 1 mmol/kg over 12 hours), calcitonin (3 to 6 U/kg IV every 24 hours), or ethelynediamine tetraacetic (EDTA) acid may also be administered.

Phosphate   Serum phosphate concentration is influenced by PTH and is inversely related to the serum calcium concentration.

Hypophosphatemia

Causes   Excessive renal phosphate losses (e.g., vitamin D–resistant rickets), phosphate-binding antacids, diabetic ketoacidosis

Complications   Neurologic symptoms (including irritability, weakness, confusion, and possible seizures)

Treatment   Oral phosphate supplements (1 to 5 g/day) every 4 hours plus vitamin D

Hyperphosphatemia

Causes   Tumor lysis syndrome, rhabdomyolysis, infants fed cow's milk, chronic renal failure

Complications   May cause refractory hypocalcemia

Treatment   Oral phosphate binder (e.g., amphogel)

Magnesium   Magnesium is an intracellular cation that activates intracellular enzyme systems and also affects protein and carbohydrate metabolism. Magnesium regulation is tied to calcium regulation and also to potassium balance.

Hypomagnesemia

Causes   Decreased magnesium intake, increased gastrointestinal losses of magnesium (e.g., malabsorption), impaired renal function (decreased renal conservation of magnesium)

Complications   May cause refractory hypocalcemia, neuromuscular irritability, and hypokalemia

Treatment   Magnesium supplementation

Hypermagesemia   Rarely a problem in PICU

Glucose   Glucose is a source of energy and is required for optimal cardiovascular and neurologic function. Infants have high glucose needs and low glycogen stores; thus they can rapidly become hypoglycemic. *Hyper*glycemia, on the other hand, may be harmful to the injured or hypoxic brain or heart (e.g., during or immediately following resuscitation).

ıse rhythms: Cardiac rhythm associ-
with loss of central pulses. Cardiac
ession must be performed until perfus-
ythm is restored. Only a few specific
ns require identification, since their
ıce influences therapeutic decisions.

*ıseless ventricular tachycardia/ ven-
ular fibrillation:* Treatment includes
ıbrillation (up to three times in rapid
cession), followed by administration
epinephrine, lidocaine, and possibly
tylium (in drug-shock-drug-shock
ern) if necessary.

ıctromechanical dissociation: Narrow
S complexes associated with absence
ıulses. Treatable causes (e.g., severe
ıoxemia or acidosis, severe hypo-
ımia, tension pneumothorax, cardiac
ıponade, profound hypothermia) must
ıdentified and eliminated.

ıstole: Provide CPR and epinephrine

ıt and Resuscitation

and outcome of cardiopulmonary
ıldren differs from that observed in
ısult, the priorities of pediatric resus-
ı from adult resuscitation. In adults
is most often a *primary* event, caused
ı arrhythmia; thus the treatment of
ıbrillation. Prompt basic life support,
and advanced life support can result
ıup to 30% or more of adult victims of
ırdiac arrest, and most survivors are
ı intact.

ı cardiac arrest is usually a *secondary*
ıg progressive deterioration in respi-
ıiovascular function and associated
ıfact, in children respiratory arrest
ımore commonly than cardiac arrest;
arrest is effectively treated, cardiac
prevented, and survival is high.

ıiac arrest occurs in children, the ter-
rhythm is most often bradycardia,
ısses to asystole; once *pulseless*
is present, survival averages 7% to
ıports, and most survivors are neuro-
ıstated. Therefore the child in car-
distress requires prompt assistance
ın and support of perfusion so that

cardiac arrest is prevented. If ventricular tachycardia or fibrillation is present, it must be identified
and treated. For further information regarding resuscitation, please see Chapter 5.

Factors Influencing Stroke Volume

Stroke volume in all ages is influenced by cardiac
preload, as well as by ventricular contractility, afterload, and compliance. Although subtle differences exist between pediatric and adult ventricular
function, the principles of treatment of shock and
manipulation of stroke volume are the same in children and adults.

- *Preload:* Presystolic stretch of ventricular
  fibers. To a point, as the fibers are stretched,
  strength of contraction increases. Preload is
  increased through volume administration to
  increase ventricular end-diastolic ("filling")
  pressure.
- *Contractility:* Strength/efficiency of myocardial contraction. Correction of hypoxemia,
  acidosis, and electrolyte imbalances and administration of inotropic agents may increase
  contractility.
- *Afterload:* Ventricular wall stress/impedance
  to ventricular ejection. Afterload can be
  reduced through administration of vasodilators and increased through administration of
  vasoconstrictors.
- *Compliance:* Distensibility of the ventricles.
  This influences the relationship between
  volume administered and ventricular end-
  diastolic pressure generated. Compliance
  may be increased with vasodilator therapy;
  thus stroke volume improves at the same
  filling pressure.

Response to Catecholamines

There are some differences between the pediatric
and adult response to catecholamine administration. However, the major factor influencing the response is the child's underlying clinical condition,
which affects receptor density and clearance of
drugs. Therefore the dose of any vasoactive drug
must be titrated at the bedside, with careful monitoring of patient response and identification of side
and toxic drug effects.

Hypoglycemia

Causes   High glucose needs and low glycogen stores may result in hypoglycemia during periods of stress in infants

Complications   Cardiovascular and neurologic compromise are complications. Tachycardia and poor perfusion may be noted. Profound hypoglycemia may produce seizures (particularly in infants).

Treatment   Treat documented hypoglycemia with glucose infusion rather than repeated glucose bolus; avoid *hyper*glycemia (may compromise neurologic outcome of resuscitation or head injury).

Hyperglycemia

Causes   Diabetes mellitus, excessive glucose administration, stress

Complications   May cause decreased neurologic responsiveness or posthypoxic injury to cells

Treatment   Insulin administration is required for diabetes and occasionally for stress-related diabetes. Glucose concentration in parenteral fluids must be increased gradually to prevent development of hyperglycemia during institution of parenteral nutrition.

Cardiovascular Function

Cardiac Output and Oxygen Delivery

Cardiac output and oxygen delivery in children are higher per kilogram of body weight than in adults, but oxygen consumption is also high (Table 1-5). As a result, infants and children have less oxygen reserve than adults. Anything that increases oxygen consumption or reduces oxygen delivery in infants or children can cause decompensation, including development of metabolic acidosis.

Absolute ca
dren. Normal ca
by m^2 body su
the same in a
L/min/m^2 BSA.
or injured, card
either *adequate*
demands rather

Heart Rate and

Cardiac output
stroke volume. S
and cardiac outp
rate. Cardiac out
heart rate, and ca
rate decreases.

The significa
mined by its eff
treatment is requ
mises systemic
rhythmias can be

1. *Bradyarrhy*
   clinical con
   hypoxia, so
   administrati
   nephrine or
   ternal pacing

2. *Tachyarrhy*
   clinical con
   cardia (SVT
   lar rate >1{
   >160 to 18(
   shock is trea
   cular or intra
   can be estat
   synchronizec

3. *Col*
   ated
   con
   ing
   rhy
   pre
   a.

b.

c.

Cardiac

The etic
arrest in
adults. A
citation
cardiac a
by vent
choice i
defibrill
in survi
prehosp
neurolo

In c
event fe
ratory
hypoxia
occurs
if respi
arrest n
Wh
minal
which
cardia
11% in
logical
diores
with v

Table 1-5
Normal Oxygen Delivery and Consumption in Children

Age	O$_2$ Delivery Index	O$_2$ Co
Newborn	665-1000 ml/min/m^2 BSA	180-27(
Infant	475-700 ml/min/m^2 BSA	160-20(
Child	425-750 ml/min/m^2 BSA	120-23(
Adult	520-720 ml/min/m^2 BSA	110-16(

Note that adult oxygen delivery index is approximately four times oxygen consumption index; adults have gre

Circulating Blood Volume

Circulating blood volume (CBV) constitutes a larger proportion of total body weight in children than in adults. However, the absolute pediatric CBV is small; thus small quantities of blood loss may be clinically significant. Calculate the CBV for all critically ill or injured patients and consider any blood lost or drawn for laboratory analysis as a percentage of that CBV:

- Infant CBV: 80 ml/kg
- Child CBV: 75 ml/kg
- Adolescent CBV: 70 ml/kg

Signs of Cardiovascular Dysfunction

Shock   Shock is present when cardiac output is inadequate to meet metabolic demands. It may be associated with low, normal, or high cardiac output. Hypovolemic shock associated with dehydration or trauma is the most common form of shock observed in children. Cardiogenic and septic shock are the other two types of shock frequently observed in the PICU. General signs of shock are similar in patients of all ages, but these signs may be very subtle or nonspecific in children. Signs include tachycardia, tachypnea, mottled color, diminished peripheral pulses, lactic acidosis, and signs of organ system failure (Box 1-1). *Hypotension develops only as a late sign of shock in children, indicating decompensation.*

Box 1-1

Signs of Poor Systemic Perfusion

Tachycardia
Mottled color, pallor
Cool skin, prolonged capillary refill
Oliguria (urine volume <1-2 ml/kg/hour)
Diminished intensity of peripheral pulses
Metabolic acidosis
Change in responsiveness
Late: Hypotension, bradycardia

From Hazinski MF: *Nursing care of the critically ill child*, ed 2, St Louis, 1992, Mosby.

Treatment of Shock   Ensure appropriate heart rate, maintain adequate intravascular volume relative to the vascular space (administer isotonic crystalloids or colloids in bolus, as needed), support ventricular contractility (inotropic therapy), and manipulate vascular resistance and ventricular compliance as needed with vasoactive agents.

Congestive Heart Failure   Signs of congestive heart failure (CHF) in patients of all ages include the following:

- Signs of adrenergic stimulation: tachycardia, peripheral vasoconstriction, oliguria, and diaphoresis
- Signs of systemic venous congestion: hepatomegaly and periorbital edema. In children jugular venous distension is difficult to appreciate; thus is not a useful sign.
- Signs of pulmonary venous congestion: tachypnea, increased respiratory effort, possible crackles.

Treatment of Congestive Heart Failure   Treatment of CHF requires elimination of excess intravascular fluid and improvement in myocardial function. Fluid administration is limited, and diuresis is provided. A digitalis derivative or other inotropic agent is often administered.

Care of Vascular Monitoring Lines

The small vascular monitoring catheters used in children require continuous irrigation. Regulate and total the volume of fluid administered to flush these catheters with an infusion pump.

Respiratory Function

Components of the Respiratory System

The child's respiratory function is immature, and decompensation can occur rapidly when pulmonary disease or injury is present. Major components of the respiratory system follow.

Central Nervous System (CNS) Control of Breathing   Any condition that depresses CNS function (neurologic injury or disease, sedation, anesthesia) may result in hypoventilation. Infants may develop apnea during periods of respiratory distress.

Airways Pediatric airways are smaller, and the upper airway differs in structure from the adult upper airway. Small pediatric airways may readily become obstructed by mucous accumulation, edema, or airway constriction. Any reduction in airway radius significantly increases airway resistance and work of breathing (Figure 1-1).

The upper airway of the child is configured differently than the upper airway of the adult, making the child more difficult to intubate. In addition, the narrowest part of the child's larynx is at the level of the cricoid cartilage—this area creates a natural seal around endotracheal tubes. Cuffed endotracheal tubes may not be used in children less than 8 years of age for this reason. Proper endotracheal tube size can be estimated from age or body size/length:

- From the child's age:

$$mm\ ET\ tube\ size = \frac{Age\ (years)}{4} + 4$$

- From the size of the child's little finger or little finger nailbed
- From the child's body length, using a length-based reference tape such as the Broselow Resuscitation Tape (marketed by Armstrong, Inc.)

Note that elective intubation of the child in respiratory distress is always preferable to urgent or resuscitative intubation.

If the tube is of proper size, an air leak should be observed following intubation when approximately 25 to 30 cm H_2O inspiratory pressure is created with hand ventilation. If no leak occurs at this pressure, the tube is probably too large; if a leak is observed at lower pressures, the tube is probably too small.

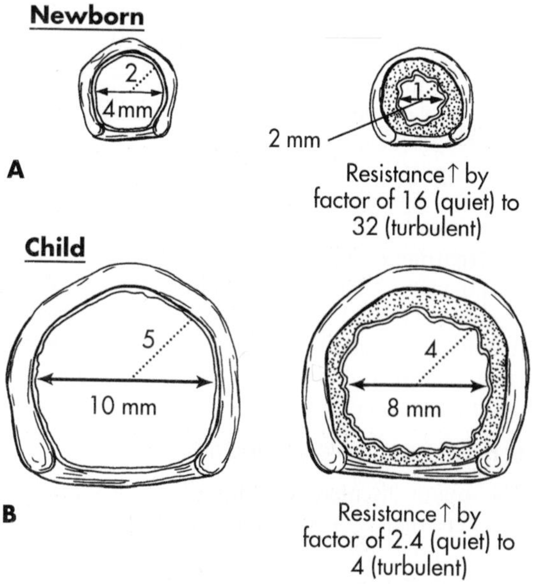

Chest Wall The child's cartilagenous chest wall is extremely compliant. It can retract inward during inspiration if respiratory disease or distress is present. Such retractions can result in a decrease in tidal volume, increased work of breathing, and fatigue.

The compliant pediatric chest should expand easily outward with positive pressure ventilation. *If the chest wall does not rise during positive pressure ventilation, the child is not being adequately ventilated.*

The child can sustain severe chest trauma without rib fractures, since the ribs often bend, rather than break. Rib fractures indicate significant chest trauma. If they are present, intrathoracic injury and pulmonary contusions should be suspected, and intentional trauma should be considered if the child is young.

Breath sounds are easily transmitted through the child's thin chest wall. As a result, adequate breath sounds may be heard despite the presence of

Figure 1-1 Effects of 1-mm of circumferential edema in neonate and young adult. **A,** The neonate possesses a larynx of approximately 4 mm diameter and 2 mm radius. If 1 mm of circumferential edema develops, it will halve the airway radius, reduce cross-section area by 75%, and increase resistance to airflow by a factor of 16 during *quiet* breathing and by a factor of 32 when air flow is turbulent (e.g., during crying or labored breathing). **B,** The young adult possesses a larynx approximately 10 mm in diameter and 5 mm in radius. The 1 mm of circumferential edema will reduce the radius by 20% (from 5 mm to 4 mm), reduce cross-section area by 44%, and increase resistance to air flow by a factor of 2.4 during quiet breathing and by a factor of 4 when air flow is turbulent (e.g., during crying or labored breathing).

atelectasis, pneumothorax, or hemothorax. Such pathology may produce a change in *pitch* of breath sounds rather than a change in intensity of the sounds—use one lung as a control and comparison for the other lung.

Respiratory Muscles   The diaphragm is the chief muscle of inspiration; thus anything that impedes diaphragm excursion in children (e.g., gastric or abdominal distension) is likely to contribute to respiratory distress. An orogastric or nasogastric tube should be inserted if gastric distension impairs ventilation. Intercostal muscles are inadequately developed before school age; thus they are unlikely to contribute to effective ventilation if diaphragm movement impaired.

Lung Tissue   Lung compliance is low in infants and increases progressively during childhood. Neonates and infants may be more susceptible to the development of atelectasis and pulmonary edema than older children. Any child with pulmonary disease or injury may be more likely to develop pulmonary edema if the fluid administration rate is generous (beyond that required to restore or maintain intravascular volume).

Signs of Respiratory Distress

Signs of respiratory distress may be subtle and nonspecific (Box 1-2). Once these signs are observed, potential respiratory failure is present, and therapy is required. If the child fails to respond to therapy or if deterioration or arterial blood gas abnormalities develop, respiratory failure is confirmed.

For further information regarding pulmonary problems and recognition and management of respiratory failure, see Chapter 6.

Neurologic Function

Neurologic Development

At birth, all major structures of the brain and all cranial nerves are present, but dendritic arborization of neurons is incomplete. The infant functions largely at a subcortical level, demonstrating brain stem functions and spinal cord reflexes. Cortical functions such as memory and fine motor coordination cannot be assessed at birth.

The skull is thin and offers inadequate protection for the brain of the infant and young child. The head of the small child is large in comparison to the body; thus, if the infant falls or is propelled (e.g., during a motor vehicle-related crash), it is likely that the head will lead and significant head injury will result.

Skull sutures are not fused until approximately 16 to 18 months of age. As a result, a gradual rise in intracranial volume (such as the development of hydrocephalus after meningitis) may produce an increase in head circumference. For this reason, the head circumference of every infant and toddler should be measured on admission. Skull sutures may separate in older children during the growth of brain tumors. However, skull expansion will not prevent the acute development of increased intracranial pressure following head trauma or an intracranial bleed.

The brain of the young child contains higher water content and less myelin than the brain of the adult, making the child's brain more homogeneous and less compartmentalized. Shear hemorrhages and diffuse brain injury are more common in children with head trauma than in adults. Signs of diffuse injury include loss of consciousness and

---

Box 1-2
Signs of Respiratory Distress and Potential Respiratory Failure

Tachypnea, tachycardia
Retractions
Nasal flaring
Grunting
Stridor or wheezing
Mottled color
Change in responsiveness
Hypoxemia, hypercarbia, decreased Hgb saturations
LATE: Poor air entry, weak cry
      Apnea or gasping
      Deterioration in systemic perfusion
      Bradycardia

From Hazinski MF: *Nursing care of the critically ill child*, ed 2, St Louis, 1992, Mosby.

fixed and dilated pupils. Although these are grim prognostic signs in adults with head injury, they may be associated with complete recovery in children if they respond to initial therapy.

Survival and recovery in children who demonstrated Glasgow Coma Scale (GCS) of 5 to 8 are higher in children than in adults with GCSs of 5 to 8. This may be explained by the fact that coma can be produced by milder injury in children or that children have greater capacity for recovery.

Spinal Cord Injury

Spinal cord injuries (SCIs) are less common in children than in adults because the pediatric spine is elastic and the vertebrae are less likely to fracture under minor stress. SCIs should be suspected in any child with head injuries and multisystem trauma, but they may not be detected with routine x-rays, since children often sustain SCIs without radiographic abnormality (SCIWORA). SCIs resulting from acceleration/deceleration forces typically result in subluxation alone or subluxation with fracture. The most common level of injury changes with patient age:

- All children: Occiput-C2 (respiratory arrest, quadriplegia)
- Infants and Toddlers: C1-C2 or C2-C3 (respiratory arrest, quadriplegia)
- Children 3 to 8 years: C3-C5 (respiratory arrest, quadriplegia)
- Children 9 to 15 years: C4-C7 injuries (high injuries: respiratory arrest, quadriplegia; lower injuries: spontaneous respirations persist, some upper extremity movement may be preserved)

For further information regarding spinal cord injury, see Chapter 12.

Neurologic Evaluation

The child's responsiveness must be evaluated in light of age and clinical condition, and changes in responsiveness over time should be particularly noted. The infant and child should always respond to parents or primary caretakers and painful stimuli—*a decreased response to painful stimulus is abnormal and should be investigated immediately.*

Ability to follow commands is assessed in children older than 2 years by asking the child to hold up two fingers or wiggle toes. These activities cannot be accomplished by reflex.

When the child is unconscious, the most important component of the GCS is assessment of motor function—the best response demonstrated should be recorded. When the child's response to painful stimulus is assessed, both *central* and *peripheral* painful stimuli are applied. A *central* painful stimulus is applied to the head or trunk above the nipple line, whereas the peripheral stimulus is applied to the medial aspect of each extremity. Note that stroking of the bottom of the foot or pinching a finger or toe can produce a withdrawal response mediated purely through a spinal reflex arc; thus it does *not* verify an intact spinal cord or higher brain functions, so should not be used for this assessment component.

Motor response is characterized as follows:

- Obeys commands: moves limb on command (motor score = 6, minimal GCS = 8)
- Localizes pain: child motions or moves toward *central* painful stimulus applied to the head, face, or the trunk above the nipple line (motor score = 5, minimal GCS = 7)
- Withdraws from pain: *peripheral* painful stimulus applied to the medial aspect of each extremity; withdrawal is demonstrated by *abduction* of each extremity (motor score = 4, minimal GCS = 6)
- Abnormal flexion: decorticate posturing in response to *central* pain stimulus (motor score = 3, minimal GCS = 5)
- Abnormal extension: decerebrate posturing in response to *central* pain stimulus (motor score = 2, minimal GCS = 4)
- F. Flaccid: no movement (motor score = 1, minimal GCS = 3)

Signs of Increased Intracranial Pressure

Signs of increased intracranial pressure (ICP) in children include a change in responsiveness, including a deterioration in ability to follow commands or in response to applied pain, and pupil dilation with decreased response to light (Box 1-3). Responsiveness should always be evaluated in light of normal response for age (e.g., a toddler

Box 1-3

Signs of Increased Intracranial Pressure in Children

Decreased responsiveness (irritability, lethargy)
Inability to follow commands
Decreased spontaneous movement
Decreased response to painful stimulus
Pupil dilation with decreased response to light
LATE: Hypertension
       Change in heart rate
       Apnea

From Hazinski MF: *Nursing care of the critically ill child,* ed 2, St Louis, 1992, Mosby.

would be expected to protest when parents leave the bedside) and the individual patient's normal response (e.g., a typically irritable child suddenly becomes lethargic).

The Cushing's triad signs of increased ICP, including hypertension, bradycardia, and apnea, may only be observed during cerebral herniation. Thus the triad should not be considered an early sign of increased ICP. Whenever any deterioration in neurologic function is detected, repeat all aspects of the neurologic evaluation described here, assess the vital signs, and notify a physician of all signs of deterioration. For further information regarding recognition and management of neurologic problems and increased intracranial pressure, see Chapter 8.

Immunologic Function

Infants are immunologically immature and are particularly susceptible to infection. The hospitalized child, particularly one enduring invasive catheterization or monitoring, is at risk for the development of nosocomial infections, which can include gram-negative, gram-positive, viral, fungal, or rickettsial organisms. Infections should be prevented with good handwashing before and after *every* patient contact by *every* member of the health care team and appropriate use of sterile and aseptic techniques during procedures. Every hospitalized child must be closely monitored to detect signs of infection or sepsis, and this monitoring must be particularly vigilant for immunocompromised or immunosuppressed children.

Suggested Readings

American College of Surgeons Committee on Trauma: *Advanced trauma life support for doctors,* ed 6, Chicago, American College of Surgeons, 1997.

Barkin RM, editor: Pediatric emergency medicine: concepts and clinical practice, ed 2, St Louis, 1997, Mosby.

Chameides L, Hazinski MF (eds), *Textbook of pediatric advanced life support,* Dallas, 1997, American Heart Association.

Deshpande JK, Tobias JD: *The pediatric pain handbook,* St Louis, 1996, Mosby.

Dipchand, AI, editor: The HSC handbook of pediatrics, ed 9, St Louis, 1997, Mosby.

Garson A Jr et al, editors: The science and practice of pediatric cardiology, ed 2, Baltimore, 1998, Williams & Wilkins.

Graef JW: *Manual of pediatric therapeutics,* ed 5, Boston, 1994, Little, Brown.

Hazinski MF: Is pediatric resuscitation unique? The relative merits of early CPR and ventilation versus early defibrillation for young victims of prehospital cardiac arrest (editorial), *Ann Emerg Med* 25:540-543, 1995.

Hazinski MF: Pediatric advanced life support. In Cummins RO, editor: *Textbook of advanced cardiac life support,* Dallas, 1997, American Heart Association.

Hazinski MF: Postoperative care of the critically ill child, *Crit Care Nurs Clin North Am* 2:599-610, 1990.

Hazinski MF: Nursing care of the critically ill child; the 7-point check, *Pediatr Nurs* 11:453, 1985.

Hellerstein S: Fluid and electrolytes: clinical aspects, *Pediatr Rev* 14:103-115, 1993.

Hirschl RB: Oxygen delivery in the pediatric surgical patient, *Curr Opin Pediatr* 6:341-347, 1994.

Meyers A: Fluid and electrolyte therapy for children, *Curr Opin Pediatr* 6:303-309, 1994.

Rudolph AA, editor: *Pediatrics,* ed 20, Boston, 1996, Appleton Lange.

2 Psychosocial Aspects of Pediatric Critical Care

Introduction

The hospitalization of a child for even a minor illness is stressful for both child and family. Life-threatening illness or injury magnifies the stress. The sensitive, empathetic nurse can mitigate some of the most frightening aspects of critical care, making the experience more positive and perhaps even growth promoting. Interventions should be aimed at enhancing individual coping skills so that the child and family can apply them to other stressful experiences and situations in the future (Box 2-1). In this chapter the term *parents* is used interchangeably with *primary caretakers*.

The critical care nurse encounters the child and family during a life-threatening illness or following a life-threatening injury, when they are emotionally vulnerable. Parents may perceive the nurses and physicians as lifelines, controlling the life of the child and access to the child. At all times, the nurse must convey sensitivity, compassion, and support to the family and must support the family as the family attempts to support the child.

Three elements can help the child to cope successfully with a crisis: (1) a resilient personality, (2) a supportive family, and (3) an outside support system. The nurse and other members of the health care team can serve as that outside support system, ensuring that the family support system is readily available to the child. The nurse can also reinforce and strengthen coping efforts of the child and family.

Emotional contagion between the child and the parents, siblings, or other relatives can either in-

---

Box 2-1

Key Elements of Family-Centered Care

- Recognizing that the family is the constant in a child's life, while the service systems and personnel within those systems fluctuate.
- Facilitating parent/professional collaboration at all levels of health care: care of an individual child; program development, implementation, and evaluation; and policy formation.
- Honoring the racial, ethnic, cultural, and socio-economic diversity of families.
- Recognizing family strengths and individuality and respecting different methods of coping.
- Sharing with parents, on a continuing basis and in a supportive manner, complete and unbiased information.
- Encouraging and facilitating family-to-family support and networking.
- Understanding and incorporating the developmental needs of infants, children, and adolescents and their families into health care systems.
- Implementing comprehensive policies and programs that provide emotional and financial support to meet the needs of families.
- Designing accessible health care systems that are flexible, culturally competent, and responsive to family-identified needs.

From National Center for Family-Centered Care: *What is family-centered care?*, Bethesda, MD, 1990, Association for the Care of Children's Health.

---

the nurse's tolerance. Instead, *the nurse should assure primary caretakers that they are welcome in the unit to help the child cope effectively and as an integral part of the child's recovery.*

To support the child effectively, each member of the health care team must understand the child's psychosocial and cognitive development, previous experience with illness, family cultural belief system, and stressors the child and family are likely to experience in the hospital (particularly the critical care unit). Such knowledge will enable each team member to best assist the child and family. This chapter summarizes psychosocial and cognitive development (including the theories of Erikson and Piaget) and the concept of death at each developmental stage. Potential stressors created by the child's hospitalization on parents, siblings, and other family members are also summarized.

Erikson identified eight crises that must be resolved at major stages of human development. In resolving each crisis, the maturing child or adult carries a balance of positive and negative aspects of that crisis into the next stage of development. This chapter summarizes these crises and their implications for psychosocial support of the critically ill or injured child.

Piaget described the five major phases in the development of logical thought. Every member of the health care team should have an understanding of these phases to communicate effectively with children and to understand the basis of their perceptions, fears, and misunderstandings.

crease the child's anxiety or contribute to the child's positive coping efforts. If the nurse supports the parents, the parents can better support and nurture the child.

Hospitalized children are likely to become upset during visits from primary caretakers, particularly when the parents depart. Parents should be assured that the child's response is normal and that the child is comforted by the presence of loved ones. Uninformed staff may feel justified in restricting visitation to avoid "upsetting" the child, but limitation of contact will only *increase* the child's anxiety. Too often, the parents are made to feel that they are "allowed" to visit contingent on

Infant

Psychosocial and Cognitive Development

Infants are not merely passive recipients of care; they normally possess the tools required to initiate social interactions. However, they vary in neurobehavioral maturity and in control and styles of behavior and communication.

Psychosocial Development

During infancy the infant and primary caretakers bond and develop the ability to signal one another. Infants learn to signal a need for food, dry clothing, or rest, and the parent or primary caretaker learns to interpret the cries and responses of the infant. Oral gratification is very important, and sucking provides comfort.

The infant's state of consciousness influences the way he or she will respond. Two sleep states and four awake states have been identified, which will influence the infant's response to stimuli. These states are as follows:

- *Deep sleep:* threshold for stimuli very high; difficult to arouse
- *Light sleep (highest proportion of infant's sleep):* some movement and irregular breathing; responsive to stimuli and arousable
- *Drowsy:* variable activity and irregular breathing, looks sleepy, will awaken to stimuli including feeding and voice
- *Quiet-alert:* wide, very bright eyes, very interested in environment and responsive
- *Active-alert:* eyes open, much body activity, very sensitive to and upset by stimuli
- *Crying:* major method of communication, increased body activity, infant may console self (suck thumb or fist) or respond to soothing

Touch is important; infants need to be caressed, stroked, cuddled, held, hugged, and loved to feel secure. A combination of verbal and tactile stimuli is generally more effective than verbal stimuli alone. The infant may also be comforted if held closely (with arms pressed close to the body), swaddled, picked up, or rocked with a pacifier. An infant who is irritable when uncovered or wrapped loosely may become calm and drowsy when swaddled.

Erikson Erikson observed that the infant must acquire a sense of basic trust while overcoming a sense of mistrust (trust vs. mistrust). To acquire trust, the infant must feel safe and develop confidence that physical needs will be met. A sense of mistrust may develop if the infant is abused or repeatedly frustrated when signaling needs or discomfort (e.g., hunger) to caretakers.

Cognitive Development

Piaget Piaget calls the period of infancy and early toddlerhood (birth to approximately 2 years) the sensorimotor phase. There are four infant stages and two toddler stages in this phase (the two toddler stages are presented in the toddler section).

- *Approximately birth to 1 month:* reflexive behavior (sucking, grasping, crying) present; cannot differentiate self from others; little tolerance for frustration or delayed gratification
- *Approximately 1 to 4 months:* reflexes replaced by voluntary activity; begins to recognize familiar objects and differentiate self from others; objects that move out of sight are forgotten; no stranger anxiety
- *Approximately 4 to 8 months:* developing sense of causality, time, deliberate intention, and separation from environment; object permanence: objects and persons exist even when out of sight—infant will begin to protest when parents leave or strangers approach
- *Approximately 9 to 12 months:* concept of object permanence further developed. Beginning of intellectual reasoning; infant begins to understand some words and gestures, jabbers expressively, will wander from primary caretaker for brief periods; may attach to transitional objects (e.g., favorite blanket or toy)

Separation Anxiety The major source of fear for infants (from approximately 6 months), toddlers, and preschoolers is separation from the parent. For this reason, primary caretakers should be encouraged to remain at the hospital and spend as much time as possible with the hospitalized infant and young child. Their presence may be particularly comforting during painful procedures. Robertson has identified three phases of separation anxiety, which may be observed when the child is separated from the primary caretaker (Box 2-2).

Death Death, per se, has no meaning for the infant. The infant's reactions to fatal illness will be based on the degree of discomfort involved and on the reactions of parents and others in the environment. Parents provide a frame of reference for the infant, and parental attitudes and feelings are clearly transmitted to the infant. If parents are helped to deal with their strong feelings, they can be calm and support the infant. Separation from the parents should be minimized, since it is the most stressful event for the infant.

Box 2-2
Separation Anxiety

Robertson described three distinct phases in the child's response to the crisis of separation. These phases do not invariably develop, nor does every child demonstrate every phase. The severity of the separation anxiety is influenced by the child's personality, the quality of the parent-child relationship, and previous experience with separation.

1. *Protest:* Child cries loudly, screams for parents, or clings to departing parent. Child may seem inconsolable and quiets only when exhausted. The nurse may successfully soothe child if the child met the nurse with the parents. Distraction and soothing behavior may comfort the child.
2. *Despair:* Child continues mourning but becomes more passive. He or she is disinterested in play or food and looks sad, lonely, and apathetic. Child may ignore returning parents or act angry but will cling to them when they begin to depart.
3. *Denial:* Child appears to have adjusted to separation, appearing friendly and interested in environment and other people. He or she will accept caretaking from several people. This behavior is not a sign of contentment but of resignation; the child has emotionally detached from the parents to escape the pain of separation. Child may react with indifference when parents return. This phase was most worrisome in early research as it was associated with the highest incidence of behavioral sequelae. Now this behavior may be seen in children who have adapted positively to frequent hospitalizations.

For further information see Robertson J: *Young children in hospitals,* New York, 1969, Basic Books.

Table 2-1
Psychosocial Development and Stressors of Hospitalization During Infancy

Psychosocial Development	Stressors of Hospitalization
Parent-infant bonding	Separation from parents
Reflex → organized responses	Inconsistent caretakers and responses
Oral gratification, sucking important	Feeding disruption, or NPO
Need for schedule, sleep	Sleep disruption, constant stimuli
	Unfamiliar environment, disrupted routines
Erikson: Trust vs. mistrust	Pain, discomfort
Piaget: Sensorimotor period	Movement restriction

imized, and parents should be encouraged to comfort and nurture the infant (e.g., participate in bath or feeding). Since oral gratification is important to the infant, a pacifier should be readily available and its use encouraged if it comforts the infant.

The critical care environment disrupts the infant's normal sleep-wake cycles and feeding routines and provides noxious and often painful stimuli. The intensive care unit (ICU) may lack *meaningful* sources of stimulation (e.g., touch, or colorful blankets or toys). The constant noxious stimulation of the ICU can interfere with quality sleep; thus the nurse must attempt to facilitate periods of reduced stimuli to enable uninterrupted rest whenever possible. Sleep deprivation or sensory overload may cause excessive irritability or lethargy that may be interpreted as physical deterioration. It may be necessary to move the infant to a quiet area of the unit and minimize noise, examinations, and handling.

Play and Preparation for Procedures

Since young infants do not comprehend explanations, they require immediate comfort after painful procedures; distraction is helpful. Older infants require time to become familiar with equipment (e.g., stethoscopes, otoscopes, or blood pressure cuffs) and should always be warned before painful procedures (Box 2-3).

Response of Infants to Critical Care

Table 2-1 summarizes major aspects of psychosocial development in the infant and lists major stressors that may be associated with hospitalization at this age. Often the most stressful aspect of critical care for the young infant is separation from parents. Therefore separation should be min-

Box 2-3

Preparation of Children and Adolescents for Procedures and Surgery*

Infants

Major fears: Separation and strangers
Preparation
  Minimize separation from parents; provide consistent caretakers; decrease parents' anxiety

Toddlers

Major fears: Separation and loss of control
Characteristics of toddlers' thinking: egocentric, primitive, magical, little concept of body integrity
Preparation
  Prepare child hours or even minutes before procedures, because preparation too far in advance produces even more intense anxiety.
  Keep explanations very simple and choose wording carefully, avoiding words with multiple meanings.
  Let the toddler play with equipment, put mask on teddy bear, and so on.
  Minimize separation from parents; keep security objects at hand.
  Recognize that any intrusive procedure is likely to provoke an intense reaction.
  Use restraints judiciously.

Preschoolers

Major fears: Bodily injury and mutilation; loss of control; the unknown; the dark; and being left alone
Characteristics of preschoolers' thinking
  Preoperational: egocentric, magical, animistic, transductive
  Highly literal interpretation of words, inability to abstract
  Primitive ideas about their bodies
  Difficulty in differentiating a "good" hurt (beneficial treatment) from a "bad" hurt (illness or injury)
Preparation
  Prepare the preschooler days in advance for major events (hours for minor ones). Tie explanations to known events (e.g., lunchtime).
  Keep explanations simple and concrete and choose wording carefully.
  Emphasize that the child will wake up after surgery, because anesthesia described as "being put to sleep" may be frightening.

Use pictures, models, actual equipment, or hospital play and behavioral rehearsal. Describe what child will feel, hear, and taste. Assess comprehension.
Repeat many times that the child has not done anything wrong and is not being punished.
Reexplain things every time they happen; do not assume the child remembers; anxiety may interfere with memory.
Do not tell the children they will feel better after surgery, because they will undoubtedly feel worse in the immediate postoperative period.
Give the child choices whenever possible.
Do not tie evaluations of the child to behavior during the procedures (e.g., he is not "a good boy" for holding still, but rather, "That was good to hold still!").
Teach the child some simple coping skills such as distraction techniques in advance of the procedure, and then guide the child in use during the procedures.
Postprocedure play sessions are important to help the child understand and integrate experience.

School-Age Children

Major fears: Loss of control, bodily injury and mutilation, failure to live up to expectations of important others, and death
Characteristics of thinking of school-age children
  Concrete operational period

From Hazinski MF: *Nursing care of the critically ill child,* ed 2, St Louis, 1992, Mosby.
*It is important to remember that the child's psychosocial developmental stage may not always match his or her chronologic age. Development may be delayed, particularly in chronically ill children. For example, an adolescent who is delayed in development may need to be approached more like a school-age child. Preparation of children and their parents should include preparation of siblings. Siblings may have fantasies about what is happening, and they may fear that they caused what happened (the illness or injury) or that the same thing will happen to them. It is vital to discuss these issues with parents who may not realize what the siblings are experiencing. Parents may not know how to approach the preparation.

Box 2-3—cont'd

Preparation of Children and Adolescents for Procedures and Surgery

Beginning of logical thought but continuing tendency to be literal

Vague, false, or nonexistent ideas about illness and body construction and function

Ability to listen attentively to all that is said without always comprehending

Reluctance to ask questions or admit not knowing something they think they are expected to know

Better ability to understand relationship between illness and treatment

Increased awareness of the significance of various illnesses, potential hazards of treatments, lifelong consequences of injury, and the meaning of death

Preparation

Prepare days to weeks in advance for major events because it is extremely important to the child's ability to cope effectively, to cooperate, and to comply with treatment; in addition, preparation gives the child a greater sense of control.

Ask children to explain what they understand.

Use body diagrams, pictures, and models; these children enjoy learning scientific terminology and handling actual equipment because their thinking is concrete (although some older school-age children object to being seen looking at a doll).

Stress that peer group contact can be maintained.

Emphasize the "normal" things the child will be able to do after hospitalization.

Give as many choices as possible to increase the child's sense of control.

Reassure the child that he has done nothing wrong and that necessary procedures and surgery are not punishments.

Standardized films, slide-tape programs, or videotapes may be helpful.

Anticipate and answer questions regarding the long-term consequences (e.g., what the scar will look like, how long activities may be curtailed)

Sessions conducted after the procedure are important to help the child "work through" and master the experience.

Adolescents

Major fears: Loss of control; altered body image; separation from peer group

Characteristics of adolescents' thinking

Beginning of formal operational thought and ability to think abstractly

Existence of some magic thinking (e.g., feeling guilty for illness) and egocentrism

Tendency toward hyperresponsiveness to pain

Little understanding of the structure and workings of the body

Preparation

Because advance preparation is vital to adolescents' ability to cope, cooperate, and comply, prepare them in advance—preferably weeks before major events.

Allow adolescents to be an integral part of decision-making about their care, because they can project the future and see long-term consequences and thus are able to understand much more.

Give information sensitively, because adolescents react not only to *what* they are told but to the *manner* in which they are told. Explore tactfully what adolescents know and what they do not know.

Stress how much adolescents can do for themselves and how important their compliance and cooperation are to their treatment and recovery; be honest about the consequences.

Allow the adolescent as many choices and as much control as possible. Respect adolescents' need to exert independence from parents, and remember that they may alternate between dependence and a wish to be independent.

Maintain contact with peer group if adolescent desires.

Modeling films or slide-tape programs may be helpful.

Teach adolescent coping techniques such as relaxation, deep breathing, self-comforting talk and/or the use of imagery.

Play enables the infant to learn about self and others. The infant engages in three forms of play:

- *Social-affective play:* interaction with and imitation of adults
- *Sense-pleasure play:* pleasure derived from sensory stimuli such as lights, colors, and motion
- *Sensorimotor activity:* motor activity and play with body and toys (e.g., objects flung from crib and retrieved by adults); once object permanence develops, peek-a-boo is enjoyable

Since infant play usually requires movement, restraints are very stressful. If sucking a favorite thumb or fist comforts the infant, attempts should be made to keep that hand free (not restrained or used for intravenous therapy). Encourage parents to bring a transitional object or toy from home, but don't lose it (list the toy on the nursing care plan and locate it after each linen change).

Toddler

Psychosocial and Cognitive Development

Psychosocial Development

The toddler is beginning to develop autonomy and self-control). Once toddlers develop upright locomotion, the hands are freed to explore the environment. Toddlers delight in discovering new things and are often liberal with expressions of affection.

This stage is also the "NO" stage—the toddler frequently uses this word as a method of control, whether or not "no" is really intended. The toddler is struggling to assert independence and gain control of the environment. Temper tantrums result from the toddler's low frustration tolerance (exacerbated by illness, pain, or sleep deprivation) and need to test the limits of acceptable behavior.

Primary caretakers represent safety and security to the toddler, and the toddler is very attached to them. During play the toddler can tolerate brief periods of separation from them, but prolonged separation is very stressful.

All children need limits to feel secure and are frightened without them. Toddlers have not yet mastered control over their emotions; thus they require consistent limits and help in channeling strong feelings into socially acceptable behavior. When control is lost, it may be necessary to remove the toddler from the situation. The toddler may be able to regain self-control during a "time out" that includes an explanation of why the precipitating behavior cannot continue and redirection toward a more acceptable activity or behavior.

Elimination and retention are important skills developed during this period. Once the toddler has developed bowel and bladder control, soiling can create stress.

Erikson   Erikson describes the life crisis of the toddler years as the resolution of autonomy vs. shame and doubt. As the toddler successfully masters control of his or her body (including behavior and sphincter control), he or she develops a sense of autonomy. However, lack of control over behavior or repeated inability to control bowel and bladder function can lead to a sense of internal stress, including shame and doubt.

Cognitive Development

Piaget   The toddler experiences the last two phases of the sensorimotor period of development, beginning to think and reason.

- *First four phases:* See Infant, p. 16.
- *Approximately 13 to 18 months:* Toddler further differentiates self from other objects and will search for objects that have disappeared. Early traces of memory are present, and toddler develops sense of causal relationships.
- *Approximately 19 to 24 months:* Egocentric and magical thinking begin. Toddlers cannot appreciate other points of view and perceive that events result from their activities and thoughts.

The toddler is extremely ritualistic and takes comfort from consistency of environment and daily activities. Changes in routine require an adjustment period. A sense of time is beginning to develop but is related to major daily activities (e.g., meals, naptime).

At approximately 2 to 4 years, preoperational thought develops. Vocabulary and language increase tremendously. However, magical thinking and egocentricity are still present. The toddler can't generalize and reasons from the particular to the particular. He or she often assigns causal relationship to things that are only related by time. Animism (endowing animate qualities to inanimate objects) is present during this stage and continues during preschool years.

Separation Anxiety Ideally hospitalization of older infants and toddlers should be avoided, since at this age the child is most likely to be adversely affected by separation from primary caretakers (see Box 2-2). Although some separation is unavoidable when the toddler is hospitalized, it should be minimized.

Death The toddler's egocentrism, poorly developed concept of time, and inability to distinguish fact from fantasy preclude true comprehension of death. Although toddlers may repeat what sounds like a definition of death, they are unable to comprehend it. Death may mean separation from love objects or disruption in routine. The dying toddler responds with fear or sadness when parents express these emotions.

Response of Toddlers To Critical Care

Table 2-2 summarizes major elements of psychosocial development in the toddler and lists major stressors that may be associated with hospitalization at this age. Toddlers are at high risk for development of emotional sequelae related to the experience of hospitalization and separation from parents or primary caretakers. The critical care unit can be especially terrifying because familiar people and routines are missing and the unit is filled with unknown people and strange sights and noises. Painful procedures may be par-

Table 2-2
Psychosocial Development and Stressors of Hospitalization During Toddler Years

Psychosocial Development	Stressors of Hospitalization
Stranger anxiety	Separation from parents, examination by strangers
Upright locomotion, autonomy	Movement restriction
Developing body image	Fear of bodily harm
Soiling → control; ability to choose	Loss of control, regression
Egocentricity	Pain-punishment relationship
Developing language	Communication may not be understood
Erikson: Autonomy vs. shame and doubt	Fear, pain, regression, shame
Piaget: Sensorimotor period	Movement restriction
	Magical, animistic thinking begins

ticularly stressful because the toddler may perceive that the procedures are intended as punishment.

The best way to minimize the toddler's anxiety is to minimize separation from primary caretakers, since their presence is crucial to the toddler. If possible, one primary support person should remain at the hospital at all times and in the unit with the toddler as much as possible.

The toddler's fears of separation and association of pain with punishment can increase anxiety. Toddlers are often unable to understand why parents cannot rescue them from discomfort. Parents should not routinely be asked to participate in painful procedures or restrain the child during procedures; however, each situation should be evaluated individually, based on the expressed wishes of the child and parents. Parents should have the opportunity to comfort the child during or immediately following procedures. The toddler should be told that he or she is "good," throughout the procedure whether or not the child is cooperative. Attempt to explain that the procedure is painful but necessary to make the toddler well. Avoid a promise that the toddler will "feel better," since the painful procedure won't feel good.

A small number of nurses should consistently care for the toddler to minimize the variety of schedules and personalities to which the child must adapt. In addition, the toddler is able to develop trust in a small number of familiar nurses and may take comfort from them when the primary caretakers are not present.

Restraints should be used as seldom as possible, although intravenous sites and catheters must be protected. Because toddlers can become frightened when forced to lie supine, they should be allowed to sit up once they are stable. This allows the toddler to look around the unit and see people approaching the bedside.

Whenever possible, schedule activities, therapies, and undisturbed sleep time and post a written schedule at the foot of the bed. Never perform painful procedures without warning; if possible, move the child to a treatment room so the bed is not the sight of the procedure. If the child is unstable, this may not be possible. Provide adequate analgesia or anesthesia.

Play and Preparation for Procedures

The toddler resists any real or perceived painful experience. Since the toddler has a poorly defined concept of body integrity, intrusive procedures (even painless ones such as measurement of blood pressure) may invoke an intense reaction.

Toddlers require very simple explanations of procedures. Prolonged or detailed explanations delivered too far in advance will only serve to frighten the toddler (see Box 2-3). When painful procedures are necessary, take the following steps:

- Provide a brief explanation and assure the child that you will be there with him or her
- Administer appropriate analgesia
- Perform the procedure as quickly as possible
- Comfort the child (and provide opportunity for caretakers to comfort child)

Most of the toddler's time is spent in play. Play enables the toddler to learn about the world, communicate feelings, overcome boredom, develop motor skills and independence, and work through anxiety. The toddler's need for play continues despite illness or injury and provides an outlet for fear, frustration, anxiety, and anger. Passive play such as music, mobiles, talking storyboards, and movies can be used in the ICU. Nurses or family members may play "for" the child, tossing washcloth "balls" into a basket or operating a talking or mechanical toy. Involve parents in play with the child. Encourage parents and other family members to make audiotapes or videotapes of goodnight stories or goodnight songs to comfort the toddler in their absence. Puppets and toys may be used to help the toddler express feelings and fears.

Preschool Child

Psychosocial and Cognitive Development

The preschooler (ages 3 to 5) demonstrates progressive development of motor, verbal, and social skills. This is a time of enthusiastic and energetic learning and exploration.

Psychosocial Development

The major task of the preschooler is development of a sense of initiative. The child's frustration tolerance is limited but better developed than during toddler years. The child may feel guilty if he or she is unable to live up to personal or parental expectations. Since a preschooler's conscience is primitive and uncompromising, right and wrong are interpreted according to the behavior modeled by parents and the reward or punishment the behavior earns. Painful treatments or separation from family are likely to be interpreted as punishment.

The process of sex-role identification begins during the preschool years. Initially the child turns toward the parent of the opposite sex and away from the parent of the same sex. During later preschool years the child begins to identify with and imitate the parent of the same sex. This may affect the choice of parental support during hospitalization.

The preschool child's coping strategies are often well established. Parents should be asked to describe how the child behaves when frightened or angry, and how the child can be comforted.

Erikson   The major developmental task described by Erikson is the resolution of the conflict between *initiative vs. guilt.* If the preschooler meets personal and family expectations, self-confidence and pride in accomplishments develops. If the preschooler fails to meet expectations, guilt and anxiety can develop.

Cognitive Development

Piaget   Preoperational intellectual development continues until approximately age 4. *Intuitive* intellectual development is present by approximately 4 to 6 years of age. Explanations are better understood than during toddler years, and the preschooler defines things or people in terms of their functions in the preschooler's life.

Cognitive Development and Interaction   Animism, magical thinking and an egocentric view of the world continue. Preschoolers continue to view illness or injury as punishment for "bad" actions or thoughts. The vivid imagination of the preschooler makes differentiation of fact from fantasy difficult. The preschooler is often frightened of the dark and imagined monsters.

Preschoolers frequently ask "Why?" to learn the reasons for everything. However, the preschooler won't always understand the answers. Preschoolers still engage in transductive reasoning (i.e., two events that occur at the same time must be related). Frequently the preschooler perceives events correctly but interprets the significance or causality of events incorrectly.

The preschooler is rigidly tied to routines. The familiar pattern of daily activities gives the preschooler security.

Separation Anxiety   The preschooler will tolerate brief separations from parents and is less frightened of strangers than the toddler. Support from parents is needed during periods of stress, however.

Death   Preschoolers probably comprehend death more than they are able to verbalize. Recent studies have documented the fact that even young children are aware of death. Fear of death may be present as early as 3 years, and health care providers should be prepared to discuss death simply and honestly in response to questions asked by the child. Lengthy explanations should be avoided.

The preschooler is aware that death exists but views it as an altered temporary and reversible form of life. Magical thinking and egocentrism dominate the preschooler's thoughts of death and lead the child to believe that misbehavior, anger, or bad thoughts are responsible for illness or pain (e.g., people get sick or die because they are bad). Provide reassurances and explanations to clarify frightening misconceptions (e.g., remind the child that a treatment is not punishment and will help the child's heart to get stronger or kidneys to work better). Reassure the child that he or she won't be alone. Preschoolers are particularly sensitive to the sadness of family members and require reassurances that they are loved and that they will not be separated from loved ones.

The child's view of death is based on experience with relatives or pets or recollections from television or movies. In fact, television presentations and experiences with community violence may lead the child to equate death with violence or murder. The experience with the death of animals may lead the preschooler to associate death with disfigurement, however, and frequent reassurances and explanations may be required. Preschoolers are very concrete, and care must be taken with word choice when discussing illness or death. Death should not be described as "going to sleep," since the preschooler may fear bedtime.

Response of the Preschooler to Critical Care

Table 2-3 summarizes major aspects of psychosocial development in the preschooler and lists major stressors that may be associated with hospitalization at this age. The critical care environment can be extremely stressful to the preschooler, who normally has difficulty separating reality from fantasy. The environment and everyone in it can seem threatening or hostile to a child who is uncomfortable, in pain, and sleep deprived. The preschooler believes that ghosts and monsters are real and may ascribe sinister explanations to sights and sounds in the crit-

Table 2-3
Psychosocial Development and Stressors of Hospitalization During Preschool Years

Psychosocial Development	Stressors of Hospitalization
Verbal means of communication	Poor comprehension of explanations, time
Expanding imagination	Heightened vulnerability (imagined fears)
	Magical and egocentric thinking present
Developing body control; body image	Fear of bodily harm
Conscience	Requires truthfulness, realistic time estimates (don't violate)
Coping, ego defenses developing	Anxiety, ego defenses may complicate care
Erikson: Initiative vs. guilt	Guilt: hospitalization as punishment
Piaget: Preoperational thought	May not comprehend as much as speech suggests, temporal relationships rather than causal relationships interpreted by child (child interprets things that occur close in time to be related)

ical care unit. The unknown and the dark are also frightening; thus the child should be reassured that the parent (or nurse) is nearby. Equipment and procedures must always be explained in simple terms.

The preschooler's primitive body image contributes to fears of mutilation and may cause misconceptions about therapies. Invasive procedures are extremely threatening, since the child often thinks that the skin is "holding in" body parts. Dressings and Band-Aids are very important at this age. The child may fear that body parts will leak out of wounds when dressings are removed; thus the child should be told the skin has healed under the dressing.

The preschooler becomes very insecure if control of body functions or emotions is lost. Whenever possible, offer the child realistic choices (e.g., when a bath will be performed, or which color bandage is preferred) to give the child some areas of control. However, do not give the child choices when none exist.

The preschooler's coping style will often be apparent during hospitalization and should be supported. Withdrawal, projection, aggression, or regression may be observed. If the child normally becomes quiet when he or she is frightened, do not press the child to speak. The child may benefit from other ways of communicating feelings or fears (e.g., through drawings or play). Regression may be observed in the hospital or following discharge. Prepare the family for the possibility and reassure them that such behavior is normal.

Play and Preparation for Procedures

Play is an important aspect of the care of the seriously ill or injured child. It can be used to demonstrate equipment or procedures on dolls before the child experiences them. Play may also help the child cope with anger or fears following procedures or surgery. The preschooler is developing a sense of time intervals and can comprehend brief explanations of procedures (see Box 2-3).

The preschooler often dramatizes stressful situations, fears, or disturbing events through verbalization or play in order to master strong feelings. This type of play enables the child to communicate what can't be spoken or augment what can be expressed and provides an acceptable outlet for negative feelings. The preschooler frequently assumes the role of parent or health care provider to gain control of situations.

Since the preschooler is very verbal, health care providers may forget how vulnerable the child feels and may tend to presume that the child understands all things discussed. It is extremely important to realize how immature the child is.

School-Age Child

Psychosocial and Cognitive Development

Psychosocial Development

The school years are ones of accomplishment and tremendous intellectual growth. The school provides a new set of peers, and the child is geared to meet the expectations of people outside of the family. This leads to critical self-appraisal and competitiveness. Rejection by the peer group or perception of being "different" or inadequate can be devastating to the school-age child.

Most peer-group interactions take place with same-sex children, and members of the opposite sex are often viewed with derision. This attitude begins to change as the child enters preadolescence.

The school-age child remains an integral part of a family and often serves important roles as sibling and son or daughter. The parent-child relationship begins to change as the child realizes that parents are not infallible. Relationships with parents and other authority figures at this age may influence the child's perception of and relationship to authority figures later in life. Parents may have difficulty relinquishing some of their control over the child as the child begins to form new relationships.

Erikson   The major crisis of the school years is the resolution of the balance between *industry vs. inferiority.* The child takes pride in the ability to assume new responsibilities and to acquire new knowledge and skills. With increasing independence comes increasing self-esteem. However, the child may develop a sense of inadequacy, or inferiority if attempts at tasks or goals repeatedly result in failure.

Cognitive Development

Piaget   At approximately 7 years of age the child enters the period of *concrete operational thought.* This marks the beginning of logical thought, although abstract notions and concepts are still difficult or impossible for the child to comprehend. The child is able to use deductive reasoning and see the relationship of parts to a whole. As a result, the child becomes more flexible (particularly during later school years) and no longer requires absolute consistency in daily routine. Magical rituals, however, still help the child cope with stressful situations.

Cognitive Development and Interaction   The child's concepts of time, space, and causality are more sophisticated and realistic. As children learn to tell time, read, and write, a whole new world

opens to them. They can understand events happening in the past and present and can postulate on events in the future.

Moral judgment is developing during this period. Young school-age children believe that rules are unalterable and imposed from above. The rightness or wrongness of any act is judged by its consequences rather than its motives. These children are likely to interpret illness or injury as punishment for wrongdoing or bad thoughts.

Older school-age children begin to understand that rules can be flexible and are maintained through social agreement. These children begin to evaluate intent as well as action to determine the rightness or wrongness of an action.

In general, the healthy child is unaccustomed to a focus on the body and possesses only a rudimentary concept of body functions.

Separation Anxiety   The school-age child is more accustomed to brief separations from primary caretakers but takes comfort and strength from their presence. Once a concept of time is well developed, the child can better tolerate separation with knowledge of the time the parent will return.

Death   Young school-age children often have a very real understanding of the seriousness of their condition, although their understanding of death is imprecise until their concept of time is well developed. Death is often personified as a ghost or the devil, and children may fear that death will come and take them away from parents and friends.

Experiences with death in the community, on television, or in movies may affect the child's view of death and dying. In general, the young school-age child has not grasped the quality of time and thus does not appreciate the finality of death. Young school-age children may believe that family members could return from the dead if they wanted to. By approximately age 7, children begin to suspect that they will die. After the age of 8 or 9 years, when the child's concept of time is more complete, a more permanent view of death develops. During this stage the child begins to understand that parents may be powerless to prevent death. The death of another child in the unit may raise questions and should be answered honestly, while respecting each child's privacy. Healthy children at this age (e.g., siblings or friends) often need clarification about the cause of death and reassurances that they are not likely to die soon.

Terminally ill school-age children are often aware of their fatal prognosis without being told. They are acutely aware of nonverbal cues and often understand much more of what they overhear than staff and parents realize. Attempts to shield the child from prognosis may isolate the child from the conversation and comfort they need. The child must be able to rely on primary caretakers and health care providers to tell the truth. Parents and primary caretakers should always be involved in discussions of death.

Response of the School-Age Child to Critical Care

Table 2-4 summarizes major aspects of psychosocial development in the school-age child and lists major stressors that may be associated with hospi-

Table 2-4
Psychosocial Development and Stressors of Hospitalization During School Age

Psychosocial Development	Stressors of Hospitalization
School environment, peers important	Loss of routine, peer support
	Concern with being "different"
Critical self-appraisal, latency years	Uncomfortable with focus on body
Reality-oriented (rules, fairness important)	Guilt associated with illness, injury
Tremendous intellectual growth	Comprehends some implications of illness or injury, but thinking still concrete
Erikson: Industry vs. inferiority	Hospitalization threatens independence, future; support of parents still needed
Piaget: Concrete operational thought	Loss of control; potential perception that treatment decisions are made by others

talization at this age. Most school-age children carry negative impressions of their experiences in the critical care unit. They are often extremely sensitive to their environment and demonstrate detailed recall of events that happened to them and other patients. Frequently the child's recollections represent distorted reality. With more liberal use of analgesics, sedatives, and amnesiacs in recent years, some children appear to have minimal recollection of the critical care experience.

School-age children have fairly realistic fears, including fear of bodily mutilation and concern about the potential benefits and hazards of therapy. Some degree of anxiety continues to result from magical thinking and fantasy, and the child's poor concept of bodily functions may contribute to misconceptions. The child requires education about illness or injury and therapy and should be allowed to participate in therapeutic decisions. Do not assume that the child understands all vocabulary used.

The hospitalized school-age child is forced to depend on others (often virtual strangers) for basic personal needs and hygiene, and this can create stress. Health care providers must respect the child's privacy and modesty and enable the child to make choices regarding personal care (e.g., child may or may not wish parents to assist in the bath and may wish to wash some body parts alone).

Parents still provide important support for the school-age child. In addition, visits from friends may assist the child's coping and help the child maintain contact with peer groups.

Play and Preparation for Procedures

School-age children understand simple explanations provided in advance of procedures and have a good concept of time intervals and the timing of events. They are better able to verbalize questions and fears and understand verbal explanations, but their thinking remains very concrete. Play is one way to assess the child's understanding of upcoming events and allows the child to reenact stressful events or procedures to master them after the fact. Role reversal during play with members of the health care team provides the child with a sense of control, and gives the staff insight into the child's perceptions about care.

Unstructured play gives the child the opportunity to gain skills and a sense of competence. It also enhances the child's feelings of control and predictability.

Adolescent

Psychosocial and Cognitive Development

Adolescence is a time of profound physiologic, physical, and psychologic change. The turmoil of adolescent years may make hospitalization particularly stressful, and the hospitalized adolescent patient may be particularly challenging. With supportive care the hospital stay may provide the following benefits: improved physical well-being and/or appearance, positive perception of self as the result of attention received from others, an expanded social network, and a respite from responsibilities.

Psychosocial Development

The major tasks of the adolescent period include separation from parents, adaptation to a rapidly changing body, the development of a sexual identity, and acquisition of a sense of identity and autonomous function.

The behavior of the adolescent is frequently inconsistent and unpredictable. During adolescence some degree of mood swings, depression, periodic regression, and mild antisocial behavior are "normal," although extremes of these behaviors should be evaluated.

Adolescence can be divided into three stages, roughly according to age, but more accurately according to behavior.

- *Early adolescence (girls: 12 to 14 or 15 years, boys: 13 to 15 or 16 years):* Body image issues predominate, and the adolescent is acutely aware of body changes and imperfections. Peer group is extremely important, a same-sex best friend is common. The parent-child relationship is intact, although the child is spending more time away from home. Concerns about illness focus on effects on appearance, function, and mobility.
- *Middle adolescence (14 or 15 to 17 years):* Conflicts over issues of autonomy, accountability, and self-determination cause tension between child and parents. Adolescents are egocentric, narcissistic, and preoccupied with appearance and attractiveness to the opposite sex. Peers set standards for appearance and behavior. Concerns about illness focus on changes in physical appearance that might make the child unacceptable to peer group.
- *Late adolescence (17 to 22 years):* The adolescent is normally fairly secure in self-esteem, independence, and sexual relationships. He or she now listens to parental advice but makes independent decisions. Concerns about illness focus on its potential for affecting the realization of career and life goals.

Erikson Erikson describes the conflict of adolescence as one of *identity vs. role diffusion.* If the adolescent is able to successfully break from childhood and develop an independent identity and role separate from primary caretakers, a sense of security and self-satisfaction develop. If the adolescent becomes confused or insecure, it may threaten his or her ability to function confidently into adulthood.

Cognitive Development

Piaget Piaget's fourth and last stage of cognitive development, *formal operations,* is attained during adolescence. The adolescent develops the ability to think abstractly and is now able to project to the future and see the potential consequences of actions.

Cognitive Development and Interaction The teenager may not be aware of basic information about body functions. Visible consequences of illness or injury may appear to generate more initial concern than functional consequences.

The adolescent is able to understand other points of view but remains preoccupied with his or her own views. Magical thinking still exists to some degree, and teenagers often think they are to blame for their illness or injuries; thus guilt and shame often result.

Death Adolescents have the capacity to understand death on the adult level, but they have difficulty accepting death as reality and often think that death can be defied. Adolescents often believe they are invincible. This attitude may be responsible for much of the self-destructive or daring behavior that causes injuries or drug use.

The magical thinking that persists into adolescence may cause guilty feelings or self-blame about a fatal illness. The adolescent should be reassured with opportunities for open discussions of feelings.

Adolescents have difficulty coping with death at the age when they are striving to establish their own identity and plans for the future. The possibility of death-before-fulfillment compounds the adolescent's stress during hospitalization. Adolescents should be involved in treatment decisions and decisions to terminate care, but they should not make these decisions alone. Although they have the *cognitive ability* to understand details about their illness, they may or may not have the *emotional maturity* to make final decisions. In addition, they should be allowed to plan for their death.

Response of Adolescents to Critical Care

Table 2-5 summarizes major aspects of psychosocial development in the adolescent and lists major stressors that may be associated with hospitalization at this age. Critical illness or injury may create a crisis for the adolescent. Initially the adolescent may feel protected in the unit, but later pain, fear, and loss of privacy may become humiliating or frightening. The major threats of hospitalization during adolescence are loss of control and of identity, change in bodily appearance/image, and separation from peer group. Critically ill adolescents may also be concerned about their survival.

Privacy is of paramount importance for the adolescent, and every effort should be made to keep the adolescent's body covered, particularly during rounds or visits from family or friends. It is traumatic for the adolescent to be surrounded by, examined by, and discussed by strangers.

Ideal sources of support may be difficult to identify for the adolescent. Some teenagers welcome separation from parents during hospitalization, whereas others draw strength from parents. The adolescent may desire visits from friends or may become embarrassed and refuse the visits.

Table 2-5
Psychosocial Development and Stressors of Hospitalization During Adolescence

Psychosocial Development	Stressors of Hospitalization
Puberty and body changes	Loss of privacy (acutely self-conscious)
Break from childhood, developing independence	Threat to independence
Ego defenses, coping style developed	May be difficult to assess level or causes of anxiety
Conflict between ideology and practicality	May be distrustful of adults
Developing individuality	Loss of clothing, privacy threaten self-concept; concern regarding effects of illness/injury on appearance
Peer group important	Separation from peers stressful
Erikson: Identity vs. role diffusion	Concern for future
Piaget: Formal operational thought	Loss of control; may feel left out of treatment decisions

Discuss these issues with the patient and family and take cues from them.

The adolescent may use a variety of coping strategies during hospitalization, including denial, regression, withdrawal, intellectualization, projection, and displacement. The staff should support the patient's attempts at mastery of the situation and augment coping attempts as much as possible. Answer the adolescent's questions and clarify misconceptions.

Play and Preparation for Procedures

Adolescents should be able to comprehend explanations of proposed treatments and procedures and should be given plenty of time to ask questions. Distraction with activities such as television, reading the newspaper, or playing video games offers adolescents temporary escape from their situation, an outlet for strong feelings, and meaningful stimulation. The adolescent may cope with stress by daydreaming (see Box 2-3).

Family Members and the Critical Care Unit

Every child is a member of a family and has roles to play as a son, daughter, brother, sister, grandson, niece, cousin, or friend; these roles continue during the child's hospitalization. The child's critical illness or injury may disrupt the family's established roles, rules, and functions. For this reason, critical care must do more than *include* the family—it must be *centered on* the family. This care must be sensitive to cultural, cognitive, and socioeconomic diversity.

Research regarding childhood injuries suggests that the risk of some injuries (particularly near-drowning) is increased during episodes of family stress; thus the family may be in crisis before the child's severe injury, and the injury then compounds the stress. The way the family responds to this disruption and potential crisis may drastically affect the outcome for both the family and the child.

It is important to understand the family's perception of the child's condition and the perceived impact of the child's hospitalization on family life. Each family must be assessed individually (Box 2-4).

Visiting policies should be liberal and geared to the requirements of the child and family. Although nurses recognize the importance of family support, they often view family visits as stressful for the child, family, and staff. The care of the child may be so emotionally taxing that the nurse has no energy left to support the family. If this is the case, the nurse should request assistance from a clinical nurse specialist, nurse manager, physician, chaplain, or social worker rather than curtail visitation.

Subjective feelings that nurses develop about family members often influence the level of the nurse's involvement with that family. However, such feelings should not be allowed to influence the quality of the care the child and family receive. The nurse is often meeting the family at their worst. Judgmental feelings about family members serve

---

Box 2-4

Suggested Questions to Include in a Family Assessment

Who are the significant family members?

Whom does the family identify as leader? Spokesman? Contact member?

Who makes the decisions regarding care for family members?

What is the family's religious and ethnic orientation? Do these play important roles in the family?

What is the developmental level of the patient and family?

What are the expected times when the family will visit?

Where does the family live in relationship to the hospital? How far must they travel?

What is the educational level of family members?

What information does the family need to or want to know?

What emotional support do the family members need?

Which significant family members need to be consulted in decision making?

Has the family experienced something like this before? How did they cope? What resources did they use?

What are the family members' expectations regarding patient outcome? What are their goals for the patient?

From Caine RM: Families in crisis: making the critical difference, *Focus Crit Care* 16:184, 1989; and Hazinski MF: *Nursing care of the critically ill child*, ed 2, St Louis, 1992, Mosby.

---

no useful purpose and may alienate the family at the time they most need support.

Classification of "traditional" family members is no longer possible. Today, nuclear family units (father, mother, and children) are less common, and nontraditional families are more common. Therefore the definition of "family" for purposes of visiting must be individualized.

Parents/Primary Caretakers

Disruption in the parent-child relationship often provokes more anxiety for parents than the child's illness or injury or the critical care unit itself. Parents may feel guilty that they failed to keep their child healthy or uninjured or failed to seek medical attention promptly. In addition, parents may feel frustrated because they perceive that they can't contribute to their child's care or survival and may feel superfluous to the child's care. Following admission of the child to the ICU, parents need to see their child to believe that the child is alive.

Age-Specific Concerns of Parents

Some of the concerns and reactions of parents of critically ill or injured children vary according to the age of the child. Some unique stresses of parents of children at different ages are summarized here.

Neonate   Parents have feelings related to their new status as parents and must resolve their dreams for the infant with potential feelings of frustration, inadequacy, failure, and guilt regarding the infant's condition. They may need help in learning their parenting roles and encouragement to touch their baby and participate in care.

Infant   The parent-infant bond may be threatened, and parents often need encouragement to touch and stroke the infant. The infant may be comforted if the parent sings a familiar song or reads a favorite bedtime story or poem.

Toddler   Parents need to be reminded of their central role in the child's life and will likely benefit if they are allowed to nurture the child in some way (e.g., help with the bath, read a story, apply lotion to the child). The parents can be valuable interpreters of the toddler's language and rituals and are crucial to the toddler's sense of security and ability to cope. Parents may blame one another if the toddler is injured or has ingested a toxic substance.

Preschoolers   Parents are the primary comforters of preschoolers and can help prepare the child for procedures or activities. The parents may be anxious if the child regresses, and they need to hear that regression may be normal during periods of stress. Parental participation in care (e.g., bathing the child) helps both the child and family.

School-Age Child   Parents should be prepared for inconsistent behavior from the child, as the child is likely to alternate between independence and regression. Parents can bring information and letters from the child's school to maintain the child's ties with the school peer group. Older children may prefer that caretaking activities (e.g., personal hygiene) be performed by the nurse rather than the parents.

Adolescent   The adolescent often demonstrates both dependent and independent behavior, which can be very confusing to parents. Any stress that existed between the adolescent and the parents may be exacerbated during the critical illness, or it may assume a role of lesser importance. Parents should be encouraged/required to include the adolescent in decisions about care. Visits from the peer group should be encouraged if the adolescent desires this.

Parental Stressors in the Critical Care Unit

Stress   *Stress* is a condition or situation that imposes demands for adjustment. Parents face many stresses when the child is hospitalized, including fears for the child's life and future and the sights and sounds of the ICU. Additional sources of stress may exist outside of the hospital, including care of siblings, lost time from work, or family problems. Of all stresses experienced by the parents, the ICU environment may be most stressful (see the following paragraphs).

Crisis   A crisis is a state of disequilibrium characterized by an inability to use coping mechanisms to deal effectively with an actual or emerging problem. The individual in crisis requires outside assistance. High stress levels may precipitate a crisis state. Factors that affect an individual's vulnerability to crisis include the following:

- *Perception of the event:* Families must have a realistic idea of the child's condition to be able to support the child and deal effectively with the child's plan of care.
- *Situational supports:* Stressed people and those in crisis are more dependent than usual and require support from family members or friends.

- *Coping strategies:* These are behaviors that an individual demonstrates when stressed; they are individualized and may be subconscious. Further stress results if previously effective coping strategies fail. The parents may require assistance dealing with the crisis in manageable parts.

Working With Individuals Under Stress   People under stress are unable to function at their usual levels. When working with families of critically ill children, it is important to understand several responses of individuals to stress (Sedgwick, 1975).

- *Reduced ability to use incoming information:* Repetition of information is often needed. Use consistent words and provide information in small amounts.
- *Decreased ability to think clearly and problem solve:* The ability to organize thoughts and draw conclusions from information is limited. Parents may appear to respond equally to small and large stresses.
- *Reduced ability to master tasks:* People in stress or crisis narrow their perception of events, making completion of some tasks (e.g., admission paperwork) almost impossible.
- *Decreased sense of personal effectiveness:* This may be reflected by feelings of loss, bewilderment, incompetence, failure, worthlessness, helplessness, or humiliation. Parents need to hear what they *can* do to help rather than what they *can't* do.
- *Reduced ability to reach effective, constructive decisions:* Events are distorted and exaggerated in the mind of the stressed individual, making it very difficult for that individual to make informed, intelligent decisions. If at all possible, allow parents time to assimilate information.
- *Heightened or decreased sensitivity:* People under stress are easily distracted and annoyed and may be generally irritable. Parents may become so focused on the child that they forget to eat or sleep.
- *Decreased sensitivity to the environment:* Stressed individuals may be oblivious to events around them, often missing cues from

staff, spouses, or other family members. Use straightforward communication whenever possible.

Parental Response to the ICU   When the child is admitted to the critical care unit, parents may demonstrate a staged response not unlike the grieving process. Initially most parents demonstrate shock, disbelief, and denial, which may last a few hours or the first day. Denial may enable the parents to cope. Although unrealistic expectations should not be supported, the staff should not immediately remove all hope. Parents must be helped to understand the child's condition, but explanations should be provided in small amounts with a great deal of compassion and repetition.

Parents may become angry, seeking to blame someone for the child's condition; the blame may be placed on health care providers and may be manifest in complaints about the child's care. Parents may become depressed as they realize the severity of the child's condition. At this time, the parent needs to be able to express frustration and help the child. Parents need opportunities to touch the child or participate in care such as bathing the child or applying lotion.

Coping with the ICU Environment   Parents should be brought to visit their child as soon after admission as possible because they need to see for themselves that their child is alive. Before the parents enter the ICU, they should receive a brief explanation of the equipment they will see and sounds they will hear in the ICU. If possible, the child and the area around the bed should be cleaned of any blood. When time is short, a clean sheet can be placed over the child or the bed. The most important function of this first visit is to reaffirm that the child still lives and needs their love and support.

Family members should always be accompanied by a staff member during the first visit. This staff member can answer questions and clarify misconceptions. At times, silent support is needed most. Family members do not need explanations about every piece of equipment. They *do* need to hear some sensitive expressions of concern about their child and reassurances that the child is being watched closely.

Coping patterns used by parents during visits to the ICU may include visual survey, withdrawal, restriction of attention (to focus on minor details), or intellectualization. The nurse must recognize these behaviors as coping patterns and answer the questions that the parents are really asking. Patience is required to allow the parents to deal with reality at their own pace. The nurse assists the parents by clarifying information and helping the parents to begin to support the child.

Potential stressors of the ICU for parents and potential adaptation of the parents to the ICU are listed in Table 2-6.

During crises, communication with primary caretakers must be frequent and clear. Key elements to effective communication include the following:

- *Communicate at frequent, predictable intervals:* If parents are told to expect the results of a test at a specific time, a health care

provider should speak to them even before that time. If test results are delayed, explain the delay before the deadline passes.
- *Use consistent terminology:* Record specific terms and risks discussed in the chart and in the nursing care plan.
- *Provide the opportunity for parents to ask questions and express feelings.*
- *Include the assistance of support personnel:* Ask the family if they would like to contact other family members or members of the clergy.

Siblings

The effects of a child's illness on other siblings in the family have only recently been appreciated. When a critical illness or injury strikes one child, the siblings in the family may feel left out or forgotten because of the large amount of time parents spend at the hospital. In addition, the siblings may feel responsible for the child's critical illness or injury, assuming that bad words or feelings may have caused the problem. The siblings may begin to demonstrate changes in behavior, sleep or eating habits, school performance, or peer relationships.

Siblings should not be isolated from family discussions of the child's critical illness or injury. Too often, adults fear that such conversation will be "upsetting" to the siblings, when isolation from the family is actually more frightening to the sibling. The advisability of sibling visitation should be evaluated on an individual basis but is usually helpful to the sibling, the parents, and the patient.

Table 2-6
Potential Stressors of the ICU and Parental Coping Strategies

Stressors	Coping Strategies
Sights and sound in the ICU	Ask questions about equipment, therapy
Child's appearance	Touch the child frequently
Child's condition	Ask questions about condition, therapy
Child's behavior and emotional reactions	Visit child on a regular basis
	Solicit information about behavior
Procedures performed on the child	Be present during procedures (if desired)
	Participate in the child's care (e.g., bathing, massage, feeding)
Limited visitation	Request visitation frequently
Lack of privacy	Request privacy, befriend other family members
Staff communication and behavior	Develop trusting relationship with caretakers

For further information, see Carter M, Miles MS: Parental environmental stress in pediatric intensive care units, *Dimensions Crit Care Nurs* 4:180, 1985.

Helping Children Deal With Unique Stresses

Suicidal Behavior

Suicidal behavior in school-age children and adolescents is increasing at an alarming rate. Too often, injuries in children are accepted as accidental, and questions regarding possible self-infliction with suicidal intent are likely to go unasked. Thus the actual prevalence of suicidal behavior in children is unknown.

If the staff suspects that injuries were self-inflicted, the child should be asked privately about the injuries. Questions to the family may reveal a history of worrisome, self-destructive or suicidal behavior (Box 2-5). If the cause of the child's injuries has not been established, the staff may ask initial nonspecific questions such as, "How were you feeling just before you fell out of that window?" If there is any question of suicidal behavior or if the child is admitted to the hospital following a suicide attempt, referral should be made to a child psychiatrist or psychologist or a psychiatric liaison nurse. Once suicidal behavior has been confirmed, the child should not be asked repeatedly for details or explanations; discussion should be deferred for the child's therapist. If the child initiates discussion, of course, the nurse should be a supportive listener and avoid any suggestion that the topic is inappropriate or somehow forbidden.

The child's treatment during initial stages of hospitalization in the critical care unit can set the tone for subsequent receptivity of the child and family to psychologic counseling. An open, caring, nonjudgmental attitude on the part of the staff will help set a positive tone.

Families may feel shocked and surprised that such a thing could happen in their family, and primary caretakers may feel guilty for failing to recognize the signs of the child's distress. They may also deny that a problem exists. Suicidal behavior may raise value conflicts or touch on special personal feelings of everyone involved with the patient. Open discussion about feelings of parents, family, and staff members should take place at appropriate times with skilled psychiatric or psychologic personnel.

Coping With Unexpected Trauma*

Ideally the child should be prepared for the hospitalization experience. However, when the hospitalization is sudden, such as after trauma, such preparation is not possible. Trauma can introduce a variety of stresses, including sudden event, injury, intense stimulation, high uncertainty, disorganization, and all the stresses associated with critical care and hospitalization. These stresses can produce a reaction similar to posttraumatic stress syndrome.

Traumatic injuries can lead to behavioral sequelae. Four characteristics can last long after the trauma:

- Repeated memories of the event
- Repetitive behavioral reenactments
- Fears related to the trauma
- Altered attitudes about people, life, and the future

Family-centered support must be provided for the child and family after trauma. The parents and child should be together as soon as possible; the parents need reassurance that the child is alive, and the child needs the support of the parents. The involvement and response of siblings must be evaluated, and the siblings supported (see Helping Children Cope with the Critical Illness of a Family Member).

Immediate Interventions for the Child

The child requires help in understanding that the traumatic event is over and that painful treatments and procedures will help him or her recover. The child will require explanations of what happened and plenty of time to ask questions.

Interventions After Stabilization

Too often, adults make the traumatic event a taboo subject, ignoring the child's attempts to discuss it, thinking the child will become upset. On the contrary, the child must have the opportunity to

---

Box 2-5

Potential Signs of Self-Destructive or Suicidal Behavior

Prolonged depression
Threats of suicide
Previous suicide attempts
Irregular eating habits
Loss of interest in life, school, or work
Giving away possessions or making final (burial)
    arrangements
Marked changes in personality or behavior

From Hazinski MF: *Nursing care of the critically ill child,* ed 2, St Louis, 1992, Mosby.

---

*Based on Lewandowski LA, Baranoski MV: Psychological aspects of acute trauma: intervening with children and families in the patient setting, *Child Adolesc Psychiatr Clin North Am* 3:513-529, 1994.

process the event through conversation and play. The child may need to hear details of the injury and care over and over again. Children need "a safe, empathic, facilitative environment in which to process the facts and meaning of the event and their response to it." The nurse can provide this environment, suggesting that the child discuss the incident, draw it, or reconstruct it through play. Through comments made by the caregiver, children learn that they can express and control their strong emotions about the event. It is helpful if the parents are present during these sessions. Psychiatric or psychologic evaluation may be needed if the child experiences severe trauma or demonstrates very strong reactions to the event.

Some children and families benefit from additional counseling after discharge. Such counseling helps each member of the family, including siblings, to cope with the impact of the child's injury and near-death.

Helping the Child Cope With Critical Illness or Death of a Family Member

Note: This information may be useful in assisting siblings to cope with the death of a pediatric patient or in helping patients cope with the death of parents, siblings, or friends (e.g., the patient survived a motor vehicle crash in which other family members or classmates died, or a parent suffered a sudden myocardial infarction and died during the child's hospitalization). Therefore in this section the assisted child may be either the patient in the critical care unit or the patient's sibling or friend.*

When the Patient Is Dying

This information is provided in Chapter 4, Care of the Dying Child.

Helping Children Cope With the Critical Illness of a Family Member

When a parent or sibling is seriously ill, the healthy children in the family must cope with the anxiety caused by the serious illness and the absence of one or both parents from the home. Thus the healthy

child may be isolated from the events that occur in the hospital and the support that is available there; loneliness is a common result. Children frequently feel guilty about the injury or illness experienced by a loved one, thinking that angry thoughts or bad behavior may have caused the problem. Healthy children worry about seriously ill parents and wonder what will happen to them and the family if the parent dies. They worry about the ill or injured sibling and the sibling's survival.

The nurse should ask parents about the children at home: how they are doing, who is caring for them, and how the children are acting. The nurse may help the parent(s) detect problems by asking specific questions regarding the eating and sleeping habits and the home and school behavior of the other children. Often these questions will reveal evidence of the children's reactions to stress.

The nurse should encourage the parent(s) to discuss the illness or injury of the family member honestly with children in the family and allow the healthy children plenty of time to ask questions and clarify information. Attempts to shield a child from the situation will likely only isolate the child, forcing the child to deal with the anxiety alone. Often the child's fears are worse than the reality of the situation. The nurse can serve as a valuable resource to the parent(s) in preparing for discussion with the child. If the discussion occurs at the hospital, the nurse may be present to support the parent(s) and the healthy child, if the parents desire this. Age-specific concerns, considerations, and possible interventions for healthy children during the critical illness of a parent or sibling are presented in Table 2-7.

When a Family Member Is Dying

The death of a loved one, whether it is sudden or expected, is an experience that can affect the child for years. The child's ability to actualize the loss is often determined by how family members and health care professionals assist the child before, during, and after the death. The information in this section is designed to assist the health care provider in supporting children who are experiencing the death of a sibling, parent, friend or other loved one.

Forming a Caring Relationship   Each person's reaction to death is affected by previous experiences with separation and loss. To serve as a re-

---

*Much of this information was contributed by Julie Wall, RN, MSN.

Table 2-7
Developmental View of Major Concerns, Considerations, and Possible Interventions for Well Children
with Critically Ill Family Members

Developmental Stage	Major Concerns	Considerations and Interventions
Infants	Separation is the major fear.	To extent possible, provide consistent caretakers in child's own home.
	Disruptions in environment cause increased upset.	Facilitate parent/caretaker understanding of child's responses by familiarizing them with the three phases of separation anxiety and ways to support infant.
		Assist parent(s) in developing a schedule for and ways of maintaining contact with well children at home.
		Help parent(s) determine when it will be alright to leave their ill spouse or child and times when it will be important for them to be present to support their ill loved one.
		Suggest parent(s) write out schedule, usual routines and likes of infant for caretaker(s) at home to provide greater consistency.
	Sensitivity to emotional climate/ reactions of primary caretakers.	Help well parent(s) to understand that their emotions and reactions will affect their infant. Help them to find ways to manage their anxiety and release intense emotions away from their infant or young child.
	Separated parents may feel sense of emptiness, guilt, and concern when separated from their infants or young children.	Suggest parent(s) make a tape of their voice (e.g., reading a story) to be played for child.
		Ask ill or well parent(s) about their children and their feelings, fears and concerns.
		Make sure ill parent or sibling receives updates and reassurances about child(ren) at home.
		Suggest well parent(s) bring in photographs of well child(ren), audio or videotapes, scribbled pictures, and so on for ill family member.
Toddlers	Still very attached to and dependent on parents, who represent safety and security; thus separations are still very difficult.	Above interventions will also be helpful for toddlers.
	May experience parental separation as punishment through abandonment and thus become terrified; inconsolable, markedly active protest.	Educate parent(s) that even these young children are aware something is wrong (e.g., that parent or sibling is away and significant others are upset) and need some reassurance.
		Help parents develop simple, concrete, and honest explanations and reassurances.
		Give child frequent reassurances that he or she is a good girl or boy and that parent(s) still love him or her very much.
		Allow child to play tapes or look at pictures of ill parent or sibling over and over if they wish, as this is child's way of gaining mastery of a situation. Giving a toddler one of parents' tangible possessions may also help him or her feel more secure.
	Disruptions in rituals and routines are very difficult.	The more rituals and routines that can be preserved, the greater the comfort and security child will feel.

From Lewandowski LA: Needs of children during the critical illness of a parent or sibling, *Crit Care Nurs Clin North Am* 4:579-581, 1992.   *Continued*

Table 2-7—cont'd
Developmental View of Major Concerns, Considerations, and Possible Interventions for Well Children with Critically Ill Family Members

Developmental Stage	Major Concerns	Considerations and Interventions
	Regression, loss of recently acquired skills may occur.	Predict to parent(s) that this may occur and should be seen as child's temporary way of responding to upset and disruption.
		Help parents understand that child should not be criticized or punished (e.g., for loss of toilet training skills) but given as much love and support as possible. Suggest that they wait until hospitalization is over and a "normal" family routine reestablished before putting additional demands on the child for independent behaviors, toilet training, and other acquired skills.
Preschoolers	May still have some concerns about separation, although they are better able to tolerate this with consistent support.	Consistent familiar caretaker(s) in child's own home is the best way to provide consistency for child and to decrease additional upset.
	Thinking egocentric and magical; ideas about causality still forming, may make faulty linkages.	Encourage parent(s)/caretakers to explore child's understanding of explanations, words, and the situation to uncover misconceptions and faulty understanding that may cause increased concerns.
	More able to understand explanations but may use words they hear from adults without really understanding meaning.	Assist parents in developing explanations consistent with their cultural and religious beliefs.
	May fear they caused the illness and separations by their bad behavior, thoughts, or wishes.	Encourage parents to acknowledge upset to child and give simple explanations and reassurances.
	Difficult (usually impossible) to shield child from upset of significant others.	Encourage caretakers to share feelings and model for child how to talk about feelings and concerns.
	May have concerns about receiving adequate caretaking or about being forgotten or "lost in the shuffle."	Suggest that parents assure their children that someone will always be there to take care of them.
		Encourage parent to inform child of what caretaking arrangements will be and when they will see or hear from parent(s) again.
		Encourage parent to inform nursery school teacher and other significant caretaker of situation so that child's reactions can be observed and better understood and child can be given increased support.
	Child may be given messages that playing, laughing, having fun, and engaging in normal activities are unacceptable.	Assist parent(s)/caretakers in understanding the critical importance and normalizing function of play for young children; that play is how children learn, grow, express their feelings, and gain understanding and mastery of difficult situations.

From Lewandowski LA: Needs of children during the critical illness of a parent or sibling, *Crit Care Nurs Clin North Am* 4:579-581, 1992.

Table 2-7—cont'd
Developmental View of Major Concerns, Considerations, and Possible Interventions for Well Children
with Critically Ill Family Members

Developmental Stage	Major Concerns	Considerations and Interventions
		Help parent(s)/caretakers understand that because a child is able to play and laugh, this does not mean child does not care about ill family member or is not profoundly affected by the situation.
		Educate parent(s) regarding the importance of normal routines to child's sense of safety and security.
School-age children	Child very concrete in thinking and cannot understand abstractions. May have need to see ill parent or sibling.	With support, preparation, and follow-up arranged allow child to visit ill parent or sibling. Explain to parent(s) that children's fantasies about how person will look and what happens in a hospital are almost always much worse than the reality.
	Although more able to understand causality and explanations, may need more concrete explanations.	Give concrete explanations using pictures, diagrams, and drawings and give the "why" and "hows" and concrete details as child wishes to hear them.
	Are able to worry and wonder at a more sophisticated level; may fear ill parent or sibling's death.	Initiate discussions of feelings and situation and take cues from child's responses. Reassure child about causality of illness and that they are not responsible.
	May experience feelings of vulnerability, uncertainty, guilt, intense emotions, and many disruptions in home and school activities.	Allow children to feel included and informed and that their feelings and activities are important.
	May get message or feel themselves that their feelings and activities are not important; may worry about causing parent(s) additional burden or concern.	When parents are unable to be available, substitute significant adults can help fill the interested and supporter role at games, school functions, and other activities.
	Children who have limited contact with ill parent, are shielded from information, and have little opportunity to discuss feelings are more likely to have physical symptoms (e.g., headaches, stomach aches, influenza).	Whenever possible, facilitate contact with peers to avert feelings of isolation.
		Encourage parent(s) to inform appropriate school personnel of situation so child can receive understanding and support at school.
		Encourage parent(s) to balance benefit of normalcy of going to school, usual activities with child's level of upset, need for support, and benefits of being involved part of family.
		Encourage visit of child to ill parent or sibling when child desires this, building in adequate preparation, support, and follow-up.
Adolescents	More able to understand illness/injury, causality, and seriousness of situation, as well as possible implications and long-term consequences.	Encourage caretakers to initiate open and honest discussions of situation with adolescent, providing support and encouragement to ask questions and acknowledging that the situation is confusing and upsetting for everyone at times.

Continued

Table 2-7—cont'd
Developmental View of Major Concerns, Considerations, and Possible Interventions for Well Children with Critically Ill Family Members

Developmental Stage	Major Concerns	Considerations and Interventions
	May not ask questions or admit that they do not understand words or explanations given. Need to feel independent (or feeling that others expect them to be) may preclude adolescents from admitting need for support and reassurance. Prior conflicts with ill parent or sibling may lead to feelings of guilt or ambivalence. May be given or assume increased responsibility for maintaining household, care of younger siblings.	Encourage parent(s) to reassure adolescent that despite conflicts, the loving relationship between them and ill parent or sibling is still there and that conflicts can be worked out after the crisis situation is over. Suggest that parent(s) encourage contact with supportive peers and significant other adult figures (e.g., coach, teacher) who adolescent trusts to discuss feelings and provide added support. If increased demands are prolonged or occur frequently, as in chronic recurring serious illness, adolescent may feel torn between family responsibility and need to pursue normal adolescent activities with friends. Suggest parent(s) acknowledge adolescent's valuable contribution and also try to make responsibilities less burdensome by using other resources, giving the message that adolescent's needs are important too. Increased responsibility can be growth experience, enhancing feelings of competence and importance if adolescent is supported and not unduly burdened. Encourage parent(s) to give adolescents an appropriate measure of control over decisions affecting them (e.g., when they will go to school and when they will come to hospital).

From Lewandowski LA: Needs of children during the critical illness of a parent or sibling, *Crit Care Nurs Clin North Am* 4:579-581, 1992.

source to grieving children, the caregiver must develop insight into personal loss experiences. Unreconciled feelings of anger, sadness, fear, or pain from a personal loss may impede the caregiver's ability to support the grieving child. Children will benefit most from an open sharing of grief; the child must know that expressions of sadness, pain, guilt, and anger are acceptable.

Well-meaning family members or caregivers often attempt to protect children from the pain of death. Occasionally protection is needed, but the child most likely requires adult help to understand that grief is a normal response to loss. If the child is discouraged from discussing the death, unanswered questions, misinterpretation of events, and unresolved feelings can cause confusion and may prevent the child from resolving the loss.

To support the child, the caregiver must develop a relationship with the child. The caregiver must demonstrate warmth, sensitivity, and acceptance of the child's feelings. The most beneficial attitude conveyed by the caregiver is one of *empathy,* expressing the sincere desire to understand the child's grief and help the child.

The Child's Potential Response to Loss   The nurse plays a key role in educating family members regarding the impact of death on a child. The adults in the family may be struggling with their own grief and find it difficult to comprehend the child's emotional responses. When the child is silent or appears to play in a carefree manner, adults may assume that the child is not affected by the death or does not realize that the death has occurred. In reality, the child may be experiencing denial, and the child's grief is still deeply felt.

When death occurs, children sense that something very significant has happened. If the child is excluded from expressions of grief, he or she may not only experience the loss of the loved one, but also feel the loss of parental support. Age-specific concerns, considerations, and possible interventions may be found in Table 2-7.

The child's expressions of grief are not identical to those of adults; thus they cannot be interpreted according to adult values or behaviors. Children often lack the ability to mourn (express grief publicly); they tend to grieve internally and intermittently. If grief is not shared, it can't be resolved.

The child's grief may be expressed in strong outbursts over a short period; the child may act out, withdraw, or "misbehave." Family members must recognize grief behavior and understand that the child may mourn in segments over several years, reliving, reworking, and (hopefully) reconciling the grief.

It should be remembered that the death of a loved one is a challenging part of life; when mastered, it can result in strengthened coping skills and enhanced self-esteem.

Concepts of Death   The child's understanding of death changes as the child masters developmental tasks. These concepts have been presented in the sections regarding major childhood age groups but are summarized briefly here.

- *Infant:* There is no understanding of death. Response to death is actually anxiety resulting from the reactions of primary caretakers.
- *Toddlers:* Toddlers will be most distressed by separation from trusted adults or disruption in routines. There is no real concept of death. They will respond to the emotional tones of others.
- *Preschoolers:* Preschoolers can comprehend more than they can verbalize and are very concrete in interpretation of words and expressions. Misinterpretations or fantasies often increase the child's anxiety. Preschool-

ers often believe that the dead can return to life. The preschooler's response is chiefly affected by the behavior of primary caretakers and family.
- *School-age child:* Death is often perceived by young school-age children as something that comes and takes a person away or as murder; it is not perceived as permanent. By approximately 7 to 9 years of age, the concept of death is becoming more accurate.
- *Adolescent:* Death is the end of life. Adolescent self-absorption often leaves little energy for fear of death. Adolescents often think of themselves as invincible and death as something that occurs in the future.

The Death of a Loved One   Whenever possible, the nurse should be available to help a child prepare for the death of a loved one before that death occurs. Children should be included in ICU visits, particularly if the visits provide the child with the opportunity to say "goodbye" to a loved one. If the family does not suggest a visit by children in the family, the nurse should raise the question. Once the visit is planned, the nurse must prepare the child for the sights and sounds of the ICU and the appearance of the loved one.

Before the Visit   Although some children will be intrigued by the ICU equipment and sounds, most will be overwhelmed by the intensity of the ICU and the visit. The role of the nurse is to temper the hostile surroundings to a manageable degree for the child. Before the visit, the nurse should speak with the child to confirm whether or not the child does wish to visit and to elicit information about the child's relationship with the (dying) family member, any previous experience the child has had with ICUs or death, and the child's typical stress behaviors. The nurse should then briefly but gently describe the unit and the appearance of the loved one to the child. It may be helpful to show pictures or demonstrate equipment for children with more concrete thought processes. A balance must be achieved in providing sufficient information to prepare the child but not so much information that the child is overwhelmed.

If the visit is a first visit or if it follows a change in the patient's condition or appearance, it is important to discuss the noticeable changes. The changes may include a description of skin color, responsiveness, sleep or awake state, or altered respiratory pattern. The presence of any new equipment in the room should be explained.

The ICU Before the child enters the unit, when possible, the nurse should attempt to cover tubes and wires with a sheet. Blood should be washed from the patient's skin. The linens should be fresh; if there is no time to change the bottom sheet, cover any stains or spills with a folded sheet. Any stained or discolored tape should be covered with a fresh layer of tape. The patient should be positioned as comfortably as possible, with hair combed. The male patient should be shaved, if possible. Any syringes or unnecessary instruments or equipment should be removed from the area. Special pictures of the child or drawings or cards made by the child should be displayed. Personal touches, such as the patient's robe, favorite book, or slippers should remain in place to offer familiarity to the child.

The Visit The child should be accompanied by a family member and the nurse, and the nurse should monitor the child's response throughout the visit. It may be necessary to remind the child that it is "okay" to touch the patient; keep in mind that the child may not be able to do more than look at the patient during the initial minutes of the visit. Although it is not always possible to determine if the patient can hear the child, it is helpful to encourage the child to talk with the patient. If the patient does respond, this response should be called to the child's attention.

The Response Children may display a variety of behaviors during a visit to the ICU. Some may focus on the equipment, some may focus on the loved one, and others may keep their distance from the bedside. It should be made clear to the child that there is no "right" or "wrong" way to visit, and the child should do what feels comfortable.

After the visit, the nurse should speak with the child and answer any questions that the child has. At this time the nurse should also clarify any misconceptions the child has about the visit or the condition of the loved one.

The Death Each child will respond differently to the death of a loved one. Some children are afraid to be alone, whereas others need time alone and space to "try on" and later incorporate their new role within the family. All children need reassurance that the family will continue in some form and that their needs will be met.

After the death of a loved one, grieving children need the permission and the opportunity to grieve and mourn, a safe individual in whom to confide, and the reassurance that they are loved. Any component of these needs that the nurse can provide will move the child and family toward reconciliation of the loss. Referral to a clinical nurse specialist or therapist may assist the child in the grieving process.

The Death of A Sibling

Each child within a family has a position in that family; when one child dies, the family structure is irrevocably altered. The position of each person changes.

Children who experience the death of a sibling also lose their parents for a time, because the parents must be involved in the hospitalization and death of the sibling, the funeral arrangements, and their own grief. Caregivers must help the remaining children cope with feelings of abandonment and guilt about surviving. It may be necessary to refocus parents on the needs of the child (Box 2-6).

Family members must be sensitive to the needs of surviving siblings. Approximately half of these siblings develop depression, fears, problems in school, or separation anxiety; psychiatric or psychologic counseling may be needed.

Siblings may be afraid to cry for fear of upsetting their parents. If the child feels isolated from the parents or feels that grief is unacceptable, the child may become a "silent griever," repressing feelings; thus grief is unresolved. Children may feel that they need to be "strong" for their parents. This is an unrealistic and unreasonable burden for them to bear.

Occasionally parents blame themselves or the surviving siblings for the death of a child. If such blame is assigned or assumed by the sibling, the result can be devastating. Often the surviving siblings misbehave or regress, requiring more parental attention at the very time that the parents have little attention to give. The siblings may also fear their own or their parents' deaths and need reassurances each time the parents leave that they will return.

Any potential problems detected by the nurse should be discussed openly and honestly with the family. Extended family members and friends may

Box 2-6

Guidelines for Parents of Grieving Siblings Following the Death of a Child

Helpful Activities

Take care of own physical needs.

Provide time for own grief.

Deal with feelings of guilt and blame.

Realize that children grieve in their own way, and support and encourage this.

Locate individuals or groups that can provide professional support for your children.

Remember your deceased child in healthy ways.

Spend time with surviving children.

Allow your surviving children independence.

Potentially Destructive or Unhelpful Activities

Trite sayings

Idealizing the deceased child

Comparing surviving siblings with the deceased child

Trying to replace the deceased child with other children

From Hazinski MF: *Nursing care of the critically ill child*, ed 2, St Louis, 1992, Mosby.

be able to help, and the family may be referred to local support groups. The hospital may offer support groups for grieving family members. A national organization, Compassionate Friends, has chapters in most major cities and offers literature and support groups to assist in the management of grief and mourning. Through support groups, children learn how to survive the death of a loved one and how to share feelings; the children learn that they can survive.

Art may help surviving children express their feelings. They may also wish to make a memory book with photographs and memorabilia from the loved one who has died.

The Death of a Parent

Bereaved children feel the loss of the deceased parent and emotional and possible physical separation from the surviving parent. In addition, the be-

reaved child may feel abandoned by the deceased parent. The child may feel unloved and worthless, and this low self-esteem may cause behavior changes. If the causes of the behavior are not appreciated, any punishment that results can reinforce the child's feelings of worthlessness.

Children may deny the death of the parent to avoid the pain of their loss. They may deny the death itself, rushing home to tell the (deceased) parent news of school. The child may also attempt to deny the pain of the loss, attempting to act as if the deceased parent were not important.

The child will be assisted in grief and mourning if supportive adults are patient and accepting of his or her expressions of loss. The child's behavior should not be labeled as "bad" or "good." Certainly limits are still required, but some flexibility is appropriate.

Assessing the Response of the Child to Death of a Loved One

Children often regress after the death of a loved one. Regression is a normal coping mechanism that allows for regrouping of strength and resources to move toward mastery of the situation. It is not uncommon for children to move in and out of periods of regressive behavior just as they move in and out of periods of grief. Each child responds uniquely to the death experience, and there are no universal norms indicating "appropriate" vs. "inappropriate" grief.

No single symptom indicates the need for professional counseling after the death of a loved one. However, a severe, uncontrollable reaction or self-destructive behavior suggests the need for consultation with the child's pediatrician. In addition, the pediatrician should be consulted if a family member or nurse instinctively feels that professional intervention is needed. The behaviors listed in the box identify potentially worrisome behavior (Box 2-7).

Every child worries at one time or another about the death of a parent. This fear is intensified in children who have experienced the death of one parent. These children may have an exaggerated (but unexpressed) fear that their remaining parent will die, leaving them without adult support.

It is not possible to promise the grieving child that the remaining parent will live forever.

However, the parent can remind the child that a second death would be unusual and is unlikely. In addition, the parent should make some arrangements for the care of the remaining children and the household in the event of such a death. The surviving children may wish to participate in the plans and decisions and may take comfort from knowing that they will not have to worry about loss of home and separation from siblings.

Following the death of a parent, sibling, or other loved one, children may appear to be handling the death quite well. However, any change or transition in life (e.g., a move to a new home or school, the remarriage of a parent, or the loss of another loved one) may cause regression. Children grieve and rework mourning intermittently as they move toward mastery of each developmental milestone.

Psychosocial Aspects of Pediatric Critical Care Nursing

A critical care unit is not only intense and stressful for parents and patients, but it can be intense and stressful for the staff who work there. If the demands, tensions, and stresses of pediatric critical care nursing are not dealt with in a constructive manner, they can escalate and lead to frustration, dissatisfaction, and increased nursing staff turnover. Nurses can prevent these problems, however, by understanding potential sources of stress and using coping strategies and stress reduction techniques.

The challenges of this specialty can create stress, but they can also provide sources of great satisfaction. The challenges include the nature of direct patient care, interpersonal relationships, and the acquisition of knowledge. It is gratifying to watch the child progress and recover, especially when the nurse has contributed to that recovery. It is equally gratifying to visit children after they have been transferred from the ICU and to see them resuming normal activities consistent with their developmental age.

The nurse shares very personal and intense feelings with the child and family as she assists them through an extremely difficult experience. If the child dies, the nurse may help ensure that the child's death is peaceful, pain free, and dignified. That same nurse is helping the family survive a potentially devastating experience. Such opportunities must be respected and can be very rewarding.

The critical care nurse is able to deliver holistic, family-centered care to one or two patients and their families. This close relationship is not always possible with large numbers of patients in less acute patient care units. The nurse often has the opportunity to take more initiative and engage in more independent decision-making in the critical care unit than is possible on the general care unit.

The close working relationships that develop among the nurses, physicians, and other co-workers in the critical care unit can also be rewarding. Teamwork is readily apparent in good units and obviously lacking in units where mutual respect is lacking. Critical care nurses and physicians are usually recognized for their specialized knowledge and competence, and each must acknowledge the unique contributions made by each member of the health care team.

Conclusions

The environment and dynamics of a pediatric critical care unit may create a great deal of stress for the child, family, and staff. This chapter has discussed some of the psychosocial and emotional considerations that are an extremely important aspect of pediatric critical care. Particular skill and attention are required to prevent these considerations from getting lost in the requirements of technology, physical care, and repetitive routines. A knowledgeable, sensitive, and caring nurse can help to turn the critical care experience from a stress-enhancing time to a growth-producing experience for the child and family.

Suggested Readings

Betz C: After the operation—postprocedural sessions to allay anxiety, *MCN* 7:260, 1982.

Bowlby J: *Attachment and loss,* vol 2, *Separation,* New York, 1973, Basic Books.

Brent DA: Depression and suicide in children and adolescents, *Pediatr Rev* 14:380-388, 1993.

Dracup K, Clark S: Challenges in critical care nursing; helping patients and families cope, *Crit Care Nurs* (suppl, Aug), 1993, pp 1-24.

Erikson EH: Children and society, ed 2, New York, 1963, WW Norton.

Gellert E, Gircus JS, Cohen J: What do I have inside of me? How children view their bodies, In Gellert E, editor: *Psychosocial aspects of pediatric care,* New York, 1978, Grune and Stratton.

Lewandowski, LA: Needs of children during the critical illness of a parent or sibling, *Crit Care Nurs Clin North Am* 4:573-585, 1992.

Lewandowski LA, Baranoski MV: Psychological aspects of acute trauma; intervening with children and families in the inpatient setting, *Child Adolesc Psychiatry Clin North Am* 3:513-529, 1994.

Miles M , Carter M: Sources of parental stress in pediatric intensive care units, *Child Health Care* 11:65, 1982.

Munn VA, Tichy AM: Nurses' perceptions of stressors in pediatric intensive care, *J Pediatr Nurs* 2:405, 1987.

Murphy LB: *The widening world of childhood: paths toward mastery,* New York, 1962, Basic Books.

Piaget J: *The origins of intelligence in children,* New York, 1952, International Universities Press.

Robertson J: Young children in hospitals, New York, 1969, Basic Books.

Sedgwick R: Psychological responses to stress, *J Psychiatr Nurs* 13:20, 1975.

Wofelt A: *Helping children cope with grief,* Muncie, Ind, 1983, Accelerated Development.

3

Analgesia, Sedation, and Neuromuscular Blockade in Pediatric Critical Care

Pearls

- Most children in the pediatric intensive care unit (PICU) experience pain and anxiety; thus the question is *which* analgesic or sedatives to administer, rather than *if* an analgesic or sedative *should* be administered.
- Consistent tools should be used to quantify severity of pain and evaluate efficacy of analgesia.
- If drugs with short half-lives are administered by continuous infusion, bolus drug administration must be provided when the infusion is initiated to enable rapid achievement of effective serum drug steady-state levels. If rapid achievement of serum drug concentrations is desired, additional bolus administration should be provided when the infusion is increased.
- Always monitor the child's cardiorespiratory function closely.
- Wean chronic or high-dose narcotic, sedative, or barbiturate drugs *gradually.*

Introduction

Pain is a complex phenomenon that received little attention in pediatrics until the late 1970s. Until recently, many health care professionals mistakenly believed that the child's immature nervous system rendered him or her incapable of feeling pain or assumed that lack of requests for analgesics indicated that the child was pain free. Several studies documented the inadequacy of analgesia provided to pediatric patients (e.g., following cardiovascular surgery). In addition, there was a lack of scientific information regarding the safety and efficacy of analgesics in young children and difficulty in identifying pain behaviors in infants and children. Clearly children can feel pain, and adequate analgesia is required in the critical care unit.

Critically ill and injured children with wounds, indwelling catheters, and tubes usually experience pain, and analgesic administration should be planned. Pain management in the critically ill child requires therapy that is both effective and *appropriate* for the condition of the patient. Effective analgesia has been shown to reduce postsurgical stress response and may obviate such complications as cardiovascular instability and increased intracranial pressure (ICP). However, virtually all agents used for sedation or analgesia may depress cardiorespiratory function; thus careful monitoring is always required.

There can be no "cookbook" guide to analgesia and sedation in pediatric critical care. Patients demonstrate wide variability in the type of drug required (sedation, analgesia, or both), the duration of therapy needed, and dosing requirements. Therefore evaluate each patient and his or her response to therapy individually.

When analgesics are ordered on an "as needed" (PRN) basis, it is often interpreted to mean "only when requested," or "as little as possible." Nurses must ensure effective pain control whether or not the child or parent requests it.

Essential Anatomy and Physiology

The transmission of pain from the skin or tissues to the central nervous system (CNS) and the modulation of pain impulses are extremely complex. Pain is an outcome of sensory, developmental, and situational factors that all contribute to the pain experience.

The system for sensation of pain develops during the second and third trimester of fetal life and continues to mature during the first 2 years of life. Beyond the toddler years, perception of pain is identical in adult and pediatric patients, although psychosocial and behavioral expressions of and responses to pain change with growth and development.

The peripheral pain system includes sensory receptors (mechanoreceptors, free nerve endings, and nociceptive receptors) in the skin and C and A-delta fibers that conduct the pain impulse to the CNS. The sensory receptors for pain and pressure in or close to the skin surface can be identified in fetal life, and their density at birth is similar to that of adults. These receptors depolarize in response to mechanical injury, chemical irritants, and inflammatory mediators (Deshpande and Tobias, 1996) and synapse with neurons in the dorsal horn of the spinal cord.

The initial pain signal is transmitted by two nerve fiber systems: the high-threshold fast fibers (A-delta fibers) and the generalized-stimulus slow fibers (C fibers). The A-delta fibers are myelinated and rapidly transmit information regarding sharp or acute pain. The C fibers respond to slow, dull, aching pain; heat; and chemical stimuli. These fibers are stimulated slowly, and they remain stimulated during chronic pain.

Cutaneous (pain or proprioception) sensation is present as early as the 7th week of gestation and reflexes to cutaneous sensory stimulation can be documented from all cutaneous and mucous surfaces by the 20th week of gestation. Release of excitatory neurotransmitters, required for transmission and modulation of painful impulses, is first noted at 12 to 16 weeks of gestation. The mechanisms of pain sensation are completely developed at birth. Although neonatal nerve fibers are not completely myelinated, they do transmit sharp or acute pain quickly to the CNS since the neonatal nerve fibers are short. In fact, nerve tracts to the brain stem and thalamus are myelinated by the 30th week of gestation, and thalamocortical tracks are myelinated by the 37th week of gestation. Therefore neonates can perceive all forms of pain.

The central pain system includes the spinal cord and brain. When peripheral nerve fibers enter the spinal cord, they converge on the dorsal horn of the cord. Development of this part of the spinal cord begins before the 13th week of gestation and is complete by approximately the 30th to the 32nd week of gestation. In the dorsal horn the pain signal is amplified or attenuated by other stimuli arriving at the dorsal horn from the brain (supraspinal centers). This intrinsic modulation of the pain signal forms the basis of some mechanisms of pain control. For example, morphine may decrease pain by stimulating areas of the brain that control descending fibers to the dorsal horn. Stimulation of alternate afferent dorsal horn peripheral nerve fibers may overwhelm the afferent system so that the unpleasant, painful sensation is blocked (the "gate" theory).

Once the pain message has been modulated at the level of the spinal cord, it is transmitted to the supraspinal centers in the brain through a variety of fibers. In the brain the pain signal is projected to the sensory, arousal, neuroendocrine, and personality areas. In short, the sensation of pain is influenced by a combination of sensory, developmental, and situational factors.

Assessment of Pain

The recognition and treatment of pain can be difficult because there are few objective quantitative measurements on which to base clinical decisions. The nurse must be able to recognize pain behaviors or specific behavioral patterns that communicate pain, including posture, motor response, and facial expressions, to evaluate the child's nonverbal cues that indicate the presence, location, and severity of pain.

Physiologic Indicators of Pain

Pain may produce evidence of adrenergic nervous system ("fight or flight") activation, including tachycardia, hypertension, pupil dilation, and diaphoresis. However, although it is clear that pain can influence these characteristics, it is unclear how to separate the effects of pain from those of critical illness or injury. Marked increases in both blood pressure and heart rate have been observed during and after painful procedures in neonates. However, these signs may be observed only during the first minutes that pain is experienced.

Chronic pain or pain of long duration may be associated with rebound signs of vagal stimulation, including a fall in heart and respiratory rates and blood pressure. However, these responses are very individualized. Therefore observe the child closely for patient-specific physiologic signs of pain.

Physical and physiologic consequences of prolonged pain can now be measured. When minimal anesthesia is administered to neonatal surgical patients or to infants after cardiovascular surgery, a marked release of catecholamines, cortisol, glucagon, aldosterone, and other catabolic hormones has been documented, which may be associated with complications such as lactic acidosis. However, these responses are not specific to pain. The incidence of postoperative complications has been shown to decrease when effective analgesia is provided.

Pediatric Pain Behavior

Children in pain are often restless and agitated and cannot be easily distracted. The child may cry or fuss, will have a short attention span, and will not be easily comforted. Infants will fail to make or hold eye contact. A facial grimace may be observed, and the child often holds or guards painful body parts rigidly. Pain may also produce sleep disturbances, anorexia, and lethargy. Unfortunately critical illness or injury, sleep deprivation, and fear produce many of the same symptoms; thus these signs are often not attributed to pain. However, when asked, children as young as 2 years may reliably provide specific information about the pain they experience.

The child's reactions to pain are affected by psychosocial factors and other stressors in the child's life. Children in pain may be frightened or conditioned by sex-role identification or parental admonishment to be stoic. Exhaustion may result in reduced response to any stimuli (including pain).

The child's physical condition also affects his or her response to and expression of pain. Expressions of pain may be difficult to appreciate in the preverbal, exhausted, frightened, intubated or unstable child. Clearly the child with alteration in level of consciousness may be unable to demonstrate signs of pain.

The parents can be valuable interpreters of the child's behavior and signs of pain. They can describe the child's normal behavior, as well as behavior when he or she is frightened or in pain.

Pain Scales

Nurses have access to a tremendous amount of information about a child's pain because nurses observe patients 24 hours a day. This information must be gathered, documented, and conveyed as objectively and professionally as possible. Pain assessment scales may be used to locate pain, quantify pain severity, and evaluate the effectiveness of pain therapy.

A number of pain assessment tools and scales have been developed for and validated with children. These scales include the Hester Poker Chips scale, the Beyer Oucher, the Eland Color Tool (Figure 3-1), the use of faces (Figure 3-2), and

---

Box 3-1

The Hester Poker Chip Pain Assessment Tool

Place 5 poker chips in front of the child and tell the child that each chip represents a "piece of hurt or pain." Separate one chip from the others and tell the child that when only one chip is present, a "little hurt" is present (ask child for an example of a little hurt). Stack all of the chips together and tell the child they represent "as much hurt as you could ever have." Ask the child to locate any little or big hurts and show you with the chips how much hurt is present. The chips enable you to rank the hurt on a scale of 0 to 5.

Modified from Hester NO: The preoperational child's reaction to immunizations, *Nurs Res* 28:250, 1979.

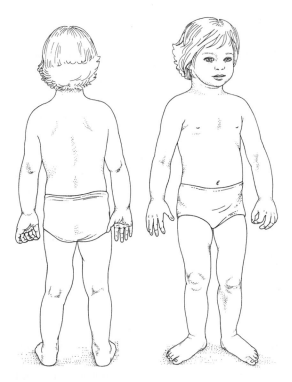

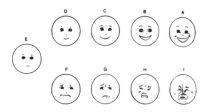

Figure 3-2 The McGrath Nine-Point Faces Scale. (From Johns Hopkins Hospital Department of Pediatrics: *Harriet Lane handbook,* ed 13, edited by Johnson KB, St Louis, 1993, Mosby.)

Figure 3-1 Human figure outlines for the Eland Color tool. Eight crayons should be presented to the child in random order. Ask the child to "pick a crayon with a color that reminds you of the most hurt (or pain) that you could possibly have"; once that crayon is selected, separate it from the others. Next, ask the child to select a crayon with a color that "reminds you of pain that is a little less than the pain we just talked about"; once the second crayon is selected, separate it from the group and place it with the first crayon selected. Ask the child to select a third crayon with a color "that reminds you of only a little pain"; separate this crayon and move it to the selected group. Finally, ask the child to select a crayon with a color that "reminds you of no hurt (or pain)" and separate that fourth color. Show the four crayons selected to the child and arrange them in order of "worst hurt (or pain)" to "no hurt (or pain)" and ask the child to show on the body outline "where the hurt is." If the child offers any verbal comments, note these. (Outlines reproduced with permission from Stevens B: Nursing management of pain in children. In Foster RL, Hunsberger MM, Anderson JJT, editors: *Family-centered nursing care of children,* Philadelphia, 1989, WB Saunders.)

the Children's Hospital of Eastern Ontario Pain Scale (Table 3-1).

A verbal child may simply be asked to locate and rank the severity of each pain on a scale of 1 to 10 (or 0 to 5). If the child is preverbal, intubated, or otherwise unable to speak, his or her behavior, facial expression, position, and movement should be evaluated to determine the presence and severity of pain.

Any assessment that is used to detect the presence of pain should be repeated to determine the patient's response to analgesics. Successful analgesia (pain reduction) includes reduction in irritability, longer periods of sleep, longer attention span, good eye contact, and willingness to participate in play.

It is unrealistic to believe that all pain can be eliminated for every child. However, reduction of severe pain is a realistic goal. If the child's pain suddenly *increases,* attempts should be made to control it and identify the cause.

Nonpharmacologic Methods of Pain Control

Although nurses frequently provide nonpharmacologic methods of pain control (e.g., a soothing backrub, touch), little research has been completed to validate these nursing interventions. Such research should be performed by pediatric critical care nurses.

Table 3-1
The Children's Hospital of Eastern Ontario Pain Scale: Behavioral Definitions and Scoring

Behavior	Score	Definition	Behavior	Score	Definition
Cry			**Torso**		
No crying	1	Child is not crying.	Neutral	1	Body (not limbs) is at rest, torso is inactive.
Moaning	2	Child is moaning or quietly vocalizing, silent cry.	Shifting	2	Body is in motion in a shifting or serpentine fashion.
Crying	2	Child is crying but the cry is gentle or whimpering.	Tense	2	Body is arched or rigid.
Scream	3	Child is in a full-lunged cry; sobbing; may be scored with complaint or without complaints.	Shivering	2	Body is shuddering or shaking involuntarily.
			Upright	2	Body is in a vertical or upright position.
			Restrained	2	Body is restrained.
Facial			**Touch**		
Composed	1	Neutral facial expression.	Not touching	1	Child is not touching or grabbing at wound.
Grimacing	2	Score only if definitive negative facial expression.	Reaching	2	Child is reaching for but not touching wound.
Smiling	0	Score only if definite positive facial expression.	Touching	2	Child is gently touching wound or wound area.
Child Verbal			Grabbing	2	Child is grabbing vigorously at wound.
None	1	Child not talking.			
Other complaints	1	Child complains but not about pain; e.g., "I want to see Mommy" or "I am thirsty."	Restrained	2	Child's arms are restrained.
Pain complaints	2	Child complains about pain.	**Legs**		
Both complaints	2	Child complains about pain and about things; e.g., "It hurts; I want Mommy."	Neutral	2	Legs may be in any position but are relaxed. Includes gentle swimming or serpentine-like movements.
Positive	0	Child makes any positive statement or talks about other things without complaint.	Squirming/kicking	2	Definitive uneasy or restless movements in the legs and/or striking out with foot or feet.
			Drawn up/tensed	2	Legs tensed and/or pulled up tightly to body and kept there.
			Standing	2	Standing, crouching, or kneeling.
			Restrained	2	Child's legs are being held down.

From McGrath PA, DeVeber LL, Heam MT: Multidimensional pain assessment in children. In Fields HL, Dubner LR, Cervero F, editors: *Advances in pain research and therapy*, New York, 1985, Raven Press.

Specific Methods

Nonpharmacologic methods of pain control are presented briefly here (for further information, see Hazinski, 1992, Chapter 3):

- *Parents:* Parents are the single most powerful nonpharmacologic method of pain relief available to the child—they often instinctively provide comfort and therapeutic touch. The child may appear more distressed when parents are present because the child feels safe expressing discomfort to the parents.
- *Play and therapeutic activity:* Play can provide a method of expression and the opportunity to reveal fear and uncertainty and to master fears. Medical equipment can be used to identify sources of pain and fear and to clarify the child's understanding of and response to therapy.
- *Touch:* All children need to be touched stroked, and held. If it is impossible for the child to be held, move a chair close to the child's bed so the parents can maintain close physical contact with the child.
- *Music and distraction:* Distraction is a powerful method of pain relief. Television or music can temporarily divert attention from pain. Classical music or the use of earphones alone may reduce extraneous noise and stimulation for the critically ill child. The child may also be distracted and comforted by audiotapes made by parents or other loved ones, particularly if they include favorite stories or songs.
- *Imagination and imagery:* The child may be assisted in relaxation by suggestions and imagery (e.g., imagine you are floating on a cloud in the sky—when you look down, you can see your favorite place—can you describe it?).
- *Hypnosis:* Hypnosis has been effective in relieving pain and nausea after chemotherapy, but it requires a trained therapist.
- *Heat and cold:* Heat or cold can provide comfort and interrupt transmission of painful stimuli. Heat promotes vasodilation, so blood flow increases to the area and may remove the byproducts of cell breakdown. Cold may slow down the transmission of pain impulses. The applied temperature and perfusion of the underlying skin must be closely monitored during thermal therapy.

- *TENS Units:* Transcutaneous electrical nerve stimulators (TENS) are small plastic units that deliver small amounts of electrical energy to the skin through two to four electrodes. TENS units may be particularly useful for treatment of myofascial pain and stiffness, skin or bone pain, or incision pain (Mannheimer and Lampe, 1984).

Treatment of Myofascial Pain

Myofascial pain is characterized by muscles that are stiff, sore, and achy. Most myofascial pain can be alleviated by stimulation of accupressure points, using one or more of the following interventions: application of heat and cold (alternate every 20 minutes); warm bath and massage; TENS on acupuncture settings for no longer than 20 minutes followed by conventional TENS settings; administration of nonsteroidal antiinflammatory drugs (NSAIDs) or muscle relaxants, and active or passive range-of-motion exercises.

Pharmacologic Measures to Relieve Pain

Pain control may be achieved by systemic or local analgesic administration. Local analgesia may be most appropriate for procedure-related or incision pain, whereas multiple sites of pain may be most effectively controlled by systemic analgesics. If the critically ill or injured child is mechanically ventilated, systemic analgesia may be appropriate. Any child receiving analgesics should be closely monitored, and the drugs must be *titrated* to achieve maximum analgesic (therapeutic) effects with minimal side effects (drug dosages are listed in Table 3-2).

Nonnarcotic Analgesics

Nonnarcotic analgesics may be extremely useful for the treatment of mild to moderate pain, particularly musculoskeletal pain. These drugs may also be useful in the treatment of moderate pain when combined with narcotics and may reduce total narcotic requirements. Most of these analgesics are prostaglandin synthetase inhibitors (see Nonsteroidal Antiinflammatory Drugs).

Text continued on p. 56

Table 3-2
Dosing and Kinetics of Analgesics, Narcotics, Sedatives, Neuromuscular Blockers, and Antagonists

Drug (Trade)	Onset/Duration	Metabolism/Excretion	Bolus Dose	Infusion Dose	Comments
Nonsteroidal Antiinflammatory Drugs (NSAIDs)					
Aspirin	PO Onset: 15-30 min Peak: 1-2 h Duration: 4-6 h T½: 1-3.5 h	Hydrolyzed in GI Tract Hepatic metabolism Renal excretion	10-15 mg/kg q4h MAX (Total): 60-80 mg/kg/24 h or 4 g/24h THERAPEUTIC LEVELS: 150-300 mg/L	N/A	**Do not administer to children or adolescents for flulike illness;** Decreases platelet number and function
Acetaminophen (Tylenol)	PO Onset: 10-30 min PO Peak: 0.5-2 h PO Duration: 4-6 h Half-life: 1-4 h	Hepatic metabolism Renal excretion Contraindicated in patients with G-6 PD deficiency	10-20 mg/kg q4h MAX: 3g/24 h or 60-80 mg/kg/24 h, 4-6 doses	N/A	Lacks peripheral antiinflammatory activity of other NSAIDS
Choline Magnesium Trisalicylates (Trilisayte)	Peak: 2 h	Hepatic hydrolyzation Renal excretion of metabolites	10-15 mg/kg/dose orally, q6-8 h (tablet or liquid)	N/A	Highly protein bound Minimal antiplatelet activity
Ibuprofen (Motrin, Advil, Nuprin, Mediprin)	PO Peak: 0.5 h Half-life: 6 h	Hepatic transformation Renal excretion	10 mg/kg q6-8h MAX: 40 mg/kg/day	N/A	Highly (90%-99%) protein bound Use with caution in patients with ASA hypersensitivity or if hepatic/renal insufficiency
Ketorolac (Toradol)	IM Peak: 50 min Half-life: 6 h	91% renal excretion	0.5 mg/kg q6h, PO or IV MAX: 40 mg/kg/day PO, 120 mg/day IV	N/A	Will prolong bleeding time but not PT, PTT DO NOT administer during febrile illness in children or if hepatic, renal dysfunction, present
Naproxen (Naprosyn, Anaprox)	Peak: 2-4 h Steady-state: 4-5 doses Half-life: approx 13 h	95% renal excretion	7 mg PO MAX: 15 mg/kg day	N/A	May cause GI bleeding, heartburn, headaches. Should be ingested with food.
Narcotics					
Alfentanil (Alfenta)	Onset: <30 sec Peak: 1 min Duration: 11-30 min Half-life: 0.1-2 h	Hepatic metabolism Renal excretion	1-50 µg/kg IV	0.5-1 µg/kg/min	

Drug	Pharmacokinetics	Metabolism/Excretion	Dose	Continuous Infusion	Comments
Butorphanol (Stadol)	Onset: 1-8 min Peak: <5 min Duration: 3-4 min Half-life: 2.5-3.5 h	Hepatic metabolism Renal excretion	20-30 μg/kg IV for children (pediatric experience limited)	N/A	Mixed opioid agonist/antagonist
Codeine	Onset: 10-30 min Duration: 3-4 h	Hepatic metabolism Renal excretion of metabolites	0.5-1 mg/kg PO q2-3 h	NOT INTENDED FOR IV USE	
Fentanyl (Sublimaze)	Onset: 1-8 min Peak: minutes (IV) Duration: 0.5-1 h Half-life: 0.3-4 h (child)	Hepatic transformation Renal excretion of 75% of metabolites	1-5 μg/kg IV Caudal epidural: 1 μg/kg Patch: 25, 50, 75, 100 μg/h Oralet: 8-12 μg/kg	1-5 μg/kg/hr (higher doses may be necessary if tolerance develops) Caudal epidural: 0.5-1.5μg/kg/h	May cause chest muscle rigidity related to high dose and rapid administration (may be avoided if neuromuscular blocker administered before fentanyl administration) May increase ICP in patients with head injury Side effects less prominent than with morphine
Hydromorphone (Dilaudid)	Onset: 5-10 min Duration: 3-4 h Half-life: 2-4 h	Hepatic glucouronidation	PO: 0.03-0.08 mg/kg/dose q4-6h MAX: 5 mg IV: 0.015 mg/kg/dose q4-6 h		
Meperidine (Demerol)	Onset: 1-10 min IV, 15-20 min IM, 20 min PO Duration: 2-4 h Half-life (child): 2-4 h	Hepatic hydrolysis; active metabolites Renal excretion of some metabolites	0.05-1.5 mg/kg IV q2-4h MAX: 100 mg	0.5-0.7 mg/kg/h	Potentiated by MAO inhibitors and phenothiazines Metabolite normeperidine can accumulate after repeated doses, causing CNS symptoms and reduced analgesia in infants and children
Methadone (Dolphine)	Onset: 5-10 min IV Duration: 4-24 h	Hepatic metabolism	IV: 0.1-0.2 mg/kg THEN 0.05-0.1 mg/kg PO: 0.2 mg/kg q6-24h MAX: 10 mg	Not recommended	

GI, Gastrointestinal; *ASA*, acetylsalicylic acid; *PT*, prothrombin time; *PTT*, partial thromboplastin time; *ICP*, intracranial pressures; *MAO*, monoamine oxidase; *CNS*, central nervous system.
From Deshpande JK, Tobias JD: *The pediatric pain handbook*, St Louis, 1996 Mosby; Marx CM: Sedation and analgesia. In Blumer JL, editor: *A practical guide to pediatric intensive care*, ed 3, St Louis, 1990, Mosby; PDR: *Physician's desk reference*, Montvale, NJ, 1995, Medical Economics Data Production Company; Skidmore-Roth L: *1993 Mosby's nursing drug reference*, St Louis, 1993, Mosby; Tyler DC: Analgesia, sedation, and paralysis in pediatric critical care. In Fuhrman B, Zimmerman J, editors: *Pediatric critical care*, St Louis, 1997, Mosby.

Continued

Table 3-2
Dosing and Kinetics of Analgesics, Narcotics, Sedatives, Neuromuscular Blockers, and Antagonists—cont'd

Drug (Trade)	Onset/Duration	Metabolism/Excretion	Bolus Dose	Infusion Dose	Comments
Morphine	Onset: 1-10 min Peak: 30 min IV Duration: 3-4 h Half-life (child): 3-4 h	Hepatic metabolism; active metabolites Renal, bile excretion	0.05-0.1 mg/kg IV (q1-2h) Caudal epidural: 75 100 µg/kg Intrathecal: 10-20 µg/kg	0.1 mg/kg/h	For patient-controlled analgesia, see Box 3-4, p. 69.
Nalbuphine (Nubain)	Onset 2-3 min Peak: 30-45 min Duration: 1-3 h Half-life (adults): 5 h	Hepatic metabolism Renal excretion	0.05-0.2 mg/kg (q1-2h) MAX: 20 mg	0.1-0.4 mg/kg/h	
Sufentanil (Sufenta)	Onset: <30 sec Peak: minutes Duration: <1 h Half-life (child): 1.5-4 h	Transformed in liver and small intestine	0.1-3 µg/kg IV	1-1.4 µg/kg/h	
Opioid Antagonist					
Naloxone (Narcan)	Onset: <2 min Duration: 1-4 h (often shorter than underlying narcotic)	Hepatic metabolism (conjugated)	FULL NARCOTIC REVERSAL <20 kg: 0.1 mg/kg IV push FULL NARCOTIC REVERSAL >20 kg: 2 mg IV push PARTIAL NARCOTIC REVERSAL: 0.005-0.01 mg IV	0.1 mg/kg/h or administer 66% of initial reversal dose/h	Repeated dosing frequently required May cause acute narcotic withdrawal, including seizures, respiratory depression
Sedatives—Benzodiazepines					
Diazepam (Valium)	Onset: 1 min Peak: 15 min Duration: 5-60 min Half-life: 12-36 h	Hepatic metabolism Renal excretion	0.04-0.3 mg/kg IV q2-4h PO or PR: 0.2-0.3 mg/kg MAX: 0.6 mg/kg over 8 hr DO NOT ADMINISTER IM	N/A	May produce cardiac and respiratory depression Administer slowly

Drug	Pharmacokinetics	Metabolism/Excretion	Dose	Continuous Infusion	Comments
Lorazepam (Ativan)	Onset: 15 min Peak: 15-20 min Duration: 8-10 h Half-life (adults): 10-20 h	Hepatic metabolism Renal excretion	0.025-0.05 mg/kg IV or PO MAX: 4 mg/dose MAY BE ADMINISTERED IM if IV access unavailable MAX DILUTION: 0.25 mg/ml	0.025-0.1mg/kg/h	Some retrograde amnesia may occur; observe for precipitation
Midazolam (Versed)	Onset: 3-5 min Peak: 30 min Duration: 5-10 h Half-life: 2-8 h	Hepatic metabolism Renal excretion	0.05-0.2 mg/kg IV NOTE: Higher doses (0.03-0.75 mg/kg) used for PO, rectal, and intranasal use	0.05-0.2 mg/kg/h	97% protein-bound May be contraindicated in patients with: high ICP, systemic or pulmonary hypertension
Benzodiazepine Antagonist					
Flumazenil (Romazicon)	Onset: 1-2 min Peak: 6-10 min Duration related to plasma concentration of benzodiazepine and dose of flumazenil	Hepatic metabolism	0.01-0.015 mg/kg IV MAX: 2 mg		Has been associated with seizures, particularly in patients who have received long-term benzodiazepine therapy or who have tricylcic antidepressant overdose
Anesthetics					
Ketamine (Ketalar)	Onset: 3-4 min IM, 30 sec IV Duration: 12-25 min IM, 5-10 min IV Half-life (adult): 2 h	Hepatic metabolism	ANALGESIA: 0.5-1 mg/kg IM ANESTHESIA: IM: 2-10 mg/kg IV: 0.5-2 mg/kg PO: 0.5-1 mg/kg	1-2 mg/kg/h	May cause hypertension respiratory depression, laryngospasm, increased ICP
Propofol (Diprivian)	Onset: 40 sec Half-life: 1-8 h	70% excreted in urine also hepatic metabolism (conjugated)	200-300 mg/kg/min	5-200 mg/kg/min (short term)	Should not be used in patients with cardiovascular compromise Prolonged use not recommended

GI, Gastrointestinal; *ASA,* acelylsalicylic acid; *PT,* prothrombin time; *PTT,* partial thromboplastin time; *ICP,* intracranial pressures; *MAO,* monoamine oxidase; *CNS,* central nervous system.

From Deshpande JK, Tobias JD: *The pediatric pain handbook,* St Louis, 1996 Mosby; Marx CM: Sedation and analgesia. In Blumer JL, editor: *A practical guide to pediatric intensive care,* ed 3, St Louis, 1990, Mosby; PDR: *Physician's desk reference,* Montvale, NJ, 1995, Medical Economics Data Production Company; Skidmore-Roth L: *1993 Mosby's nursing drug reference,* St Louis, 1993, Mosby; Tyler DC: Analgesia, sedation, and paralysis in pediatric critical care. In Fuhrman B, Zimmerman J, editors: *Pediatric critical care,* St Louis, 1997, Mosby.

Continued

Table 3-2
Dosing and Kinetics of Analgesics, Narcotics, Sedatives, Neuromuscular Blockers, and Antagonists—cont'd

Drug (Trade)	Onset/Duration	Metabolism/Excretion	Bolus Dose	Infusion Dose	Comments
Barbiturates					
Pentobarbital (Nembutal)	Onset: nearly immediate Peak: minutes Duration: 1-4 h Half-life: 14-50 h	Hepatic metabolism Renal excretion of metabolites	IV: 1-4 mg/kg PO, PR: 2-4 mg/kg IM injection painful	1-4 µg/kg/h	35%-45% protein-bound May cause vasodilation and may depress myocardial contractility
Sodium Thiopental (Pentothal)	Onset: 30-40 sec Peak: rapid Duration: <30 min Half-life: 3-8 h	Redistributes rapidly in tissues	2-6 mg/kg IV	N/A	See above
Chloral Hydrate					
Chloral Hydrate (Noctec)	Onset: 30 min Peak: 60 min Duration: 1-2 h IV Half-life (neonate): 8.5-64 h	Metabolized in liver and erythrocytes and kidney Renal excretion of metabolites	Sedation: 25-50 mg/kg PO or PR Hypnotic: 75-100 mg/kg MAX: 2 g/24 h		35%-41% protein-bound May cause GI irritation, paradoxic excitement, vasodilation
Neuromuscular Blocking Agents					
Atracurium	Onset: 2 min Duration: 20-30 min Half-life: 2 min	Hoffman degradation inactivation): potentially active metabolites	0.3-0.6 mg/kg	0.3-0.6 mg/kg/h	Do not mix with alkaline solutions Metabolites may produce CNS complications, including seizures at high levels

Drug	Pharmacokinetics	Major elimination	Dose	Infusion	Comments
Doxacurium	Peak block: 3-9 min; Duration to 25% recovery: 55-160 min	Major elimination: unchanged in urine	Children 2-12 yr: 0.03-0.5 mg/kg IV, followed by 0.005-0.01 mg/kg 30-45 minutes later	N/A	
d-Tubocurarine	Onset: 15 sec; Peak: 2-3 min; Duration: 35-45 min; Half-life: 1-3 h	60% renal excretion, also 10%-40% hepatic and renal degradation	0.5 mg/kg	N/A	Inject slowly; rapid infusion may produce hypotension
Mivacurium	Onset: 2-3 min; Peak: 1½-8 min; Duration:5-30 min	Plasma cholinesterases hydrolyze rapidly	IV: 0.2 mg/kg	5-30 µg/kg/min	
Pancuronium	Onset: 30-45 sec; Peak: 3-5 min; Duration: 50-60min	80% renal	0.05-0.1 mg/kg	0.05-0.1 mg/kg/h	Vagolytic, so may result in an increase in heart rate, mean arterial pressure, cardiac output
Succinylcholine	Onset: 0.5-1 min (IV); Peak: 2-3 min (IV); Duration: 4-5 min	Plasma cholinesterase Hydrolyzed in urine	*Infants:* IV: 2 mg/kg IM: 4.0 mg/kg *Children:* 1-1.5 mg/kg	N/A	May produce arrhythmias (especially bradycardia), increased intracranial pressure, hyperkalemia. See Box 3-2.
Rocuronium (Zemuron)	Onset: <1 min; Duration: 20-40 min	Primarily hepatic	0.6-1mg/kg	N/A	
Vecuronium	Onset 1.5 min; Duration: 25-30 min	70%-80% Hepatic; active metabolites 20%-30% renal	0.5-0.1 mg/kg	0.06-0.1 mg/kg/h	

GI, Gastrointestinal; *ASA*, acetylsalicylic acid; *PT*, prothrombin time; *PTT*, partial thromboplastin time; *ICP*, intracranial pressures; *MAO*, monoamine oxidase; *CNS*, central nervous system.
From Deshpande JK, Tobias JD: *The pediatric pain handbook*, St Louis, 1996 Mosby; Marx CM: Sedation and analgesia. In Blumer JL, editor: *A practical guide to pediatric intensive care*, ed 3, St Louis, 1990, Mosby; PDR: *Physician's desk reference*, Montvale, NJ, 1995, Medical Economics Data Production Company; Skidmore-Roth L: *1993 Mosby's nursing drug reference*, St Louis, 1993, Mosby; Tyler DC: Analgesia, sedation, and paralysis in pediatric critical care. In Fuhrman B, Zimmerman J, editors: *Pediatric critical care*, St Louis, 1997, Mosby.

A second group of nonnarcotic analgesics includes the alpha-2 agonists (e.g., clonidine) and drugs such as anticonvulsants or tricyclic antidepressants. Both groups of drugs have other primary indications but do have analgesic effects. These drugs are not reviewed further here, but the reader is referred to more comprehensive sources (Tobias, 1995).

Aspirin

Aspirin should not be used for routine analgesia for children who have flulike symptoms because of its possible association with Reye's syndrome. For older children aspirin may be an effective analgesic and antiinflammatory drug if it is used alone or in combination therapy. Aspirin depresses platelet number and function; thus it should not be administered in the presence of thrombocytopenia or coagulopathies.

Acetaminophen

Acetaminophen is a potent analgesic that is useful in the treatment of fever or pain in younger children. It has no antiinflammatory effect. Acetaminophen does not produce the platelet dysfunction or the increased risk of Reye's syndrome that is associated with aspirin.

Nonsteroidal Antiinflammatory Drugs

Most drugs in this category inhibit the synthesis of mediators that stimulate free nerve endings in the peripheral nervous system; they may exert effects on central prostaglandin synthesis. NSAIDs have superior antiinflammatory properties when compared with aspirin or acetaminophen. They are most effective in combination with narcotics for treatment of mild or moderate pain, particularly postoperative pain, and often reduce narcotic requirements. Side effects of NSAIDs include platelet dysfunction, gastrointestinal bleeding, peptic ulcer formation, and hepatic dysfunction. NSAIDs inhibit renal prostaglandins; thus they should be used with caution in patients with renal failure because the NSAIDs may exacerbate existing compromise in renal blood flow and glomerular filtration rate. Alterations in glomerular filtration are most likely to occur if NSAIDs are administered in combination with other nephrotoxic drugs or in the presence of profound hypovolemia.

Ibuprofen *Ibuprofen* (Advil, Mediprin, Motrin, Nuprin) is a NSAID that is thought to inhibit prostaglandin synthesis. It is available in liquid or tablet form (dosage: 10 mg/kg every 6 hours, maximum 40 mg/kg/day in 3 to 4 doses) and is rapidly absorbed from the gastrointestinal (GI) tract. Ibuprofen is highly protein bound; thus it may displace other drugs from proteins. It prolongs bleeding time, and concomitant use with anticoagulants potentiates the anticoagulant effects. It should not be used in children with coagulopathies, lupus, or GI disease. Ibuprofen is transformed in the liver and excreted in the urine, so should not be used for children with hepatic or renal failure.

Choline Magnesium Trisalicylate *Choline magnesium trisalicylate (Trilisayte)* is a relatively old analgesic that inhibits prostaglandin. Recently this drug has been successfully used for the treatment of advanced pediatric cancer pain. It may be superior to other NSAIDs for these patients because it does not interfere with platelet function. It should not be administered during febrile illness in children.

Indomethacin and Ketorolac Most NSAIDs are available only in oral preparations, but *indomethacin* and *ketorolac tromethamine* (0.5 mg/kg every 6 hours, maximum of 60 mg/kg/day) may be administered by parenteral route. Ketorolac is an antiinflammatory agent, an antipyretic, and an analgesic. It has proven to be valuable alone and in combination with other drugs in the treatment of postoperative pain in children and adolescents. It has several advantages over other NSAIDs. When ketorolac is administered following surgery in children, total opioid requirements, pain scores, and adverse effects may be decreased. It produces less nausea and vomiting and renal impairment than reported with other NSAIDs. This drug is not thought to produce sedation, respiratory depression, or physical and psychologic dependence. Although this drug does prolong bleeding time, it does not affect platelet count, prothrombin time, or partial thromboplastin time.

Corticosteroids

Corticosteroids are not analgesics. They can relieve pain through an antiinflammatory effect; thus they are generally administered in combination with a narcotic and a nonnarcotic to produce analgesia. Joint pain and pain from bone metastases, nerve pressure, hepatomegaly, and brain tumors may be relieved through the antiinflammatory effect of corticosteroid administration.

Narcotics/Opioids

Narcotic analgesics remain the single most important group of drugs for the relief of moderate to severe pain. The choice of a narcotic agent should be based on pharmacokinetic considerations, the side-effect profile of the drug, available routes of administration, and receptor specificity. Administration of narcotics requires decisions regarding: (1) the route of administration: intravenous (IV), intramuscular (IM), oral, subcutaneous, transmucosal, or transdermal; (2) the choice of narcotic; and (3) the method of administration (fixed interval, continuous, or patient-controlled analgesia). This section provides information regarding narcotic choice, including potential routes of administration and delivery options (see also Table 3-2).

Narcotic/Opioid Receptors

Narcotic action is governed by a variety of independent receptors that can be used to classify narcotic action (Table 3-3). The *mu (μ) receptor* and the *delta (δ) receptor* produce supraspinal analgesia, occurring in the brain. These mu and delta effects are those most commonly associated with narcotic drugs, including euphoria and potential respiratory depression. *The kappa (κ) receptor* is believed to govern analgesia below the level of the brain in the spinal cord pain control fibers. Kappa receptor activation produces pinpoint pupils and some sedative side effects. *Sigma (σ) receptor* stimulation is associated with unpleasant side effects, including hallucinations, and cardiorespiratory stimulation.

Morphine and Morphine Agonists

Morphine is the prototype for the mu and kappa receptor agonist narcotics. Other drugs in this category include methadone, hydromorphone (Dilaudid), meperidine (Demerol), and fentanyl and its derivatives. These drugs differ principally in their side-effect profile and pharmacokinetics. The natu-

Table 3-3
Subdivisions of Opiate Receptors and Clinical Effects

Receptor Type	Drugs	Clinical Effects
(μ)	Morphine Fentanyl Codeine Naloxone	Supraspinal analgesia, euphoria, respiratory depression, physical dependence
(δ)	Enkephaline	Supraspinal analgesia, euphoria, respiratory depression, physical dependence
(κ)	Mixed agonist/ antagonist	Spinal analgesia, sedation, miosis, hypothermia
(σ)	Phencyclidine	Psychotomimetic effects, hallucinations, dysphoria, respiratory and vasomotor stimulation

Deshpande JK, Tobias JD: *The pediatric pain handbook,* St Louis, 1966, Mosby; and Koren G, Maurice L: Pediatric uses of opioids, *Pediatr Clin North Am* 36(5):1141, 1989.

rally occurring opioids have long plasma half-lives but may produce tachycardia and hypotension. The synthetic opioids (fentanyl, sufentanil, and alfentanil) have short plasma half-lives and are often given by continuous infusion. In general, these synthetics have minimal cardiovascular effects; thus they may be ideal for the unstable patient. Sufentanil can cause severe bradycardia; thus its use is often avoided in patients with cardiovascular dysfunction. Fentanyl may increase the ICP in patients with head injury (Sperry et al, 1992; Tobias, 1992).

Morphine   Morphine remains an effective agent for the treatment of moderate or severe pain. Note that, if cardiovascular function or intravascular volume is compromised, the venodilation produced by morphine may result in a decrease in blood pressure or systemic perfusion. As with other opioids, morphine is metabolized in the liver, and metabolites are excreted in the urine. As a result, if renal failure is present, some morphine metabolites such as morphine-6-glucuronide may accumulate and produce respiratory depression. Analgesia may be achieved with intermittent doses because the plasma half-life of morphine is 2 to 8 hours, but it is longer in the newborn than in the older infant or adult.

Morphine is the drug most commonly used for patient controlled analgesia. In general, a basal infusion rate may begin at 0.01 to 0.02 mg/kg/hr. Recent pediatric studies suggest that even a very low dose basal infusion (0.004 mg/kg/hr) can provide analgesia and improved sleep at night with minimal side effects in children. A high morphine patient-controlled analgesia (PCA) basal infusion rate is undesirable for several reasons. It increases the likelihood of adverse effects (nausea and vomiting, respiratory depression, sedation), with negligible improvement in analgesia. In addition, a high basal rate removes the theoretic safety mechanism of PCA (i.e., the patient with too much narcotic will be too sleepy to activate the PRN bolus).

Methadone Methadone is an extremely long-acting narcotic that may only require a single dose daily. Continuous infusion is not required, and therapeutic serum concentrations may be achieved by repeated doses administered every 6 to 12 hours (e.g., 0.1 mg/kg every 6 hours for 24 hours, then 0.1 mg/kg every 8 hours for 24 hours, then 0.1 mg/kg every 12 hours thereafter), although 72 hours or more will be required to achieve steady-state drug concentrations. Alternatively an initial IV dose of 0.1 to 0.2 mg/kg may be administered slowly, then 0.05 mg/kg every 10 to 15 minutes until analgesia is achieved. Once therapeutic drug levels are achieved, the drug may be administered every 4 to 24 hours (0.05 to 0.1 mg/kg every 4 to 12 hours by *slow* IV push is typical). This drug is effective for chronic pain control and may also be used to taper narcotic therapy in children who have developed tolerance to high-dose infusions of agents such as fentanyl. In these children a daily dose of methadone is calculated as equivalent to the total daily fentanyl dose (divided into 2 doses). It may permit a switch from IV to oral therapy, eliminating the need for IV access.

Hydromorphone (Dilaudid) Hydromorphone is a morphine derivative that is much more potent than morphine. It has no active metabolites, so it may be a drug of choice for patients with renal failure. It may cause fewer complications related to histamine release (e.g., pruritus) than morphine or other opioids; thus it may be particularly useful for patients with graft-vs.-host disease, burns, or other skin problems. If pruritus continues to be a problem, consider fentanyl. Onset of action may be within 5 minutes of an IV dose and 20 to 30 minutes of an oral dose.

Meperidine (Demerol) Meperidine is a poor choice for postoperative analgesia because it is associated with several potential CNS complications, including dysphoria, restlessness, agitation, and seizures. This toxicity results from the accumulation of the metabolite normeperidine, which is a CNS stimulant with analgesic properties and a long serum half-life. Normeperidine accumulation is particularly likely when the drug is administered over several days, when it is co-administered with phenobarbital or other agents that increase hepatic microsomal enzymes, or when it is administered to patients with impaired renal function.

Fentanyl and Derivatives (Sufentanil and Alfentanil) These drugs constitute the synthetic opioids. They produce fewer cardiovascular side effects and less histamine release than morphine and other natural opioids, but have very short serum half-lives (1.5 to 4 hours). As a result, these drugs are frequently administered by continuous infusion with intermittent supplemental boluses.

Bolus fentanyl administration may produce a rise in ICP and a fall in mean arterial blood pressure in children with head injury, so use with caution in these patients. Chest muscle rigidity occasionally associated with fentanyl is dose-related and may be prevented by slow infusion of the fentanyl, or reversed with naloxone or interrupted with neuromuscular blocking agents.

Fentanyl, sufentanil, and alfentanil differ in kinetics and potency but are otherwise similar. They all undergo tissue redistribution. Clearance of fentanyl is similar for full-term neonates, infants and children, although clearance is significantly reduced in premature neonates. An increased volume of distribution and reduced renal clearance cause lower plasma clearance of fentanyl in premature neonates.

Sufentanil is approximately 10 times as potent as fentanyl. Alfentanil has a shorter duration of action and more rapid onset than fentanyl but is much less potent; thus it is often used for short procedures.

Fentanyl and its derivatives are most commonly administered intravenously. However, oral and intranasal forms of these drugs may be used for premedication and postoperative analgesia. The Food and Drug Administration has recently approved a raspberry-flavored lozenge or "oralet" form of the drug, oral transmucosal fentanyl citrate (OTFC), which is available in 200, 300, and 400 μg doses. Sedation results from absorption of fentanyl across the buccal mucosa; thus the effectiveness of the lozenge is diminished if the lozenge is chewed and swallowed rather than sucked.

Transdermal fentanyl patches deliver 25, 50, 75, or 100 μg/hr. These patches eliminate the need for IV access. However, dosage selection and control are limited, particularly for smaller patients, preventing use of these patches in young patients. In addition, analgesic serum levels may not be achieved for up to 12 hours after patch application. The manufacturer cautions against use in children younger than 12 years of age because of concern regarding respiratory depression. Respiratory function must be monitored closely when any narcotic is administered.

Codeine Codeine may be used to treat mild or moderate pain. Although it may be administered by oral or IV route, the oral route is used most commonly in children. In fact, IV codeine has been associated with histaminic-induced hypotension; thus IV codeine administration is not recommended for children. Codeine is often administered in a dose of 0.5 to 1 mg/kg in combination with 10 mg/kg of acetaminophen, resulting in potentiation of the analgesic effects of each drug. Codeine can produce respiratory depression, delayed gastric emptying, nausea, vomiting and constipation.

Mixed Agonists/Antagonists

These drugs consist of nalbuphine (Nubain), pentazocine (Talwin), and butorphanol (Stadol). These drugs have been developed in an attempt to target very specific receptors; they exert effects at one opioid receptor (typically the kappa or delta receptor) and antagonize a second receptor (typically the mu receptor). The theoretic benefit of the mixed agonist/antagonist action is a limitation of potential side effects (such as respiratory depression), but the price paid is the limitation of pain relief. These mixed drugs can actually produce the same respiratory depression, sedation, and GI symptoms as an equipotent dose of morphine (Deshpande and Tobias, 1996). The limitation of analgesic effect of these mixed agonists/antagonists and the fact that they limit the analgesic effects of concurrently administered opioids may make them less desirable for use in the ICU.

Nalbuphine (Nubain) Nalbuphine is a mu-antagonist but is a partial sigma-receptor agonist and a partial agonist at the kappa-receptor. Therefore it produces analgesia with minimal respiratory depression. Nalbuphine has the highest therapeutic index and therefore is the safest parenteral narcotic when mild to moderate analgesia is desired.

Because nalbuphine may block mu receptors, it may compete with other narcotics such as fentanyl or morphine and may actually increase the respiratory drive. This is desirable if extubation is the goal. Nalbuphine should not routinely be combined with morphine, since it will block the analgesic effects of the morphine. During chronic narcotic administration, nalbuphine may precipitate withdrawal if substituted for morphine, fentanyl, or similar drugs.

Pentazocine (Talwin) Pentazocine is a sigma-receptor agonist that alters ascending pain pathways in the CNS and also alters pain perception. IV administration has rapid onset, with a duration of 4 to 6 hours. It may cause drowsiness, headaches, hallucinations, nausea, vomiting, and cardiorespiratory depression. This drug may not be mixed in solution with barbiturates.

Butorphanol Tartrate (Stadol) Stadol is a potent narcotic analgesic that is effective in the relief of moderate to severe pain. It is thought to exert its analgesic activity in subcortical areas of the CNS, possibly the limbic system. Stadol may produce respiratory depression, which is reversible by naloxone. The severity of the respiratory depression is independent of dose, but the duration is dose related. This drug increases pulmonary artery pressure, pulmonary artery occlusion pressure, and pulmonary vascular resistance and may increase cerebrospinal fluid and ICP. This drug should be used with caution in children with organ system failure and may precipitate withdrawal in the narcotic-dependent patient.

Opioid Antagonist

Naloxone (Narcan)   Naloxone is a mu and kappa receptor antagonist and is used to reverse narcotic effects. Because it is a competitive inhibitor of the narcotic, the naloxone dose (1 to 4 µg/kg) must be tailored to the amount of the narcotic present rather than to the patient weight, and the timing and frequency of the doses and method of naloxone delivery must consider the half-life of the narcotic to be antagonized. *Since naloxone has a shorter duration of action than the majority of narcotics it reverses, a continuous infusion or repeated doses of naloxone will likely be required to provide lasting reversal in severe overdoses.* Rapid naloxone reversal of profound analgesia (such as that produced by fentanyl) may produce dramatic clinical effects, including hypertension and occasional pulmonary edema. Carefully titrated doses of naloxone can reverse the adverse effects of narcotics without reversing the analgesic properties. Naloxone may precipitate acute narcotic withdrawal in addicted individuals. *If respiratory depression is present, respiratory support must be provided until clear and consistent reversal of narcotic effects has been achieved.*

Sedatives and Anesthetics

Sedatives are important adjuncts to pain control in the PICU since they can eliminate the emotional aspects of pain by decreasing anxiety, inducing sleep, and eliminating the memory of painful or frightening events. The drugs used most commonly as sedatives in the PICU include the benzodiazepines, the barbiturates, and chloral hydrate.

Benzodiazepines

These drugs act in the limbic system, causing anterograde amnesia (prevention of memory of new information) without loss of memory (retrograde amnesia). They have no intrinsic analgesic proper-

ties; thus they must be administered with analgesics if pain is present. They produce few cardiovascular effects but may depress respirations and produce apnea, particularly after bolus or high doses. Reversal can be accomplished with flumazenil (8 to 15 µg/kg intravenously every 30 to 60 minutes); seizures can result. Prolonged administration of benzodiazepines may result in physical dependence, and an abstinence syndrome may be induced by abrupt withdrawal. Therefore taper the IV dose slowly. All three of the currently available benzodiazepines may be administered orally, rectally, or intravenously. Midazolam and lorazepam may be administered intramuscularly, and midazolam may be administered intranasally. Note that these drugs differ in onset of action; this difference must be considered when switching from one drug to the other in clinical use.

Diazepam (Valium)   Diazepam is the oldest of the benzodiazepines in common clinical use. It is available in oral and parenteral solutions but cannot be given intramuscularly. It is insoluble in water; thus it must be administered in a solution of preservative, making this drug undesirable for neonatal use and incompatible with most IV solutions. Diazepam has a long elimination half-life, and active metabolites may have even longer half-lives that produce hypnotic effects. Diazepam has minimal cardiovascular effects unless the patient is hypovolemic, but it may produce respiratory depression (particularly when used in the treatment of seizures).

Midazolam (Versed)   Midazolam has become the most popular of the benzodiazepines because it has a rapid onset of action and a short half-life and the IV form is water-soluble. It may be administered by intermittent or continuous infusion. Better sedation is usually achieved with lower drug doses if continuous infusion rather than bolus therapy is used. Bolus administration is ideal to achieve sedation during short procedures. Because the IV drug is water-soluble, it is compatible with most intravenous solutions. It may be administered by IV or IM routes and may also be administered intranasally, orally, sublingually, or subcutaneously.

The combination of midazolam with fentanyl or nalbuphine provides deep analgesia and sedation with potent effects on memory for the duration of the infusion. Active metabolites may result from the metabolism of this drug. The effects of midazolam may be potentiated by the alteration in metabolism or a decrease in protein binding. Since the drug is metabolized through the P450 hepatic system, any drug that may affect hepatic blood flow or the P450 system specifically may alter the effects of midazolam. Cimetidine decreases blood flow to the liver and competes for the P450 enzymes; thus cimetidine prolongs the effects of midazolam. Some anticonvulsants such as phenobarbital induce the P450 enzyme system and thus decrease midazolam effects, whereas others inhibit the enzyme system and prolong the midazolam effects. The major disadvantage of this drug is its cost.

Lorazepam (Ativan) Lorazepam is currently available in several generic forms. Its onset of action is slower, and it has a longer duration of action than midazolam; thus it may be administered by intermittent, demand dosing, as well as continuous infusion. Its hepatic metabolism does not use the P450 system; thus metabolism of lorazepam is less likely to be affected by concurrent drug administration or hepatic failure.

Anesthetics

Ketamine Ketamine is an IV anesthetic agent that provides both amnesia and analgesia—it produces a dissociative state. Low doses (0.5 to 1 mg/kg) provide analgesia of the skin muscle and bone, whereas higher doses (1 to 2 mg/kg) produce general anesthesia. In general, the drug has minimal cardiovascular or respiratory depressant effects, although it may produce an increase in heart rate and blood pressure and possibly hypotension in children with myocardial dysfunction. Ketamine has minimal effect on respiratory function, although the child's airway protective mechanisms and ventilation must be closely monitored. Ketamine is a bronchodilator, and it may increase pulmonary vascular resistance. Hallucinations associated with the drug are dose related and may be prevented by administration of lorazepam or midazolam 5 minutes before ketamine administration.

This drug may be administered by continuous infusion, although bolus administration may be useful during procedures.

Propofol (Diprivan) Propofol is a short-acting, sedative-hypnotic agent and an IV anesthetic agent with no analgesic properties. It has rapid onset, rapid clearance, and no active metabolites. This drug should not be used in patients with cardiovascular compromise, since it has vasodilatory and negative inotropic effects (will decrease myocardial contractility) and vagal effects that may produce bradycardia. Continuous infusion for prolonged sedation is no longer recommended for children less than 12 years of age, following reports of fatal cardiac failure and unexplained metabolic acidosis.

However, this drug has become increasingly popular for *short-term* anesthesia and procedural anesthesia (dose: 200 to 300 µg/kg/min). Potential complications include metabolic acidosis, neurologic dysfunction, hypothermia, respiratory depression, and liver dysfunction. Propofol is not water soluble; it is suspended in oil. It can be very painful when injected, unless the injection site is pretreated with IV lidocaine. Because the drug has such a short duration of action, repeated dosing is required if bolus therapy is provided (Pepperman and Macrae, 1997). Continuous infusion is used in the operating room for short procedures.

Barbiturates

Barbiturates are potent anticonvulsants and have been used to induce coma in patients with severe head injury and increased ICP or status epilepticus unresponsive to other anticonvulsants. These agents may also be effective sedatives and amnesiacs, particularly when used in conjunction with benzodiazepines. They may be particularly useful for sedation during extracorporeal membrane oxygenation therapy. The available barbiturates differ in pharmacokinetics, and they can be separated into four classes based on duration of action. They all have dose-related effects on respiratory drive and airway protective mechanisms; high doses may produce apnea and hypotension. Most depress normal sleep patterns. All undergo hepatic metabolism; thus liver failure affects duration of action.

Sodium Thiopental This drug is an ultra short–acting barbiturate (5 to 10 minute duration of action following IV administration) that is often used during induction of anesthesia. It has significant myocardial and respiratory depressant effects. Its negative inotropic and vasodilator effects can produce hypotension, particularly in the presence of hypovolemia.

Pentobarbital This intermediate-acting barbiturate (45- to 60-minute duration of action) has favorable pharmacokinetics for use in the PICU for sedation and nonpainful procedures. It may be used to rapidly induce coma or suppress seizure activity. Myocardial depression and vasodilation produced by the drug may result in hypotension and compromise in systemic perfusion; these effects may be modulated by concurrent volume administration and vasoactive drug therapy. The drug is generally administered intravenously or rectally; IM injection is painful and not recommended.

Phenobarbital Long-acting drug with potent anticonvulsant effects but fewer sedative properties. Not used for sedation.

Chloral Hydrate

Chloral hydrate is a sedative-hypnotic agent that may be administered by oral or rectal routes (no IV form available) and is well-absorbed from the GI tract. It produces sedation *but not analgesia* and is most appropriately used for sedation during brief, nonpainful procedures such as a computed tomography scan (75 mg/kg administered rectally). Chloral hydrate has several undesirable side effects, including gastric irritation, apnea, respiratory depression, and depression of normal sleep patterns. This drug is metabolized in the liver and metabolites may accumulate, producing such complications as neonatal hyperbilirubinemia. For this reason, it is no longer recommended for infants less than 3 months of age and should not be used in children with hepatic dysfunction. Chronic use may produce tolerance and physical dependence, and sudden discontinuation can induce withdrawal symptoms.

Neuromuscular Blocking Agents

Neuromuscular blocking agents (NMBAs) interfere with the normal transmission of impulses from nerves to muscles, producing muscle paralysis. Most are nondepolarizing agents that antagonize effects of the neuromuscular transmitter, acetylcholine, at the receptors to prevent muscle depolarization. Succinylcholine is the only depolarizing neuromuscular blocker: it binds to the acetylcholine receptors and produces depolarization of the sarcolemma.

NMBAs may be used to facilitate mechanical ventilatory control, control ICP, reduce myocardial oxygen requirements, or facilitate procedures or diagnostic studies. These drugs are never administered alone; they must be used in conjunction with sedatives. Adequate airway and ventilatory support must always be ensured during the use of these agents.

There can be tremendous variability in NMBA dose requirements and effects based on the patient's clinical condition and concurrent drug therapy. NMBAs may be antagonized by some drugs (e.g., theophylline or anticonvulsant therapy), inhibited by some clinical conditions (e.g., hyperkalemia, burn injuries), and enhanced by other conditions (e.g., hyperkalemia, renal or hepatic failure, some antibiotics).

Excessive blockade may result in prolonged recovery times; thus these drugs must be carefully titrated. A transcutaneous nerve stimulator can be used to evaluate the degree of neuromuscular blockade, enabling dose adjustment (see later paragraphs).

NMBAs may be administered by fixed interval dosing or continuous infusion with PRN bolus. Regardless of the administration method, patient response must be constantly evaluated.

Pancuronium (Pavulon) Pancuronium is a long-acting neuromuscular blocker with a steroid nucleus. It produces full relaxation in approximately 2 to 4 minutes, with a duration of 45 to 60 minutes. Beta-adrenergic and anticholinergic effects may produce tachycardia and hypertension. Elimination occurs primarily (80%) through the kidneys; thus this drug should be avoided in patients with renal failure.

To titrate a continuous pancuronium infusion, a nerve stimulator is placed on the ulnar nerve once the bolus dose (0.1 mg/kg) is administered. Every 2 hours a standard "train of four" stimulus is monitored. Once the first twitch is observed, the continuous infusion is begun at 0.05 mg/kg/hour. The dose is adjusted in increments of 0.01 mg/kg/hour to maintain 1 to 2 twitches every 2 hours. If an increase in the infusion rate is required, a bolus equivalent to the current hourly rate is also administered before the infusion is increased. This procedure enables precise titration of the pancuronium to patient response (Tobias et al, in press).

Vecuronium (Norcuron) Vecuronium is an intermediate-acting steroidal neuromuscular blocker, with potency similar to pancuronium but a shorter duration of action (25 to 30 minutes). This drug may be preferred for use in children with cardiovascular compromise, since it does not cause release of histamine and has no vagolytic effects. Elimination occurs primarily (70% to 80%) through the liver, but metabolites that are excreted by the kidneys do exert weak neuromuscular blockade. Therefore prolonged effects may be seen in patients with renal failure.

Atracurium (Tracrium) Atracurium is a nonsteroidal intermediate-acting neuromuscular blocker that is eliminated by nonenzymatic Hoffmann degradation; thus its elimination is independent of renal and hepatic function. However, hepatic metabolism is required for excretion of drug metabolites. One metabolite, laudanosine, can cause seizures in high concentrations, but this has not been reported clinically. Histamine release is a prominent effect of this drug; thus its use is usually avoided in children with asthma. Typical doses (0.6 mg/kg) do not affect heart rate or blood pressure.

Rocuronium Bromide (Zemuron) Rocuronium is a nondepolarizing neuromuscular blocking agent with rapid-to-intermediate action. It competes for cholinergic receptors at the motor end-plate, and its action is antagonized by acetylcholinesterase inhibitors. It is an ideal drug for intubation, particularly when there are contraindications to succinylcholine administration. Average time to completion of intubation in children following administration is 1 minute. Renal impairment may result in a small reduction in drug clearance, although tissue redistribution accounts for approximately 80% of the initial dose.

Doxacurium This new nondepolarizing muscle relaxant has a duration of action similar to that of pancuronium and few cardiovascular effects. The duration of action in children may be shorter than that of adults. This drug does not contain steroids.

Mivacurium This short-acting nondepolarizing agent enables rapid recovery (within approximately 10 minutes) because it is metabolized by plasma cholinesterases. Hemodynamic effects are minimal.

Succinylcholine Succinylcholine is a depolarizing neuromuscular blocker with an extremely rapid onset of action (30 to 45 seconds). Because the drug is metabolized by pseudocholinesterase in the plasma, its duration of action is approximately 4 to 6 minutes. It can produce transient bradycardia and other bradyarrhythmias, as well as negative inotropic effects. There are contraindications to succinylcholine administration, including several conditions in which the drug may produce an exaggerated hyperkalemic response (Box 3-2).

There have been rare reports of acute rhabdomyolysis with hyperkalemia followed by ventricular arrhythmias, cardiac arrest, and death after administration of succinylcholine to apparently healthy children who are later found to have undiagnosed skeletal muscle myopathy, most often Duchenne's muscular dystrophy. Children 8 years of age and younger are most commonly affected, although this complication has been reported in adolescents. This syndrome should be suspected when any child develops peaked T waves and cardiac arrest immediately after receiving succinylcholine. Immediate treatment of hyperkalemia is required, including administration of IV sodium bicarbonate (2.5 mEq/kg over 30 to 60 minutes), calcium gluconate (0.6 to 1 ml/kg of 10% solution over 2 to 4 minutes), and glucose plus insulin (1 to 2 ml/kg of 25% dextrose plus 0.02 to 0.04 U regular insulin/kg). For further information, see Hyperkalemia, Chapter 7.

Box 3-2

Conditions Associated With Increased Risk of Succinylcholine-Induced Hyperkalemia

Metabolic

Hyperkalemia
Renal failure
Malignant hyperthermia

Tissue Destruction

Burns (>15% BSA, from 48 hours to 2 to 3 months following thermal injury)
Massive trauma, especially crush injuries (for 5 to 15 days after injury)

Central Nervous System Injury with Muscle Wasting (risk persists for approximately 3 to 6 months)
Stroke
Myotonias
Muscular dystrophy
Gullian-Barré syndrome
Spinal cord injury
Diffuse head injury
Encephalitis

Muscle immobilization and atrophy
Muscle denervation
Upper or lower motor neuron lesions

Miscellaneous Conditions Possibly Associated With Risk

Clostridial infections
Severe prolonged infections (>1 week)
Anterior horn cell disease
Insecticide poisoning (organophosphates, carbamates)
Nerve gas poisoning
Family history of decreased succinylcholine clearance

From Deshpande JK, Tobias JD: *The pediatric pain book*, St Louis, 1996, Mosby; Keyes W: Neuromuscular blockade. In Holbrook PR, editor: *Textbook of critical care*, Philadelphia, 1993, Saunders; and Kelly JS, MacGregor DA: Drugs acting at the cholinergic receptor. In Chernow B, editor: *The pharmacologic approach to the critically ill patient*, ed 3, Baltimore, 1994, Williams & Wilkins.

Rapid and Modified Rapid Sequence Induction

Rapid sequence induction is most commonly performed to facilitate rapid control and intubation of the airway. Before administration of any medications, the patient is preoxygenated. All equipment is checked and ready so intubation can be accomplished smoothly once pharmacologic sedation and paralysis is induced (Box 3-3).

Succinylcholine is frequently used during rapid sequence induction. Contraindications to its use include conditions in which the drug may produce hyperkalemia. These are listed in Box 3-2.

Regional Therapy

Regional analgesics and anesthetics are becoming increasingly popular. They enable extremely effective analgesia with fewer systemic effects such as respiratory depression. These analgesics require placement of catheters to enable injection of local anesthetics and narcotics into the pleural or epidural space or to block peripheral nerves. Complications of these therapies include those of catheter placement, narcotic effects, and local anesthetic toxicities (see Complications). These therapies should be used with caution in neonates.

Local Anesthetics

Local anesthetics may be used to minimize sensation in an isolated area before needle or catheter insertion or wound debridement or to provide regional anesthesia (e.g., epidural anesthesia). The most common local anesthetics include lidocaine (concentration of 0.5% to 2%, dose of 5 to 7 mg/kg), bupivacaine (concentration of 0.25% to 0.5%, dose of 1.5 to 2.5 mg/kg) and cocaine (topical dose of 1 to 2 mg/kg).

Spinal (Epidural or Intrathecal) Anesthesia

Local anesthetics and narcotics may be administered into the epidural space (between the dura and the ligamentum flavum) to provide selective anal-

Box 3-3

Rapid and Modified Rapid Sequence Induction

I. Rapid Sequence Induction

Rapid sequence induction is designed to induce loss of consciousness and muscle relaxation so control of the airway and intubation can be accomplished within seconds. This requires preoxygenation of the patient, assembly of all drugs and equipment at hand, and establishment of cardiorespiratory monitoring. The following steps occur sequentially:

1. Establish cardiorespiratory monitoring (ECG, pulse oximetry, noninvasive blood pressure monitoring)
2. Preoxygenate with 100% oxygen.
3. Atropine: 0.02 mg/kg (minimum: 0.1 mg) may be administered to prevent bradycardia (especially for children <7 years). Alternative: glycopyrrolate (Rubinul, 0.01-0.02 mg/kg).
4. Provide cricoid pressure and administer 100% oxygen by "blow by" technique.

The following drugs (Nos. 5 and 6) are administered in rapid sequence by intravenous push:

5. Thiopental: 3-5 mg/kg IV (unless patient hypotensive or in status asthmaticus) Alternatives: Midazolam: 0.1 mg/kg IV (Maximum dose: 5 mg) plus fentanyl
6. Succinylcholine: 1-2 mg/kg IV
   Pancuronium 0.01 mg/kg IV may be administered to reduce fasciculations (for children >12 years)
   Alternative: Vecuronium: 0.15-0.2 mg/kg IV (effects will last up to 60 minutes) or rocuronium (0.6-1.5 mg/kg, very rapid onset)
7. Intubate and maintain cricoid pressure while tube placement is verified.
8. Release cricoid pressure.
9. Tape endotracheal tube in place and reverify placement (including chest radiograph).

NOTE: The preceding sequence should not be used if head injury and increased ICP are present. Patients with increased ICP should be hyperventilated, and succinylcholine use is controversial because it will increase cerebral blood flow and ICP. Medical contraindications to the use of succinylcholine are provided in Box 3-2.

II. Modified Rapid Sequence Induction

This procedure is recommended if head injury and increased ICP are present.

1. Establish cardiorespiratory monitoring (ECG, pulse oximetry, noninvasive blood pressure).
2. Preoxygenate with 100% oxygen.
3. Atropine
4. Lidocaine: 1.5 mg/kg IV if severe head injury present (wait 2 minutes before administering succinylcholine–see No. 7).
5. Apply cricoid pressure while continuing to deliver 100% oxygen.
6. Thiopental: 3-5 mg/kg IV (unless patient hypotensive or in status asthmaticus) Alternatives: Midazolam: 0.1 mg/kg IV (Maximum dose: 5 mg) plus fentanyl.
7. Hyperventilate and continue to hyperventilate.
8. Succinylcholine: 2 mg/kg IV
   Alternative: Vecuronium: 0.2 mg/kg IV (effects will last up to 60 minutes)
9. Intubate when full muscle relaxation achieved.
10. Check tube placement with auscultation while maintaining cricoid pressure.
11. Release cricoid pressure.
12. Tape tube and reverify proper position (including chest radiograph).

Sources:

1. Pediatric Emergency Medicine Committee of the American College of Emergency Physicians, Gerardi MJ et al: Rapid-sequence intubation of the pediatric patient, *Ann Emerg Med* 28:55-74, 1996
2. Deshpande JK, Tobias JD, editors: *The pediatric pain handbook*, St Louis, 1996, Mosby.
3. Fitzmaurice LS: Approach to multiple trauma. In Barkin RM, editor: *Pediatric emergency medicine: concepts and clinical practice*, St Louis, 1992, Mosby.

gesia along the entire spinal axis. These drugs affect the spinal cord, dorsal root ganglia, and spinal nerve roots. The local anesthetics bind the neuron sodium channels and prevent depolarization; this blocks nerve impulse conduction and results in sensory blockade with minimal effects on sympathetic or motor function. The opioids bind to receptors in the dorsal horn of the spinal cord and block transmission of local pain impulses to the brain (Deshpande and Tobias, 1996). Epidural analgesia can provide excellent postoperative analgesia for children undergoing thoracic, abdominal, perineal and lower extremity surgery and may reduce total narcotic and analgesia use and need for postoperative mechanical ventilation. Typically a combination of a local anesthetic (e.g., bupivacaine) and a narcotic (fentanyl) is administered (Table 3-4).

Adverse effects of epidural analgesia include complications of catheter placement (e.g., epidural hematoma or spinal headache), those of narcotic administration (e.g., respiratory depression) and those of local anesthetic toxicity (e.g., vasodilation or respiratory muscle paralysis—see Complications). Systemic toxicity (primarily seizures) has been reported with the use of continuous epidural infusions of local anesthetics. Epidural catheters are not placed in patients with severe coagulopathies, systemic infections, or progressive or degenerative CNS diseases.

Side effects of narcotic administration may include respiratory depression, which is particularly likely if hydrophilic narcotics (e.g., morphine) are used. Such narcotics enter the cerebrospinal fluid and may travel to the respiratory center, producing respiratory depression as long as 12 to 24 hours after drug administration. Respiratory depression is less likely if lipophilic narcotics (e.g., fentanyl or derivatives) are used. Respiratory depression associated with any of these narcotics may be reversed with naloxone. Pruritus may develop and may also be reversed with naloxone.

Complications related to the local anesthetic are prevented by verification of catheter placement. An initial test dose of local anesthetic containing epinephrine is provided, and the catheter is aspirated before any drug is administered. The total amount of drug administered is also limited; large-bolus dosing and high continuous infusion doses

Table 3-4
Epidural Doses and Infusions of Bupivacaine and Fentanyl

Single Bolus With Bupivacaine (0.25% With Epinephrine)

Caudal	
Midthoracic block	1.3 ml/kg
Low thoracic block	1.0 ml/kg
Lumbar/sacral	0.5-0.75 ml/kg (max 25 ml)
Lumbar	0.5-0.75 ml/kg (max 20 ml)
Thoracic	0.3-0.5 ml/kg (max 12 ml)

Infusions With Bupivacaine 0.1% With 2-5 μg/ml of Fentanyl*

Caudal†	
Neonates	0.2-0.25 ml/kg/hr
<30 kg	0.4 ml/kg/hr
>40 kg	15 ml/hr
Lumbar†	
Neonates	0.2-0.25 ml/kg/hr
<30 kg	0.3-0.4 ml/kg/hr
>40 kg	15 ml/hr
Bolus dose	1/3 of hourly rate every 1 hr PRN
Thoracic‡	
<30 kg	0.3 ml/kg/hr
>40 kg	12 ml/hr
Bolus dose	1/3 of hourly rate every 1 hr PRN

Reproduced with permission from: Rasmussen GE: Epidural and spinal anesthesia and analgesia. In Deshpande JK, Tobias JD, editors: *The pediatric pain handbook*, St Louis, 1996, Mosby, page 97.
*Regardless of the site of administration, the dose of bupivacaine should not exceed 0.4 to 0.5 mg/kg/hr in patients older than 3 months of age and 0.2 to 0.25 mg/kg/hr in patients younger than 3 months of age. If opioids are added to the solution for neonates, the starting dose should be one third to one half that used in older patients.
†For lumbar/caudal administration, the starting fentanyl concentration is 2.5 μg/ml with an infusion rate of 0.4 ml/kg/hr resulting in a fentanyl dose of 1 μg/kg/hr. In patients >40 kg the infusion is maintained at 15 ml/hr while the fentanyl concentration in the solutions is increased as needed to deliver 1.0 μg/kg/hr.
‡For thoracic infusions the starting fentanyl concentration is 2 μg/ml with an infusion rate of 0.3 ml/kg/hr, resulting in a fentanyl dose of 0.6 μg/kg/hr. In patients >40 kg the infusion is maintained at 12 ml/hr while the fentanyl concentration in the solution is increased as needed to deliver 0.6 μg/kg/hr.

are avoided. If local anesthetic toxicity develops, the administration of the drug is immediately interrupted; support of airway, intubation, and ventilation with 100% oxygen are provided; and heart rate and cardiac output are supported (with cardiopulmonary resuscitation initiated as needed). Anticonvulsant therapy, defibrillation, and antiarrhythmic therapy are provided as needed (Deshpande and Tobias, 1996).

Single-shot caudal blockade (so-called "Kiddie-Caudals") has produced effective analgesia associated with perineal and lower extremity procedures and surgery.

Interpleural Anesthesia

Interpleural anesthesia (IPA) involves the placement of a catheter in the paravertebral space between the visceral and parietal pleurae to block intercostal nerves and relieve pain following thoracotomy or chest trauma. Intermittent or continuous infusion of a local anesthetic via the catheter (bupivacaine 1.25 to 2.5 mg/kg/hour) may reduce (but not eliminate) the need for systemic narcotics. IPA provides less complete analgesia than epidural administration and may produce local anesthetic toxicity, including seizures, hypotension, and arrhythmias (see Complications).

Peripheral Nerve Blockade

Administration of a local anesthetic via a catheter placed in the neurovascular sheath of peripheral nerves may interrupt pain impulse transmission and may be extremely effective in preventing postoperative pain. The most common sites of peripheral nerve blockade include the intercostal nerves (following rib fractures or thoracotomy), brachial plexus (arm pain), lumbar plexus (leg pain), or femoral nerve (for femoral fracture pain). Intermittent administration of anesthetic may provide pain relief for up to 8 hours, and continuous administration may also be provided.

Topical Anesthetic Ointment

Topical analgesic ointments containing tetracaine, adrenaline, and cocaine (TAC) or lidocaine and prilocaine (Eutectic Mixture of Local Anesthetics, or EMLA) may be applied over wounds, veins, or arteries to reduce the pain of suturing, venipuncture, or arterial puncture. The procedure or puncture should not be attempted for 20 to 60 minutes after application to enable the ointment to be effective. Use of these topical ointments has recently been extended to additional procedures such as lumbar punctures and bone marrow aspirations.

TAC requires approximately 20 minutes to be effective, and EMLA cream requires approximately 60 minutes to be effective, so planning is required to ensure adequate time for the agent to produce effective analgesia before the painful procedure. A dilute form of TAC (1% tetracaine, 1:4,000 adrenalin, and 4% cocaine, dosed at 1.5 ml/10 kg) is available that produces effective analgesia but minimal side effects. EMLA cream is available in patches (equivalent to 2.5 g cream).

Maximizing Effectiveness of Drug Therapy

The most effective pain control attempts to prevent pain; thus the patient's need for analgesia must be *anticipated*. Effective analgesia also requires titration of the optimal drug dose and involves consideration of drug pharmacokinetics.

The *pharmacokinetics* of a drug refers to the relationship between the administered dose and the systemic drug levels achieved. It is influenced by the patient's age (e.g., neonates demonstrate decreased drug excretion since renal and hepatic drug function are limited) and clinical condition (e.g., hepatic and renal function, additional drugs administered). The following information applies to the critically ill infant and child; additional dosage adjustments may be required when analgesia (particularly by continuous infusion) is provided to the very premature neonate.

Continuous Infusion   To optimize pain control, a continuous level of analgesia should be maintained to prevent a "roller coaster" effect of pain and pain relief. The use of continuous infusion provides a rational approach to continuous analgesia but may require both bolus and continuous administration of the drug to achieve and maintain drug steady-state concentrations.

All drugs administered by continuous infusion gradually accumulate in the body to achieve steady-state concentrations in five half-lives. Most sedatives and analgesic drugs have a 1- to 4-hour half-life; thus steady-state concentration requires 5 to 20 hours or longer to achieve (see Table 3-2), unless a bolus dose of the drug is provided.

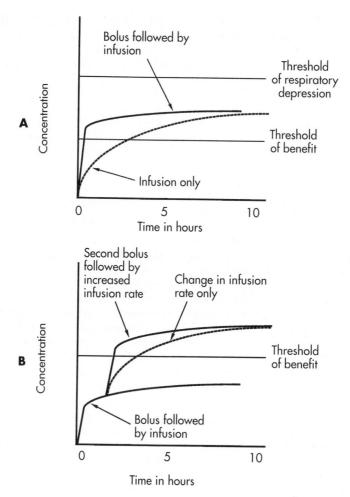

Figure 3-3   Pharmacokinetics of bolus plus continuous infusion. **A,** Drug levels achieved with bolus vs. bolus plus infusion. This relationship applies to drugs such as morphine with a 2- to 3-hour half-life. Note that therapeutic levels are not achieved for several hours following initiation of infusion unless a bolus dose also is provided. **B,** Bolus followed by infusion with additional bolus and increased infusion rate. Simply increasing the infusion rate will probably delay pain control further. The ideal method of adjustment includes provision of a second bolus dose, as well as an increase in the infusion rate so a steady-state therapeutic drug level is achieved quickly. (From Hazinski MF: *Nursing care of the critically ill child,* ed 2, St Louis, 1992, Mosby.)

A bolus dose of the analgesic or sedative should be administered when a continuous infusion is begun to ensure rapid achievement of steady-state drug concentration (Figure 3-3, *A*). *If inadequate analgesia or sedation is achieved, an additional bolus of the drug should be administered each time the infusion rate is increased*—if the drug infusion rate is increased *without* provision of the drug bolus, 5 half-lives of the drug will be required before the new dose results in steady-state concentrations (Figure 3-3, *B*). Too often, if continuous infusion therapy is inadequate, the infusion rate is repeatedly increased without bolus therapy and before any one dose has reached steady state. This practice may result in toxicity once the drug concentration finally reaches steady state.

Patient-Controlled Analgesia Superior pain relief has been achieved through the use of PCA. This method of delivery uses small, computerized infusion pumps that deliver a specific amount of the analgesic (most often morphine) continuously. Bolus administration of the drug is provided when the PCA is initiated. The patient may also press a button to administer a small bolus of medication to treat breakthrough pain (Box 3-4). Lockout periods and dose limits can be programmed. This method of analgesia requires an alert cooperative patient who is able to comprehend the delivery system. Although PCA is extremely effective in the management of severe or chronic pain in the school-age child (≥7 years of age), children 4 to 6 years of age may require encouragement to administer the small bolus doses during painful procedures. The role of these devices in the care of very young patients (≤5 to 7 years of age) may be limited.

A high basal infusion rate of morphine during PCA may be associated with increased side effects and negligible improvement in analgesia. If the basal infusion rate is sufficiently low, side effects should be prevented and the child may experience more effective analgesia (see Morphine).

Alternative Routes of Administration If IV therapy is not possible or if drug compatibilities complicate IV administration, alternative routes of drug administration should be considered. These include transdermal, mucosal, or subcutaneous routes.

Avoidance of Intramuscular Route of Administration The IM route of administration is undesirable for the critically ill child for several reasons: (1) altered tissue perfusion leads to unpredictable drug absorption and patient response, (2) the number of injection sites is limited, (3) injections cannot be performed in children with thrombocytopenia, (4) children hate them, and (5) nurses hate to administer them. For these reasons, IM injections should be avoided.

Box 3-4

Typical Morphine Doses for Patient-Controlled Analgesia

Loading dose: 0.01-0.03 mg/kg every 5 minutes to achieve desired level of analgesia
Basal Infusion: 0.004-0.01 mg/kg/hour
PRN Bolus: 0.01-0.03 mg/kg (lock-out maximum: no more frequently than every 6-10 minutes, and maximum of 4-6 boluses/hr)

Potential Complications of Pharmacologic Pain Control

Dosing Errors

Whenever a narcotic or sedative is administered, the nurse should double-check the original physician order against the drug or nursing card to prevent errors in dosing. In general, the nurse should verify any pediatric dose (other than preparations of continuous infusions of drugs such as pentobarbital) that requires more than one vial to prepare. If unit dosing is provided, the labeling on the syringe should be checked against the original order.

To prevent errors in transcription of verbal orders, the nurse should repeat the verbal order in the presence of a second nurse, and two nurses should co-sign the verbal order.

Cardiorespiratory Depression

Most analgesics and sedatives have the potential for producing cardiorespiratory depression. Cardiovascular effects may result from vasodilation and will be exacerbated if the patient is hypovolemic; fluid administration may correct the problem. Some sedatives, analgesics, and anesthetics depress myocardial function and should be used with caution in patients in shock; concurrent administration of vasoactive drugs may be required. Respiratory depression may be caused by CNS depression; the patient's respiratory function should be closely monitored, particularly if the patient is breathing spontaneously.

Complications of Local Anesthetics

Adverse reactions may be associated with administration of local anesthetics. The drugs themselves can produce CNS complications (including seizures, sedation, and paresthesias) and cardiovascular complications (including myocardial depression, hypotension, and arrhythmias). These complications are especially likely if high doses of local anesthetics are administered or if the local anesthetics are absorbed systemically (e.g., during intrapleural administration). Epidural administration of local anesthetics can produce hypotension (related to venous pooling) or muscle weakness. Inadvertent intrathecal injection of local anesthetics during epidural anesthesia may produce total spinal blockade or respiratory muscle paralysis.

Abstinence/Dependence/Withdrawal Syndromes

Long-term administration of narcotics and sedatives may produce increased drug tolerance, necessitating increased drug dosage over time; as a result, high doses of these drugs are ultimately delivered. If narcotic therapy has been continuously provided for 4 to 5 days or longer or if high doses have been administered, caution must be taken when the drug is discontinued. Abrupt cessation of narcotic administration may produce a classic narcotic abstinence (withdrawal) syndrome, including agitation, diaphoresis, decrease in oxygen saturation, and nausea and vomiting. Naloxone or nalbuphine may also produce abrupt withdrawal if administered to the child receiving chronic narcotic therapy. Although the complication is not life threatening, it is extremely uncomfortable for the patient and may disrupt attempts at weaning ventilatory support. All narcotics and sedatives administered for 5 days or more should be gradually weaned to prevent this complication.

This abstinence/withdrawal/dependence syndrome *should not be confused with drug addiction.* When the drug is administered to control pain or sedate the patient, this effect does not produce *psychologic* dependence with potential for later withdrawal. Instead, physical effects resulting from abrupt withdrawal of high or chronic doses of the drug are created. It is important that the word *ad-*

diction be avoided, since it is inaccurate and may frighten the parents or the child. If the drug dose is gradually reduced, the physical symptoms of abstinence or withdrawal are minimized. There is no evidence that children receiving narcotics or sedatives for medicinal purposes are at risk for the development of drug addiction at a later time.

Gradual weaning of *narcotics* involves a decrease in the dose by approximately 5% to 10%/day (or 25% every 3 to 4 days). During weaning of the IV narcotic, an oral drug such as methadone may be provided. Methadone doses may begin at the same dose as the narcotic (morphine or fentanyl), although lower doses may be effective. Methadone allows tapering of the IV narcotic; then the methadone dose is tapered approximately 10% to 20%/week.

Sedatives should also be weaned gradually if they have been administered for several days. Abstinence/withdrawal syndrome resulting from benzodiazepine therapy may be associated with movement disorders and occasional seizure activity. Substitution of alternative benzodiazepines or oral diazepam or lorazepam may be used to enable gradual reduction in the IV dose. Flumazenil is a benzodiazepine antagonist that may be used to reverse the effects of diazepam and midazolam—however, it may precipitate withdrawal.

Abrupt discontinuation of *barbiturates* also can produce profound symptoms of abstinence, including severe cardiovascular dysfunction and seizure activity. Gradual dose reduction is advisable following long-term or high-dose therapy.

Critical Illness Polyneuropathy/Myopathy

Polyneuropathy and myopathy have been described in both adults and children following critical illness. This complication is described as a syndrome of muscle weakness that may include tetraplegia or prolonged dependence on mechanical ventilation. When electrophysiologic testing has been performed, it has documented distal axonal nerve degeneration and denervation and atrophy of muscle. Once this syndrome develops, intensive physical therapy is needed, and recovery, if it occurs, may require a year or longer.

The precise etiology of this problem is unclear. Although initially described in association with prolonged mechanical ventilation and sepsis, this syndrome has been reported in association with many conditions necessitating critical care and prolonged mechanical ventilation. Most patients who develop this neuromyopathy have required prolonged bed rest and have received neuromuscular blockade (most often vecuronium); and many have received additional drugs that may exert synergistic effects on the neuromuscular junction. Many, but not all, have developed sepsis in the course of their critical illness.

High-dose steroids have been shown to cause severe muscle atrophy and thus may contribute to the development of a neuromyopathy associated with neuromuscular blockade. The risk of neuropathy may be increased if the neuromuscular blockade is induced with aminosteroids such as pancuronium and vecuronium. Aminoglycoside antibiotics may potentiate effects of the neuromuscular blockade and contribute to the development of a neuromyopathy, because these antibiotics have intrinsic neuromuscular blocking effects of their own. Drugs such as furosemide and the benzodiazepines (midazolam and diazepam) also act synergistically with neuromuscular blocking agents. Impaired renal function may contribute to the problem, resulting in reduced drug clearance. It is also likely that an initial insult (e.g., trauma, surgery, infection) causes release of cytokines and alters perfusion to the neuromuscular junction, rendering this unit more susceptible to the effects of drugs such as steroids or aminoglycosides.

The best way to treat this neuromyopathy of critical illness is to prevent it. If administration of neuromuscular blockade is anticipated, all medications the child is receiving should be reviewed, and, if possible, additional drugs likely to contribute to the neuromyopathy should be avoided. Although it may not be practical to avoid *all* such drugs, modification of drug selection or dosing regimen may be attempted. If concurrent steroid administration is required (e.g., for a child with asthma or chronic lung disease), aminosteroid neuromuscular blocking agents (specifically pancuronium and vecuronium) should probably not be used, and agents such as doxacurium or atracurium that do not contain steroids should be considered instead. Paralyzing agents should be titrated to patient response, and use of peripheral nerve stimulators and "train of four" response (see preceding paragraphs) should be used to prevent excessive administration of neuromuscular blockade. Passive range-of-motion exercises should be performed during periods of pharmacologic paralysis, and active range-of-motion exercises begun as soon as the patient is awake. It is important to note that this neuromyopathy of critical care may develop despite all attempts to prevent it. Aggressive physical therapy should be initiated as soon as the diagnosis is suspected.

Conclusions

This chapter has summarized applicable pain physiology and some practical approaches to assessment and management of pediatric pain. Although drug preferences and methods of pain control vary widely throughout the country, principles of drug administration and risk-benefit profiles are consistent. There is no question that effective analgesia can result in marked improvement in patient progress and reduction in complications.

Suggested Readings

American Pain Society: Principles of analgesic use in the treatment of acute pain and chronic cancer pain, Washington, DC, 1988, American Pain Society (free: 1615 L Street, NW, Washington DC 20036).

Berde CB: Toxicity of local anesthetics in infants and children, *J Pediatr* 122:S14-S20, 1993.

Bergman I et al: Reversible neurologic abnormalities associated with prolonged intravenous midazolam and fentanyl administration, *J Pediatr* 119:644-649, 1991.

Bolton CF: Sepsis and the systemic inflammatory response syndrome: neuromuscular manifestations, *Crit Care Med* 24:1408-1416, 1996.

Committee on Drugs, American Academy of Pediatrics: Guidelines for monitoring and management of pediatric patients during and after sedation for diagnostic and therapeutic procedures, *Pediatrics* 89:1110-1115, 1992.

Coté CJ: Sedation for the pediatric patient; a review, *Pediatr Anesth* 41:31-58, 1994.

Coté CJ: Sedation protocols—why so many variations (editorial), *Pediatrics* 94:281-283, 1994.

Deshpande JK, Tobias JD: *The pediatric pain handbook,* St Louis, 1996, Mosby.

Eland JM: Pain in children, *Nurs Clin North Am* 25:871-884, 1990.

Gooch JL et al: Prolonged paralysis after treatment with neuromuscular junction blocking agents, *Crit Care Med* 9:1125-1131, 1991.

Hazinski MF: *Nursing care of the critically ill child,* ed 2, St Louis, 1992, Mosby.

Hoyt JW: Persistent paralysis in critically ill patients after the use of neuromuscular blocking agents, *New Horizons* 2:48-55, 1994.

Jacox A et al: Management of cancer pain; clinical practice guidelines, AHCR Publication No. 94-0592. Rockville, Md, Agency for Health Care Policy and Research, US Department of Health and Human Services, Public Health Service.

Katz R, Kelly HW, His A: Prospective study on the occurrence of withdrawal in critically ill children who receive fentanyl by continuous infusion, *Crit Care Med* 22:763-767, 1994.

Mannheimer JS, Lampe GN: *Clinical transcutaneous electrical nerve stimulation,* Philadelphia, 1984, FA Davis.

Marx CM et al: Optimal sedation of mechanically ventilated pediatric critical care patients, *Crit Care Med* 22:163-170, 1994.

McCaffery M, Beebe A: Pain: clinical manual for nursing practice, St Louis, 1989, Mosby.

Pediatric Emergency Medicine Committee of the American College of Emergency Physicians, Gerardi MJ et al: Rapid-sequence intubation of the pediatric patient, *Ann Emerg Med* 28:55-74, 1996.

Pepperman ML, Macrae D: A comparison of propofol and other sedative use in paediatric intensive care in the United Kingdom, *Paediatric Anaesth* 7(2):143-153, 1997.

Reimche LD et al: Chloral hydrate sedation in neonates and infants—clinical and pharmacologic considerations, *Dev Pharmacol Ther* 12:57-64, 1989.

Rossiter A et al: Pancuronium-induced prolonged neuromuscular blockade, *Crit Care Med* 19:1583-1587, 1991.

Schechter NL, Berde CB, Yaster M, editors: *Pain in infants, children and adolescents,* Baltimore, 1993, Williams & Wilkins.

Segredo V et al: Persistent paralysis in critically ill patients after long-term administration of vecuronium, *N Engl J Med* 327:524-528, 1992.

Sladen RN: Neuromuscular blocking agents in the intensive care unit: a two-edged sword, *Crit Care Med* 23:423-431, 1995.

Sperry RJ et al: Fentanyl and sufentanil increase intracranial pressure in head trauma patients, *Anesthesiology* 77:416-410, 1992.

Taddio A et al: Efficacy and safety of lidocaine-prilocaine cream for pain during circumcision, *N Engl J Med* 336:1197-1201, 1997.

Tobias JD: Increased intracranial pressure after fentanyl administration in a child with closed head trauma, *Pediatr Emerg Care* 10:89-90, 1994.

Tobias JD: Sedation and anesthesia for pediatric bronchoscopy, *Curr Opin Pediatr* 9(3):198-206, 1997.

Tobias JD: Sedation and analgesia for children in the pediatric intensive care unit, *J Intensive Care Med,* In Press.

Tyler DC et al: Toward validation of pain measurement tools for children: a pilot study, *Pain* 52:301-309, 1993.

Yaster M et al: Local anesthesia in the management of acute pain in children, *J Pediatr* 124:165-176, 1994.

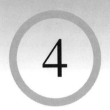

The Dying Child in the Intensive Care Unit

Pearls

- If it is impossible to save the child's life, the health care team must attempt to ensure that the child's death is peaceful and pain free.
- The death of a child is extremely stressful for parents and family, and each will respond in a unique way.
- If in doubt about what to say—*listen*.
- The health care staff may grieve for the child but must always be able to support the family.
- Siblings and extended family members should not be neglected when the child is dying.

Additional Helpful Chapters

Chapter 2: Psychosocial Aspects and Helping Children Deal With Unique Stresses
Chapter 3: Management of Pain
Chapter 5: Cardiopulmonary Resuscitation
Chapter 6: Respiratory Failure

Introduction

The nurse caring for the dying child faces many challenges. The child's physical care must continue, and the child's and family's emotional and psychologic needs must also be addressed. This chapter explores the needs of the dying child and the child's family in the intensive care unit (ICU) setting and presents nursing interventions designed to meet the needs of the patient and family.

Despite many advances in technology, approximately 3% to 18% of critically ill children admitted to pediatric intensive care units die there. Some of these deaths are anticipated as the child with terminal or chronic illness succumbs to organ failure. However, many deaths occur within hours of admission to the ICU, when the staff and family have little time to prepare.

Unexpected (sudden) death always creates unique stresses for the family. If the death occurs soon after admission, the parents and family must absorb a great deal of information in a few hours and may be overwhelmed. The ICU staff must provide intensive psychosocial support during the time they are fighting for the child's life. If the child dies during surgery, the family may be devastated that they weren't able to be with the child at the time of death. If the hospitalized child suddenly deteriorates, the parents may think that they should have prevented the death.

Although death may not be unexpected in the child with chronic or terminal illness, the time of the death may surprise the parents. The trajectory of chronic illness is so unpredictable that it is difficult to suspect which complication will be fatal.

Fatally ill children occasionally make dramatic recoveries. If the child recovers after the family begins to grieve, the family may feel anger at the medical team or guilt for abandoning the child.

Many families may benefit from psychologic counseling after the death of a child. Families should be encouraged to seek such counseling if they demonstrate difficulty coping with the child's death, resolving feelings of anger or helplessness, or dealing with the remaining family and responsibilities (see Chapter 2).

Care of the Dying Child

Admission To The Intensive Care Unit

The Terminally Ill Child

The most common condition requiring ICU admission for *terminally* ill children is respiratory distress or failure. Ideally terminally ill children are not intubated unless the respiratory distress is thought to be a temporary condition (e.g., pneumonia). Occasionally the child deteriorates before the wishes of the child and family can be determined.

If at all possible *before* intubation, determine the child's and the family's feelings about intubation, mechanical ventilatory support, and cardiopulmonary resuscitation. Record this information in the chart and discuss it with the child's physician so unwarranted therapy is prevented. If the child is conscious and can remain *unintubated,* encourage him or her to express concerns, fears, questions, and preferences regarding care. Involve parents in these discussions.

The Acutely Ill or Injured Child

The conscious child with life-threatening medical illness or injury will probably be very frightened about the ICU environment, ICU equipment, and proposed interventions (e.g., intubation, catheterization). If the child has been unconscious but regains consciousness, the nurse must explain events necessitating the ICU admission, the equipment present, and the care provided. Reassurance is always necessary.

The conscious intubated child must be taught how to communicate with the nursing staff. Call bells, computers, or alphabet and phrase boards may be used. Assure the child that the staff is working to help the child feel better and that the

child's parents and nurses will be nearby at all times. Such communication is important, even if the child appears to be unconscious.

It is important to talk with the child and offer explanations for movement or therapy and preparation for any painful procedures. At all times, *assume that the child can hear you,* even if the child does not show signs of response.

Talking About Death

Children are often aware of and anxious about impending death, whether or not they have been informed of the fatal prognosis. In general, if the child is sufficiently mature to ask if he or she is dying, the child is old enough to discuss the possibility of death in some form. Discussions of death must be at a level appropriate to the child's cognitive and psychosocial development (Table 4-1).

It is very difficult to instill hope in the child and family and at the same time allow the child to share concerns and fears about dying. Watch the child closely for behavioral cues that may indicate his or her need to discuss death. If possible, postpone the administration of sedatives until the child's questions are answered and fears are addressed (Table 4-2).

The child's parents are often the best people to talk to the child about death, but they will require assistance from health care professionals. Discussions of death between parent and child should generally be initiated by the child, and the child should be allowed to set the pace and tone of the discussions. Children who are dying often express anxiety about pain, loneliness, separation from parents, and loss of control; these issues should be addressed.

The child's questions must be answered honestly while maintaining an element of hope. It is extremely important to clarify and then answer the *child's* questions rather than the questions anticipated by the nurse or parents. Observe the child's responses closely and help the child communicate concerns.

The child may become angry with parents or hospital staff; this anger may reflect a response to painful therapy, or it may indicate the child's perception that his or her questions and concerns are being ignored or avoided. The child may also fear

Table 4-1
The Child's Concept of Death

Age Group	Concept of Death	Major Fears
Infant	No real concept	Separation from parents
Toddlers	No real concept	Separation from parents, disruption in routines, painful procedures
Preschoolers	Death as temporary or involves mutilation	Separation from parents, painful death or mutilation (fantasies); sensitive to parental cues, may assume guilt for illness
School-age	Concept more accurate by 7 to 9 years; death known to be permanent by 8 to 9 years	Very sensitive to nonverbal cues—often detects bad prognosis before discussion, so may feel isolated if it is not discussed truthfully; death often thought of as being "taken away"; needs reassurance that he or she won't be alone and that child was not responsible for fatal illness or injury
Adolescence	Able to comprehend death, but may not accept death as reality (invincibility)	Loss of control and privacy, separation from peer group (and possibly parents); magical thinking may cause denial, guilt

Table 4-2
Potential Responses to Frequent Questions or Statements From the Child Who Is Dying

Question/Comment	Response
Am I dying?	You are very sick and I am worried about you. It is possible that you might die, but we are doing everything we can to help you. Are you afraid of dying? Depending on the child's answer, the nurse can continue to explore the child's specific fears.
I'm afraid to die.	What does dying mean to you? The nurse can then explore the child's perceptions of death and reinforce the positive concepts and reduce the negative concepts. The child should know that he or she won't be alone: someone will always be present.
I don't want to die.	I can understand that—I don't want to die either. What is the worst thing about dying to you? The nurse can then explore the child's concerns.

being isolated or abandoned. The family should remain with the child as much as possible to communicate their love and support and reassure the child that he or she will not be alone.

Some families are unable to discuss death with the child because of their anxiety, grief, fear, and coping strategies. Determine the specific information that has been provided to the dying child and to other family members and help the family support the child.

A consistent physician and primary nurse or clinical nurse specialist must be available to help the child and family. The nurse must keep the family and the health care team informed about information provided to or by the child. It is also important to help the child understand the reaction of family members; too often, the child interprets the family's anxiety and depression as rejection or loss of love.

Physical Care

The reduction or elimination of pain is often the single most important aspect of physical care for the dying child. Both pharmacologic and psychologic measures are used (see Chapter 3). Although administration of analgesics may hasten death, pain relief should be the most important physical consideration when death is inevitable.

Comfort measures are important for the dying child. These may include soothing baths and backrubs, opportunities to be held, and diversionary activities such as television and pleasant music. Such activities can reduce anxiety and pain and provide valuable time for the child and family to be together.

Posting a daily schedule can ensure that the child and family have adequate time to visit and rest. In addition, nursing care activities can be planned around important visitation times.

Give careful attention to skin care, positioning of the child, hygiene, and the preservation of optimal bowel and bladder function. If bowel or bladder control is lost, immediate attention to hygiene is important for the child's self-esteem and comfort.

Family Visitation

All children need to be with their families; this is particularly true when the child is dying. Encourage the parents to remain with the child as much as

is feasible and to bring siblings to the hospital. Alter visiting regulations (if needed) to enable visitation by those important to the child.

Preparation and Support of the Family

Assessment of Family Stressors and Strengths

It may be difficult to characterize and anticipate the expected course of dying. As a result, the parents of children with serious health care problems often are uncertain about their child's prognosis.

The nurse must assess the impact of the child's illness and admission to the ICU on the parents and the family. Information about the parents' coping strategies and data about decision-making and treatment choices are vital pieces of information that can be obtained by a relatively short, directed nursing interview (Box 4-1).

Cultural and religious factors that influence the

Box 4-1

Alterations in Parenting: Nursing Assessment Interview

Parenting is defined as the ability of a nurturing figure(s) to create an environment that promotes the optimum growth and development of a child. When the child is dying, parents need to feel that they have an essential and irreplaceable role to play in the child's care and preparation for death. Nurses can facilitate a working relationship with the parents by meeting the parents' expressed and demonstrated needs. This guide suggests areas to explore during a parental interview and must be *individually tailored*.

I. **Nondirected recall:** What are the parents' experiences related to the child's illness and condition?

II. **Perceptions About the Child's Illness:** What do the parents know and how do they feel about it?

III. **Impact of the Child's Illness on the Child:** What does the child know and feel?

IV. **Experiences as a Parent:** How has the child's condition affected the parents' ability to nurture the child? What has been most difficult?

V. **Family Impact:** How has the child's illness affected family life? Ask about other family members.

VI. **Coping:** What has been most helpful or least helpful to the parents? Inquire about family support systems.

VII. **Nurse/Parent Relationship:** How can the nurses best help the parents? How much do the parents wish to participate in their child's care? What are the expectations regarding family visitation (who will be visiting, when)?

Based on Miles MS: In Carpentino LS, editor: *Handbook of nursing diagnosis,* Philadelphia, 1987, JB Lippincott.

family's ability to cope with death and loss must be identified. Publications available from the Park Ridge Center are particularly helpful resources.

Potential Parental Responses

Anticipatory Grief

Anticipatory grief is a coping mechanism that may be used when the death of a loved one is expected; the grieving process may begin before the death occurs in anticipation of that loss. However, when a child dies suddenly, parents are unable to prepare. If these parents can be helped to understand the gravity of the child's condition, they may have a brief time to anticipate the child's death.

Parental anticipation of the child's death is evident when the parents talk about the seriousness of the child's illness, the possibility of death, memories of the child's life, and what life will be like without the child. These discussions indicate that the parents may be accepting the reality of the child's death and preparing emotionally for that death.

Anger and Guilt

Grief responses of parents may also include expressions of anger and guilt about the child's impending death. The nurse and the health care team must help the parents understand that their grief response is normal.

Denial

Some parents cope with their child's illness by denial. This coping strategy may prevent decisions regarding termination of therapy and inhibit discussions of death with the child. The health care team must gently and firmly convey the severity of the child's condition. The nurse may note observable changes in the child's status (e.g., deterioration in color or respiratory pattern). Argumentative or confrontational tactics must be avoided, however, because they can undermine the parents' confidence in the health care team.

Withdrawal and Avoidance

Some parents may withdraw and simply avoid visiting the child. When parents decrease their visiting time, it is important to assess their coping strategies and talk to them about the child's need for support.

Parents should be assisted in finding time to rest and to eat, since they must be strong if they are to support their child and each other.

Support of Siblings

If possible, the parents should prepare the siblings for the death of the child. Siblings of approximately preschool age or older should be given the opportunity to come to the hospital to say good-bye and be with the parents during the final visit after the child's death. Toddlers may also be brought to visit with the dying child, particularly if the dying child wishes to see the toddler. Decisions regarding the presence of the sibling must be individualized, but even very young siblings (e.g., infants) may provide comfort to the parents and the dying child during this time.

Parents may neglect the important needs of siblings during their support of the dying child. Encourage the parents to discuss the child's impending death with the siblings. If the parents lose control and avoid such discussion, the siblings are forced to deal with grief and fear alone.

Frequently the sibling may feel responsible for the child's death or guilty for surviving when the child died. Inform the parents of these potential sibling responses.

As a rule, if the sibling is old enough to know and love the child who has died, he or she should probably be allowed to attend the funeral. Exclusion from the funeral may isolate the sibling and affect his or her ability to cope with the child's death.

The siblings may benefit from involvement in group therapy with other children who have experienced the death of a family member. Such groups may be sponsored by the local chapter of Compassionate Friends or the hospital (see Chapter 2).

Treatment Decisions

Decisions to Withhold or Withdraw Treatment

The health care team often helps parents make decisions about withholding treatment or resuscitation or withdrawing therapy. Nurses play a vital role in these discussions in advocating for the child and parent and in expressing a personal point of view. However, if the nurse assumes a spokesperson role for the child or parents, he or she is obligated to speak *only for the child and family.* Personal opinion must be clearly separated from the expressed preferences of the child and family.

Discussions of treatment limitations or withdrawal or establishment of "do not attempt resuscitation (DNAR)" orders may be difficult. However, unless such decisions are made and appropriate orders written, the child may be subjected to futile resuscitation or forced to endure uncomfortable procedures. Often these very treatments carry the risk of the most feared aspects of death: pain, loneliness, separation from parents, and loss of control.

The health care team is not obligated to offer treatment that is futile; thus *withholding* futile treatment is widely accepted. Although courts have not generally differentiated between withholding and withdrawing therapy, some states may require that a court order be obtained to *withdraw* treatment such as ventilatory support. The hospital legal counsel and ethics committee may be consulted at this time.

Court orders are never required to remove ventilatory support when a child has been pronounced "brain dead." These patients have died, and treatment is discontinued. Mechanical ventilation may be continued for a few hours to enable the family to say good-bye. Of course, it will be continued if solid organ donation is planned.

Limitation (or prevention) of resuscitation attempts requires a written order by a physician, which must often be renewed at regular intervals (Figure 4-1). In the absence of a written DNAR order, resuscitation must be initiated in the event of a patient respiratory or cardiac arrest. Unsuccessful resuscitation can be discontinued at any time by the physician in charge of the resuscitation.

Organ Donation

Discussion of organ donation is required by law if the child becomes an eligible potential donor. If solid organ transplantation is desired, the patient must be declared "brain dead" before these organs can be used.

When the child dies suddenly, it may be diffi-cult for parents to focus on decisions regarding organ donation. Whenever possible, introduce the idea early to give the parents sufficient time to make a decision. This has the added benefit of separating ("uncoupling") the request from final decisions about the child's care.

The concept of brain death is poorly understood by the general public, so discussions with the family must be precise. The parents are not asked to *agree* to brain death pronouncement; the pronouncement of brain death is based on clinical examination, not consensus. The ventilator is not "life support," since the child's life has ended when brain death is pronounced.

Solid organ donation requires several hours of preparation and surgery, and incisions are made in the child's body. Typical funeral arrangements are not delayed, however. Contact a coordinator from the local organ procurement agency whenever a potential organ donor is identified. These coordinators can be extremely valuable resources for the hospital staff and family, and they can later keep the family informed in general terms of the results of organ transplantation. Many parents have stated that donation of their child's organs helped them to find meaning in their child's death.

Organ donation should not interfere with the parents' need to see and hold their child for a final time. It is a vital step in grief resolution.

Interventions at the Time of Death

Support During Resuscitation

When cardiopulmonary resuscitation is performed, information should be provided to the parents at regular intervals. A staff member must communicate with and support the parents and keep the resuscitation team aware of the parents questions.

The parents may wish to be present during resuscitation. Communicate the request to the health care team and evaluate each request individually. If CPR is underway when the parents arrive at the hospital, the resuscitation may be the only time the parents are able to be with the child before death is

❤ Vanderbilt University Medical Center

PHYSICIAN'S ORDER TO LIMIT CARDIOPULMONARY RESUSCITATION

THIS FORM MUST BE COMPLETED IN FULL, INCLUDING LEGIBLE SIGNATURE.

STEPS:
1. Be familiar with Vanderbilt University Hospital policy for Do Not Resuscitate/Do Not Intubate/Limited Cardiopulmonary Resuscitation (Hospital Policy 20-06).
2. Discuss resuscitation options, rationale for recommended option, and expected consequences of recommended option with patient, family, and/or surrogate as well as other appropriate health care providers.
3. Attending must document above discussions and rationale for limitation of therapeutic measures on Code Status Progress Note form (MC 3834).
4. Complete orders below and sign. An order written by housestaff at the direction of the attending physician must be countersigned by the attending within 24 hours.
5. Notify and explain resuscitation status to nursing staff.
6. This order must be re-evaluated every 14 days, or if the patient's condition warrants change, or when the patient is transferred to a new service or to a different level of care, which ever occurs first. If code status changes to anything other than full resuscitation status, new Physician's Order to Limit Cardiopulmonary Resuscitation and Code Status Progress Note forms must be completed and signed.

CODE STATUS:

❑ **DO NOT RESUSCITATE** – In the event of cardiac or respiratory arrest, all cardiopulmonary resuscitative efforts should be withheld.

❑ **DO NOT INTUBATE** – In the event of cardiac or respiratory arrest, tracheal intubation and mechanical respiration/ventilation should be withheld. All other medically appropriate resuscitative, therapeutic, and/or palliative efforts should be provided.

❑ **LIMITED CARDIOPULMONARY RESUSCITATION** – In the event of cardiac or respiratory arrest, the following specified measures should be withheld. All other medically appropriate resuscitative, therapeutic, and/or palliative efforts should be provided.

❑ Withhold Antiarrhythmics	❑ Withhold Ventilation by Mask
❑ Withhold Intravenous Vasoactive Drugs	❑ Withhold Endotracheal Intubation
❑ Withhold Defibrillation/Cardioversion	❑ Withhold Mechanical Ventilation
❑ Withhold Chest Compression	❑ Withhold Other (specify) _____

_____

_____

_____   _____
Signature of Resident (if applicable)   Date/Time
(Requires Attending Physician's Cosignature Within 24 Hours)

❑ Order Cancelled

_____   _____
Attending Signature   Date/Time

Attending Signature   Date / Time

Implementation (By Responsible Nurse)
❑ Sticker Placed   ❑ Tabs Placed

Discontinuation (By Responsible Nurse)
❑ Sticker Removed   ❑ Tabs Removed

Signature   Time   Date

Signature   Time   Date

(Re-evaluation signatures on back)   © Vanderbilt University Medical Center 1995

Figure 4-1 Sample "Do Not Attempt Resuscitation" order sheet. (Modified from Vanderbilt University Medical Center, Copyright 1995. Reproduced with permission.)

pronounced. If parents are present, they will require information throughout the resuscitation.

Ask if the parents would like anyone contacted such as clergy or members of the family. During this time, make a telephone available to the family.

One of the major challenges in communicating with parents of the critically ill child is the need to balance hope with realism. Statements about the child's condition must be direct and sensitive, using carefully chosen terms and avoiding medical jargon. If the child fails to respond quickly to resuscitation, prepare the parents for the child's death—this may be accomplished in stages. The following sequence of information offered in parts separated by several minutes may be used to prepare parents in stages for a poor resuscitation outcome:

1. The child stopped breathing, but the nurse immediately provided breaths, using a mask and bag and oxygen (or cardiopulmonary resuscitation [CPR]).
2. The heart slowed and stopped beating. This is usually a sign that the heart is suffering from lack of oxygen, despite the help of the nurses and doctors (or CPR).
3. The heart has not restarted even after emergency drugs and CPR, and the doctors are worried that the heart will not start beating on its own. At such a time, the parents often voice concerns about the futility of the resuscitation or the likelihood that the child has suffered damage to all organs. By the time resuscitative efforts are discontinued, the parents are somewhat prepared to hear that the child died.

Support During Expected Death

Preparation for Imminent Death

If the child is allowed to die without resuscitation or other intervention, the health care team must describe to the parents the ways the child's breathing and appearance may change just before death. Discuss the amount of sedation and analgesia the child will receive with the child and parents. If possible, ensure effective pain control while leaving the child as alert as possible.

If possible, move the child and family to a private area of the unit. However, this privacy should not isolate the child from the constant attendance of the nursing staff. The parents should have access to a telephone, restroom, and shower facilities.

The parents must be encouraged to continue to eat and rest to maintain physical strength. However, do not pressure parents to leave the bedside if they are reluctant to do so. If the parents do leave the bedside, assure them that they will be summoned back if the child's condition changes.

When the child's death is imminent, the family may ask that a member of the clergy be summoned. In addition, the nurse must be sure that the child is comfortable. A nurse should remain with the child and family. Silence cardiac monitoring alarms if at all possible. When the child dies, a physician should be present to confirm that the child has died (to pronounce death), to offer support to the family, and to answer the parents' questions.

Informing Parents of the Child's Death

When the parents are told of the child's death, empathy and compassion must be used. If the parents cannot be at the child's side, the news of the death should be relayed by a physician and nurse whom the parents already know and trust. If possible, tell the parents in a private room.

Ideally the parents are not told of the child's death over the telephone. If telephone notification is absolutely necessary, the parents should be prepared for bad news. If possible, ensure that supportive friends or family are with the parents.

If the child dies peacefully, in no apparent pain, it is important to share this information with the parents. This usually comforts the family.

Support After Death

The Final Visit After Death

Parents and other family members should have an opportunity to see the child after death. This final visit with the child may enable the parents to say good-bye, to begin to realize that the child has really died, and to begin the grief process. Many parents who fail to see their child for a final visit may experience difficulty believing that the child is actually dead.

Before the final visit, clean and prepare the room and the child's body so the child will look as good as possible for the parents. This final preparation of the body also provides the nursing staff with an opportunity to say good-bye to the child. A priest or a family member may wish to participate in this final bath. All blood, povidone-iodine (Betadine), or adhesive is removed; and lotion may be applied. Change the bed linens and the child's pajamas. Wash or brush the child's hair neatly. Cover incisions and wounds with clean, dry dressings.

If organ donation will occur, mechanical ventilation and intravenous therapy must continue. If a postmortem examination is to be performed, it may be necessary for invasive catheters and tubes to remain in place; if the tubes must remain, use fresh tape to cover any bloodstained or discolored tape. If a postmortem examination will not be performed and organ donation is not possible, remove equipment as appropriate.

If the child sustained severe, visible injuries, describe his or her appearance to the parents before their visit. Unless the child's head and face are seriously injured, most injuries can be effectively covered by dressings and sheets.

The parents may need privacy or support while seeing their child after death. If possible, ask the parents if they would like to hold their child.

Support of the Parents Immediately After the Child's Death

Parents must have the opportunity to express their pain and sorrow in a private place with health care professionals. The responses of the parents will be determined by the family's unique method of coping with the child's death.

Most health care professionals feel insecure about what to say to parents who are deeply distressed and grieving. Listening is often the most important form of support provided.

Avoid platitudes—don't tell parents, "I know how you feel"; such a remark appears to minimize the parents' pain. Avoid religious pronouncements such as, "It was God's will," since it is presumptuous to interpret the meaning of life or death for the family.

Members of the health care team may cry with the parents when the child dies. Expression of emotion is appropriate, and helps the parents realize that their child's death has touched many people. However, such emotions are excessive if the nurse is unable to continue to function as a support to the parents.

The behavioral and emotional responses of parents are determined by the personality and cultural background of each parent, the role of the child in the family, and the circumstances of the death. Some parents may act shocked and immobilized. Other parents demonstrate a temporary lack of affect, denying their deep and painful feelings. Other emotions, including anger, rage, frustration, and guilt, may overwhelm the parents. Behavioral responses are quite varied and might include intense crying, wailing, hysteria, physical acting out, or stoicism. Although it is difficult, the nurse should remain with family members who are expressing strong emotions or who have lost control. Too often, when the parents express strong emotion, they are chastised or offered medication.

Parents may remember only selective things about the day their child died. However, they usually remember in minute detail how they were told of the child's death and how they were treated by the nursing staff, health care team, and even hospital support personnel. Both positive and negative responses are recalled for months and years.

Parents may share their feelings of helplessness and begin to explore the unanswerable question, "Why?" Do not discourage these questions or negate them. The nurse should listen to the parents' concerns and indicate that guilt feelings are normal. In addition, reinforce the positive aspects of the parents' role. The nurse may make observations about the child such as, "Everyone has mentioned that Jimmy was always smiling and happy—he certainly must have known he was loved."

Parents need support and guidance related to the many decisions required after the child's death (e.g., autopsy consent, informing friends and relatives, and funeral and burial decisions). The nurse or a social worker may provide valuable assistance.

Some parents may want to leave the hospital immediately after the final paperwork is completed. On the other hand, if the child has been hospitalized for a long time, the parents may be reluctant to leave, since they feel that the hospital staff shares common recent memories of the child. Departure from the hospital for these parents may represent the final separation from their child.

Parents have reported that it is very traumatic to receive their child's possessions because this action symbolizes the full reality of the child's death. Too often, a plastic garbage sack is the most readily available container, but use of such a sack is insensitive and possibly offensive to the parents. Special containers should be available for this purpose.

Grief After Death

The grief response observed in the hospital is only the beginning of a long phase of sorrow and pain. As the shock and numbness dissipate, parents and other family members grieve for months and even years.

Parents report a sense of emptiness, yearning, and loneliness and the intense desire to hold, caress, touch, and talk with the child who has died. There may be preoccupation with thoughts about the child or a sense of the child's presence in the room. It may be painful for the parents even to walk past the child's room. The parents should be warned about these experiences, since they may be particularly stressful.

Parents should know that memories of the child can be therapeutic. Suppression of these memories deprives the parents of a potential source of comfort.

Parents are often devastated because they were unable to protect their child from death. This feeling is based on the parental protective role in society and often produces feelings of intense helplessness and guilt. Guilt is one of the most painful and persistent emotions experienced by bereaved parents.

Helplessness may cause anger about the child's death. Targets of anger may include health care professionals. If the child died following trauma, the drunken driver or the municipality that failed to deal with an unsafe intersection may also be targets

for anger. Anger may also be directed toward family members and friends who fail to understand and those who do not support the parents adequately. Anger at God can lead to confusion regarding religious beliefs, compounding the grief.

Grieving parents often become disorganized in daily life and work activities. They have difficulty concentrating, are unable to make decisions, and may be depressed. Job performance often deteriorates. This disorganization may be most evident months after the child's death. At this time, counseling may be particularly helpful.

Bereaved parents are gradually helped by the passage of time and the concern of others who listen to their pain. In time the pain becomes less intense, although it can be reawakened by unexpected memories. Anniversaries of the child's birth and death are painful for many years.

Grief following the death of a child is intense, with long-lasting effects on parents and other family members. Someone from the health care team must be available to and responsible for contacting the parents after the child's death. This contact person can provide reference material and information about bereavement support groups (Box 4-2). The family often wishes to return to the hospital for visits and counseling sessions and may wish to discuss postmortem findings with the child's physician.

Conclusion

Professionals who work in critical care settings have a vital contribution to make in supporting dying children and their families. The care of dying children is challenging and emotionally draining, and the family requires a great deal of support. Societal attitudes about childhood death reinforce the feeling of failure when the child's life cannot be saved. This can have a tremendous impact on the professional staff. If the staff are not able to deal with their own feelings, they may not be able to adequately help parents in this tragic experience.

Box 4-2
Bereavement Support Groups

AMEND: Association of Mothers Experiencing
   Neonatal Death
4324 Berrywick Terrace
St Louis, MO 63128
(314) 487-7582

Compassionate Friends
PO Box 3696
Oak Brook IL 60522-3696
(312) 323-5010

Griefbusters
Hospice of the Central Coast
100 Barnet Segal Lane
Monterey, CA 93940
(831) 649-1772

ILLOWA Chapter of Guilds for Infant Survival
923 Central Park Avenue
Davenport, IA 52804
(319) 487-7582

National Hospice Organization
1901 N. Moore St., Suite 901
Arlington, VA 22209
(703) 243-5900

National Sudden Infant Death Syndrome
   Foundation
1314 Bedford Ave.
Suite 210
Baltimore, MD 21208
(800) 221-SIDS

Parents of Murdered Children
100 E. 8th St., B-41
Cincinnati, OH 45202
(513) 721-5683
(888) 818-POMC

SHARE: Pregnancy and Infant Loss, Inc.
St. Joseph's Health Center
300 First Capitol Drive
St. Charles, MO 63301
(314) 947-6164

Suggested Readings

Betz CL: Death, dying and bereavement: a review of the literature, 1970-1985. In Krulik T, Holaday B, Martinson IM, editors: *The child and family facing life-threatening illness,* Philadelphia, 1987, JB Lippincott.

Bluebond-Langner M: *The private worlds of dying children,* Princeton, NJ, 1978, Princeton University Press.

Bluebond-Langner M: *In the shadow of illness; parents and siblings of the chronically ill child,* Princeton, NJ, 1996, Princeton University Press.

Chesler MA, Paris J, Barbarin OA: "Telling" the child with cancer: parental choices to share information with ill children, *J Pediatr Psychol* 11:496, 1986.

Clarmont P et al: *A joyful journey,* Grand Rapids, 1997, Zondervan.

Eickhorn DJ, Meyers TA, Guzzetta CE: Letting the family say good-bye during CPR, *Am J Nurs* 95(3): 60-63, 1995.

King NMP, Cross AW: Children as decision-makers; guidelines for pediatricians, *J Pediatr* 115:10, 1989.

Krulik T, Holaday B, Martinson IM, editors: *The child and family facing life-threatening illness,* Philadelphia, 1987, JB Lippincott.

Randolph AG et al: Factors explaining variability among caregivers in the intent to restrict life support functions in a pediatric intensive care unit, *Crit Care Med* 15:435-439, 1997.

Schiff HS: *The bereaved parent,* New York, 1977, Penguin Books.

Wass H, Corr CA, editors: *Childhood and death,* New York, 1984, Hemisphere Publishing.

For lists of helpful readings for siblings and parents, see Hazinski MF: *Nursing care of the critically ill child,* ed 2, St Louis, 1992, Mosby, pp 115-116.

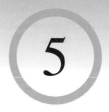

5 Cardiovascular Disorders

Introduction

Assessment and support of cardiopulmonary function is essential for every critically ill patient, and monitoring of heart rate is performed for virtually every intensive care unit (ICU) patient. Tachycardia is often observed in the seriously ill or injured child; it may signal stress, pain, or fever. It may also be observed in conjunction with cardiorespiratory or neurologic deterioration. The most common cause of bradycardia is hypoxia; thus a fall in heart rate is an ominous sign in the critically ill patient. Careful monitoring and therapy can often prevent the development of decompensated shock and cardiac arrest.

Essential Anatomy and Physiology

The cardiovascular system is designed to deliver oxygenated blood to the tissues and organs and to carry metabolic wastes from the tissues to the heart for eventual elimination by the lungs. Adequate systemic perfusion requires an appropriate heart rate, adequate intravascular volume relative to the vascular space, effective myocardial function, and appropriate arterial and venous tone and tissue utilization of oxygen.

Cardiovascular Development

Etiology and Epidemiology of Congenital Heart Disease

Most fetal cardiac development occurs between the fourth and seventh weeks of fetal life. The heart is most susceptible to teratogenic (harmful) influences during this time. Congenital heart disease (CHD) occurs in approximately 0.8% of all live births. Most (90%) of CHD is thought to be caused by multifactorial (or polygenic) inheritance; this means that there is a genetic predisposition *and* an adverse response to environmental teratogens during cardiac development. In the presence of a strong genetic predisposition, even a mild teratogenic influence can contribute to the development of CHD. Alternatively, if there is no genetic predisposition, very few factors can produce CHD. Recurrence risks for CHD average 2% to 4% in most families once one child with CHD is born, although they may be much higher with some forms of CHD or if a parent (particularly the mother) has CHD.

Environmental factors (teratogens) alone account for only approximately 1% of all CHD, and only a few maternal diseases or conditions have been consistently linked with CHD. Approximately 5% to 8% of CHD is associated with chromosomal anomalies or syndromes (Table 5-1).

Extracardiac anomalies are present in 20% to 45% of children with CHD. Gastrointestinal anomalies (including tracheoesophageal fistula or diaphragm hernia), renal anomalies (renal malformation or agenesis), and coagulopathies have been associated with CHD. Complex cyanotic heart disease (including anomalous systemic and pulmonary veins, transposition of the great vessels, and pulmonary stenosis) and malposition of the abdominal viscera may be part of an *asplenia syndrome*. Since asplenia increases the patient's vulnerability to infection (particularly from encapsulated organisms), asplenia should be ruled out by abdominal ultrasound in neonates and young infants with complex cyanotic heart disease. The following precautions are required if asplenia is present:

- Irradiation of all blood products before administration
- Preoperative and postoperative administration of antibiotic prophylaxis

- Pneumococcal vaccine before the child enters school (see Chapter 11)

Polysplenia may also be associated with cyanotic CHD and malposition of abdominal viscera. In polysplenia the child has multiple nodules of functioning splenic tissue rather than a single spleen. No spleen is visible on abdominal ultrasound, but the risk of infection is not increased because functioning splenic tissue is present.

Development of the Heart and Great Vessels

The cardiovascular system is the first system to function in the embryo. At approximately the twenty-first day of fetal life, two endocardial heart tubes begin to fuse and become surrounded by a layer of mesenchymal tissue (which will become the myocardium and epicardium). Expansion, elongation, and dilation of portions of the heart tube result in coiling of the tube to the right (this is normal dextro-looping, or D-looping), resulting in the formation of a common atrium, common ventricle, and truncus arteriosus.

The coiled heart tube is divided by septa into the right and left atria, the right and left ventricles, and the pulmonary artery and aorta (Figure 5-1). When the great vessels are in normal position, they are characterized as follows:

- *D-related great vessels:* The aorta is to the right (dextral) of the pulmonary artery.
- The normal aortic valve is located posterior and to the right of the pulmonic valve.

If the great vessels are transposed but the ventricles are not, this is referred to as *D-transposition*. With this form of transposition, the *ventricles* have looped normally during development, but the great vessels are transposed; thus the aorta arises from the right ventricle and receives systemic venous blood, and the pulmonary artery arises from the left ventricle and receives pulmonary venous blood. This form of transposition is also referred to as transposition of the great arteries (TGA).

The atrioventricular (AV) valves develop in association with specific ventricles. If the mitral valve develops, it will be associated with the morphologic (structural) left ventricle, wherever that ventricle is located. If the tricuspid valve develops,

Table 5-1
Cardiac Anomalies Associated with Genetic or Maternal Health Factors

Chromosomal Disease or Syndrome	Associated Cardiac Anomaly
Trisomy 13 (Patau's syndrome)	Patent ductus arteriosus and/or ventricular septal defect with pulmonary hypertension
Trisomy 18 (Edward's syndrome)	Ventricular septal defect; patent ductus arteriosus
Trisomy 21 (Down's syndrome)	Endocardial cushion defect; ventricular septal defect; patent ductus arteriosus
Turner's syndrome	Coarctation of the aorta
Mosaic Turner's syndrome (XO/XY)	Pulmonary valvular stenosis
Marfan's syndrome	Aortic or mitral valve abnormalities; dissecting aortic aneurysms; myocardial disease
Holt-Oram syndrome	Atrial septal defect or single atrium; severe pulmonary vascular disease; total anomalous pulmonary venous return; arrhythmias
Ellis–van Creveld syndrome	Single atrium or large atrial septal defect
Williams elfin facies syndrome	Supravalvular aortic stenosis; peripheral pulmonary stenosis
Laurence-Moon-Bardet-Biedl syndrome	Aortic or pulmonary valvular stenosis; tetralogy of Fallot; ventricular septal defect
Hunter's syndrome	Abnormalities of the mitral or tricuspid valves or coronary artery obstruction
Hurler's syndrome	Abnormalities of the mitral or tricuspid valves or coronary artery obstruction
Friedreich's ataxia	Cardiomyopathy
Neurofibromatosis	Pulmonary valvular stenosis
DiGeorge's syndrome	Interrupted aortic arch
Rubella syndrome	Patent ductus arteriosus; peripheral pulmonary stenosis

Maternal Health Factors	Associated Cardiac Anomaly
Fetal alcohol syndrome	Ventricular septal defect; atrial septal defect; tetralogy of Fallot
Maternal thalidomide ingestion	Tetralogy of Fallot; truncus arteriosus
Fetal trimethadione syndrome	Ventricular septal defect; tetralogy of Fallot
Maternal diabetes (insulin dependent)	Transposition of the great vessels; ventricular septal defect

From Hazinski MF: *Nursing care of the critically ill child,* ed 2, St Louis, 1992, Mosby. Modified from Noonan JA: Syndromes associated with cardiac defects. In Engle MA, editor: *Pediatric cardiovascular disease, cardiovascular clinics,* vol 11, Philadelphia, 1981, FA Davis; and Reynolds DW, Stagno S, Alford CA: Chronic congenital and perinatal infections. In Avery GB, editor: *Neonatology: pathophysiology and management of the newborn,* ed 3, Philadelphia, 1988, WB Saunders.

it will be associated with the morphologic (structural) right ventricle, wherever that ventricle is located.

Malrotation during looping of the cardiac tube can cause the tube to coil to the left, resulting in *L-transposition,* also called corrected transposition. Systemic venous blood still flows into the pulmonary circulation, and pulmonary venous blood flows into the systemic circulation. The term *ventricular inversion* should probably be used, since it is the position of the *ventricles* and their associated AV valves that is reversed. Systemic venous blood flows through a *mitral* valve and a structural *left*

ventricle to enter the pulmonary circulation, and pulmonary venous blood flows through a *tricuspid* valve and a structural *right* ventricle to enter the systemic circulation. Although the position of the great vessels is abnormal (they are in l-position), they will receive the appropriate venous blood.

Classification of Complex Cardiac Malpositions and Malformations

Although simple descriptive terms are used for the most common forms of CHD (e.g., atrial septal defect, truncus arteriosus, tricuspid atresia), some cardiac malpositions and malformations are fairly

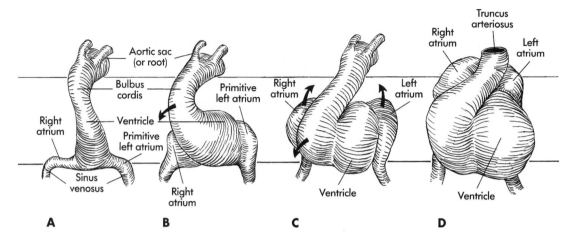

Figure 5-1 Cardiac embryologic development—coiling of the heart tube. At approximately the twenty-first to the twenty-second day of fetal life, the two lateral endothelial heart tubes fuse to form a single endocardial tube. **A,** Between the twenty-second and twenty-eighth days of life, the heart tube thickens. **B** and **C,** The tube then coils to the right. **D,** By approximately the twenty-eighth day of fetal life, the tube is completely coiled, and major chambers can be identified. At this time, blood is flowing through the heart, and septation of the heart and great vessels can occur. (Illustration by Marilou Kundemueller.)

complex. These include malpositions of the abdominal organs or viscera, as well as malposition of the ventricles and possibly the great vessels. Complex CHD may be classified according to the system of Van Praagh, with modifications proposed by Anderson. This system uses a three-letter system in brackets ({A,B,c}) to characterize the positions of the patient's viscera (first letter, capitalized), the ventricular loop (second letter, capitalized), and the great vessels or arteries (third letter, not capitalized). The cardiac chambers are identified by morphology (structure and appearance) and then are characterized as *concordant* (consistent in position) or *discordant* (inconsistent in position). The normal heart is characterized as {S,D,d-normal}. This classification is summarized in Box 5-1.

Fetal Circulation

Fetal circulation is anatomically and physiologically different from postnatal circulation in several important ways. In the fetus oxygenation of the blood occurs in the placenta, which is a relatively inefficient oxygenator of the blood. Fetal blood is hypoxemic when compared with postnatal blood. The fetal Po_2 is approximately 20 to 30 mm Hg but is 60% to 70% saturated because fetal hemoglobin binds oxygen more readily than "adult" hemoglobin. Oxygen delivery is adequate in the fetus because the hemoglobin saturation is relatively high and the cardiac output is approximately four times that of the adult per kilogram of body weight.

Fetal circulation is designed to direct the best oxygenated blood from the placenta to the fetal brain and to divert blood away from the nonfunctional lungs and pulmonary circulation. The *ductus venosus* diverts placental blood through the liver into the inferior vena cava (IVC). As the blood enters the right atrium, it is diverted toward the atrial septum, where the flapped *foramen ovale* allows this placental blood to enter the left atrium so that it can pass through the left side of the heart into the aorta to the fetal brain. Blood returning from the superior vena cava (SVC) flows through the right atrium and ventricle but is diverted away from the pulmonary artery through the *ductus arteriosus* into the descending aorta. Half of this descending aortic blood returns directly to the placenta.

Fetal *pulmonary vascular resistance(PVR)* is high because the fetal alveoli are fluid-filled and hypoxic, and alveolar hypoxia stimulates pulmonary vasoconstriction. Fetal *systemic vascular*

Box 5-1

Classification System for Complex Cardiac Malpositions and Malformations, Based on Van Praagh

Position of Abdominal Viscera and Atria (S, I, or a)

The orientation of the right and left atria is usually consistent (concordant) with the orientation of the abdominal viscera. The structural right atrium is usually identifiable because it is joined to the suprahepatic portion of the inferior vena cava. S, I, or A is used to classify visceral position as *situs Solitus, situs Inversus,* or situs ambiguous:

S *(situs Solitus):* Abdominal organs are in normal position (with liver on the right, stomach and spleen on the left). The structural right atrium is on the right, and the structural left atrium is on the left, joined to the pulmonary veins. The lung in right chest is trilobed; the lung in left chest is bilobed.

I *(situs Inversus):* Mirror-image location of body organs, with the liver on the left and the stomach and spleen on the right. The lung in left chest is trilobed, whereas the lung in right chest is bilobed. The structural right atrium (joined to the vena cavae) is located on the left side, and the structural left atrium (joined to the pulmonary veins) is located on the right side.

A *(situs ambiguous):* Atrial structure is indeterminate, and viscera are mixed in orientation. Asplenia or polysplenia syndromes are classified in this way. Asplenia is associated with bilateral right-sided viscera (both lungs are trilobed, the liver is horizontal with equal lobes, and both atria are structurally right atria). Polysplenia is associated with bilateral left-sided viscera (both lungs are bilobed, the stomach and liver are often central, and malrotation of the bowel is often present). Both atria are structurally left atria, which usually results in the presence of a nonsinus pacemaker.

Description of the Ventricular Loop (D or L)

A dextral-loop, or D-loop (normal), is present if the structural right ventricle is located on the right and the structural left ventricle is located on the left. An L-loop has occurred if the structural right ventricle is on the left and the structural left ventricle is on the right.

Position of the Great Vessels (d-Normal or d- or l-Transposition)

The position of the great vessels is characterized by the relationship of the semilunar valves:

d-*normal:* The aortic valve is posterior and to the right of the pulmonary valve. This may also be called the *Solitus* position, indicated by a capital letter *S.*

d-*transposition:* The aortic valve is located to the right but anterior to the pulmonic valve.

l-*transposition:* The vessels are located abnormally, and the aortic valve is located to the left of the pulmonic valve.

---

resistance *(SVR)* is low, since a significant portion of systemic venous blood enters the placenta, which is a low-resistance pathway.

Normal Perinatal Circulatory Changes

At birth, the normal neonate switches from placental to pulmonary oxygenation of the blood, and the placenta is eliminated from the circulation. Ventilation expands the lungs, immediately improving alveolar oxygenation. The fluid in the alveoli is absorbed into the pulmonary capillaries. As a result, alveolar hypoxia is eliminated, PVR falls, and blood flow into the lungs increases dramatically. At sea level, PVR falls by approximately 80% immediately after birth and normally reaches adult levels during the first weeks of life if the ductus closes normally.

Fetal shunts normally close after birth. The umbilical arteries and vein and the ductus venosus constrict when the umbilical cord is cut; these vessels eventually undergo fibrous infiltration. The flapped foramen ovale closes when right atrial pressure falls below left atrial pressure. This opening may remain probe patent in some patients

Table 5-2
Calculation of Pulmonary Vascular Resistance

Calculations

$$PVR \text{ (Wood units)} = \frac{\text{Mean PA pressure} - \text{Mean LA pressure}}{\text{Cardiac output (liters/min)}}$$

$$PVR \text{ (index units)} = \frac{\text{Mean PA pressure} - \text{Mean LA pressure}}{\text{Cardiac index (liters/min/m}^2 \text{ BSA)}}$$

$$PVR \text{ (dynes-sec-cm}^{-5}) = \frac{\text{Mean PA pressure} - \text{Mean LA pressure (mm Hg)} \times 80}{\text{Cardiac output (liters/min)}}$$

NOTE: To obtain PVR index in dynes-sec-cm^{-5}, substitute cardiac index for cardiac output in denominator.

Normal Values in Infants and Children

Age	PVR (Wood Units)	PVR (Index Units)	PVR (dynes-sec-cm^{-5})
Young infant	25-40	7-10	2000-3200 (indexed: 560-800 dynes-sec-cm^{-5}/m^2)
Child	0.5-4	1-3	40-320 (indexed: 80-240 dynes-sec-cm^{-5}/m^2)

Potential Causes of Elevated PVR
Alveolar hypoxia and pulmonary artery constriction: Consider all potential causes of alveolar hypoxia, including hypoventilation, endotracheal tube obstruction, and pneumothorax
Increased blood flow (cardiac output) in the face of unchanged vascular tone
Obstruction to flow: pulmonary venous obstruction, mitral valve stenosis, or severe left ventricular failure

From Hazinski MF: Pediatric evaluation and monitoring considerations. In Darovic GO, editor: *Hemodynamic monitoring, invasive and noninvasive clinical applications,* ed 2, Philadelphia, 1995, Saunders.

into adult years, but it should be functionally closed within hours.

The rise in oxygenation of the newborn blood is a potent stimulus for constriction of the ductus arteriosus within 10 to 24 hours after a full-term birth. Neonates born prematurely may lack constrictive muscle in the ductus; thus closure may be prevented or delayed. Ductal closure may also be delayed in patients who are relatively hypoxemic at birth. This includes infants living at high altitudes, because the relatively low inspired oxygen tension produces a mild hypoxemia. Ductal constriction may also be delayed in neonates with pulmonary disease.

PVR normally falls progressively during the first weeks of life (Table 5-2). During the neonatal period the pulmonary arteries remain very reactive and can constrict in response to alveolar hypoxia, acidosis, hyperexpansion (overdistension) of the alveoli, or hypothermia. These factors must be avoided in infants or children with pulmonary hypertension, particularly following cardiovascular surgery.

Pulmonary vasodilation can be promoted by maintaining alveolar oxygenation, an alkalotic pH, appropriate alveolar expansion, and analgesia. This is accomplished by providing supplemental inspired oxygen and mechanical ventilation with positive end-expiratory pressure (PEEP) as needed. In addition, a mild alkalosis is maintained through mild hyperventilation, administration of sodium bicarbonate, or both (bicarbonate administration increases carbon dioxide production; thus hyperventilation is required). During mechanical ventilation, the tidal volume must be appropriate and barotrauma prevented. Finally, adequate analgesia must be provided and excessive stimulation avoided.

At the time of a full-term birth, the *preacinar pulmonary arteries* (those accompanying airways as small as the terminal bronchioles) have a thick muscle coat. Immediately after birth, this muscle layer begins to thin, and it continues to regress during the first days of life. Although the muscle layer thins, it does extend into smaller and smaller pulmonary arteries with age. During infancy and childhood the muscle layer extends into the arteries accompanying the respiratory bronchioles, into the alveolar ducts, and finally into those arteries surrounding the alveoli, the *interacinar arteries*.

SVR begins to rise as soon as the placenta is separated from the neonatal circulation (Table 5-3), and systemic arterial pressure and left ventricular pressure rise.

Alterations in Normal Pulmonary Vascular Development

Altitude, prematurity, alveolar hypoxia, lung disease, and CHD may affect normal postnatal pulmonary vascular development. Patients living at

---

Table 5-3
Calculation of Systemic Vascular Resistance

Calculations

$$\text{SVR (Wood units)} = \frac{\text{Mean arterial pressure} - \text{Mean RA pressure}}{\text{Cardiac output}}$$

$$\text{SVR (Index units)} = \frac{\text{Mean arterial pressure} - \text{Mean RA pressure}}{\text{Cardiac index}}$$

$$\text{SVR (dynes-sec-cm}^{-5}) = \frac{\text{Mean arterial pressure} - \text{Mean RA pressure}}{\text{Cardiac output}} \times 80$$

NOTE: To determine SVR index in dynes-sec-cm^{-5}, substitute cardiac index for cardiac output in denominator.

Normal Values for Infants and Children

Age	SVR (Wood Units)	SVR (Index Units)	SVR (dynes/sec/cm^{-5})
Infant	35-50	10-15	2800-4000 (indexed: 800-1200 dynes-sec-cm^{-5}/m^2)
Toddler	25-35	20	2000-2800 (indexed: 1600 dynes-sec-cm^{-5}/m^2)
Child	15-25	15-30	1200-2000 (indexed: 1200-2400 dynes-sec-cm^{-5}/m^2)

NOTE: The numerical value of indexed measurements decreases with age because body surface area is very low in infants and gradually increases with growth.

Factors Causing Changes in SVR
Increased
Compensatory vasoconstriction associated with low cardiac output
Administration of vasoconstrictive agents
Adrenergic stimulation

Decreased
Sepsis, the systemic inflammatory response syndrome (SIRS)
Anaphylaxis
Administration of vasodilatory agents
Sympathetic nervous system blockade (spinal anesthesia, barbiturate overdose), or damage or transection to the spinal cord

From Hazinski MF: Pediatric evaluation and monitoring considerations. In Darovic GO, editor: *Hemodynamic monitoring, invasive and noninvasive clinical applications,* ed 2, Philadelphia, 1995, Saunders.

high altitudes characteristically demonstrate a delayed postnatal fall in PVR because a low inspired oxygen tension creates a mild alveolar hypoxia.

If the infant is born prematurely, several factors can affect PVR. The medial muscle layer of the pulmonary arteries may be incompletely developed; thus it may regress in a shorter time after birth. As a result, the very premature infant may demonstrate a significant fall in PVR and symptoms of a congenital heart defect with a left-to-right (or aorta–to–pulmonary artery) shunt, such as patent ductus arteriosus, within hours after birth.

Perinatal alveolar hypoxia (e.g., caused by respiratory distress syndrome) may stimulate pulmonary vasoconstriction and may delay the normal fall in PVR. As a result, when the premature infant has lung disease and CHD, symptoms of the left-to-right shunt from the CHD may not develop until the lung disease begins to resolve and PVR falls.

Prenatal and perinatal alveolar hypoxia have been implicated in the development of persistent pulmonary hypertension of the newborn (PPHN), also known as persistent fetal circulation (PFC). This disease is associated with abnormal extension of the pulmonary arterial muscle layer into the smallest pulmonary arteries, with a resultant increase in PVR.

CHD, which produces an increase in pulmonary blood flow, can stimulate pulmonary vasoconstriction and persistence of the pulmonary artery medial muscle layer, which normally thins immediately after birth. Thus the full-term infant with CHD may demonstrate a delayed fall in PVR and may not demonstrate signs or symptoms of a left-to-right shunt for 4 to 12 weeks after birth.

Gross Anatomy

Right Side of the Heart

Systemic venous blood returns to the right atrium through the SVC and IVC. The *sinoatrial (SA) node* is the normal pacemaker of the heart and is located near the junction of the SVC and the right atrium. Rapid conduction between the SA node and the AV node can occur along any one of three *internodal conduction pathways.* Although the anterior pathway is usually dominant, injury to any of these pathways (e.g., during cardiovascular surgery) can produce AV conduction block.

The *tricuspid valve* is normally the anterior AV valve, separating the right atrium from the right ventricle. Each of its three valve leaflets is attached to several chordae tendineae, which are in turn attached to one of three papillary muscles in the right ventricle (Figure 5-2).

The right ventricle is normally the most anterior of the four cardiac chambers, and its inferior border forms most of the left inferior cardiac border on a standard (anterior-posterior [AP]) chest radiograph. The right ventricle receives blood from the right atrium and pumps blood into the pulmonary artery. Because PVR is low, the right ventricle normally generates low pressure to eject blood into the pulmonary circulation. The right ventricle is morphologically or structurally different from the left ventricle. The right ventricle contains muscle bundles, called trabeculations, which are not present in the left ventricle. The right ventricle has a thinner wall and smaller lumen than the left ventricle.

The right ventricle is functionally divided into an inflow and an outflow portion by the *crista supraventricularis,* a ridge formed by two muscle bands that extend from the anterior wall of the right ventricle to the tricuspid valve. The pulmonary outflow tract is also referred to as the pulmonary infundibulum. The pulmonary valve is a semilunar valve that is normally located above, in front of, and to the left of the aortic valve.

Left Side of the Heart

Oxygenated blood returns from the lungs via four pulmonary veins to the left atrium. The left atrium is normally the most posterior of the four cardiac chambers and normally does not contribute to the cardiac border on AP chest radiographs.

Pulmonary venous blood normally flows from the left atrium across the mitral valve into the left ventricle. The *mitral valve* consists of two leaflets of unequal size: the smaller septal leaflet and the larger posterior leaflet. The mitral leaflets attach to several chordae tendineae, which in turn attach to two groups of papillary muscles.

The left ventricle is located behind the right ventricle; thus it may not form a distinct part of the cardiac border on AP chest radiographs. The left ventricle is characterized by a thick wall, a large lumen, and smooth walls. The septal leaflet of the mitral valve divides the left ventricle into an inflow

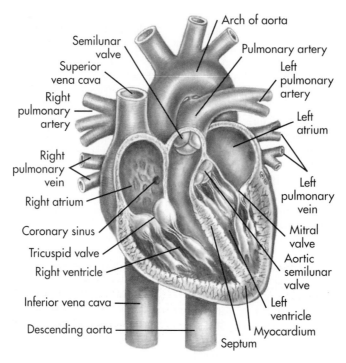

Figure 5-2   Frontal schematic view of the heart. (From Thompson JM et al, editors: *Mosby's clinical nursing*, ed 3, St Louis, 1993.)

and an outflow chamber when the mitral valve is open (during diastole).

The aortic valve is a semilunar valve. The cusps of this valve are labeled based on their relationship to the coronary arteries, which arise immediately above the valve. The cusps are labeled as the left coronary cusp, the right coronary cusp, and the noncoronary cusp.

Normal Cardiac Function

Cardiac Cycle

The heart receives systemic venous blood and ejects it into the lungs, and receives pulmonary venous blood and ejects it into the body. These circulations are normally separate but occur simultaneously; thus the heart functions as a two-sided pump. Blood is propelled by sequential relaxation and contraction of the atria and sequential relaxation and contraction of the ventricles.

Systemic venous blood enters the right atrium through the SVC and IVC. This blood is joined by coronary sinus blood in the right atrium (Figure 5-3). Complete mixing of this blood is accomplished in the right ventricle; thus the pulmonary artery is the first place to obtain a mixed venous sample of blood. Normally, approximately 75% of the hemoglobin is saturated with oxygen in a mixed venous oxygen sample.

During atrial and ventricular diastole (relaxation), the tricuspid and mitral valves are open, and systemic and pulmonary venous blood flows into the right and left ventricles, respectively. Approximately 75% of ventricular filling occurs during this time. Mean right atrial pressure is approximately equal to mean right ventricular end-diastolic pressure (RVEDP), and mean left atrial pressure is approximately equal to mean left ventricular end-diastolic pressure (LVEDP).

Atrial systole contributes the final 25% to 30% of ventricular filling. Normally, this portion is in-

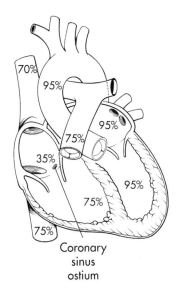

70%
95%
95%
75%
95%
35%
95%
75%
75%

Coronary
sinus
ostium

Figure 5-3 Normal oxygen saturations in the pediatric heart; catheterization data.

that is properly positioned in the lung (in a segment posterior and inferior to the heart), the pulmonary artery occlusion, or wedge, pressure should equal the left atrial pressure. In the absence of mitral valve disease, the left atrial pressure should equal the LVEDP. Therefore pulmonary artery occlusion/wedge pressure is normally equal to LVEDP. Several conditions can prevent this equalization so that the pulmonary artery occlusion/wedge pressure does *not* equal left atrial pressure and LVEDP. These are included in Box 5-2.

Coronary Circulation

Coronary artery blood flow constitutes a very small but significant portion of total cardiac output, because it perfuses the "pump." The normal distribution of the coronary arteries is identical in infants, children, and adults, although the structure of the arteries changes with age. Coronary artery flow occurs predominantly during ventricular diastole. Left ventricular coronary artery flow occurs *only* during ventricular diastole, whereas right ventricular coronary flow occurs during ventricular systole and diastole. Perfusion of the heart occurs from epicardium through myocardium to endocardium.

Coronary artery flow increases in response to a rise in myocardial oxygen consumption or a significant fall in arterial oxygen content (e.g., hypoxemia or severe anemia). If coronary blood flow or oxygen content is compromised, myocardial oxygen supply may initially be maintained by an increase in myocardial oxygen *extraction;* oxygen extraction can be increased from the normal 50% to 60% range to as high as 75% of oxygen delivered.

Coronary blood flow is regulated by the coronary artery and arteriole diameters, which are controlled by the autonomic nervous system and by vasoactive substances released from cardiac tissue. Constant adjustment in vessel diameter helps to maintain constant coronary artery flow over a wide range of conditions.

Coronary artery blood flow is affected by *coronary artery perfusion pressure.* Coronary artery perfusion pressure is the difference between systemic arterial diastolic pressure and ventricular end-diastolic pressure (VEDP). If systemic arterial diastolic pressure falls significantly (e.g., with hypotension, aortic insufficiency, or extreme vasodi-

consequential. However, if ventricular dysfunction is present, loss of atrial systole, which occurs with heart block or atrial fibrillation, may produce a significant fall in stroke volume and cardiac output.

Ventricular contraction begins immediately after atrial contraction. Initially the contraction is *isovolumetric*—it occurs without ejection of blood. Once right ventricular pressure exceeds right atrial pressure and left ventricular pressure exceeds left atrial pressure, the tricuspid and mitral valves close (nearly simultaneously). Then right and left ventricular pressures rise rapidly until they exceed pulmonary artery and aortic pressures, respectively. At this point the pulmonary and aortic valves open and the ejection phase of ventricular contraction, the *isotonic* phase, occurs.

Blood entering the pulmonary circulation passes through pulmonary arteries into the alveolar capillary bed, where it receives oxygen and surrenders carbon dioxide. Oxygenated blood enters the pulmonary veins and flows into the left atrium. Unless an intrapulmonary shunt is present, this blood is almost fully saturated with oxygen. There are no valves in this pulmonary venous system. As a result, if a balloon-tipped pulmonary artery catheter is wedged into a small pulmonary artery

---

Box 5-2

Factors Affecting the Relationship of Pulmonary Artery Occlusion Pressure to Left Ventricular End-Diastolic Pressure

Conditions That May Make Pulmonary Artery Occlusion/Wedge Pressure Fail to Equal Ventricular End-Diastolic Pressure

Extreme tachycardia, which can abbreviate diastolic time so that pressures cannot equalize

Pulmonary venous constriction or obstruction (will create a pressure gradient, making pulmonary artery occlusion/wedge pressure higher than left atrial pressure)

Mitral valve stenosis or insufficiency

Incorrect catheter placement: the catheter tip should be located in a posterior segment of the lung, inferior to the heart (West zone III.)

High positive end-expiratory pressure (can increase alveolar pressure)

Mechanical balloon problems: eccentric balloon occlusion, overwedging

Improper monitoring system setup (e.g., zeroing, leveling, and calibration of the transducer is faulty)

Influence of Location of Pulmonary Artery Catheter Tip in Lung: West Zones

Zone I: Superior segments (High PEEP may create function Zone I.)
Alveolar pressure > arterial pressure > pulmonary venous pressure
PAOP > LVEDP

Zone II: Middle segments (High PEEP may create functional Zone II.)
Arterial pressure > alveolar pressure > pulmonary venous pressure
PAOP > LVEDP

Zone III: Inferior segments (below the heart)
Arterial pressure > pulmonary venous pressure > alveolar pressure
PAOP = LVEDP

---

lation) or VEDP rises significantly, coronary artery perfusion pressure will fall. Initially, the coronary arteries will dilate to maintain flow, but once the vessels are maximally dilated, coronary blood flow will be directly related to coronary artery perfusion pressure and will fall if the perfusion pressure falls further.

Coronary artery disease is uncommon in children, although it can develop as a result of rejection following cardiac transplantation. Several conditions may, however, compromise coronary artery perfusion. *Anomalous origin of the coronary artery from the pulmonary artery* is an uncommon congenital defect that can produce ischemic heart disease and myocardial infarction during childhood. The anomalous coronary artery arises from the pulmonary artery. The pulmonary artery pressure is much lower than the aortic pressure perfusing the normal coronary artery. As a result, a "steal" of blood from the remaining normal coronary artery occurs. Blood shunts from the normal coronary artery through collateral vessels into the abnormal coronary artery and retrograde into the low-pressure, low-resistance pulmonary artery. This shunting of blood away from the normal coronary artery circulation creates inadequate myocardial perfusion, ischemia, and possibly infarction.

Severe *left ventricular outflow tract obstruction* or severe left ventricular failure may produce inadequate coronary artery perfusion and myocardial ischemia for a variety of reasons. If LVEDP is extremely high, coronary artery perfusion pressure will fall, and coronary blood flow will be reduced. In addition, when severe left ventricular outflow tract obstruction or severe left ventricular failure is present, the left ventricle will require a prolonged ejection time; when systolic time requires a greater portion of the cardiac cycle, diastolic time and coronary artery perfusion time are compromised. Episodes of *tachycardia* will further compromise perfusion because diastolic filling time is reduced and myocardial oxygen consumption is increased.

Several congenital heart defects (e.g., patent ductus arteriosus or aortic insufficiency) may affect coronary artery blood flow by producing a fall in systemic arterial diastolic pressure. If any of these conditions are present, particularly in association with a compromise in cardiac output or the myocardial oxygen supply-demand ratio, the patient must be monitored closely for signs of myocardial dysfunction, possible myocardial ischemia, and possible ventricular arrhythmias.

Cellular Physiology

The heart contains muscle, connective tissue, and conductive tissue. The myocardium and conductive tissue transmit electrochemical impulses, or *current.* Current is generated by the flow of electrons across the cell membrane.

Muscle and nerve cells have a *membrane* (also known as *transmembrane*) *potential,* which is the difference in electrical charge between the inside and the outside of the cells. The inside of the cell is negatively charged (−70 to −90 mV) with respect to the outside of the cell. This membrane potential is generated by concentration gradients for potassium and sodium across the cell membrane.

At rest, the concentration of potassium is higher *inside* the cell than outside the cell, and the concentration of sodium is higher *outside* the cell than inside the cell. These concentration gradients favor potassium exodus from the cell and sodium entry into the cell. The resting cell membrane is relatively impermeable to sodium, and an active pump transports sodium out of the cell and allows potassium to enter the cell.

When the myocardium is stimulated sufficiently, a change in intracellular electrical charge, called an *action potential,* develops. The sodium permeability of the sarcolemma membrane increases dramatically, and permeability to potassium is temporarily reduced. When the positively charged sodium ions rush through fast channels into the cell, a *current* flow (flow of electrons) is generated, and the inside of the cell becomes positively charged with respect to the outside of the cell. This also means that the outside of the cell becomes negatively charged with respect to the inside of the cell (Figure 5-4). This current flow, which occurs during myocardial depolarization, can be measured from the surface of the body in the electrocardiogram (ECG).

Depolarization of the myocardial cell occurs in a fraction of a second. The fast sodium channels are then quickly closed, but slow channels to calcium then open. This calcium influx prolongs the duration of the action potential and prevents immediate repolarization of the cell, and is unique to myocar-

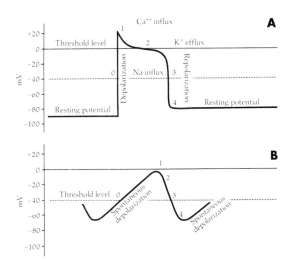

Figure 5-4 Cardiac action potentials. **A,** Action potential phases 0 to 4 of nonpacemaker cardiac cells. **B,** Action potential of pacemaker cell. (From Thompson JM et al: *Mosby's clinical nursing,* ed 3, St Louis, 1993, Mosby.)

dial cells. Membrane permeability to potassium is then restored, and the slow calcium channels close. The cell becomes repolarized by an exodus of potassium from the cell and eventual restoration of sodium and potassium gradients by the sodium-potassium pump.

All myocardial cells are self-excitable to some degree. Pacemaker cells can depolarize spontaneously and at a rate that is faster than that of other myocardial cells. The configuration of the pacemaker action potential is different than that of other myocardial cells. The resting membrane potential of the pacemaker cell is less negative than typical myocardial cells, and a *prepotential* or gradual reduction in the pacemaker membrane potential begins to develop almost as soon as the pacemaker cell is repolarized. This prepotential is caused by slow inward movement of sodium ions, which is unique to pacemaker cells. As a result of the prepotential, pacemaker cells are capable of depolarizing more frequently than other normal myocardial cells, and the pacemaker cells can then stimulate other myocardial cells to depolarize.

Once any part of a pacemaker or myocardial cell becomes depolarized, the action potential becomes propagated throughout the cell. It then quickly spreads from cell to cell in the heart through low-resistance connections called *intercalated disks.*

Hypoxia, electrolyte imbalances, and other myocardial injury can alter the generation and conduction of action potentials. Myocardial cells that are hypoxic or suffer other injury can depolarize more frequently than usual, creating arrhythmias such as premature ventricular contractions or ventricular tachycardia. Electrolyte imbalances, particularly significant alterations in serum (extracellular) potassium, can influence myocardial excitability and contractility.

Vagal (parasympathetic) stimulation reduces excitability of myocardial cells and can reduce the spontaneous pacemaker firing rate. Alternatively *sympathetic stimulation increases excitability* of the cells and can increase the pacemaker firing rate.

Electrical depolarization of the myocardium should result in mechanical contraction. However, there is no guarantee that effective *electrical* depolarization of the myocardium will result in adequate *mechanical* function. The child's cardiac function and systemic perfusion must always be closely monitored, even in the presence of a normal heart rate and ECG.

The myocardium consists of interconnected myocardial cells, or *myocytes,* surrounded by the sarcolemma membrane. Each myocyte contains *myofibrils,* which contain the *sarcomeres,* the contractile element of the myocardial cell. The sarcomeres contain overlapping protein filaments of *actin* and *myosin.* Contraction occurs when the myocardium depolarizes and intracellular ionized calcium increases. The calcium reacts with sites on the actin and myosin, stimulating the formation of cross-linkages between the filaments, pulling them together and causing myocardial shortening or contraction. This contraction requires energy, using adenosine triphosphate (ATP) and magnesium.

Factors Influencing Ventricular Function

Myocardial performance can be affected by changes in oxygenation, perfusion, serum ionized calcium concentration, acid-base and electrolyte balance, sympathetic or vagal stimulation, and drugs. These factors can affect cardiac output by altering either heart rate or ventricular stroke volume.

Sympathetic nervous system beta-adrenergic stimulation increases myocardial calcium release and influx; thus myocardial contraction is enhanced. In addition, because calcium reuptake is more rapid, the ventricular systolic time is shorter. This results in prolongation of the diastolic filling time at the same heart rate; thus stroke volume is increased. Beta-adrenergic stimulation also increases heart rate. Many of these effects are mediated by cyclic adenosine monophosphate (cAMP), an intracellular messenger that promotes phosphorylation of sarcolemmal proteins and increases the opening of calcium channels in myocardial cell membranes. Phosphodiesterase then converts the cAMP to an inactive compound, ending the cAMP and sympathetic effects. *Phosphodiesterase inhibitors* (such as amrinone) prevent the inactivation of cAMP; thus they prolong any adrenergic effects that are mediated by cAMP.

Contractility is enhanced by any conditions or factors that increase intracellular calcium. Alpha-adrenergic stimulation and cardiac glycosides all increase intracellular ionized calcium. The intracellular sodium concentration can influence the free calcium levels in the myocyte because sodium and calcium ions share storage sites and compete for space in the sodium-potassium pump. When the intracellular sodium concentration is increased (e.g., during digitalis therapy), sodium occupies space in the exchange pump; thus calcium ions accumulate in the myocardial cell, and myocardial contractility increases.

Three terms borrowed from the physiology laboratory have been used to describe several important factors influencing myocardial function. These terms—*preload, contractility,* and *afterload*—have been defined precisely in the physiology laboratory using isolated normal myocardial preparations. Their application to the clinical setting, however, where it may be impossible to separate the effects of each factor, has been less precise. The common usage and clinical application of these terms are provided here.

Ventricular Preload and Compliance

Preload   Preload is the amount of stretch that is present in the ventricular myocardial fibers before contraction. Frank and Starling worked with isolated heart preparations and showed that, to a point, the tension generated by myocardial fibers during contraction is directly related to the stretch placed on the fibers *before* contraction. The tension generated by the fibers will increase if the stretch on the fibers is increased before contraction. Their observations became known as the Frank-Starling Law of the Heart.

In the clinical setting, since we have no convenient way of determining the presystolic stretch of myocardial fibers, we measure the VEDP. Because we cannot measure the tension generated by the myocardial fibers during contraction, we evaluate the stroke volume or cardiac output.

The VEDP can be measured in the clinical setting. RVEDP is equal to right atrial pressure unless tricuspid valve stenosis is present. Central venous pressure (CVP) should equal right atrial and RVEDP unless central venous obstruction is present. The CVP can be estimated clinically to some degree. Hepatomegaly is present once the CVP exceeds approximately 6 to 8 mm Hg. However, other conditions, including hepatitis and cirrhosis, can also increase the liver size and cloud the clinical estimation of CVP. The presence of edema is not a reliable indicator of high venous pressures. Systemic edema will be present when the CVP is high, but this edema may also be present at a low CVP if capillary leak (e.g., with sepsis) or hypoalbuminemia is present.

The LVEDP is equal to left atrial pressure unless mitral valve disease is present. The pulmonary artery wedge pressure (PAWP, also known as pulmonary artery occlusion pressure [PAOP]) can equal the left atrial pressure if the catheter tip is appropriately placed and wedged and the measurement system is appropriately zeroed, leveled, and calibrated. The LVEDP can be difficult to evaluate clinically. If the LVEDP is high (>25 mm Hg), pulmonary edema will be present. However, pulmonary edema will also be present at lower pressures if pulmonary capillary permeability is increased. The LVEDP may differ significantly from the RVEDP, particularly in the presence of severe pulmonary hypertension, sepsis, or some forms of CHD. Therefore *the CVP reflects RVEDP and may be very different from the LVEDP and PAOP.*

To a point, as the right or left VEDP is increased, the ventricular fibers are stretched, and the stroke volume or output of that ventricle is increased (Figure 5-5). VEDP is increased by bolus intravenous (IV) volume administration. The most significant improvement in stroke volume and cardiac output is likely to be observed when a CVP or PAOP ≤5 mm Hg is increased to approximately 10 to 15 mm Hg.

The ideal VEDP associated with optimal cardiac output must be determined individually and may change from day to day, particularly if myocardial dysfunction is present. When fluid is administered to optimize ventricular myocardial preload and VEDP, the fluid should be carefully titrated and patient response, including assessment

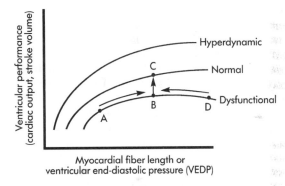

Figure 5-5 Frank-Starling curve. In the laboratory, Frank and Starling used isolated *normal* heart muscle strips to demonstrate that stretching the myocardial fibers before they contracted increased the tension the fibers generated with contraction. Thus the original Frank-Starling curve is depicted as a normal curve, demonstrating the relationship between myocardial fiber length and ventricular performance. In the clinical setting, the ventricular end-diastolic pressure *(VEDP)* is substituted for the myocardial fiber length; the VEDP is manipulated through volume administration (*A to B*) and diuresis (*D to B*). A dysfunctional ventricle is characterized by a depressed and flatter Frank-Starling curve; dysfunctional ventricles demonstrate only modest improvement in performance with volume administration and typically require volume titration, as well as inotropic support, vasodilator therapy, and correction of any conditions that are depressing function to maximize cardiac output and performance at a given VEDP (*B to C*). If the patient's ventricles are hyperdynamic, cardiac output will be high even at low VEDP. (Illustration courtesy William Banner, Jr MD.)

of systemic/organ perfusion, must be carefully evaluated.

The VEDP cannot be increased indefinitely without some consequences. If pulmonary capillary permeability is normal, an LVEDP and pulmonary capillary pressure of 25 mm Hg will be associated with the development of pulmonary edema. Pulmonary edema will develop at lower pressures if pulmonary capillary permeability is increased (e.g., in sepsis or acute respiratory distress syndrome). Therefore volume administration has probably been maximized once the VEDP reaches approximately 15 to 18 mm Hg. At that point, further improvement in cardiac output should probably be accomplished through titration of inotropic and possibly vasodilator drugs.

Studies of newborn lambs in the 1970s suggested that neonates could not increase stroke volume or cardiac output in response to volume administration. However, more recent research suggests that neonates *are* capable of increasing stroke volume in response to volume therapy, provided that ventricular function is adequate and the aortic pressure and ventricular afterload do not rise precipitously.

Compliance   The patient's VEDP is not linearly and directly related to volume administration. The relationship between the VEDP and volume administration is affected by ventricular *compliance. Compliance is the distensibility of the ventricle. It is defined as the change in ventricular volume (in milliliters) for a given change in pressure (in millimeters of mercury),* or $\triangle V/\triangle P$. If the ventricle is extremely compliant, a large volume of IV fluids may be administered in a short period of time without substantially increasing the VEDP.

The opposite of compliance is stiffness. If the ventricle is noncompliant, or stiff, even a small amount of IV volume administration may increase the VEDP. Dysfunctional or hypertrophied (thick) ventricles tend to be noncompliant. They have a higher VEDP even at rest and typically require a somewhat higher VEDP than normal to optimize ventricular performance, stroke volume, and cardiac output.

Vasodilator therapy will improve ventricular compliance. This means that a greater volume can be present in the ventricle at the end of diastole without much increase in VEDP. Thus at the same VEDP, stroke volume is increased. Constrictive pericarditis and tamponade reduce ventricular compliance because they prevent ventricular expansion during diastole.

Contractility

Contractility refers to the strength and efficiency of ventricular contraction; it is the force generated by the myocardium, independent of preload and afterload. Contractility is estimated by the velocity of fiber shortening; if myocardial function is good, the fibers will shorten rapidly. This shortens systole at the same heart rate; thus the ventricle has longer time to fill (diastole), and stroke volume increases.

A compromise in ventricular contractility should be suspected if cardiac output and systemic perfusion are inadequate despite the presence of an adequate cardiac preload (CVP and pulmonary artery wedge/occlusion pressure ≥8 to 12 mm Hg). Other clinical signs of myocardial dysfunction may include diminished peripheral pulses, oliguria, narrowing of the pulse pressure, and possible peripheral vasoconstriction.

Contractility is not easily measured at the bedside. The most common method used is echocardiographic evaluation of ventricular fiber shortening times and measurement of the shortening fraction of the left ventricular diameter (calculated by the difference between the end-diastolic and end-systolic dimensions, divided by the end-diastolic dimension). The normal shortening fraction is approximately 28% to 44% in children.

If a pulmonary artery catheter with thermodilution cardiac output thermistor is in place, a bedside ventricular function curve can be created by graphing the cardiac output (on the vertical axis) at various pulmonary artery wedge/occlusion pressures (representing the LVEDP on the horizontal axis). If cardiac output improves with no change in the LVEDP, ventricular contractility or compliance has improved. Other parameters to calculate and monitor in the child with potential myocardial dysfunction include stroke volume and stroke index, left and right ventricular stroke work index, and arteriovenous oxygen content difference (a-v $\dot{D}O_2$). These parameters are summarized in Table 5-4.

Several other methods of describing ventricular performance require cardiac catheterization or

Table 5-4
Measured and Calculated Hemodynamic Variables in Infants and Children

Variable	Formula	Normal Range
Cardiac index	Cardiac output/m^2 body surface area (BSA)	3.0-4.5 L/min/m^2 BSA
Systemic vascular resistance (SVR)	Index units: $\dfrac{\text{Mean arterial pressure} - \text{Mean RA pressure}}{\text{Cardiac index}}$	Index units Infant: 10-15 Toddler: 20 Child: 15-30
	Wood units: $\dfrac{\text{Mean arterial pressure} - \text{Mean RA pressure}}{\text{Cardiac output}}$	Wood units Infant: 35-50 Toddler: 25-35 Child: 15-25
	Dynes-sec-cm^{-5}: $\dfrac{\text{Mean arterial pressure} - \text{Mean RA Pressure} \times 80}{\text{Cardiac output}}$	Dynes-sec-cm^{-5} Infant: 2800-4000 (indexed: 800-1200) Toddler: 2000-2800 (indexed: 1600) Child: 1200-2000 (indexed: 1200-2400)
	NOTE: To determine SVR index in dynes, substitute cardiac index for output in denominator	
Pulmonary vascular resistance (PVR)	Index units: $\dfrac{\text{Mean PA pressure} - \text{Mean LA pressure}}{\text{Cardiac index}}$	Index units Young infant: 7-10 Child: 1-3
	Wood units: $\dfrac{\text{Mean PA pressure} - \text{Mean LA pressure}}{\text{Cardiac output}}$	Wood units Young infant: 25-40 Child: 0.5-4
	Dynes-sec-cm^{-5}: $\dfrac{\text{Mean PA pressure} - \text{Mean LA pressure} \times 80}{\text{Cardiac output}}$	Dynes-sec-cm^{-5} Young infant: 2000-3200 (indexed: 560-800) Child: 40-320 (indexed: 80-240)

Data from Hazinski MF: Pediatric evaluation and monitoring considerations. In Darovic GO, editor: *Hemodynamic monitoring: invasive and noninvasive clinical applications*, Philadelphia, 1996, WB Saunders; Katz RW, Pollack MM, Weibley RE: Pulmonary artery catheterization in pediatric intensive care. In Barnes LA: *Advances in pediatrics: intensive care*, St Louis, 1984, Mosby; and Perloff WH: Invasive measurements in the PICU. In Fuhrman BP, Zimerman JJ, editors: *Pediatric critical care*, St Louis, 1998, Mosby.

Continued

Table 5-4
Measured and Calculated Hemodynamic Variables in Infants and Children—cont'd

Variable	Formula	Normal Range
Stroke volume index	$\dfrac{\text{Cardiac index}}{\text{Heart rate}}$	30-65 ml/beat/m² BSA
LV stroke work index	SI × MAP × 0.0136	56 ± 6 g-m/m²
RV stroke work index	SI × MPAP × 0.0136	0.5 ± 0.06 g-m/m²
Arterial oxyhemoglobin saturation	Obtained by pulse oximetry or co-oximeter	96%-100%
Mixed venous oxyhemoglobin saturation	Estimated by pulmonary artery oximeter, evaluated by co-oximeter from pulmonary artery blood sample	65%-80% (see Figure 5-6, A-H)
Oxygen delivery ($\dot{D}o_2$)	Cardiac index (in ml) × Cao_2 Cao_2 = Arterial oxygen content (ml O_2/dl of blood) Cao_2 = (Hgb × 1.34 ml O_2/L × Hgb saturation) + Pao_2 × 0.003	425-750 ml/min/m²
Oxygen consumption ($\dot{V}o_2$)	Cardiac index (in ml) × $Av\dot{D}o_2$ $Av\dot{D}o_2 = Cao_2 - C\bar{v}o_2$ $C\bar{v}o_2$ = Mixed venous oxygen content (ml O_2/dl blood from PA) $C\bar{v}o_2$ = (Hgb × 1.34 ml O_2/L × Mixed venous Hgb saturation) × $P\bar{v}o_2$ × 0.003	120-230 ml/min/m²
Cardiac output (Fick)	$\dfrac{\dot{V}o_2}{Cao_2 - C\bar{v}o_2}$	Cardiac output averages 200 ml/kg/min in newborns and 100-150 ml/kg/min in infants and children
O_2 extraction ratio	$\dfrac{Av\dot{D}o_2}{Cao_2}$	

Data from Hazinski MF: Pediatric evaluation and monitoring considerations. In Darovic GO, editor: *Hemodynamic monitoring: invasive and noninvasive clinical applications*, Philadelphia, 1996, WB Saunders; Katz RW, Pollack MM, Weibley RE: Pulmonary artery catheterization in pediatric intensive care. In Barnes LA: *Advances in pediatrics: intensive care*, St Louis, 1984, Mosby; and Perloff WH: Invasive measurements in the PICU. In Fuhrman BP, Zimerman JJ, editors: *Pediatric critical care*, St Louis, 1998, Mosby.

nuclear imaging. These include calculation of end-diastolic volume, ejection fraction, and systolic output.

Although evaluation of contractility considers the effectiveness of ventricular *systolic* function, ventricular filling, stroke volume, and cardiac output may also be impaired by a compromise in ventricular *diastolic* function. Diastolic function can be evaluated by echocardiography, but this evaluation will also be influenced by heart rate, ventricular preload, and ventricular systolic function.

Afterload

Afterload is any impediment to ventricular ejection. It is the sum of all forces opposing ventricular emptying and is described as ventricular *wall stress*. If ventricular wall stress is increased, there will be a significant impediment to ventricular ejection and the ventricle will be required to generate higher pressure to eject the same amount of blood. If the higher pressure cannot be generated, the amount of blood ejected by the ventricle will fall. With any increase in afterload, oxygen consumption and the work of the ventricle increase. Even a normal afterload may be excessive when myocardial function is poor.

The major determinants of ventricular afterload or wall stress are: ventricular lumen radius, ventricular wall thickness (note that hypertrophy decreases afterload), and the ventricular intracavitary ejection pressure. In the absence of left ventricular outflow tract obstruction, left ventricular ejection pressure will be equal to aortic and systemic arterial pressure. In the absence of right ventricular outflow tract obstruction, right ventricular ejection pressure will be equal to pulmonary arterial pressure. Systemic and pulmonary artery pressures in turn are determined by blood flow and resistance. Therefore, *in the absence of ventricular outflow tract obstruction or significant alterations in ventricular size or wall thickness, ventricular afterload will be determined primarily by the impedance provided by the pulmonary and systemic arterial circulations.*

The ventricle of the infant or child can usually adapt to increases in ventricular afterload, provided that the increases are neither severe nor acute. For example, if the left ventricular muscle thickness increases and the diameter of the left ventricular chamber is reduced, wall stress (afterload) may be normalized. If, however, afterload increases severely or acutely, such as occurs with acute, reactive pulmonary vasoconstriction in response to severe alveolar hypoxia, cardiac output may fall.

Afterload cannot be measured in the clinical setting. Resistances in the pulmonary and systemic circulations can be *calculated* using a thermodilution pulmonary artery catheter. SVR may also be calculated using estimations of cardiac output obtained by Doppler calculations, and PVR may be estimated using echocardiography. It is important to note that, at best, SVR and PVR are *calculated* or *estimated* numbers, not measurements.

Oxygen Delivery, Cardiac Output, and Oxygen Consumption

Oxygen Delivery

The ultimate function of the heart and lungs is to deliver oxygenated blood to the tissues. Systemic oxygen delivery ($\dot{D}o_2$) is the volume of oxygen (in milliliters per minute) delivered to the tissues (Figure 5-6, *A,* and Box 5-3) in 1 minute. $\dot{D}o_2(I)$ is the volume of oxygen delivered to the tissues in 1 minute indexed to body surface area (BSA), provided in milliliters per minute per square meter. $\dot{D}o_2$ is the product of arterial oxygen content (the amount of oxygen in arterial blood in milliliters per deciliter), the cardiac *output* (in liters per minute), and the factor 10. $\dot{D}o_2(I)$ is the product of arterial oxygen content (in milliliters per deciliter), the cardiac *index* (in liters per minute per square meter), and the factor 10.

If either arterial oxygen content or cardiac output falls without a commensurate and compensatory increase in the other component, oxygen delivery will fall (Figure 5-6, *B to H,* and Box 5-4). For example, if arterial oxygen content falls (e.g., caused by a fall in hemoglobin concentration or its saturation), oxygen delivery can be maintained by a commensurate rise in cardiac output. If cardiac output falls, oxygen delivery will fall in direct correlation, since there is no way for arterial oxygen to increase commensurately.

If oxygen delivery falls significantly, the sympathetic nervous system attempts to redistribute

---

Box 5-3

Calculation of Arterial Oxygen Content and Oxygen Delivery

Arterial Oxygen Content

= O_2 bound to hemoglobin (Hgb) + Dissolved O_2

= (Hgb concentration in g/dl) $\times$ 1.36 ml O_2/g $\times$ Hgb saturation + 0.003 $\times$ Pao$_2$

Normal is 18-20 ml O_2/dl blood

Oxygen Delivery (Indexed to Body Surface Area)

= Arterial O_2 content $\times$ Cardiac index $\times$ 10

= Normal 18-10 ml O_2/dl blood $\times$ 3.0-4.5 L/min/m^2 BSA $\times$ 10

Normal in infants and children is approximately 750 ml/min/m^2 BSA

---

blood flow to vital organs. In addition, tissue oxygen extraction increases. If these compensatory mechanisms fail to maintain adequate blood flow or oxygen delivery, anaerobic metabolism will result in a lactic acidosis.

Oxygen Content

Oxygen content is the total amount of oxygen (in milliliters) carried in each deciliter of blood. Because oxygen is carried primarily in the form of oxyhemoglobin, the arterial oxygen content essentially is determined by the hemoglobin concentration and its saturation, although a small amount of oxygen is carried dissolved in the blood (see Box 5-3).

Arterial oxygen content will be decreased by anemia or a fall in the oxyhemoglobin saturation. For this reason, anemia should be avoided in the patient with compromised cardiorespiratory function, and transfusion therapy to a hemoglobin concentration of approximately 12 to 15 g/dl should be considered if anemia develops.

There is no "magic" hemoglobin concentration that is perfect for all patients. A low hemoglobin value decreases the oxygen-carrying capacity of the blood. An extremely high hemoglobin value is also undesirable because it increases blood viscosity and resistance to blood flow in small vessels. In the presence of sluggish systemic, pulmonary, or cerebral perfusion, the hemoglobin may be maintained at 10 to 11 g/dl, despite the fall in oxygen content that results.

The oxyhemoglobin saturation will fall in the presence of an intrapulmonary shunt or a right-to-left intracardiac shunt (cyanotic CHD). If an intra-

---

Box 5-4

Factors Affecting Oxygen Delivery

Factors Compromising Arterial Oxygen Content

Hemoglobin concentration (e.g., anemia)

Hemoglobin saturation (e.g., hypoxemia, caused by pulmonary disease or cyanotic heart disease)

Factors Compromising Cardiac Output

Inadequate cardiac preload (e.g., dehydration, hypovolemia)

Myocardial dysfunction (e.g., congenital heart disease, cardiomyopathy, drug toxicity, sepsis)

Inappropriate afterload (e.g., severe pulmonary or aortic stenosis, pulmonary hypertension)

Maldistribution of blood flow (e.g., sepsis)

Potential Consequences of Anemia or Hypoxemia on Oxygen Delivery

Compensated: Arterial oxygen content falls. If cardiac output increases commensurately, oxygen delivery can be maintained at normal or near-normal levels.

Not compensated: If arterial oxygen content falls and cardiac output fails to increase commensurately, oxygen delivery will fall.

Potential consequences of Low Cardiac Output on Oxygen Delivery

Compensated: No compensation is possible.

Not compensated: When cardiac output falls, oxygen delivery falls.

Text continued on p. 111

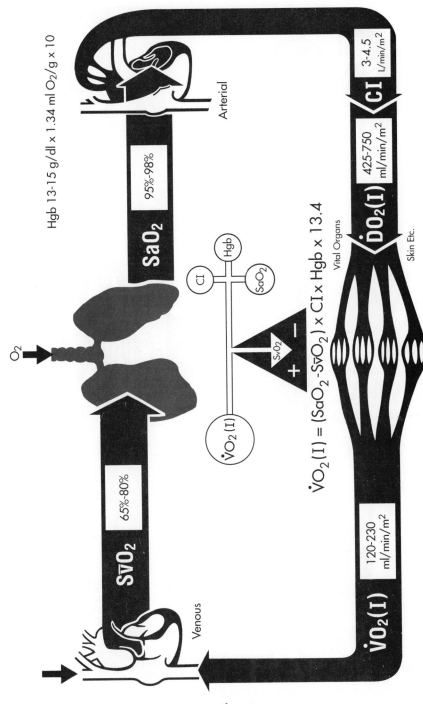

$$\dot{V}O_2(I) = (SaO_2 - S\bar{v}O_2) \times CI \times Hgb \times 13.4$$

Hgb 13-15 g/dl × 1.34 ml O_2/g × 10

Figure 5-6 Oxygen delivery and balance. **A,** Normal. (Courtesy Abbott Critical Care Laboratories, Mountain View, Calif.)

Continued

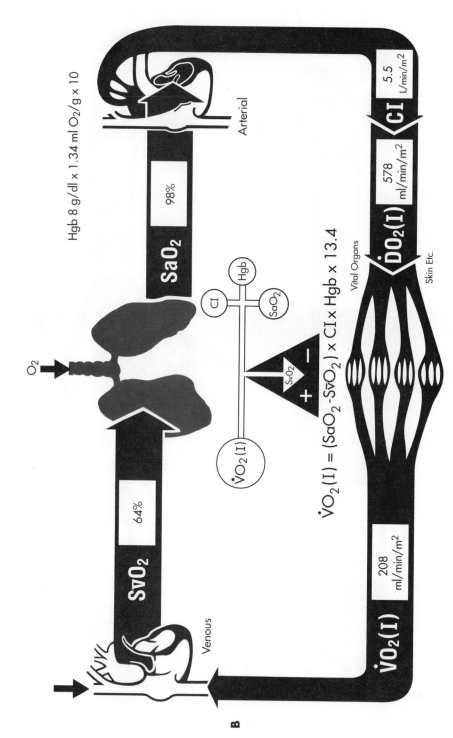

Hgb 8 g/dl × 1.34 ml O_2/g × 10

$$\dot{V}O_2(I) = (SaO_2 - \bar{S}\bar{v}O_2) \times CI \times Hgb \times 13.4$$

Figure 5-6, cont'd   Oxygen delivery and balance. **B**, Compensated anemia (increased cardiac output).   (Courtesy Abbott Critical Care Laboratories, Mountain View, Calif.)

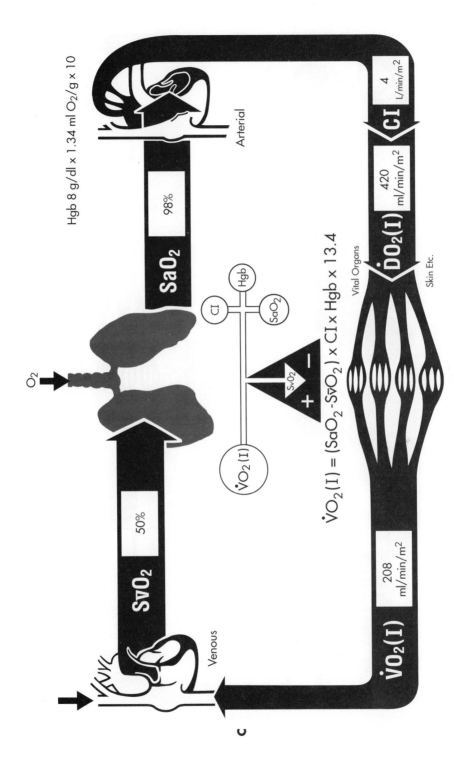

Hgb 8 g/dl × 1.34 ml O_2/g × 10

Figure 5-6, cont'd Oxygen delivery and balance. **C,** Uncompensated anemia (normal cardiac output).

$$\dot{V}O_2(I) = (SaO_2 - S\bar{v}O_2) \times CI \times Hgb \times 13.4$$

Continued

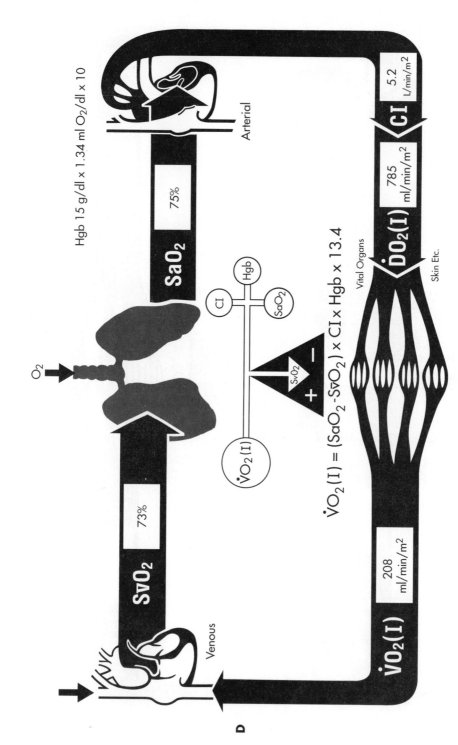

Figure 5-6, cont'd Oxygen delivery and balance. **D**, Compensated hypoxemia (increased cardiac output). (Courtesy Abbott Critical Care Laboratories, Mountain View, Calif.)

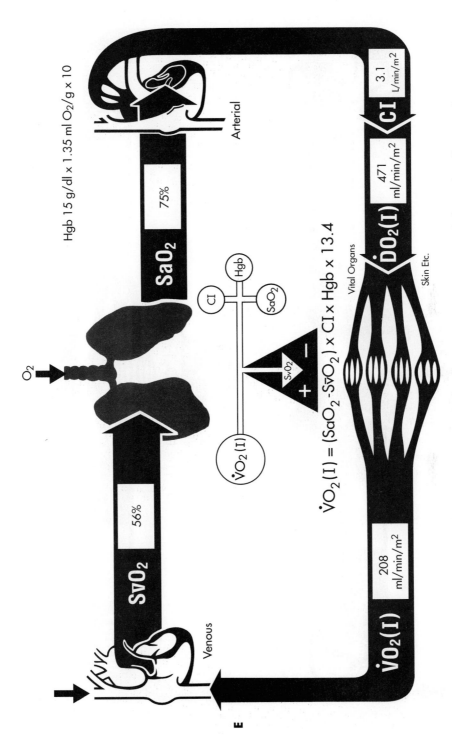

$$\dot{V}O_2(I) = (SaO_2 - S\bar{v}O_2) \times CI \times Hgb \times 13.4$$

Hgb 15 g/dl $\times$ 1.35 ml O_2/g $\times$ 10

Figure 5-6, cont'd   Oxygen delivery and balance. **E,** Uncompensated hypoxemia (normal cardiac output).

Continued

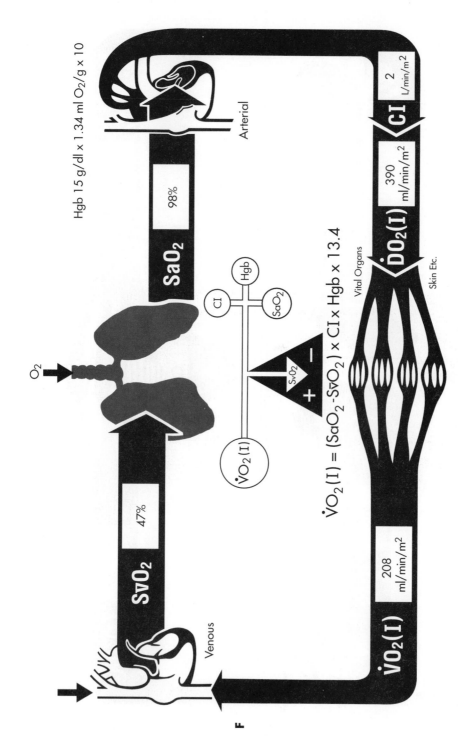

Figure 5-6, cont'd Oxygen delivery and balance. **F,** Shock with low cardiac output. (Courtesy Abbott Critical Care Laboratories, Mountain View, Calif.)

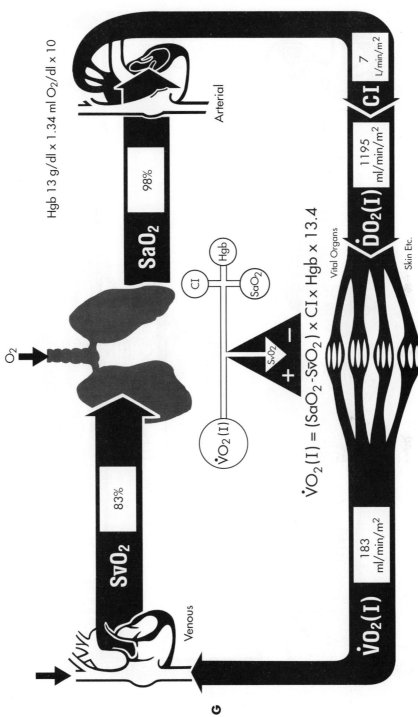

$Hgb\ 13\ g/dl \times 1.34\ ml\ O_2/dl \times 10$

$\dot{V}O_2(I) = (SaO_2 - S\bar{v}O_2) \times CI \times Hgb \times 13.4$

Figure 5-6, cont'd   Oxygen delivery and balance. **G,** Sepsis with low oxygen extraction (high oxygen delivery).

Continued

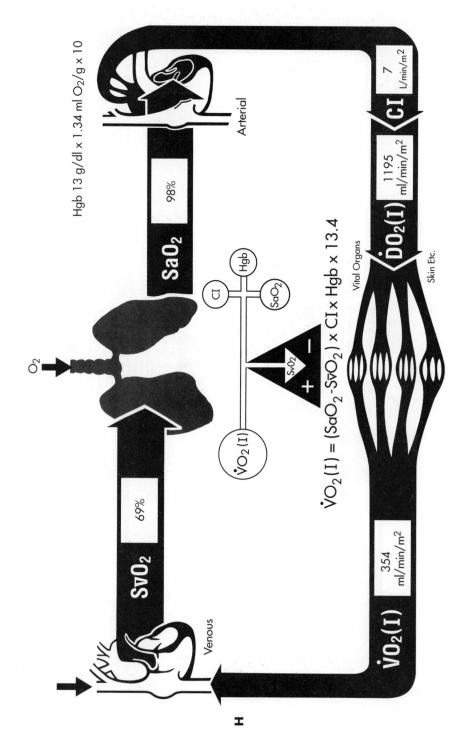

Hgb 13 g/dl × 1.34 ml O_2/g × 10

SaO_2 98%

SvO_2 69%

Arterial

Venous

O_2

CI   Hgb SaO_2

$\dot{V}O_2(I)$

SvO_2

+   −

$\dot{V}O_2(I) = (SaO_2 - SvO_2) \times CI \times Hgb \times 13.4$

Vital Organs

Skin Etc.

$\dot{D}O_2(I)$ 1195 ml/min/m²

CI   7 L/min/m²

$\dot{V}O_2(I)$ 354 ml/min/m²

H

Figure 5-6, cont'd   Oxygen delivery and balance. **H,** Sepsis with improved oxygen extraction (treated sepsis with high oxygen delivery). (Courtesy Abbott Critical Care Laboratories, Mountain View, Calif.)

pulmonary shunt is causing the hypoxemia, the oxyhemoglobin saturation and the arterial oxygen content can usually be increased through the administration of supplemental inspired oxygen. It may be necessary to provide mechanical ventilation with PEEP to maximize oxyhemoglobin saturation hypoxemia (see Chapter 6).

The child with cyanotic CHD is always hypoxemic. As a compensatory mechanism, these children develop polycythemia; thus their arterial oxygen content may be near normal despite oxyhemoglobin desaturation. These children cannot tolerate a fall in hemoglobin concentration such as may occur following a minor surgical procedure, since it will result in a significant fall in oxygen content. If possible, in these children the hemoglobin concentration should be maintained at approximately 15 to 18 g/dl. The child with cyanotic CHD and polycythemia cannot be allowed to become dehydrated and hemoconcentrated. Once the hemoglobin concentration exceeds 20 to 25 g/dl and the hematocrit exceeds 60% to 70%, the blood becomes too viscous, and the risk of thromboembolic complications is high. Pheresis (removal of whole blood and replacement of the volume with plasma, albumin, or normal saline) is generally recommended at this point.

Arterial oxygen content can be calculated by multiplying the hemoglobin concentration, 1.34 ml O_2/g Hb, and the arterial oxyhemoglobin saturation, and adding this number to 0.003 times the arterial oxygen tension. The arterial oxyhemoglobin saturation can be evaluated using arterial blood gas analysis, and it can be monitored noninvasively using pulse oximetry.

If the patient's hemoglobin concentration is stable (e.g., hemorrhage or other sources of blood loss have been ruled out and volume resuscitation is not producing a hemodilution), *trends* in the pulse oximeter readings of oxyhemoglobin saturation will reflect *trends* in the arterial oxygen content. However, the hemoglobin saturation does *not* equal the arterial oxygen tension, A few important numbers should be noted:

- At a normal pH, a hemoglobin saturation of 97% correlates with a PaO_2 of 95 mm Hg.
- At a normal pH, a hemoglobin saturation of 90% correlates with a PaO_2 of 60 mm Hg.

The arterial oxygen content can be estimated by multiplying the oximeter hemoglobin saturation by the known hemoglobin concentration and 13.66 ml O_2/dl. This estimate will not be accurate if the patient's hemoglobin concentration is varying widely (e.g., during hemorrhage or transfusion therapy). Pulse oximetry will *not* accurately reflect hemoglobin saturation in the presence of methemoglobinemia or carbon monoxide poisoning.

Cardiac Output

Cardiac output is the volume of blood ejected by the heart in 1 minute. *Cardiac output is the product of heart rate and stroke volume.* Cardiac output may be recorded in liters per minute or milliliters per minute, although in children it is often normalized to BSA and recorded as the cardiac index (in milliliters per minute per square meter). Normal cardiac index averages 3 to 4.5 ml/min/m^2 BSA (Table 5-5).

The child's cardiac output or index should be evaluated in light of the clinical condition to determine if the cardiac output/index is *adequate* or *inadequate* to maintain oxygen and substrate delivery and aerobic metabolism. Inadequate cardiac output/index results in tissue and organ ischemia, with the development of a metabolic acidosis. Cardiac output can be inadequate even if the calculated cardiac output/index is "normal" or "elevated" if it is maldistributed (e.g., sepsis) or if metabolic demands are high (e.g., malignant hyperthermia).

Cardiac output can be affected by factors that alter heart rate or stroke volume. If either factor decreases without a commensurate and compensatory increase in the other factor, cardiac output will fall. If the heart rate falls, stroke volume may not increase sufficiently; thus bradycardia often produces a fall in cardiac output. Tachycardia is an efficient method of increasing cardiac output during episodes of stress such as fever, pain, or cardiorespiratory failure. In fact, tachycardia *should* be present under these conditions. However, an extremely rapid heart rate (ventricular rate exceeding 180 to 200 beats/min) can produce a fall in cardiac output if ventricular filling time is severely compromised.

Stroke volume averages 1.5 ml/kg. Stroke volume will be influenced by heart rate and by ven-

Table 5-5
Normal Cardiac Output, Oxygen Delivery, and Oxygen Consumption in Children

Age (weight/BSA)	Cardiac Output (ml/min)*	Heart Rate	Normal Stroke Volume (ml)	Oxygen Delivery ($\dot{D}o_2$)†		Oxygen Consumption ($\dot{V}o_2$)	
				(ml/min)	(ml/min/m²)	(ml/min)	(ml/min/m²)
Newborn (3.2 kg/0.2 m²)	700-800	145	5	133-200	665-1000	36-54	180-270
6 mo (8 kg/0.42 m²)	1000-1600	120	10	200-280	476-667	70-100	167-238
1 yr (10 kg/0.5 m²)	1300-1500	115	13	260-300	520-600	85-110	170-220
2 yr (13 kg/0.59 m²)	1500-2000	115	18	300-400	508-678	91-123	154-208
4 yr (17 kg/0.71 m²)	2300-2375	105	27	460-475	648-669	110-150	155-211
5 yr (19 kg/0.77 m²)	2500-3000	95	31	500-600	649-779	115-170	149-221
8 yr (28 kg/0.96 m²)	3400-3600	83	42	680-720	708-750	150-208	156-200
10 yr (35 kg/1.1 m²)	3800-4000	75	50	760-800	690-727	190-250	122-227
15 yr (50 kg/1.4 m²)	5000-6000	70	85	1200	857	300-400	120-200

From Hazinski MF: Anatomic and physiologic differences between children and adults. In Terra DL, Morris F: *Essentials of pediatric intensive care,* St Louis, 1997, Quality Medical Publishers.

NOTE: Cardiac index $= \dfrac{\text{Cardiac output}}{\text{m}^2 \text{ BSA}}$

*Cardiac index for children: 3.0-4.5 L/min/m².
†Assuming a hemoglobin concentration of 15 g/dl normal arterial oxygen content.

tricular preload, contractility, and afterload. These factors have been described.

Clinical Assessment of Cardiac Output Cardiac output is evaluated clinically through assessment of systemic and organ perfusion and function. When cardiac output is inadequate to maintain sufficient oxygen delivery and aerobic metabolism, signs of poor systemic perfusion, metabolic acidosis, and organ system failure develop. These include tachycardia, mottled or pale color, decreased urine output, alteration in the quality of peripheral pulses, and metabolic (lactic) acidosis. The child's responsiveness and level of consciousness may be compromised.

If *hypovolemic* or *cardiogenic* shock is present, adrenergic compensatory mechanisms will attempt to redistribute blood flow, diverting it away from the skin, gut, and kidneys to maintain vital blood flow to the heart and brain. This diversion results in peripheral vasoconstriction with cooling of the extremities and delayed capillary refill, and diminished peripheral pulses.

When *distributive* shock is present, compensatory diversion of blood flow cannot occur; thus the skin may remain warm, and peripheral pulses may actually be bounding. However, shock is still present, because some tissue beds have excessive blood flow, whereas others have inadequate blood flow.

Cardiac output can be calculated using a pulmonary artery catheter with a thermistor probe. The cardiac output can be continuously evaluated if the pulmonary artery catheter contains an oximeter for continuous evaluation of pulmonary artery (mixed venous) oxyhemoglobin saturation. Cardiac output can also be estimated using Doppler studies of flow through the aorta.

Relationship of Mixed Venous Oxygen Saturation to Cardiac Output The mixed venous oxygen saturation is the saturation of blood in the pulmonary artery following mixing of systemic venous blood from the SVC, IVC, and coronary artery circulations. The mixed venous oxygen saturation can be continuously monitored through the use of a pulmonary artery catheter with a pulmonary thermistor. *If hemoglobin concentration and saturation and oxygen consumption/extraction are stable* (these assumptions often can *not* be made about the critically ill patient!), *the mixed venous oxygen saturation will vary directly with the cardiac output.*

Box 5-5

Fick Cardiac Output Calculation

$$\text{Fick cardiac output (L/min)} = \frac{\text{Oxygen consumption (ml/min)}^*}{\text{Arterial O}_2 \text{ content} - \text{Mixed venous O}_2 \text{ content (ml/L)}\dagger}$$

To Convert the Fick Cardiac Output to Cardiac Index

$$\text{Cardiac index (L/min/m}^2) = \frac{\text{Fick cardiac output (L/min)}}{\text{Body surface area (m}^2)}$$

Most Likely Sources of Error in Fick Cardiac Output Determination

Determination or estimation of oxygen consumption

If right atrial sample used for mixed venous sample, preferential sampling of SVC, IVC, or coronary sinus blood may yield erroneous results

Mathematical error

Intracardiac or great vessel shunt—a left-to-right shunt can raise the mixed venous oxygen saturation and result in falsely high cardiac output calculation

From Hazinski MF: *Nursing care of the critically ill child,* ed 2, St Louis, 1992, Mosby.
*Determination of oxygen consumption:
  Measurement by calorimeter
  Estimation: 5-8 ml/kg/min *OR* 150-160 ml/min/m² for child (and 120-130 ml/min/m² for the young neonate)
  Child must be in steady state
†Calculation of arterial and venous oxygen content:
  Arterial oxygen content = Cao$_2$ (in ml O$_2$ per L blood)
  Cao$_2$ = (Hgb concentration in g/dl) × 1.34 ml O$_2$/g × oxyhemoglobin saturation × 10
  Mixed venous oxygen content = C$\bar{v}$o$_2$ (in ml O$_2$ per L blood)
  C$\bar{v}$o$_2$ = (Hgb concentration in g/dl) × 1.34 ml O$_2$/g × oxyhemoglobin saturation × 10
  To add dissolved oxygen to these figures, multiply 0.003 × Pao$_2$ and add to arterial oxygen content and multiply 0.003 × P$\bar{v}$o$_2$ and add to mixed venous oxygen content

---

If cardiac output falls and hemoglobin concentration and saturation are unchanged, oxygen delivery falls. In the absence of any change in oxygen consumption/extraction, this will produce a fall in the amount of oxygen returning to the heart in the venous circulation, and the mixed venous oxygen saturation will fall.

If cardiac output rises and hemoglobin concentration and saturation are unchanged, oxygen delivery will rise. In the absence of any change in oxygen consumption/extraction, there will be more oxygen returning to the heart in the venous circulation, and the mixed venous oxygen saturation will rise.

In many critically ill patients the relationship between cardiac output and mixed venous oxygen saturation is not simple, because cardiac output rises as a compensatory response when anemia or hypoxemia develops, or oxygen extraction is affected by oxygen delivery and perfusion (see Figures 5-6, *B* to *H*).

Fick Calculation of Cardiac Output If a mixed venous (pulmonary venous) oxygen sample can be obtained, the cardiac output can also be calculated using the Fick equation (Box 5-5). This calculation requires determination of the oxygen consumption and simultaneous sampling of the arterial and mixed venous blood to determine the arterial and mixed venous oxygen contents (using the equation in Box 5-3). Substitution of a right atrial blood sample for the mixed venous blood sample may introduce significant error into the Fick calculation, since the right atrial blood sample may contain blood preferentially drawn from the coronary sinus (extremely low hemoglobin saturation and oxygen content), the IVC (highest hemoglobin saturation

---

Box 5-6

Factors Affecting Accuracy of Thermodilution Cardiac Output Calculation

Factors Causing Falsely High Cardiac Output Calculation

1. *Inappropriate calibration constant or programming of bedside computer or monitor.* The following errors can produce falsely high cardiac output calculations:
   a. Inaccurate catheter size and type
   b. Injectate volume *lower* than that programmed
   c. Injectate temperature *warmer* than that programmed (e.g., room temperature injectate used when computer is programmed for iced injections; iced temperature injections [<10° C]) should be used for 3-ml or 5-ml injections
2. *Inaccurately low injectate volume* (loss of injectate volume at a loose connection or from imprecise aspiration into injectate syringe)
3. *Prolonged or inconsistent injection time* (>2-4 sec)
4. *Large-volume infusion into pulmonary artery catheter sleeve or right atrium* (will warm injectate)
5. *Excessive dead space between injectate port and injectate syringe* (will result in loss of thermal indicator into tubing)

Factors Causing Falsely Low Cardiac Output Calculations

1. *Inappropriate calibration constant or programming of bedside computer or monitor.* The following errors can result in falsely low cardiac output calculations:
   a. Inaccurate catheter size and type
   b. Injectate volume *higher* than that programmed
   c. Injectate temperature *colder* than that programmed (e.g., iced injectate used when monitor is programmed for room temperature injections)
2. *Inaccurately high injectate volume*
3. *Prolonged or inconsistent injection (>2-4 sec)*

---

and oxygen content of all venous sources), or the SVC (lower hemoglobin saturation and oxygen content than the IVC).

If the child's cardiorespiratory function and metabolism are relatively stable, the oxygen consumption can be estimated at 5 to 8 ml/kg/min, or at 140 ml/min/m^2 for use in the Fick equation. However, since oxygen consumption can vary widely in the presence of cardiorespiratory failure, head injuries, burns, fever, or sepsis, estimations of oxygen consumption may introduce significant error in the Fick calculation (see Box 5-5).

Thermodilution Cardiac Output Calculation

The thermodilution cardiac output calculation is a form of indicator dilution. The indicator used is cool (room temperature or iced) fluid injected into the right atrium. This fluid mixes with the right ventricular output and is ejected into the pulmonary artery. A thermistor records the temperature change over time in the pulmonary artery, and a computer calculates the area under the time/temperature curve. *The cardiac output is inversely related to the area under the time/temperature curve.* If the temperature change is large and persists for a relatively long period of time, this means that right ventricular output must be small, since it does not succeed in warming the injectate. If the temperature change is small and does not persist, this means that right ventricular output is large, since it rapidly warms the cold injectate. *Error in the thermodilution calculation can be introduced by anything that artificially increases or decreases the magnitude of the temperature change in the pulmonary artery.* These factors are listed in Box 5-6. Therefore the injection technique must be standardized so that error is eliminated or standardized (Box 5-7).

Oxygen Consumption and Extraction

Oxygen consumption ($\dot{V}o_2$) is the volume of oxygen consumed by the tissues per minute. It is the product of the amount of oxygen extracted from each milliliter of blood and the cardiac output. Normally, oxygen consumption is approximately 25% of oxygen delivery; thus mild reductions in oxygen delivery can be tolerated.

Oxygen consumption is normally independent of oxygen delivery. Many conditions are characterized by an increase in tissue oxygen demand; pain,

Box 5-7

Thermodilution Cardiac Output Injection Technique

1. Verify appropriate tubing connections. Injection system should be joined directly to right atrial injection port without any excess tubing dead space between them.
2. Ensure that injectate fluid is iced appropriately if 3-ml or 5-ml injections are used.
3. Verify catheter tip position (pulmonary artery waveform should be visible).
4. Verify programming of bedside computer or monitor for:
   a. Patient size, weight, length, body surface area
   b. Catheter size and type
   c. Injectate volume
   d. Injectate temperature
5. Turn on computer or select cardiac output calculation function on monitor.
6. Turn injection syringe stopcock *closed* to patient and *open* to waste syringe. Aspirate appropriate injectate volume into injectate syringe and inject it beyond temperature probe into waste syringe.
7. When injectate temperature <10°-15° C is detected, prepare for cardiac output calculations.
8. Signal computer or monitor that injection will be performed; watch for "ready" indicator. If necessary, interrupt large-volume infusions into pulmonary artery catheter sheath or right atrium.

9. Turn injection syringe stopcock *open* to patient and right atrial injection port and *closed* to waste syringe.
10. When computer or monitor displays a "ready" indicator, quickly aspirate exactly 3-ml (or 5-ml) volume into injection syringe.
11. Depress "start" button on computer or monitor if necessary and inject the fluid into the proximal right atrial injection port within 2-4 sec *during patient end-expiration.*
12. Note cardiac output/index displayed and view and record graphic representation of the time/temperature curve.
13. Repeat steps 8 to 12 two more times. The first injection result is typically discarded, since it will typically yield a result higher than subsequent injections (most of the cold indicator has remained in the catheter to "prime" it). The second and third injections are averaged, provided that they do not differ by more than 10% and the graphic representation of the time/temperature curve is similar. If the second and third injections vary by more than 10%, perform a fourth injection.

Remember: Iced injectate should be used when injection volume of 3 ml or 5 ml is used. Small errors in technique or injectate volume or temperature can produce significant changes in cardiac output calculation.

---

burns, head injury, and, in neonates, cold stress all increase oxygen demand. These conditions should be avoided or promptly treated in the critical care unit, since the patient's ability to deliver oxygen may be limited. During times of increased oxygen demand, oxygen delivery often increases; for example, cardiac output and oxygen delivery increase during exercise.

If *oxygen delivery is reduced,* oxygen consumption will initially be maintained through an increase in tissue oxygen extraction. Capillary diffusion parameters for oxygen are altered by the opening of previously closed capillaries and reduction in the velocity of blood traversing the capillary bed, resulting in increased time available for oxygen diffusion. In addition, tissue acidosis can

alter the red blood cell (RBC) 2,3-diphosphoglycerate, shifting the oxyhemoglobin dissociation curve to the right, so that hemoglobin releases oxygen more readily to tissues.

If *oxygen delivery is significantly compromised,* oxygen consumption will ultimately fall. At this point, oxygen consumption becomes *supply dependent,* determined by the amount of oxygen delivered, rather than by the tissue need for oxygen. Tissue ischemia, anaerobic metabolism, and acidosis result. The treatment of this problem is to improve oxygen delivery to the point where consumption is no longer linked to delivery.

Some diseases are characterized by supply-dependent oxygen consumption. In these diseases, such as acute respiratory distress syndrome or sepsis, oxygen consumption is linearly related to oxygen demand. Any decrease in oxygen delivery (e.g., pulmonary edema compromises oxygenation, or cardiac output falls) results in a proportional decrease in oxygen consumption. Increasing oxygen delivery, through improvement in oxygenation and cardiac output, will result in an increase in oxygen consumption. Therapy for these diseases is directed at maximizing oxygen delivery and minimizing those factors that unnecessarily increase oxygen demand (e.g., fever, pain, work of breathing). There is no evidence, however, that increasing oxygen delivery to "super-normal" levels will improve outcome.

Clinical Determination of Oxygen Consumption

Oxygen consumption may be estimated from normative values: it normally averages 5 to 8 ml/kg/min, or 120 to 230 ml/min/m² BSA (see Table 5-5). However, a variety of clinical conditions, including severe respiratory or congestive heart failure or sepsis, can alter oxygen consumption dramatically, rendering normative estimates inaccurate.

Calculation of oxygen consumption requires determination of cardiac output and arterial and mixed venous oxygen saturations, as well as hemoglobin concentration. Oxygen consumption is then the product of cardiac output and the difference between arterial and venous oxygen content (Box 5-8).

A common variable used to evaluate the relationship between oxygen delivery and oxygen consumption is the *arteriovenous oxygen content difference* (a-v $\dot{D}o_2$), which is normally approximately 3 to 5 ml/dl (approximately 25% of the total oxygen delivery of 18 to 20 ml O_2/dl blood). Because oxygen consumption is maintained at a fairly constant level over a broad range of clinical conditions, cardiac output is usually inversely proportional to the a-v $\dot{D}o_2$. If cardiac output falls, blood flow to the tissues is decreased and the tissues must extract more oxygen from each milliliter of blood perfusing them. If cardiac output rises, blood flow to the tissues is increased and the tissues can extract a smaller amount of oxygen from each milliliter of blood perfusing them. Conditions such as sepsis can alter the

***

Box 5-8

Estimation of Oxygen Consumption

Oxygen consumption = Cardiac output × Arteriovenous oxygen content difference × 10
= CO × ([Arterial saturation − Mixed venous saturation] × [Hgb concentration × 1.36 ml/g]) × 10

Oxygen consumption in infants: 10-14 ml O_2/kg/min

Oxygen consumption in children: 5-8 ml O_2/kg/min

Oxygen consumption averages 150-160 ml/min/ m² body surface area.

From Hazinski MF: *Nursing care of the critically ill child,* ed 2, St Louis, 1992, Mosby.

***

relationship between the a-v $\dot{D}o_2$ and the cardiac output, since the diseases alter the ability of tissues to extract and utilize oxygen (see Figure 5-6, *F* to *H*).

Oxygen consumption may be measured through use of a calorimetry circuit. This circuit may be used in spontaneously breathing patients by joining it to a mouthpiece, face mask, or head hood. It may also be joined to a mechanical ventilator circuit. During calorimetry calculations, all expired air must be collected by the circuit; thus air leak around the mouthpiece, face mask, head hood, or endotracheal tube must be eliminated during the study.

Autonomic Nervous System

The autonomic nervous system controls visceral functions of the body, including blood pressure, cardiovascular function, gastrointestinal motility, and temperature. Autonomic centers are located in the hypothalamus, brain stem, and spinal cord. These centers receive signals from chemoreceptors and baroreceptors and transmit signals through two major systems—the sympathetic and parasympathetic nervous systems—to maintain homeostasis.

Sympathetic Nervous System

The sympathetic nervous system (SNS) influences are mediated through innervated fibers, as well as through circulating catecholamines. The SNS nerves originate in the spinal cord between the first thoracic and second lumbar vertebrae. They pass to a chain of sympathetic ganglia located adjacent to the spinal column and then synapse (connect) with other terminal neurons that transmit signals to effector organs such as the heart, adrenal medulla, and all arterioles in all systemic organs to control blood flow and pressure.

Cardiac SNS nerve fibers are distributed to all chambers of the heart, including branches near the SA node, and branches accompanying the coronary vessels to innervate the myocardium. Fibers to the adrenal medulla stimulate epinephrine and small amounts of norepinephrine secretion to produce systemic effects. The classical effects associated with SNS stimulation include the "fight or flight" response: tachycardia; increased cardiac contractility; redistribution of blood flow away from the gut and kidneys and flow toward the heart, brain and muscle; diaphoresis; and pupil dilation.

Adrenergic Neurotransmitters *Norepinephrine* is the SNS neurotransmitter released from the sympathetic nerves at the neuromuscular junction. It is synthesized by the sympathetic nerve fiber and stored in vesicles near the nerve membrane. When the nerve is depolarized, norepinephrine is released into the tissue to exert its effects for a few seconds and then is taken back up by nerve endings or inactivated by enzymes.

Epinephrine is released chiefly by the adrenal medulla following SNS stimulation. The epinephrine, along with a small amount of norepinephrine, is secreted into the bloodstream and mediates the stress response. The hemodynamic effects of the epinephrine are similar to but more significant than the local effects produced by the norepinephrine.

Adrenergic Receptor Types and Densities Neurotransmitters, as well as exogenous (administered) catecholamines, stimulate the effector organs by binding with receptors on the surfaces of cells. Adrenergic receptors are glycoproteins associated with the cell membrane, which have high specificity and biding affinity for certain catecholamines. Activation of the adrenergic receptor alters intracellular function. There are four major SNS receptor types that are described in clinical practice: beta-1 and beta-2 receptors, alpha receptors, and dopaminergic receptors. Each is described separately below.

When norepinephrine is secreted, it stimulates only beta-1 (innervated) receptors. A more diffuse stress response, involving activation of the adrenal medulla, will result in more diffuse stimulation of all adrenergic receptors. IV administration of exogenous adrenergic drugs can stimulate all adrenergic receptors, including beta-1, beta-2, alpha-adrenergic, and dopaminergic receptors, according to drug characteristics.

The density of adrenergic receptors on the cell surface is not static; it is affected by a variety of clinical conditions. *Down-regulation* of a receptor means that there is a decrease in the number of that type of receptor on the cell surface, making the cell less capable of responding to endogenous or exogenous catecholamine stimulation. Beta-adrenergic myocardial receptors are down-regulated in patients with severe congestive heart failure. Therefore the patient may be less responsive to endogenous or administered catecholamines. Alpha-adrenergic receptors are down-regulated in patients with sepsis; thus vasodilation occurs.

Up-regulation of a receptor means that there is an increase in the number of that type of receptor on the cell surface. When a receptor is up-regulated, the cell is more capable of being stimulated by circulating or administered catecholamines. For example, up-regulation of cardiac beta receptors occurs in patients with mild heart failure or hyperthyroidism.

Beta-Adrenergic Receptors All beta receptors produce intracellular effects through stimulation of adenyl cyclase, which causes formation of cAMP. The cAMP acts as an intracellular messenger, promoting phosphorylation of sarcolemmal proteins and increased opening of calcium channels in myocardial and vascular cell membranes. Phosphodiesterase then converts the cAMP to an inactive compound, ending the cAMP and sympathetic effects. *Phosphodiesterase inhibitors* (such as amrinone) prevent the inactivation of the cAMP; thus they prolong any adrenergic effects that are mediated by cAMP. Beta-adrenergic receptors can be subdivided into beta-1 and beta-2 subtypes.

The *beta-1* receptor is the predominant adrenergic receptor in the human heart. Since beta-1 receptors are innervated, they are activated preferentially by neuronally released norepinephrine. Beta-1 receptor activation results in an *increase in heart rate, AV conduction velocity, and ventricular contractility*. Beta-1 innervation to the newborn myocardium is incomplete during the first weeks of life; as a result, the newborn is less capable of demonstrating maximal heart rate and contractility response during endogenous catecholamine stimulation.

Beta-2 adrenergic receptors are not innervated; they are activated only by circulating catecholamines (predominantly epinephrine). Beta-2 receptor activation produces *peripheral vasodilation and bronchial dilation.*

Alpha-Adrenergic Receptors   Alpha-adrenergic receptors can be subdivided into alpha-1 and alpha-2 subtypes. Activation of alpha-1 receptors affects intracellular function by increasing transcellular calcium flux. Activation of alpha-2 receptors stimulates adenyl cyclase and increases intracellular production of cAMP. Endogenous epinephrine and norepinephrine stimulate both alpha-receptor cell types, whereas synthetic (administered) catecholamines may preferentially affect one or the other.

Alpha-adrenergic stimulation results in constriction of vascular and bronchial smooth muscle. This *produces peripheral vasoconstriction, including constriction of the skin, mesenteric (gut), and renal arteries*. Venoconstriction also occurs.

Dopaminergic Receptors   Dopamine is an endogenous catecholamine that is present in terminal sympathetic nerves as a precursor of norepinephrine. *Activation of dopaminergic receptors results in renal, coronary, mesenteric, and cerebral artery dilation*. Since renal arterial dilation produces an increase in glomerular filtration, urine output generally increases. Renal sodium excretion also increases.

Exogenous dopamine administration can decrease aldosterone secretion, inhibit secretion of thyroid-stimulating hormone, and reduce insulin secretion. These effects should be considered when dopamine is administered to critically ill patients.

Parasympathetic Nervous System

The parasympathetic nervous system is a totally innervated system that consists of a series of nerves arising from cell bodies located in the brain stem and the second through fourth sacral segments of the spinal cord. The parasympathetic nerve *fibers* arise from the third, seventh, ninth, and tenth cranial nerves, as well as from the sacral spinal cord. Approximately 75% of all parasympathetic nerve fibers are located in the vagus nerves.

Acetylcholine is the neurotransmitter of parasympathetic fibers; thus parasympathetic fibers are referred to as cholinergic fibers. Acetylcholine is synthesized in the nerve body and transmitted to vesicles at the end of the nerve fiber. Stimulation of the parasympathetic nerve results in the liberation of acetylcholine, which binds with a receptor site on the effector organ. Among other effects, acetylcholine reduces intracellular levels of cAMP and can accelerate its breakdown. This will reduce beta-adrenergic effects. In addition, acetylcholine release may inhibit norepinephrine release from sympathetic fibers, with the most significant effect at the SA node.

Parasympathetic nervous system effects are consistent with "rest and repair." Parasympathetic nervous system stimulation produces a decrease in heart rate, an increase in intestinal motility, and increased enzymatic secretion. Bladder contraction and sphincter relaxation also occur with cholinergic stimulation.

Common Clinical Conditions

Congestive Heart Failure

Etiology

Congestive heart failure (CHF) indicates a set of clinical signs and symptoms indicative of myocardial dysfunction and cardiac output inadequate to meet the metabolic demands of the body. CHF in children may be caused by increased workload (congenital heart disease [CHD] or severe anemia), impaired cardiac contractility, an alteration in the sequence or rate of cardiac contraction, or a combination of these factors. CHD is the most common cause of CHF during childhood, particularly during infancy. In fact, causative CHD is suggested by the timing of onset of the CHF (Box 5-9). Uncompli-

---

Box 5-9

Causes of Congestive Heart Failure Based on Onset of Symptoms

At Birth

Hypolastic left heart syndrome (HLHS)
Volume overload lesions (e.g., severe Tricuspid regurgitation [TR] or pulmonary regurgitation [PR], large systemic arteriovenous [AV] fistula)

First Week

Transposition of the great arteries
Pulmonary ductus arteriosus (PDA) in small premature infants
HLHS (with more favorable anatomy)
Total anomalous pulmonary venous connection (TAPVC), particularly those with pulmonary venous obstruction
Critical aortic stenosis (AS) or pulmonary stenosis (PS)
Others: systemic AV fistula

1-4 Weeks

Coarctation of the aorta (with associated anomalies)
Critical AS
Large left-to-right (L-R) shunt lesions (e.g., ventricular septal defect [VSD], PDA) in premature infants
All other lesions listed above

4-6 Weeks

Some L-R shunt lesions, such as endocardial cushion defect (ECD)

7 Weeks-4 Months

Large VSD
Large PDA
Others: anomalous left coronary artery from the pulmonary artery

Modified from Park MK: *The pediatric cardiology handbook*, ed 2, St Louis, 1997, Mosby.

---

cated septal defects typically do not produce signs of CHF until pulmonary vascular resistance (PVR) falls at approximately 6 weeks to 4 months of age. If signs of CHF appear before that time, a complicating defect (e.g., left heart or aortic obstruction) or condition is likely to be present.

Surgical correction of CHD often produces signs of CHF, since pressure, flow, and resistance relationships are often altered during the surgery. If the surgical procedure requires a ventriculotomy incision, conduit insertion, or significant ventricular muscle resection (e.g., correction of truncus arteriosus), postoperative CHF is almost inevitable.

CHF may be associated with low or high cardiac output. High-output CHF can be caused by a left-to-right shunt and high pulmonary blood flow, arteriovenous malformation, or severe anemia (with hemoglobin concentration <5 g/dl and hematocrit <15%; symptoms may appear at milder levels of anemia if structural heart disease is present).

Low-output CHF may be observed in children with severe left heart or aortic obstruction (such as critical aortic stenosis or hypoplastic left heart syndrome), cardiomyopathy, or tachyarrhythmias. This form of CHF is associated with poor left ventricular function, poor systemic perfusion, or both. Low-output CHF may also be observed in children with high right atrial pressures following correction of tricuspid atresia or single ventricle or with severe right ventricular failure (e.g., as a result of severe pulmonary stenosis or pulmonary hypertension or following surgery involving a right ventriculotomy cardiac incision).

Pathophysiology

The general pathophysiology of CHF is a cycle of inadequate cardiac output, which stimulates several compensatory mechanisms designed to maintain cardiac output and redistribute circulating blood volume so that oxygen delivery is maintained to the heart and brain. These responses, part of the adrenergic "fight or flight" response, may initially maintain adequate tissue perfusion. However, they cannot be sustained indefinitely.

Sympathetic Nervous System Compensation and Redistribution of Blood Volume   Heart rate and ventricular contractility increase. Alpha-adrenergic effects result in vasoconstriction and reduction of blood flow to the skin, gut, and kidneys, with diversion of blood flow toward the brain and heart. This vasoconstriction should improve coronary perfusion pressures and venous return to the heart.

Respiratory muscles normally use a tiny portion of cardiac output and oxygen consumption. During episodes of severe respiratory distress, such as severe CHF, the child's work of breathing increases and may cause redistribution of as much as 20% of cardiac output to respiratory muscles. This further compromises systemic perfusion.

Renal and Humeral Factors Affecting Blood Volume and Distribution   When vasoconstriction reduces renal blood flow, the renin-angiotensin-aldosterone mechanism is activated, producing renal sodium and water retention. This water retention should increase circulating blood volume, systemic venous return, and cardiac output. It may, however, worsen the clinical picture of children with CHF associated with severe anemia, since it further dilutes the hemoglobin and hematocrit.

Renin release catalyzes the production of angiotensin I, which is converted to angiotensin II, a potent vasoconstrictor. This vasoconstriction may contribute to improvement in venous return and organ blood flow.

Ventricular Dilation and Hypertrophy   Compensatory ventricular hypertrophy and dilation may enable maintenance of stroke volume and effective systemic perfusion despite myocardial dysfunction. Ventricular dilation may improve stroke volume by stretching ventricular fibers, but it also increases ventricular wall stress (afterload) and myocardial oxygen consumption and reduces myocardial efficiency.

Biochemical Alterations   Binding and release of calcium and calcium entry into the sarcolemma may be impaired. These changes cause abnormalities of excitation-contraction coupling and result in decreased ventricular contractility. Some patients with CHF develop enhanced calcium influx, prolonged calcium binding, and impaired calcium uptake. This may compromise relaxation (diastole), reducing ventricular filling and stroke volume (so-called "diastolic" failure).

Effects on Oxygen Delivery and Utilization   If cardiac output is compromised significantly or oxygen requirements increase, oxygen and nutrient flow to organs—including the heart—may be insufficient to meet metabolic demands. CHF can certainly compromise oxygen delivery. In addition, adrenergic stimulation and increased work of breathing will increase oxygen requirements. Because the young infant has limited oxygen reserves, this compromise in the oxygen supply-demand ratio may result in rapid deterioration.

When oxygen delivery is compromised, tissue oxygen extraction can increase. However, extreme compromise in oxygen delivery will result in tissue hypoxia.

Chronic or severe CHF may result in myocardial energy and substrate depletion, and further myocardial dysfunction and deterioration. Extreme or prolonged compromise in the oxygen and energy supply-demand ratio will result in the development of cardiogenic shock.

Clinical Presentation

Pediatric CHF is most commonly observed during infancy and immediately after cardiovascular surgery. Classic clinical presentations associated with CHF result from adrenergic stimulation and redistribution of blood flow and from the effects of systemic or pulmonary venous congestion. Occasionally children develop signs of poor systemic perfusion and low cardiac output; if these appear, shock is present.

Cardiomegaly is usually present on chest radiographs, and pulmonary interstitial edema is often observed. A third heart sound or summation gallop may result from rapid filling of a noncompliant ventricle. These extra heart sounds may be difficult to discern during tachycardia. An ECG and echocardiogram are helpful in establishing the cause of the CHF (e.g., CHD, myocarditis).

Adrenergic Stimulation   Adrenergic stimulation produces tachycardia and redistribution of blood flow, with reduction in skin, gut, and kidney blood flow. The increase in heart rate may initially help maintain cardiac output despite a reduction in stroke volume or ventricular function. However, tachycardia reduces ventricular diastolic filling time and left coronary artery perfusion time and increases myocardial oxygen consumption.

The child with CHF often has cool and pale or mottled extremities. Urine volume is typically <0.5 to 1 ml/kg/hr despite adequate fluid intake. Urine sodium concentration is typically low, and microscopic hematuria is often present. Diaphoresis is often observed, particularly over the head and neck.

Systemic Venous Congestion Right ventricular dysfunction is associated with an increase in right ventricular end-diastolic pressure (RVEDP), right atrial pressure, and central venous pressure (CVP), with systemic venous congestion. Portal venous hypertension develops, and the liver sinusoids become engorged with blood; thus the liver enlarges and becomes palpable below the right costal margin. This *hepatomegaly* is one of the earliest signs of CHF in infants and children. Another common sign of systemic venous congestion observed in children is *periorbital edema.*

Jugular venous distension is difficult to perceive in the short, fat neck of infants and children. Ascites is the accumulation of proteinaceous fluid that is lost from the surface of the liver, gut, or mesentery into the abdominal cavity as a result of portal venous hypertension. However, it is uncommon in children with CHF and, when present, indicates that the CVP is extremely high (e.g., following correction of tricuspid atresia or single ventricle). Ascites may also indicate the presence of complicating metabolic problems such as hypoalbuminemia or cirrhosis of the liver.

If ascites does develop, the child's abdominal girth will increase, the abdomen will appear full, and the skin will be taut and shiny. If two examiners are present, a fluid wave may be elicited, and areas of shifting dullness may be noted during percussion (see Chapter 10).

If the CVP is extremely high, a pleural effusion or chylothorax may develop. These complications will produce a decrease in the intensity or a change in pitch of the breath sounds over the involved hemithorax. Chest expansion will be decreased, and hypoxemia may be noted (see Chapter 7 for indicators of a pleural effusion on the chest radiograph).

Pulmonary Venous Congestion Signs of respiratory distress are often the first and most noticeable signs of CHF in the infant and young child. Left ventricular failure results in a rise in left ventricular end-diastolic pressure (LVEDP) and an increase in left atrial and pulmonary venous pressures. Once the pulmonary venous and capillary pressures reach 20 to 25 mm Hg, pulmonary edema develops. In fact, pulmonary edema can develop at lower pressures if pulmonary capillary permeability is increased (e.g., with associated sepsis). Children with CHF typically develop pulmonary *interstitial* edema. This edema is visible on chest radiographs but may not produce rales, since it is rapidly cleared by the lymphatics when tachypnea is present. The pulmonary edema reduces lung compliance and increases respiratory rate and effort. Wheezes may be heard, particularly if the child has a large left-to-right shunt, and lobar emphysema or atelectasis may result from cardiac compression of the larger airways.

The infant or child with CHF is tachypneic with increased work of breathing. Nasal flaring and intercostal, subcostal, sternal, supraclavicular, or suprasternal retractions may be observed. "Head bobbing" may be observed in infants, and older children may demonstrate use of accessory muscles of respiration, such as use of the scapular muscles and the sternocleidomastoid muscle. Grunting is a sign of increased respiratory effort. It represents the patient's attempt to generate positive end-expiratory pressure (PEEP) by expiring against a closed glottis. This grunting may help prevent atelectasis and maintain small airway patency, but it also indicates that support of ventilation may be required.

Fluid and Electrolyte Imbalance and Nutrition The child with CHF retains free water and usually gains weight. Free water retention also produces a dilutional fall in serum sodium and hemoglobin concentrations.

The infant with CHF may be poorly nourished. Tachypnea and increased respiratory effort interfere with feeding. Prolonged feeding times are often required, and the infant may suck poorly and take only a small amount of formula. The infant often sucks a lot of air during feedings, requiring frequent "burping," and possibly causing vomiting. Frequently the infant falls asleep during feeding, exhausted before taking adequate nourishment. The high energy requirements caused by the increased respiratory rate and effort and the poor caloric intake often lead to wasting, which is masked by the weight gain associated with fluid retention. Occasionally the young infant with CHF will develop hypoglycemia between feedings, because metabolic needs are high and glycogen stores are minimal.

Congestive Heart Failure Associated With Anemia
Clinical signs of anemia-induced CHF include lethargy, weakness, and fatigue. The child is often pale and may demonstrate a systolic flow murmur. Signs of high cardiac output failure, including tachycardia (with a gallop), pulmonary edema, and hepatosplenomegaly usually develop once the hematocrit is <15% and the hemoglobin <5 g/dl. In chronic anemia, intravascular volume is maintained but hemoglobin oxygen-carrying capacity is diminished. Anemia may complicate hemorrhagic shock if acute blood loss is replaced with crystalloids.

Anemia may be caused by increased RBC destruction or decreased RBC production. Elevated bilirubin, lactic dehydrogenase (LDH) and reticulocyte counts will be present if anemia is caused by accelerated RBC destruction, whereas the reticulocyte count will be inappropriately low if RBC production is compromised.

Management

Goals of care for the child with CHF:

- Improve cardiac function.
- Eliminate excess intravascular fluid.
- Support and maximize oxygen delivery.
- Minimize oxygen demands.
- Eliminate treatable causes of CHF.

Improve Cardiac Function: Digitalis Digitalis (typically administered as digoxin in children) is the most widely used drug in the treatment of CHF in children, although its use in premature neonates is controversial. The principal effect of digoxin in older children is an inotropic one; it improves the force and velocity of ventricular contraction. It also reduces excitability of myocardial cells; thus it slows the heart rate. In addition, pediatric digoxin therapy (particularly during infancy) also appears to relieve some symptoms of CHF through effects on oxygen consumption.

Therapeutic Effects Digoxin compromises the energy supply of the sodium-potassium pump;

thus intracellular sodium accumulates. Sodium then competes with calcium for sites on the sodium-calcium exchange mechanism. Ultimately, intracellular calcium levels rise, and myocardial contractility improves. Digoxin also encourages sarcolemmal sequestration of calcium.

Digoxin slows the heart rate by a variety of mechanisms. It lowers the resting membrane potential, increases parasympathetic activity, slows SA node firing, and increases AV node recovery time. It also reduces sensitivity to norepinephrine. Digoxin may contribute to ectopic rhythms, however.

Digoxin may produce variable effects in infants. Clinical improvement is often observed without ECG evidence of improved contractility. This effect is probably related to reduction in myocardial oxygen consumption and improved match between oxygen supply and demand. Digoxin administration to *premature* neonates remains controversial and is probably not useful because positive effects are difficult to document and the incidence of clinical toxicity is high.

Dose To initiate digoxin therapy, several loading or "digitalizing" doses are administered to achieve therapeutic serum levels; maintenance doses are then provided to replace estimated daily renal excretion of the drug (Table 5-6). The total oral digitalizing dose (TDD) is calculated and then modified according to patient condition. The IV TDD may be calculated at 67% of oral TDD, although this reduction is probably not justified by bioavailability studies.

The TDD is reduced or administered over a longer period of time in the presence of inflammatory cardiac diseases, chronic hypoxemia, or decreased renal tubular function. The dose is also reduced for postoperative patients. Hypokalemia, hypomagnesemia, and hypocalcemia should be corrected, since these conditions may predispose to digitalis toxicity. Several drugs, including quinidine, amiodarone, verapamil, diltiazem, spironolactone, and indomethacin, can all increase serum digoxin levels; thus the digoxin dose should be reduced in the presence of these drugs, and serum levels should be monitored.

Once the TDD is calculated, it is administered in two to four doses (or more, if indicated by the clinical condition) over 24 to 48 hours (or longer).

Table 5-6
Pediatric Digoxin Therapy and Treatment of Digitalis Overdose

Digitalization and Maintenance Doses

Age	Total Digitalization Dose (TDD)*	Maintenance Dose
Premature neonate	IV/PO†: 10-20 µg/kg (0.010-0.020 mg/kg)	5 µg/kg/day (0.005 mg/kg/day)
Full-term neonate	IV/PO†: 30-40 µg/kg (0.030-0.040 mg/kg)	5-10 µg/kg/day (0.005-0.010 mg/kg/day)
Infant <2 yr	IV/PO†: 35-50 µg/kg (0.035-0.050) mg/kg)	10-15 µg/kg/day (0.010-0.015 mg/kg/day)
Child >2 yr	IV/PO†: 25-50 µg/kg (0.025-0.050 mg/kg) (Maximum: 1.0-2.0 mg TDD)	5-10 µg/kg/day (0.005-0.010 mg/kg/day) (Maximum: 500 µg/day)
Child >20 kg	IV or PO: 1.0-2.0 mg	IV or PO: 0.125-0.250 mg/day

Treatment of Cardiac Glycoside Intoxication With Digoxin-Specific Fab Antibody Fragments (Digibind)
Two formulas may be utilized; the proper drug dose can then be estimated using the estimated amount of drug ingested or administered, or the serum concentration.
A. Fab dose based on serum concentration of digoxin:

$$\text{Body burden} = \frac{\text{Serum digoxin concentration (ng/ml)} \times 5.6 \times \text{weight (kg)}}{1000}$$

Fab dose = 40 Fab fragments per 0.6 mg digoxin in body

NOTE: This formula may be inaccurate following ingestion, because the serum concentration may be only transiently elevated.
B. Fab dose based on estimated dose of digoxin ingested:
Estimated 80% absorption of orally ingested digoxin

Fab dose = 40 mg Fab fragments per 0.6 mg digoxin in body

C. For example: If serum digoxin level is 5 ng/ml in 10-kg infant:

$$\text{Body burden} = \frac{(5 \text{ ng/ml}) \times 5.6 \times 10 \text{ kg}}{1000}$$

Body burden = .28 mg
Fab dose = 40 mg/0.6 mg digoxin body burden

$$= 40 \text{ mg} \times \left(\frac{.28}{0.6}\right)$$

$$= 40 \text{ mg} \times 0.46$$
Fab dose = 18.4 mg for the 10-kg child

Therefore, if serum digoxin level is 5-15 ng/ml, Fab dose will be 1.8-5.6 mg/kg

From Hazinski MF: *Nursing care of the critically ill child,* ed 2, St Louis, 1992, Mosby. Data from Banner W Jr, Orsmond GS: Cardiac glycoside intoxication. In Grossman M, Dieckmann RA, editors: *Pediatric emergency medicine: a clinician's reference,* Philadelphia, JB Lippincott; Friedman WF, George V: Management of congestive heart failure in infants and children, *Pediatr Cardiovasc Rounds* 1:1, 1984; and Talner NS: Heart failure. In Adams FH, Emmanouilides GC, Riemenschneider TA, editors: *Moss' heart disease in infants, children, and adolescents,* ed 4, Baltimore, 1989, Williams & Wilkins.
*TDD typically is administered in three divided doses: 50% of TDD, 25% of TDD 8 hours later, and the final 25% of TDD administered 8 hours after the second dose, assuming no arrhythmias are detected (often a rhythm strip is obtained before third dose). TDD is reduced if myocarditis, renal failure, or hypothyroidism is present, or if digoxin is administered concurrently with quinidine, verapamil, or amiodarone.
†Although some physicians adjust the IV digitalizing dose to total approximately 70% of oral digitalizing dose, bioavailability studies suggest that the same dose may be administered for oral and parenteral digitalization.

An ECG or cardiac rhythm strip is usually obtained before the final loading dose to rule out digoxin-related arrhythmias such as heart block or ectopy. If any arrhythmias are detected, the final dose is withheld and a physician notified. Digoxin is expected to prolong the PR interval.

The maintenance dose is calculated at approximately one eighth (12%) of the TDD, given twice a day, or one fourth (25%) of the TDD given daily. Note that *the appropriate dose of digoxin is the minimum dose necessary to produce therapeutic effects,* since there may be only a small difference between therapeutic and toxic levels. In the hospital the child's heart rate is checked before administration of digoxin. If bradycardia is detected, the dose is usually withheld until a cardiac rhythm strip or ECG is obtained to rule out second- or third-degree heart block or arrhythmias.

Digoxin Levels   A serum digoxin level may be monitored when digoxin therapy is initiated, when the child's response to therapy is suboptimal, when toxicity is suspected, or when the dose is changed. The level should be drawn at least 6 hours after the last dose:

- Therapeutic serum levels are 0.8 to 2.2 ng/ml.
- Toxic levels are generally >2 to 3.5 ng/ml.

Serum digoxin levels should be interpreted with caution. Hypokalemia, hypomagnesemia, and hypercalcemia can aggravate digoxin cardiotoxicity even in the presence of "normal" serum digoxin levels. Some children also exhibit endogenous digitalis-like substances that can influence serum digoxin levels. Finally, premature neonates can demonstrate toxic bradyarrhythmias even when serum digoxin levels are normal. For these reasons, *the presence of clinical symptoms compatible with digoxin toxicity should be interpreted more strongly than the serum digoxin level alone.*

Digoxin Toxicity   Arrhythmias, particularly bradycardia, represent the most common toxic effect of digoxin in children. Heart block, atrial and ventricular premature contractions, and ventricular fibrillation have also been reported. Virtually any new arrhythmias observed after initiation of digoxin therapy may be caused by digoxin toxicity.

Less specific signs of digoxin toxicity in infants and children include drowsiness and lethargy.

Anorexia, nausea, vomiting, and diarrhea may also be observed.

If digoxin toxicity is suspected, notify a physician and withhold further digoxin doses. Send a blood sample for analysis of the serum digoxin level.

- *Toxic serum digoxin levels in asymptomatic child:* Monitor closely for arrhythmias. If large amounts of digoxin have recently been ingested or administered orally, induced vomiting may enable recovery of a significant portion of the drug. Vomiting, however, should only be induced if the child is alert with an intact cough and gag reflex. If massive amounts of the drug have been ingested, temporary transvenous pacing wires should be inserted *before* the development of symptoms.
- *Symptomatic digoxin toxicity:* Support cardiovascular and pulmonary function (including treatment of arrhythmias), prevent further drug absorption, and enhance digoxin excretion. Bradycardia is treated with atropine or pacing. Phenytoin (2 to 5 mg/kg IV) is often effective in the treatment of digoxin-induced bradycardia because it increases the SA node conduction rate and reduces automaticity. Lidocaine does not affect atrial activity but may be effective in treatment of ventricular tachyarrhythmias. Propranolol or procainamide may also be used to treat ventricular arrhythmias. *Synchronized cardioversion should not be performed* for treatment of ventricular tachycardia caused by digoxin toxicity, since it may convert ventricular tachycardia to ventricular fibrillation or asystole.

The half-life of digoxin is normally approximately 30 to 40 hours; thus the serum digoxin level should be expected to fall within that time if renal function is normal and no additional digoxin is administered. If renal function is compromised, the digoxin level may remain elevated for several days.

- *Life-threatening toxicity:* Patients with malignant arrhythmias, hypotension, and poor systemic perfusion are treated with digoxin-specific Fab antibody fragments, which bind and inactivate the digoxin. The dose of Fab provided is determined by the total body exposure to digoxin, determined by the serum digoxin concentration (for dosage, see Table 5-6) or amount of digoxin ingested. Digoxin elixir is assumed to be completely absorbed, whereas absorption of tablets is calculated at 80%. Approximately 40 mg of purified digoxin-specific Fab will bind approximately 0.6 mg of digoxin.

Parent Instruction Parents must be taught how to administer the digoxin, including what to do if a dose is omitted or if the child vomits after a dose. It is helpful to provide a schedule of administration (e.g., 8 AM and 8 PM) and relate specific instructions to that schedule. For example, if a dose is forgotten but remembered by 12 noon or midnight, it can be administered, but it should be omitted if it is remembered after those times. If parents are unsure if a specific dose was administered, it should be omitted. If the child vomits after receiving the digoxin, the dose should probably not be repeated. If more than one dose is omitted or if vomiting continues, a physician should be notified.

Parents are usually not taught to check the child's pulse before digoxin administration. The parents will be more likely to detect digoxin toxicity if they monitor the child's overall condition, appetite, and responsiveness.

Remind the parents that digoxin overdose may cause serious arrhythmias or death. The drug should be stored out of reach of children.

Improve Cardiac Function: Inotropic Agents
Several inotropic agents may improve myocardial contractility during the treatment of CHF. Each of these drugs may produce peripheral vascular effects that must be considered during drug selection and administration. For further information see Shock, Medical and Nursing Management.

Improve Cardiac Function: Vasodilator Therapy
Although peripheral vasoconstriction and redistribution of blood volume may be positive compensatory mechanisms early in the course of CHF, persistent or severe vasoconstriction increases myocardial work and may further compromise myocardial function. Vasodilator therapy may improve myocardial function by altering both ventricular preload and afterload. Venodilation reduces cardiac preload, displacing blood into venous capacitance vessels. Arterial dilation reduces cardiac afterload. Ventricular compliance is improved through administration of vasodilators.

Beneficial effects of vasodilators must be balanced with potential detrimental effects of reduction in venous return and a possible fall in blood pressure. Hypovolemia should be treated *before* initiation of vasodilator therapy, and volume expanders should be readily available during therapy. The child's systemic perfusion should be monitored and supported as needed.

For further information about the dose, administration, and effects of vasodilators, see Shock, Management.

Reduce Intravascular Volume Limitation of fluid intake and improvement in systemic perfusion and blood distribution may increase renal perfusion sufficiently to prompt a diuresis. However, administration of diuretics is often required to eliminate excess intravascular fluid (see Table 5-7 for doses and effects).

Loop Diuretics The most common pediatric diuretics are *loop diuretics,* which block sodium and chloride reabsorption in the ascending limb of the loop of Henle. These drugs include furosemide, bumetanide, torsemide, and ethacrynic acid. Hyponatremia and hypochloremia may result from the increased sodium and chloride excretion produced by loop diuretics, and hypokalemia may result from enhanced potassium excretion in the distal nephron.

Hypochloremia or hypokalemia complicating diuretic therapy can produce a metabolic alkalosis, because renal hydrogen ion excretion will be increased in exchange for reabsorbed chloride and potassium. For every hydrogen ion excreted, a bicarbonate is resorbed by the kidneys, producing the hypochloremic, hypokalemic metabolic alkalosis. Treatment is replacement of potassium and chloride losses. If the metabolic alkalosis persists, administration of ammonium chloride (75 mg/kg/day in divided doses) or acetazolamide (Diamox, a carbonic anhydrase inhibitor, administered 5 mg/kg PO or IV once daily) may be indicated. Concurrent administration of a potassium-wasting and a potassium-sparing diuretic may enable effective

Table 5-7
Diuretic Therapy for Children

Drug (Trade Name)	Peak Effect	Action	Dosage	Effect on Serum (K⁺)
Acetazolamide (Diamox)	2 hr	Carbonic anhydrase inhibitor	5 mg/kg/24 hr per day or every other day	$\downarrow\downarrow$
Amiloride (Midamor)*	3-4 hr PO	Inhibits sodium reabsorption in distal convoluted tubule, cortical collecting tubule, and collecting duct	0.3-0.45 mg/kg/24 hr with hydrochlorazide	Potassium is "saved"
Bumetanide (Bumex)	15-30 min IV, 1-2 hr PO	Inhibits Na⁺ reabsorption in loop of Henle; also blocks Cl⁻ reabsorption	0.25-0.5 mg/dose q6-12h IV; 0.02-1.0 mg/dose PO	$\downarrow\downarrow$
Chlorothiazide (Diuril)	2-4 hr	Inhibits tubular reabsorption of Na⁺ in distal tubule and loop of Henle; also inhibits water reabsorption loop	20-40 mg/kg/day PO divided bid	$\downarrow\downarrow$
Ethacrynic acid (Edecrin)	5-10 min IV, 0.5-8 hr PO	Same as furosemide (see below)	0.5-2 mg/kg/IV dose; 2-3 mg/kg/PO dose	$\downarrow\downarrow\downarrow$
Furosemide (Lasix)	5-20 min IV, 1-2 hr PO	Inhibits NaCl transport in loop of Henle and proximal and distal tubules	1-2 mg/kg/IV dose; 1-4 mg/kg/PO dose	$\downarrow\downarrow\downarrow$
Hydrochlorothiazide (Esidrix, HydroDiuril, Oretic)	2-4 hr	Inhibits Na⁺ reabsorption in distal tubule and loop of Henle and inhibits water reabsorption in loop	2-3 mg/kg/day PO in 2 divided doses (q12h)	$\downarrow\downarrow$
Hydrochlorothiazide plus spironolactone (Aldactazide)	2-4 hr (prolonged effects)	Hydrochlorothiazide functions as above; spironolactone functions as aldosterone antagonist and inhibits exchange of Na⁺ for K⁺ in distal tubule	1-2 mg/kg/24 hr <6 mo: 2-3 mg/kg/24 hr	Approximately unchanged
Mannitol	5-10 min IV	Osmotic diuretic, inhibits tubular reabsorption of water and electrolytes	0.75 mg/kg/dose over 20-25 min	Approximately unchanged
Metolazone (Zaroxolyn)	2 hr (prolonged effects)	Inhibits Na⁺ reabsorption at cortical diluting site and in proximal convoluted tubule; results in approximately equal Na⁺ and Cl⁻ excretion; may increase K⁺ excretion (increased delivery of Na⁺ to distal tubule and Na⁺/K⁺ exchange)	0.2-2.5 mg/day PO given in divided doses (q12h)	$\downarrow\downarrow$
Spironolactone (Aldactone)	1-4 days (prolonged effects)	Aldosterone antagonist; inhibits exchange of Na⁺ for K⁺ in distal tubule; typically administered in combination with other diuretics	1.3-3.3 mg/kg/day PO	K⁺ is "saved"
Torsemide (Demadox)	10 min IV, 1 hr PO	Inhibits Na⁺/K⁺/Cl⁻ transport carrier system in loop of Henle	0.1-0.3 mg/kg/day IV or PO†	$\downarrow\downarrow$
Triamterene (Dyrenium)	2-4 hr PO	Increases urinary excretion of Na⁺, Cl⁻ and water; does not alter GFR	4-6 mg/kg/24 hr, divided bid, tid or qid	K⁺ is "saved"

*Limited use in children.
†Experience in children limited.

diuresis without the need for extremely high daily potassium supplementation.

Ototoxicity is a potential complication of loop diuretics. In addition, the child's renal function must be closely monitored. These drugs are usually held if the blood urea nitrogen (BUN) or serum creatinine level rises significantly.

Major loop diuretics include:

- *Furosemide (Lasix):* Most popular loop diuretic due to rapid onset of action following IV administration. It usually produces significant diuresis. It may also be administered intramuscularly (IM) or orally. It should not be administered to children who are allergic to sulfonamides. Potassium replacement is often required.
- *Bumetanide (Bumex):* Extremely potent at small doses. Its rapid onset of action and effects are similar to those of furosemide at the loop of Henle. It will increase the glomerular filtration rate through renal and peripheral vasodilation. Diuretic effects may be blunted by indomethacin, and patients with sulfonamide allergy may be sensitive to this drug.
- *Torsemide (Demadex):* Similar in action to furosemide. It inhibits the sodium, potassium, and chloride transport system in the ascending limb of the loop of Henle. This increases urinary excretion of sodium, chloride, and water but does not affect the glomerular filtration rate.
- *Ethacrynic acid (Edecrin):* Similar in action to furosemide with rapid onset. The frequency of gastrointestinal side effects and ototoxicity make this drug less popular for children.

Thiazide Diuretics   The *thiazide drugs* are a second classification of diuretics that act at the cortical diluting segment, preventing sodium chloride and water reabsorption. Potassium loss can result from use of these diuretics, but not to the degree seen with loop diuretics.

Thiazide diuretics include:

- *Chlorothiazide (Diuril):* Most popular of the pediatric thiazide diuretics. It is administered orally.

- *Hydrochlorothiazide (Hydrodiuril, Esidrix, Oretic):* Inhibits sodium reabsorption in the distal tubule and loop of Henle and inhibits water reabsorption in the cortical diluting segment of the ascending limb of the loop of Henle. It is administered orally.
- *Metolazone (Zaroxolyn or Diulo):* Has a relatively rapid (2-hour) onset of action, and it may be particularly useful when administered in combination with furosemide. Relatively small doses may be used.

Aldosterone Inhibitors   Aldosterone inhibitors prevent sodium reabsorption while inhibiting potassium and hydrogen ion loss. These drugs are known as "potassium sparing" because potassium loss is minimal. The onset of these drugs is gradual, and their action will not peak for several days; thus the need for dosage adjustment should be anticipated. Ensure that the child's fluid and electrolyte balance are well regulated before the child is sent home with these drugs.

Aldosterone inhibitors include:

- *Spironolactone (Aldactone):* May be administered once daily. It is most effective when administered in conjunction with another diuretic with a different renal site of action.
- *Hydrochlorothiazide and spironolactone (Aldactazide):* Can produce extremely effective diuresis on a chronic basis. The spironolactone component may prevent the development of hypokalemia or the need for significant potassium supplementation. Since the drug has a very gradual onset and is not maximally effective for several days after institution of therapy, it will likely be necessary to gradually taper administration of other short-acting diuretics.

Nursing Implications   When the child receives diuretics, the nurse must monitor the child's response to therapy and assess for evidence of complications. The time of diuretic administration should be noted on the flow sheet, as well as the timing and quantity of the child's diuretic response. It may be helpful to highlight the diuretic response with an asterisk or circle so that it is easily identified. *Notify a physician immediately if the child* *fails to respond to a previously effective diuretic dose, since this may indicate worsening of the heart failure, development of renal failure, or inadequate fluid intake.* Once the child is relatively stable, attempt to schedule diuretic doses so that diuresis occurs during waking hours and the child's sleep is not constantly interrupted.

Monitor fluid and electrolyte balance closely. If cardiovascular function is extremely unstable, the margin between excessive intravascular volume requiring diuresis and inadequate intravascular volume associated with hypovolemia and poor perfusion may be very narrow. Aggressive fluid restriction and diuresis may result in hemoconcentration, which is particularly undesirable in the child with cyanotic CHD.

When systemic perfusion is poor, absorption of oral diuretics may be compromised. Parenteral diuretics may be required until systemic and gastrointestinal perfusion improve.

Electrolyte balance, particularly serum potassium and chloride concentrations, must be closely monitored. Hypokalemia should be prevented, since it may precipitate arrhythmias and potentiate digoxin toxicity. Potassium-wasting diuretics should not be administered in the presence of hypokalemia or even a "low-normal" serum potassium level until a potassium supplement is administered. Conversely, potassium-sparing diuretics should not be administered in the presence of hyperkalemia. Maintain acid-base balance and prevent hypochloremic or hypokalemic metabolic alkalosis.

In preparation for discharge, instruct the parents regarding the purpose of the diuretics, technique of administration, flexibility (or lack of it) in the administration schedule, importance of electrolyte supplements, and signs of drug complications. Indications for contacting a physician or nurse should also be reviewed.

Fluid Therapy and Nutrition Accurate measurement and recording of the child's daily weight and intake and output is imperative. Weigh the child at the same time of day on the same scale so that weight gain or loss can be evaluated. Report significant weight changes (>50 g/24 hr in infants, >200 g/24 hr in young children, or >500 g/24 hr in older children and adolescents) to a physician.

Normal urine output should average 1 to 2 ml/kg/hr if fluid intake is adequate. All sources of fluid loss should be measured, when possible, and recorded. All sources of IV fluid, including fluid used to flush monitoring lines or dilute medications, should be totaled. Sources of fluid loss that cannot be measured should also be considered; these include excessive diuresis, evaporative losses during fever, and fluid losses associated with tachypnea.

Evaluate the child's intravascular *fluid balance:*

- *Signs of hypovolemia:* Decreased urine output, dry skin and mucous membranes, flat or sunken fontanelle in infants under 18 months of age, decreased or normal tearing, and weight loss. The central venous and pulmonary artery occlusion pressures are typically <5 to 8 mm Hg, although they may be higher in the face of ventricular dysfunction. If inadequate systemic perfusion is associated with these signs, fluid administration may be required.
- *Signs of hypervolemia:* Mucous membranes are moist, signs of systemic venous congestion (e.g., hepatomegaly, periorbital edema) and pulmonary venous congestion (e.g., tachypnea, increased respiratory effort) are observed, and the central venous and pulmonary artery occlusion pressures are typically >12 to 18 mm Hg. If an endotracheal tube is in place, the presence of pink frothy sputum indicates pulmonary edema. If these signs are present, additional diuresis and additional support of cardiovascular function (e.g., inotropic support or vasodilator therapy) may be required.

Adequate nutritional support is essential. The child's daily maintenance caloric requirement should be calculated (Table 5-8) and total caloric intake recorded to determine if adequate caloric intake is being provided. If the infant is breathing at a rate of more than 60 respirations/min, it may be very difficult for that infant to ingest sufficient calories orally. It may be necessary to provide formula by gavage until the CHF is resolved.

Restriction of fluid intake to less than maintenance fluid requirements is generally indicated during initial therapy for CHF (Table 5-9). To

Table 5-8
Calculation of Pediatric Daily Caloric Requirements

Age	Daily Requirements*
High-risk neonate	120-150 Calories/kg
Normal neonate	100-120 Calories/kg
1-2 yr	90-100 Calories/kg
2-6 yr	80-90 Calories/kg
7-9 yr	70-80 Calories/kg
10-12 yr	50-60 Calories/kg

From Hazinski MF: *Nursing care of the critically ill child,* ed 2, St Louis, 1992, Mosby.
*Ill children (with disease, surgery, fever, or pain) may require additional calories above the maintenance value, and comatose children may require fewer calories (because of lack of movement).

Table 5-9
Calculation of Pediatric Maintenance Fluid Requirements

Weight	Formula*
Body Weight Daily Maintenance Formula	
Neonate (<72 hr)	60-100 ml/kg
0-10 kg	100 ml/kg
11-20 kg	1000 ml for first 10 kg + 50 ml/kg for kg 11-20
21-30 kg	1500 ml for first 20 kg + 25 ml/kg for kg 21-30
Body Weight Hourly Maintenance Formula	
0-10 kg	4 ml/kg/hr
11-20 kg	40 ml/hr for first 10 kg + 2 ml/kg/hr for kg 11-20
21-30 kg	60 ml/hr for first 20 kg + 1 ml/kg/hr for kg 21-30

Body Surface Area Formula
1500 ml/m^2 body surface area/day

Insensible Water Losses
300 ml/m^2 body surface area

From Hazinski MF: *Nursing care of the critically ill child,* ed 2, St Louis, 1992, Mosby.
*The "maintenance" fluids calculated by these formulas must only be used as a starting point to determine the fluid requirements of an individual patient. Children with cardiac, pulmonary, or renal failure or increased intracranial pressure should generally receive *less* than these calculated "maintenance" fluids (if intravascular volume is adequate). The formula utilizing body weight generally results in a generous "maintenance" fluid total.

ensure adequate nutrition within restricted fluid allotment, the caloric content of all fluid ingested should be maximized. It may be necessary to supplement formula to increase the caloric content to 26 to 30 kcal/oz.

Restriction of sodium intake is occasionally necessary. Low-sodium formulas are available, but their increased cost should be considered when preparing the infant for discharge. For older children, foods high in sodium should be avoided, especially if the CHF is severe. If a low-sodium diet at home is absolutely necessary, a dietitian should be consulted and the child's primary caretaker included in the dietary planning.

Comfort Measures and Thermoregulation The child with CHF is usually most comfortable in the semi-Fowl's or sitting position. This enables abdominal contents to drop away from the diaphragm; thus work of breathing is reduced.

If CHF is severe, stimulation of the infant or young child should be minimized to prevent needless increases in oxygen demand. Uninterrupted periods of sleep are essential.

Premature infants and neonates have difficulty maintaining body temperature when the environmental temperature is low, because the young infant cannot shiver to generate heat. If the young infant is subjected to cold stress, the infant will break down brown fat to generate heat. This process, called "nonshivering thermogenesis" will result in an increase in oxygen consumption by 40% to 100%. To avoid this increase, attempt to maintain a neutral thermal environment for the neonate and prevent drafts near the infant's bed. Keep the infant warm during procedures and diagnostic studies.

Abdominal Compression When severe right ventricular failure or high right atrial pressure is present, pulmonary blood flow and cardiac output may be enhanced by the application of abdominal compression. Mast trousers may be used to compress the abdomen and lower extremities, enhancing venous return. Alternatively, an elastic wrap may be used to secure a 1- to 2-L ventilator reservoir bag to the abdomen, and an infant mechanical ventilator may be used to periodically inflate this reservoir bag. Such abdominal compression may enhance the forward flow of blood and improve cardiac output.

Transfusion Therapy to Treat Severe Anemia   If CHF is associated with severe anemia, transfusion is usually necessary. However, blood is administered carefully to avoid development of hypervolemia and cardiovascular decompensation.

Administer packed RBCs at a rate of 3 ml/kg/hr. Administer IV furosemide during the transfusion. If CHF is severe and cardiovascular function is precarious, transfusion may be administered through partial exchange, with simultaneous removal of RBC-poor blood and replacement with packed RBCs. Immune-mediated hemolytic anemia may not respond to transfusion therapy; steroid administration or splenectomy may be required (see Chapter 11).

Evaluation of Therapy   Cardiorespiratory function should improve with treatment of CHF. Improvement in response to therapy will be indicated by gradual return of heart rate to normal levels for age and level of activity, reduction in severity of systemic and pulmonary venous congestion, return of respiratory rate and effort to more appropriate levels, improvement in urine output, improvement in skin perfusion, and ability to tolerate oral feedings (for infants).

Signs and symptoms of worsening CHF include continued tachycardia, increased severity of peripheral vasoconstriction, decreased urine output (including potential failure to respond to diuretics), hepatomegaly, inability to feed in infants, and increased respiratory rate and effort. Development of a compromise in systemic perfusion, including deterioration in color, prolongation of capillary refill, deterioration in level of consciousness and responsiveness, and development of lactic acidosis are all signs of shock and require urgent therapy.

Shock

Etiology

Shock is a condition of sustained and progressive circulatory dysfunction that results in inadequate delivery of substrates to meet tissue metabolic demands. It may also be characterized by a compromise in tissue utilization of oxygen. Shock is most often the end result of:

- Severe dehydration
- Hemorrhage
- Progressive heart failure
- Sepsis

It may also complicate pulmonary failure (cor pulmonale), drug toxicity, electrolyte or acid-base imbalance, arrhythmias, or multiple organ failure.

Shock may be associated with normal, high, or low cardiac output and oxygen delivery, but in all forms of shock, the cardiac output is *inadequate* to sustain aerobic metabolism and organ function. If adequate oxygen delivery and distribution of blood flow are not restored and maintained, organ system failure and death can result. Unfortunately, organ system failure may progress despite restoration of effective perfusion, because cells have been primed to release inflammatory mediators that produce progressive cellular and organ damage.

Shock is typically classified according to etiologic mechanism, since this classification makes initial decisions regarding therapy obvious. The most common causes of shock are:

- *Hypovolemic shock:* Inadequate intravascular volume relative to the vascular space
  Causes: dehydration, hemorrhage, or plasma loss from the vascular space (e.g., capillary leak, or "third spacing" of fluid)
- *Cardiogenic shock:* Impaired myocardial function
  Causes: CHD (e.g., hypoplastic left heart syndrome, severe aortic stenosis), surgical correction of CHD, cardiomyopathy, myocarditis, or arrhythmias
- *Septic/distributive/neurogenic shock:* Maldistribution of blood flow resulting from alterations in vascular tone and permeability, causing some tissue beds to receive excessive blood flow while others receive inadequate blood flow
  Causes: infection, drug reaction (e.g., anaphylaxis, such as penicillin reaction), or spinal cord injury (Septic shock is a *clinical* rather than a culture or laboratory diagnosis—a causative organism is isolated in less than half of patients with clinical signs of sepsis.)

This classification system represents an over-simplification of shock, since most forms of shock include elements of all of these problems. For example, if hypovolemia is severe or sustained, myocardial dysfunction will develop; thus restoration of intravascular volume alone may be inadequate to restore effective perfusion. If cardiogenic shock is present, myocardial function must be supported, but intravascular volume is also manipulated to ensure adequate cardiac preload while avoiding excessive intravascular volume. Administration of vasodilators may be required to ensure adequate distribution of blood flow. In septic shock, vasodilation and capillary leak produce both a relative and an absolute hypovolemia, myocardial dysfunction reduces ejection fraction, and massive vasodilation produces maldistribution of blood flow, with the result that some tissue beds are inadequately perfused. Therefore treatment must include volume administration, support of myocardial function, and possible administration of vasopressors.

Shock refers to a condition of inadequate blood flow and oxygen delivery rather than inadequate blood pressure. Shock may be present in the child with normal, low, or high blood pressure, but the blood pressure may be used to further classify the shock:

- *Compensated shock:* Blood pressure is normal because compensatory mechanisms are redistributing blood flow or maintaining vascular tone.
- *Decompensated shock:* Blood pressure is low (hypotension). Decompensation has occurred; cardiopulmonary arrest may be imminent.

Pathophysiology

Hypovolemic and Cardiogenic Shock In the early stages of hypovolemic and cardiogenic shock, compensatory mechanisms are activated to redistribute blood flow and retain intravascular volume to maintain perfusion of the heart and brain. These compensatory mechanisms include the following:

- *Adrenergic response and redistribution of blood flow:* Tachycardia and peripheral vasoconstriction divert blood flow away from the skin; constriction of the splanchnic circula-

tion diverts blood flow away from the gut and kidneys.
- *Renal salt and water retention:* Renin-angiotensin-aldosterone system produces sodium, chloride, and water retention.
- *Baroreceptor activation:* Fall in mean arterial pressure or pulse pressure, or a reduction in stretch of the right and left atria increases baroreceptor firing, causing further adrenergic response.

Initially these compensatory mechanisms may restore intravascular volume and constrict the vascular space sufficiently so that blood pressure and essential blood flow and oxygen delivery are maintained. These compensatory mechanisms come at a price, however, and cannot continue indefinitely. Adrenergic vasoconstriction increases left ventricular afterload and myocardial oxygen consumption, and compromises gut and kidney blood flow. Extreme tachycardia may impair subendocardial blood flow and increase myocardial oxygen requirements. Eventually, tissue ischemia and organ failure will contribute to progressive deterioration in myocardial function, oxygen delivery, and possible multiple organ dysfunction syndrome. When cardiac output and oxygen delivery fall below critical levels, myocardial perfusion is so compromised that myocardial function deteriorates further, and progressive, irreversible shock can result.

In summary, if shock is severe or sustained, the compensatory mechanisms that were initially constructive and protective eventually become destructive and contribute to the development of profoundly inadequate (low) cardiac output and oxygen delivery and decompensated shock.

Septic/Distributive/Neurogenic Shock Septic or distributive shock represents a biochemical and a physiologic cascade, which occurs in response to an infectious organism, a hypoxic insult, or poisoning, and results in massive disruption of cardiovascular regulatory systems (Figure 5-7). Activation of exogenous toxins (such as endotoxin) and endogenous mediators (such as tumor necrosis factor or many of the interleukins) stimulates a diffuse inflammatory response consisting of vasodilation and capillary leak. In addition, sepsis upsets the balance between proinflammatory and antiinflammatory

Septic Cascade

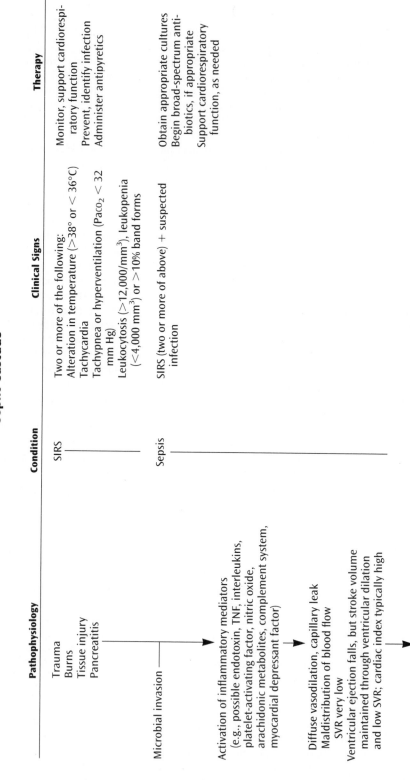

Pathophysiology	Condition	Clinical Signs	Therapy
Trauma Burns Tissue injury Pancreatitis	SIRS	Two or more of the following: Alteration in temperature ($>38°$ or $<36°C$) Tachycardia Tachypnea or hyperventilation ($Paco_2 < 32$ mm Hg) Leukocytosis ($>12,000/mm^3$), leukopenia ($<4,000$ mm^3) or $>10\%$ band forms	Monitor, support cardiorespiratory function Prevent, identify infection Administer antipyretics
Microbial invasion	Sepsis	SIRS (two or more of above) + suspected infection	Obtain appropriate cultures Begin broad-spectrum antibiotics, if appropriate Support cardiorespiratory function, as needed

Activation of inflammatory mediators (e.g., possible endotoxin, TNF, interleukins, platelet-activating factor, nitric oxide, arachidonic metabolites, complement system, myocardial depressant factor)

Diffuse vasodilation, capillary leak
Maldistribution of blood flow
SVR very low
Ventricular ejection falls, but stroke volume maintained through ventricular dilation and low SVR; cardiac index typically high

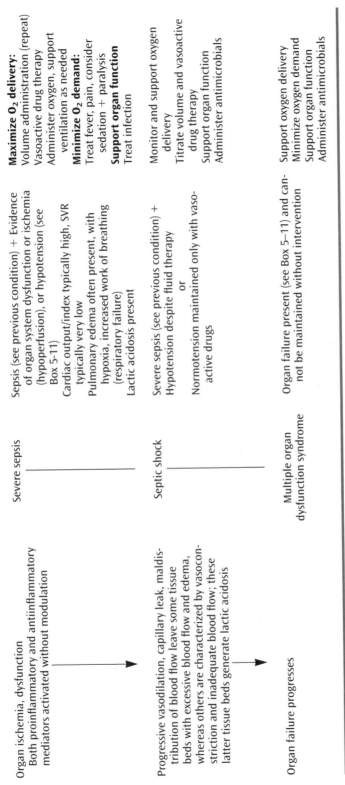

Severe sepsis

Organ ischemia, dysfunction
Both proinflammatory and antiinflammatory mediators activated without modulation

Sepsis (see previous condition) + Evidence of organ system dysfunction or ischemia (hypoperfusion), or hypotension (see Box 5-11)
Cardiac output/index typically high, SVR typically very low
Pulmonary edema often present, with hypoxia, increased work of breathing (respiratory failure)
Lactic acidosis present

Maximize O₂ delivery:
Volume administration (repeat)
Vasoactive drug therapy
Administer oxygen, support ventilation as needed
Minimize O₂ demand:
Treat fever, pain, consider sedation + paralysis
Support organ function
Treat infection

Septic shock

Progressive vasodilation, capillary leak, maldistribution of blood flow leave some tissue beds with excessive blood flow and edema, whereas others are characterized by vasoconstriction and inadequate blood flow; these latter tissue beds generate lactic acidosis

Severe sepsis (see previous condition) +
Hypotension despite fluid therapy
or
Normotension maintained only with vasoactive drugs

Monitor and support oxygen delivery
Titrate volume and vasoactive drug therapy
Support organ function
Administer antimicrobials

Multiple organ dysfunction syndrome

Organ failure progresses

Organ failure present (see Box 5-11) and cannot be maintained without intervention

Support oxygen delivery
Minimize oxygen demand
Support organ function
Administer antimicrobials

SIRS, Systemic inflammatory response; *TNF,* tumor necrosis factor; *SVR,* systemic vascular resistance.

Figure 5-7 The septic cascade. Sepsis and its complications, including septic shock, represent a biochemical and physiologic cascade that may evolve over days or be telescoped into a few hours. The clinical signs result from an imbalance between proinflammatory and antiinflammatory forces, which results in maldistribution of blood flow and the development of areas of ischemia, despite high cardiac output and oxygen delivery. Treatment focuses on maximization of oxygen delivery and minimization of oxygen demand.

systems, so that massive vasodilation and capillary leak are present in some tissues and intense vasoconstriction is present in others (Box 5-10 and Table 5-10). Systemic vascular resistance (SVR) is typically very low. The net result is a maldistribution of blood flow; some tissue beds receive excessive blood flow, whereas others are not perfused at all.

Although septic shock is associated with high cardiac output, myocardial dysfunction is present. Circulating myocardial depressant factors result in a fall in ventricular ejection fraction. Stroke volume is maintained in survivors of septic shock through compensatory ventricular dilation; this maintains stroke volume and contributes to high cardiac output despite the fall in ejection fraction. This dilation will only be effective, however, if intravascular volume is maintained through administration of IV fluids.

Cardiac output/index and oxygen delivery are typically much higher than normal during the first 24 hours after the onset of signs of septic shock.

Box 5-10

Microcirculatory Changes in Sepsis and Septic Shock

The microcirculation changes dramatically in sepsis; vasodilation, hypoperfusion, and diversion of blood flow to bypass some capillary beds contributes to progressive tissue and organ ischemia and dysfunction.

1. Vasodilation causes peripheral pooling of blood and compromised flow to some essential tissues.
2. Disseminated intravascular coagulation (DIC) may develop and is associated with deposition of fibrin and microthrombosis in some tissues.
3. Red blood cells, normally very deformable, become rigid; thus they cannot easily pass through small vessels. This leads to stagnation and sludging of blood in small vessels and compromise of oxygen delivery and metabolic support to tissues distal to the obstruction.
4. Microvascular permeability increases, resulting in fluid loss from the vascular space into the interstitial space, and edema formation.
5. Intravascular pooling occurs in some tissue beds, such as the intestinal bed.
6. Congestion and hemorrhage occurs in some tissue beds. Bacteria may become trapped in areas of circulatory compromise; thus they multiply unchecked.
7. Microvascular blood flow and vascular resistance are altered.
8. Adrenergic responses are abnormal.
9. Blood viscosity is altered. White blood cell aggregation plus red blood cell rigidity contribute to obstruction of small vessels.

10. Organ blood flow is redistributed. Hypoperfusion of the gut and some other tissue beds occurs very early in sepsis/septic shock. Early in sepsis, cardiac output/index often increases by 20% or more, but small intestine blood flow may decrease nearly 30%.
11. Arteriovenous shunts open. The blood that shunts past tissue beds returns to the systemic venous circulation well saturated with oxygen. This is why the mixed venous oxygen saturation is high and calculated oxygen extraction ratio is low.
12. Endothelium modulates vascular tone and contributes to the development of vasodilation. It also controls local blood flow and allows leakage of fluids and proteins and extravasation of white blood cells into the tissue.
13. Platelet activating factor contributes to aggregation of platelets in some small vessels, leading to obstruction.
14. Cardiopulmonary pathology includes myocardial mitochondrial edema and accumulation of intramyocardial granules. Ventricular ejection fraction decreases, and ventricular dilation develops in an attempt to maintain stroke volume in the face of a fall in ejection fraction (see Figure 5-10).

Modified from Hinshaw LB: Sepsis/septic shock: participation of the microcirculation; an abbreviated review, *Crit Care Med* 24:1072-1078, 1996.

Table 5-10
Mediators of the Septic Cascade

Type	Source	Main Functions
Interleukins (IL)		
IL-1 (α and β)	Predominantly macrophages	↑ Immune response; inflammatory mediator; activates T cells; activates phagocytes; ↑ prostaglandin production; induces a fever
IL-2 (T-cell growth factor [TCGF])	Predominantly helper T lymphocytes; natural killer (NK) cells	↑ T lymphocytes and NK cells; ↑ growth and ↑ T cells
IL-3 (multiple colony-stimulation factor [CSF])	T lymphocytes, mast cells, NK cells	Hematopoietic growth factor for immature hematopoietic precursor cells, ↑ NK cells
IL-4 (B cell growth factor [BCGF])	T lymphocytes, mast cell	Growth factor for T cells, activated B cells, and mast cells; macrophage-activating factor, ↑ IgE reactions
IL-5	T lymphocytes, macrophages	↑ Growth and proliferation of activated B cells, ↑ eosinophils, ↑ T-cell production
IL-6	Monocytes, T and B lymphocytes, fibroblasts, endothelial cells	B cell stimulatory and differentiation factor; ↑ hematopoiesis, ↑ inflammatory response, fever
IL-7	Bone marrow, thymus	↑ Lymphoid cells
IL-8 (monocyte-derived neutrophil chemotactic factor)	Macrophages, monocytes, endothelial cells	Triggers chemotactic activity of neutrophils and lymphocytes
IL-9	Helper T cells	T-cell and mast cell growth factor; maturation of erythroid progenitors
IL-10	Helper T cells	↓ Proliferation of helper T cells; ↑ cytotoxic T cell differentiation; induces major histocompatibility complex antigen expression, ↓ cytokines
IL-11	Fibroblasts	↑ Monocyte and B-cell function, ↓ some inflammatory cytokines
IL-12	Macrophages	↑ Helper T cells and production of other lymphocytes and cytokines
IL-13	Activated T cells	↑ Gene expression in nerve and intestinal cells, ↑ osteoclasts, ↑ progenitor cells in bone marrow
IL-14	T cells	B-cell growth factor
IL-15	Macrophages	Activity identical to that of IL-2
IL-16	CD8+ T cells	Chemotactic factor and growth factor for CD4+ T cells, chemotactic for eosinophils
IL-17	Helper T cells	↑ IL-6 and IL-8
Interferon (IFN)		
IFN-α	T and B lymphocytes, macrophages	Provides antiviral protection; ↓ B-cell proliferation; ↓ IL-8, ↓ tumor growth, ↑ NK cell
IFN-β	Fibroblasts, macrophages, epithelial cells	Provides antiviral protection; ↑ IL-6, ↓ IL-8
IFN-γ	T lymphocytes, NK cells	Activates macrophages, ↑ B-cell differentiation and NK cell activity, ↓ tumor growth

From Rote NS: Inflammation. In McCance, KL, Heuther SE, editors: *Pathophysiology: the biological basis for disease in adults and children,* ed 3, St Louis, 1998, Mosby.
↑, Increased; ↓, decreased.

Continued

Table 5-10
Mediators of the Septic Cascade—cont'd

Type	Source	Main Functions
Tumor Necrosis Factor (TNF)		
TNF-α	Macrophages, lymphocytes, fibroblasts, endothelial cells	$\uparrow$ Cytokines, $\uparrow$ inflammatory and immune responses
TNF-β	T cells	Cytotoxic to tumor cells, $\uparrow$ phagocytosis by macrophage and neutrophil, $\uparrow$ macrophages, $\uparrow$ B-cell proliferation
Colony-Stimulating Factors (CSF)		
G-CSF	Monocytes, fibroblasts	Myeloid growth factor
GM-CSF	T cells, fibroblasts, monocytes, endothelial cells	Myelocytic growth factor
M-CSF	Monocytes, lymphocytes, fibroblasts, endothelial and epithelial cells	Macrophage growth factor
Transforming Growth Factor (TGF-β)		
	Lymphocytes, macrophages, platelets, bone	Chemotactic for macrophages, $\uparrow$ IL-1 production; stimulates fibroblasts for wound healing; inhibits immune response; potentially inhibits mitotic division in other cells

From Rote NS: Inflammation. In McCance, KL, Heuther SE, editors: *Pathophysiology: the biological basis for disease in adults and children*, ed 3, St Louis, 1998, Mosby.
$\uparrow$, Increased; $\downarrow$, decreased.

The high cardiac output/index and high oxygen delivery are supported by the tachycardia, normal or near-normal stroke volume, and very low SVR. Survivors of septic shock typically demonstrate a return to normal heart rate, cardiac output/index, oxygen delivery, and SVR within 24 hours after the onset of shock.

Sepsis may result from community-acquired or nosocomial infections. Examples of community-acquired infections in children include meningococcal sepsis. In children nosocomial infections are a common complication of critical care. The risk of nosocomial infection increases with increased length of stay, invasive devices, and wounds.

The most common sites of nosocomial infections are as follows: lower respiratory tract (35%), sepsis (21%), genitourinary tract (21%), gastrointestinal tract (9%), skin/soft tissues and wound (7%), and pneumonia (5%). Gram-negative bacteria are responsible for approximately half of all nosocomial infections in children, whereas gram-positive bacteria account for approximately 27% and fungi account for approximately 9% of nosocomial infections in children (Singh-Naz, 1996). The remaining nosocomial infections are caused by viral or rickettsial infection.

Sepsis may be caused by an infection, or it may be initiated by translocation of gram-negative bacteria or endotoxin across the gastrointestinal mucosal membrane. This membrane is normally impermeable, but many conditions associated with critical care, including infection, acute respiratory distress syndrome, total parenteral nutrition (and any condition in which the gut is not used), shock, and hypotension have all been linked with increased gastrointestinal permeability and translocation of gram-negative bacteria or endotoxin in the gut. Such translocation can contribute to the development of signs of gram-negative sepsis, even in the absence of any infection.

Neurogenic shock represents loss of vasomotor tone, with resultant massive vasodilation. This effectively increases the vascular space and produces a relative hypovolemia, as well as a hypotension.

Clinical Presentation

Clinical signs of all forms of shock in children include nonspecific signs of distress or deterioration (child "looks bad"), plus signs of inadequate tissue perfusion. These latter signs are usually associated with signs of organ dysfunction. Classic signs of shock include:

- "Looks bad"—deterioration in color (skin appears mottled, or nailbeds are pale), irritability or a decrease in responsiveness, reduced level of activity. *A decreased response to painful stimulus is abnormal in the child of any age and often indicates severe cardiorespiratory or neurologic compromise.*
- Signs of inadequate tissue perfusion and organ function. Lactic acidosis and oliguria (urine output <1 ml/kg/hr despite an adequate fluid intake) both indicate inadequate tissue perfusion. Potential signs of organ failure are listed in Box 5-11.
- Diminished peripheral pulses and delayed capillary refill despite a warm ambient temperature.
- Hypotension is typically only a *late* sign of decompensated shock in children.

Vital Signs Vital signs should be evaluated in light of the age and clinical condition (see inside front cover). If the child has been seriously ill or injured, signs of distress may be present before shock develops, and vital signs may or may not change when signs of shock appear. Tachycardia should be present as a nonspecific sign of distress and adrenergic response. *Absence of tachycardia in a child with poor perfusion is an ominous sign and may indicate that cardiorespiratory arrest is imminent.*

Tachypnea is a nonspecific sign of distress if the child is breathing spontaneously. If shock is associated with myocardial failure or increased capillary permeability and pulmonary edema, respiratory effort or ventilatory support requirements will increase. Pink frothy sputum may be suctioned from the endotracheal tube if pulmonary edema is present.

Blood pressure is often normal in children with shock. In fact, the presence of hypotension indicates that *decompensated* shock is present. *Hypotension is present in the child beyond a year of age if the systolic blood pressure is less than 70 mm Hg plus two times the age in years.*

Automated oscillometric blood pressure measurement devices may overestimate blood pressure in the presence of severe hypotension in children or may fail to reflect a rapidly falling or very low blood pressure. Auscultated blood pressures may be difficult to obtain when shock is present because the Korotkoff sounds may be muffled or impossible to hear. Intraarterial blood pressure monitoring is the most accurate method of monitoring blood pressure in the unstable patient, provided that the transducer is leveled, zeroed, and calibrated appropriately and the catheter and tubing system provide an uninterrupted fluid column between the patient and the transducer.

Core body temperature may be normal, low, or high in the child with shock. If shock is associated with low cardiac output and significant peripheral vasoconstriction, extremities may be cold but core body temperature may be high (≥38° C), since heat cannot be eliminated through the skin. The child with sepsis caused by infection may demonstrate fever, and the infant with sepsis may demonstrate fever (>38° C) or hypothermia (<36° C). Functioning neutrophils must be present for fever and signs of inflammation to develop; thus fever and other classical signs of infection (such as redness or pus over a wound) may be absent in the neutropenic child.

Skin Perfusion Skin blood flow, color, and temperature are often altered in shock. When hypovolemic or cardiogenic shock is present, the skin is typically cool, and extremities will cool in a peripheral to proximal direction. Capillary refill time is sluggish despite a warm ambient temperature, and the skin may become pale, mottled, or gray. Peripheral pulses may be diminished in intensity. By comparison, excessive skin blood flow may be present in children with septic/distributive or neurogenic shock. The skin may have a ruddy appearance with brisk or normal capillary refill.

Signs of Potential Organ System Failure in Children

Central Nervous System

Acute change in mental status or responsiveness (confusion, agitation or lethargy) *OR*
Decrease in Glasgow coma scale score by 1 point from previous status

Pulmonary System

Unexplained hypoxemia with suspected sepsis or hypoxemia despite therapy with suspected sepsis:
  Pao_2/Fio_2 ratio <175-200 mm Hg
  Oxygenation index (OI) >10:

$$OI = \frac{\text{Mean airway pressure} \times Fio_2 \times 100}{Pao_2}$$

Rising alveolar-arterial oxygen gradient (A-a Do_2):

$\text{A-a } Do_2$ = Alveolar partial pressure of O_2　　　　　 − Arterial partial pressure of O_2
　　　 = PAo_2　　　　　　　　　　　　　　　　　− Pao_2
　　　 = $Fio_2 \times$ (Barometric pressure − 47 mm Hg) − Pao_2
　　　 = Should be <25-50 mm Hg

Bilateral pulmonary infiltrates with pulmonary artery occlusion pressure (PAOP) <18 mm Hg
Deterioration from baseline (see above and add increasing requirements for inspired oxygen to maintain Pao_2 80-100 mm Hg, or increasing ventilatory support requirements)

Cardiovascular System

Evidence of inadequate organ perfusion:
  Metabolic acidosis
  Hypotension
  Decreased ejection fraction unrelated to underlying cardiac disease
Hypotension
Evidence of decreased ejection fraction

Renal (Not Prerenal) System

Oliguria (urine output <0.5 ml/kg/min) despite adequate fluid intake
Increase in serum creatinine from normal with urine sodium <40 mmol/L
Rise in serum creatinine by 2 mg/dl in presence of preexisting renal insufficiency

Hepatobiliary System

Elevation in liver function enzymes to twice normal
Serum bilirubin >2 mg/dl

Gastrointestinal System

Paralytic ileus
Gastrointestinal bleeding

Coagulation

Confirmatory test for disseminated intravascular coagulation (fibrin degradation products >1:40 or D-dimers >2)
Thrombocytopenia or fall in platelet count by 25%
Elevated prothrombin time and partial thromboplastin time
Clinical evidence of bleeding

Modified from Hazinski MF: Shock, multiple organ dysfunction syndrome, and burns in children. From McCance KL, Huether SE, editors: *Pathophysiology: the biological basis for disease in adults and children,* ed 3, St Louis, 1998, Mosby.

Hypovolemic Shock Clinical signs are those of inadequate systemic perfusion associated with evidence of intravascular fluid loss (such as dehydration or hemorrhage). If compensatory mechanisms are functioning, they will produce tachycardia, peripheral vasoconstriction, delayed capillary refill (despite a warm ambient temperature), cool extremities, and oliguria. Capillary refill time is generally prolonged beyond 3 seconds in the presence of >10% isotonic dehydration or significant acute blood loss (≥20% to 25% acute intravascular volume loss).

The CVP and pulmonary artery wedge pressure/pulmonary artery occlusion pressure (PAWP/PAOP) are ≤5 to 8 mm Hg, and the cardiac silhouette is typically small (not enlarged) on chest radiographs. Pulmonary edema is absent unless capillary leak is present.

Clinically significant dehydration is associated with weight loss. The child with dehydration has dry mucous membranes, a sunken fontanelle (in infants), and poor skin turgor. The serum BUN and urine specific gravity are usually elevated. The serum osmolality and sodium concentration may be low, normal, or high, based on the type of dehydration present (hypotonic, isotonic, or hypertonic).

Shock With Isotonic Dehydration With isotonic dehydration, sodium loss is proportional to loss of water; thus the serum sodium level is normal, and fluid loss is proportional in the intravascular and interstitial compartments. Signs of peripheral circulatory failure (cool extremities but normal blood pressure) in the child with isotonic dehydration indicates a moderate deficit of approximately 100 ml/kg or a 10% weight loss in the infant or child. If hypotension is present, the deficit is severe: approximately 150 ml/kg or a 12% to 15% weight loss in the infant or child.

Shock With Hypotonic/Hyponatremic Dehydration With hypotonic dehydration, sodium loss is proportionately greater than the loss of water; thus the serum sodium level is low. In these patients fluid loss is predominantly from the intravascular compartment; thus signs of shock will be more severe at only moderate fluid deficit. Signs of peripheral circulatory failure will be observed at only a mild deficit of approximately 50 ml/kg or a 5% weight loss in the infant or child. Hypotension may develop

at only a moderate deficit of approximately 100 ml/kg or a 10% weight loss for the infant or child.

Shock With Hypertonic Dehydration With hypertonic dehydration, loss of water is proportionately greater than the loss of sodium; thus the serum sodium level is high. This hypernatremia helps maintain intravascular water, so that signs of shock will not be observed until the fluid deficit is severe. If signs of peripheral circulatory failure are present, the fluid deficit will be severe: approximately 150 ml/kg, with a weight loss of 12% to 15% for the child.

Hemorrhagic Shock When blood loss occurs, initial signs of shock may be subtle; thus there must be a strong index of suspicion, particularly when the blood loss is not immediately visible (e.g., with retroperitoneal or abdominal hemorrhage in the unconscious child). Hypotension often is not apparent until approximately 20% to 25% of the blood volume has been lost acutely. The hemoglobin and hematocrit values may not fall acutely until blood loss is replaced with crystalloid. To estimate the percentage of blood lost, circulating blood volume should be estimated (Table 5-11).

Cardiogenic Shock Cardiogenic shock produces signs of inadequate systemic perfusion despite the presence of adequate intravascular volume or even a relative hypervolemia. This form of shock is generally associated with low cardiac output. Adrenergic compensatory mechanisms divert blood flow from the kidneys, gut, and skin in an attempt to maintain effective blood flow to the heart and brain. The child's extremities will typically be cool to the touch, with delayed capillary refill despite a warm ambient temperature. The skin may have a

Table 5-11
Estimation of Pediatric Circulating Blood Volume

Age of Child	Blood Volume (ml/kg Body Weight)
Neonate	85-90
Infant	75-80
Child	70-75
Adolescent	65-70

From Hazinski MF: *Nursing care of the critically ill child*, ed 2, St Louis, 1992, Mosby.

mottled appearance. Peripheral pulses are usually diminished in intensity.

Since the heart is the limiting factor in the cardiovascular system, signs of high CVP (>12 to 18 mm Hg) are generally present, including hepatomegaly and periorbital edema. Evidence of pulmonary edema may be noted on chest radiographs or clinical assessment (including tachypnea and signs of respiratory distress, reduced lung compliance during hand ventilation or frothy pink sputum suctioned from an endotracheal tube). The PAWP/PAOP may be >12 to 18 mm Hg.

The cardiac silhouette is typically enlarged on chest radiographs. Occasionally children with viral myocarditis or cardiomyopathy present with vomiting and dehydration; under these conditions, the myocardial failure may not be apparent until rehydration is accomplished.

If myocardial function is severely compromised, peripheral pulses may be diminished in intensity (dampened) or may vary in intensity (pulsus alternans). If a pulmonary artery catheter enables calculation of cardiac output, a fall in cardiac output may be detected. Continuous monitoring of mixed venous oxygen saturation may reveal a fall in the $S\overline{v}O_2$ in the absence of any fall in arterial oxygen content.

Cardiac Tamponade   Signs of low cardiac output and cardiogenic shock may be identical to signs of cardiac tamponade. Although some "classic" signs of tamponade may be observed, including muffled heart tones or pulsus paradoxus, these signs may be difficult to appreciate if peripheral perfusion is poor and cardiac output and blood pressure are low. Therefore, if cardiogenic shock is suspected in the postoperative cardiovascular surgical patient or in any child at risk for the development of pericardial effusion or tamponade, tamponade should be ruled out through use of echocardiography.

Septic Shock   The clinical signs produced by septic shock typically include massive vasodilation, low SVR, capillary leak, evidence of organ failure, and lactic acidosis despite a high cardiac output/index. The high cardiac output can usually be maintained, provided that the child's intravascular volume is supported through generous fluid administration. Systemic and pulmonary edema are usually present, and organ ischemia and organ system dysfunction may develop.

If the $S\overline{v}O_2$ is monitored, it will usually be high during untreated sepsis, since oxygen delivery is high and a significant portion of cardiac output is shunting through tissue beds, which have plethoric blood flow and compromised oxygen use. When both oxygen delivery and the $S\overline{v}O_2$ are high, the oxygen extraction ratio (oxygen delivery divided by oxygen utilization) is abnormally low (e.g., 15%). The $S\overline{v}O_2$ should fall during therapy, and the oxygen extraction ratio should increase, signifying better tissue perfusion and better utilization of oxygen.

The clinical progression of sepsis in the adult patient has been described and defined by a consensus panel of physicians, and the consensus terms have been validated in adult patients. Although these terms have not been validated in the pediatric patient, most can be adapted with little difficulty (Box 5-12).

Management

Early recognition and therapy are the keys to the successful management of pediatric shock. Therefore signs of poor systemic perfusion should be identified as soon as they appear, and supportive therapy should be provided to optimize each aspect of cardiovascular and pulmonary function.

The goals of therapy are maximization of oxygen delivery and minimization of oxygen demand. Oxygen delivery is maximized by supporting arterial oxygen content, as well as cardiac output:

- *Optimize arterial oxygen content:* Support hemoglobin concentration and saturation (support airway, oxygenation, and ventilation).
- *Optimize cardiac output:* Support appropriate heart rate for clinical condition and ensure adequate cardiac preload, maximal contractility, and ideal afterload.
- *Control oxygen demand:* Treat pain and fever, prevent cold stress, and eliminate needless sources of stress.

Each of these components of therapy is included in the shock algorithm (Figure 5-8) and is summarized in the text below.

An essential aspect of care of the child in shock is *reassessment.* The child should be reevaluated

---

Box 5-12

Consensus Terminology for Clinical Progression of Sepsis and Septic Shock

Systemic Inflammatory Response Syndrome (SIRS)

Two or more of the following (as acute change):
Fever (>38° C) or hypothermia (<36° C)
Tachycardia
  Adults: >90 beats/min
  Newborns: >140 beats/min
  Infants: >120 beats/min
  Children: >90-100 beats/min
Tachypnea or hypocarbic respiratory alkalosis ($Paco_2$ <32 mm Hg with spontaneous breathing
  Adults: rate >20 breaths/min
  Infants: rate >50 to 60 breaths/min
  Children: rate >40 breaths/min
Leukocytosis (white blood cell count >12,000/mm^3), leukopenia (white blood cell count <4000/mm^3), or >10% band forms

Sepsis

SIRS (two or more of above) plus suspected infection

Severe Sepsis

Sepsis plus signs of organ dysfunction, hypoperfusion, or hypotension; signs of organ dysfunction or hypoperfusion may include lactic acidosis, oliguria, or acute alteration in mental status

Septic Shock

Severe sepsis plus hypotension despite vigorous volume administration/resuscitation, or normotension maintained with vasopressors
Adults: Fall in systolic blood pressure by 40 mm Hg or more, systolic pressure <90 mm Hg, diastolic pressure <70 mm Hg
Children (older than 1 yr): Fall in blood pressure from baseline values or systolic pressure <70 mm Hg + (2 × age in years)

Modified from Hazinski MF: Shock, multiple organ dysfunction syndrome, and burns in children. From McCance KL, Huether SE, editors: *Pathophysiology: the biological basis for disease in adults and children,* ed 3, St Louis, 1998, Mosby. Data from American College of Chest Physicians/Society of Critical Care Medicine Consensus Conference Committee: *Crit Care Med* 20:864, 1992; and Hazinski MF et al: *Am J Crit Care* 2:224, 1993.

---

constantly to determine response to therapy, identify the need for changes in therapy, and detect any signs of further deterioration.

Airway and Ventilation   The child's airway must be protected. This may require positioning of an unconscious child, suctioning of the airway, or endotracheal intubation. Elective intubation should be performed to support ventilation *before* severe respiratory deterioration or arrest occurs—this is always preferable to urgent intubation during resuscitation. Too often, advanced therapy is sabotaged by neglect of relatively simple but significant aspects of therapy—support of oxygenation and ventilation.

Indications for intubation include:

- Inadequate central nervous system control of ventilation (e.g., coma, increased intracranial pressure, sedation)
- Actual or potential airway obstruction (e.g., child with facial trauma or burns)
- Loss of protective airway reflexes (e.g., loss of consciousness)
- Excessive work of breathing with potential for deterioration (e.g., child with sepsis and pulmonary edema)
- Need for mechanical ventilation and/or PEEP
- Need for prolonged transport or diagnostic studies

These indications should always be considered in light of the child's clinical condition.

Provide supplementary oxygen as needed by mask, head hood, bag-valve-mask, or mechanical ventilation. The child in shock is, by definition, unstable; thus oxygen administration should be titrated to maintain 99% to 100% saturation of hemoglobin.

Whenever mechanical ventilatory support is provided, its effectiveness must be closely moni-

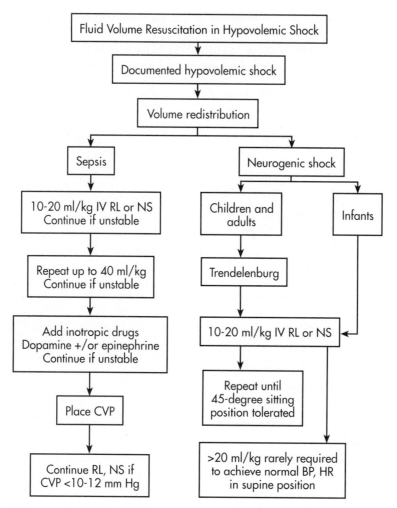

Figure 5-8   Treatment algorithm for fluid resuscitation in hypovolemic shock. *RL,* Ringer's lactate; *NS,* normal saline; *BP,* blood pressure; *HR,* heart rate; *CVP,* central venous pressure. (From Nichols DG et al: *Golden hour: the handbook of advanced pediatric life support,* ed 2, St Louis, 1996, Mosby.)

tored. The child's chest should rise equally and ad-equately bilaterally, and breath sounds should be equal and adequate bilaterally. Causes of acute de-terioration in the intubated child include tube *Dis*placement, tube *O*bstruction, *P*neumothorax, and *E*quipment failure ("DOPE").

Hemoglobin Concentration   There is no single ideal hemoglobin concentration. Inadequate hemo-globin concentration and anemia will reduce blood oxygen-carrying capacity and require a higher

cardiac output to maintain oxygen delivery. There-fore anemia should be avoided if at all possible if cardiac function is compromised. Although trans-fusion therapy does introduce the risk of blood-borne infection, it should be considered to replace acute blood loss or to treat severe anemia, particu-larly in the presence of cardiac dysfunction.

Extremely high hemoglobin concentration is undesirable, since a high hemoglobin concentra-tion will increase blood viscosity and shear stresses on small vessels, potentially causing microvascular occlusion and a compromise in tissue perfusion. In general, polycythemia produces symptoms of hyperviscosity once the is ≥70%, and pheresis (replacement of blood with serum, albumin, or crystalloid) should be considered to reduce the hemoglobin concentration if the high hematocrit is not caused by dehydration and hemoconcentration.

Support of Heart Rate   Monitor the child's heart rate continuously, and evaluate the heart rate in light of the child's clinical condition. Tachycardia is generally appropriate when the child is critically ill or injured or in pain or afraid, and a *normal* heart rate under such conditions is usually inadequate. The three most common types of symptomatic arrhythmias observed in critically ill children are bradyarrhythmias, tachyarrhythmias, and collapse rhythms (for further information see Cardiopulmonary Arrest and Cardiopulmonary Resuscitation and Arrhythmias).

Bradyarrhythmias   Bradycardia is the most common terminal rhythm observed before cardiac arrest. Since it is most often caused by hypoxia, oxygenation and ventilation must be evaluated and supported. Treatment includes:

- Ensure effective oxygenation and ventilation.
- Administer chest compressions if extreme bradycardia (e.g., heart rate <60/min) is associated with poor systemic perfusion.
- Administer epinephrine.
- Consider additional potential sympathomimetic drugs: dopamine or dobutamine. Isoproterenol may be particularly helpful in the presence of heart block, since this drug will stimulate the ventricular rate.
- Eliminate any treatable causes of the bradycardia (including acidosis, electrolyte imbalance, or vagal stimulation).
- Consider administration of atropine (0.02 mg/kg, minimum 0.1 mg).
- Consider isoproterenol (0.1 μg/kg/min), particularly if heart block is present.
- Consider pacing (esophageal pacing will pace the atria and can be effective unless heart block is present; external or transvenous pacing may be required if heart block is present).

Tachyarrhythmias   *Sinus tachycardia* may be present in the child with shock. This rhythm requires no treatment and is in fact a symptom of stress. Treatment of the cause of the shock and improvement in systemic perfusion should enable the heart rate to return to normal.

Supraventricular tachycardia (SVT) may produce signs of CHF or shock. Extremely rapid ventricular rates (exceeding approximately 220 to 240 beats/min in infants and 160 to 180 beats/min in children) compromise ventricular diastolic filling time; thus stroke volume can fall. In addition, such extremely rapid rates reduce coronary artery perfusion time; thus myocardial ischemia may develop and compromise ventricular contractility. Tachyarrhythmias may be tolerated for several hours in the child with normal cardiovascular function but may produce immediate signs of deterioration in the child with myocardial dysfunction. The treatment of choice for SVT associated with poor systemic perfusion is administration of IV or intraosseous adenosine (see Arrhythmias). If no IV access is readily available, synchronized cardioversion is performed.

Junctional ectopic tachycardia (JET) is an extremely rapid heart rate initiated by junctional tissue. This rhythm is most commonly observed following cardiovascular surgery and may be fatal if not controlled. The treatment of choice is overdrive pacing, digoxin plus amiodarone, or surface cooling. Cardioversion is usually not effective.

Ventricular tachycardia *with pulses* requires urgent treatment because it may deteriorate into ventricular tachycardia without pulses. The treatment of choice is synchronized cardioversion and lidocaine. Bretylium may also be considered.

Collapse Rhythms   The collapse rhythms include pulseless ventricular tachycardia, ventricular fibrillation (VT/VF), and electromechanical dissociation (EMD) or pulseless electrical activity (PEA). Treatment of pulseless VT/VF includes cardiopulmonary resuscitation (CPR) with cardiac compressions and defibrillation. EMD/PEA may result from severe hypovolemia (e.g., the trauma patient), tension pneumothorax, cardiac tamponade, and electrolyte imbalance. Treatment includes CPR and elimination of the cause.

Volume Resuscitation   Volume resuscitation is designed to restore intravascular volume relative to the vascular space and to optimize ventricular preload. To begin shock resuscitation, reliable IV access must be established. If IV access cannot be achieved in children younger than 6 years of age, insert an intraosseous needle and provide fluid through that route.

Fluid Selection The type of fluid administered will be determined by the child's clinical condition. In general, *isotonic crystalloids* (lactated Ringer's or normal saline) or *colloids* (protein-containing fluids such as albumin) or blood will be administered. *Hypotonic fluids are avoided,* since the portion that is water will be distributed throughout the total body water and thus will not increase intravascular volume and can contribute to cellular edema. Glucose-containing fluids are also avoided during resuscitation unless hypoglycemia has been documented with a bedside glucose analysis. Hyperglycemia during traumatic and cardiopulmonary resuscitation has been linked with poor neurologic outcome.

Crystalloid boluses of *20 ml/kg are administered over 5 to 10 minutes* and are repeated as necessary. If multiple boluses are administered, colloids are occasionally combined with crystalloids in a 2:1 or 3:1 (crystalloid-colloid) ratio.

Blood or blood component therapy is reserved for replacement of blood loss or correction of coagulopathies (Table 5-12). If hypovolemia is caused by hemorrhage, blood should be administered, generally in the form of packed RBCs, in boluses of 10 ml/kg. Traumatic fluid resuscitation utilizes both crystalloids and colloids in a 3:1 or 4:1 (crystalloid-colloid) ratio. Type-specific blood is administered when available; O-negative blood may be used under emergency conditions with a physician's order.

Transfusion therapy for the child with severe chronic anemia and CHF or shock should be accomplished slowly. Packed RBCs are administered at a rate of 3 ml/kg over several hours. Diuretics may be administered before, during, or after the transfusion. If severe myocardial dysfunction is present, an exchange transfusion may be required.

Evaluation of Patient Response During volume therapy, the child's systemic perfusion and evidence of organ perfusion and function should improve. A positive response to volume administration includes correction of hypotension and im-

provement in the temperature of extremities, the quality of peripheral pulses, the child's general color, and the briskness of capillary refill. The child's urine output should increase and level of consciousness should improve. If the child's neurologic function fails to improve or deteriorates during shock resuscitation, neurologic complications may be present.

During volume resuscitation, attempt to determine the CVP (and pulmonary artery wedge or occlusion pressure) associated with optimal systemic perfusion and urine output. This optimal pressure may change during the course of therapy as myocardial function changes.

Systemic and pulmonary edema may develop during volume resuscitation, particularly when crystalloids are used or when capillary permeability is increased (e.g., during septic shock). The development of edema does not signal the need to cease volume resuscitation, however, since the volume is required to maintain *intravascular* volume. Pulmonary edema usually compromises pulmonary function; so be prepared to provide oxygen therapy, assist with intubation, and initiate mechanical ventilation with PEEP as needed.

If the patient's systemic perfusion does not improve sufficiently with fluid therapy alone, complicating factors should be identified and treated. These factors may include tension pneumothorax, pericardial tamponade, sepsis, or acid-base or electrolyte imbalances. In addition, support of myocardial function with inotropes or vasodilators is required.

Correction of Acid-Base and Electrolyte Imbalances Hypoxia, metabolic acidosis, and electrolyte imbalances will depress myocardial function; thus they must be corrected. Hypoxia and documented metabolic acidosis in the child with shock are most effectively treated by restoration of effective systemic perfusion and support of effective oxygenation and ventilation. Administration of sodium bicarbonate may occasionally be necessary if acidosis is severe or is not corrected with volume therapy.

Correction of Acidosis The role of metabolic acidosis in the development of an acidotic pH can be calculated from the arterial blood gas results

Table 5-12
Pediatric Blood Component Therapy

Problem	"Classic" Coagulation Panel Abnormalities	Blood Component	Quantity
Acute blood loss	Hematocrit <40 (infants) <30 (children)	Whole blood	To replace loss or 10-20 ml/kg
		Packed RBCs	10 ml/kg should raise hematocrit 10 points
Chronic anemia	Hematocrit <15% to 20% Hemoglobin <5-7 g/dl Patient symptomatic	Packed RBCs If frequent or multiple transfusions required, or history of febrile reactions, consider leukocyte-poor RBCs (buffy coat removed to prevent reactions with WBCs)	Administer *slowly:* 3 ml/kg/hr (consider diuretics)
Anemia in child with T-cell immune deficiency	Hematocrit <40 (infants) <30 (children) (Consider patient baseline)	If time and patient condition allows, consider irradiated RBCs	As above (See Acute Blood Loss)
Thrombocytopenia	↓ Platelets (isolated) ↑ Template bleeding time Clot formation but lack of clot retraction	Platelets	1 U/5 kg (Maximum 10 U)
Thrombocytopathia	Normal or only slightly decreased platelet count template bleeding time Clot formation but lack of clot retraction	Platelets	1 U/5 kg (Maximum 10 U)
Disseminated intravascular coagulation (DIC)	↓ Fibrinogen and platelets (lower than expected) ↑ PT, PTT ↑ Fibrin split products	Treat cause: If fibrinogen <50, cryoprecipitate plus fresh frozen (FFP) plasma should be given If fibrinogen >50 FFP plasma alone may be effective	FFP: 10 ml/kg Cryoprecipitate: 1 bag/5 kg Titrate to achieve improvement in fibrinogen and platelet count
DIC with purpura fulminans	As above with evidence of peripheral embolic phenomena	Administer FFP to restore levels of antithrombin III, then heparin	FFP: 10 ml/kg Heparin: Load: 25 U/kg IV: 10-15 U/kg per hr Titrate to achieve rise in fibrinogen and platelet count and fall in PTT
Hemophilia A	Bleeding ↓ Factor VIII activity	Purified factor VIII	Severe life-threatening bleeding or major surgery: 50 U/kg or continuous infusion of 2 U/kg/hr to maintain factor VIII activity at 100% Minor bleeding: 25 U/kg

From Hazinski MF: *Nursing care of the critically ill child,* ed 2, St Louis, 1992, Mosby. *Continued*

Table 5-12
Pediatric Blood Component Therapy—cont'd

Problem	"Classic" Coagulation Panel Abnormalities	Blood Component	Quantity
Lack of coagulation factors in general*	↑ PT, PTT, thrombin time ↓ Fibrinogen Slow clot formation	FFP	10 ml/kg
Heparin excess†	↑ ↑ PTT, thrombin time, and template bleeding time PT may be slightly ↑ Platelet count normal (initially) Slow clot formation	Protamine sulfate (titrated to correct thrombin time)	1 mg/kg (slowly)
Protamine sulfate excess†	↑ ↑ PTT, thrombin time, and template bleeding time PT may be slightly ↑ Platelet count normal (initially) Slow clot formation	When protamine is titrated and thrombin time does not improve, heparin may be administered	Heparin IV: 50 U/kg Infusion: 10-15 U/kg/hr
Effects of aspirin (ASA)	↑ Template bleeding time	Platelets	1 U/5 kg (Maximum: 10 U)

From Hazinski MF: *Nursing care of the critically ill child*, ed 2, St Louis, 1992, Mosby.
*Usually, this condition results from a complex function of dilution and lack of replacement during surgery, inability of the liver to compensate, and occasionally from excessive loss of plasma protein (large proteins) via chest tubes.
†The only way to distinguish between these two problems is through protamine sulfate titration—see third column.

Box 5-13

Assessment of Severity of Metabolic Acidosis From pH and $Paco_2$ in the Hypercarbic Child

1. Subtract 40 from the child's $Paco_2$.
2. Multiply difference obtained in step 1 by 0.008.
3. Subtract number obtained in step 2 from 7.4; this yields the pH predicted from the hypercarbia. Acidosis greater than that predicted is metabolic in origin. If acidosis is less than predicted, some metabolic compensation for the respiratory acidosis must have occurred.
4. To calculate base deficit, subtract predicted pH (from step 3) from the child's actual pH and multiply this difference by 67. A base deficit more negative than −2 indicates the presence of metabolic acidosis, and a base excess more positive than +2 indicates the presence of a metabolic alkalosis.

Modified from Hazinski MF: *Nursing care of the critically ill child*, ed 2, St Louis, 1992, Mosby.

(Box 5-13). Three types of buffering agents can be administered to correct metabolic acidosis:

- Sodium bicarbonate: 1 mEq/kg (may be diluted) or calculated from: base deficit × 0.33 × kg body weight = approximate mEq $NaHCO_3$ required to correct approximately half of base deficit (ventilation must be effective).
- Tromethamine (THAM) does not generate carbon dioxide during buffering; thus it may be administered in the presence of a combined respiratory and metabolic acidosis. However, it can produce hyperkalemia and hypoglycemia.
- Salts of organic acids (e.g., lactate contained in lactated Ringer's solution) may also act as buffers. However, since these buffers must be metabolized to be effective, they may not be useful in shock resuscitation.

Correction of Hypoglycemia Young infants have high glucose needs and low glycogen stores; thus they may rapidly become hypoglycemic during episodes of stress, such as shock. However, empirical treatment with glucose is not advisable, since it may create hyperglycemia and will cause an acute rise in serum osmolality. Documented hypoglycemia can be treated with 5% glucose (2 to 4 ml/kg/hr) after an initial bolus of hypertonic glucose.

Correction of Potassium Imbalances Alterations in serum potassium concentration can affect myocardial contractility and conduction. However, children are far less sensitive than adults to minor changes in serum potassium concentration.

The serum potassium concentration can change with changes in acid-base balance. Acidosis or a fall in serum pH is associated with a rise in serum potassium (potassium shifts into the vascular space). Alkalosis or a rise in serum pH is associated with a fall in serum potassium (potassium shifts intracellularly). These shifts should be considered when evaluating the serum potassium, particularly if therapy will alter the pH. For example, when treating the child with diabetic ketoacidosis, expect the serum potassium to fall as the acidosis is corrected. Plan to provide a potassium supplement if the serum potassium is low or even normal when therapy is initiated.

Hypokalemia can result from dilution of the potassium, excessive potassium loss in the urine (e.g., following administration of furosemide, carbenicillin, or amphotericin), inadequate potassium administration, or a rise in pH. Treatment of hypokalemia is achieved through potassium administration, typically 0.5 to 1 mEq/kg, diluted in IV fluids and administered over several hours.

Hyperkalemia in the range of 7 to 7.5 mEq/L can be associated with malignant ventricular arrhythmias. It can result from reduced potassium excretion (e.g., renal failure), potassium accumulation during hemolysis or tissue necrosis, or a fall in serum pH. Correction of hyperkalemia includes:

- Administration of calcium gluconate, 60 to 100 mg/kg, *or* calcium chloride, 20 to 25 mg/kg IV, to stabilize myocardial membranes
- Administration of sodium bicarbonate, 1 to 2.5 mEq/kg, to increase serum pH and shift potassium back into cells (A 2.5 mEq/kg dose should reduce serum potassium approximately 2 mEq/L.)

- Administration of sodium polystyrene sulfonate (Kayexalate), a cation exchange resin, to promote exchange of sodium for potassium in the gut (A dose of 1 g of resin/kg should reduce serum potassium approximately 1 mEq/L.)
- Administration of hypertonic glucose (1 to 2 ml/kg of 25% glucose) or glucose plus regular insulin (1 U/kg) to carry potassium into cells
- Dialysis
- Exchange transfusion

Correction of Calcium Imbalances Hypocalcemia can impair myocardial function and produce arrhythmias. Both total and ionized calcium concentration should be monitored and hypocalcemia treated. The serum ionized calcium is often low in septic shock and may be low following administration of citrate-phosphate-dextran (CPD)–preserved blood. The serum ionized calcium concentration also falls when the pH rises. Other causes of hypocalcemia include a low serum magnesium concentration or a high serum phosphate concentration (such as may develop during tumor lysis syndrome). Hypocalcemia is treated with administration of calcium chloride, 20 to 25 mg/kg (0.2 to 0.25 ml/kg of 10% solution), administered no faster than 100 mg/min. Calcium should not be routinely administered during CPR, since hypercalcemia may also be present as a result of calcium release from hypoxic myocardial cells.

Hypercalcemia is occasionally observed in children with some malignancies, including acute lymphocytic leukemia, lymphomas, and soft tissue sarcomas. These malignant cells secrete a parathormone-like substance that stimulates bone reabsorption and release of calcium and rapid cell turnover. In the presence of an extremely high serum calcium concentration, the kidneys are unable to concentrate urine, and a profound diuresis may produce hypovolemia. Hypercalcemia is treated with hydration (normal saline infusion) and diuretic therapy. Calcitonin administration (3 to 6 MRC U/kg IV or IM every 6 hours) may be required.

Vasoactive Inotropic Drug Therapy If shock persists despite appropriate oxygenation, ventilation, heart rate, and intravascular volume, vasoactive drug therapy is indicated. Inotropic agents are not helpful in the treatment of hypovolemic shock unless or until intravascular volume has been restored. These drugs are extremely useful in the treatment of cardiogenic and distributive shock or in any condition in which myocardial function is impaired. Since most inotropic drugs have chronotropic effects at some doses, these drugs can be useful to optimize heart rate. It is important to consider potential therapeutic, as well as side and toxic, effects of these drugs when drug therapy is initiated.

The goals of vasoactive drug therapy in the treatment of shock are:

- To increase heart rate if it is too slow for clinical condition
- To increase cardiac output if it is inadequate
- To increase cardiac contractility
- To redistribute cardiac output
- To manipulate vascular resistance

These drugs may improve systemic perfusion and organ function by increasing or redistributing blood flow with or without an improvement in blood pressure. However, if hypotension is significant, the drugs should be titrated to improve blood pressure.

Before any vasoactive drug is administered, review the proposed effects of the drug, the clinical or physiologic criteria that will be used to monitor the effectiveness of therapy (e.g., titrate to increase heart rate or urine output), and potential undesirable side effects that may limit use of the drug (e.g., tachyarrhythmias). This information should be noted on the nursing Kardex. Regardless of the ordered dose of vasoactive drug, the nurse is expected to assist in the titration of a proper drug dose. If the prescribed dose is not producing the desired effect, contact the physician and discuss altering the drug dose. In many pediatric intensive care units (PICUs), nurses are authorized to wean or increase the dose of vasoactive drugs based on general guidelines (e.g., titrate to maintain mean arterial pressure at 70 mm Hg).

Administration Because vasoactive drugs have a very short half-life, they are administered by continuous IV or intraosseous infusion. The drugs may be diluted to either standard concentrations (e.g., everyone uses a dilution of 100-, 200-, 400-, or 800 µg/ml) or to concentrations that vary according to the patient's body weight (e.g., 6 × child's weight in kilograms is the number of milligrams per deciliter dilution). Use of standard concentrations reduces the likelihood of dilution errors, since consistent concentrations are always mixed. However, when standard concentrations are used, the dose delivered to each patient must be calculated individually. When variable concentrations of the drug are used, the dose can be easily calculated (Box 5-14). However, the concentration

---

Box 5-14

"Rule of Sixes" for Preparation of Variable Concentrations of Vasoactive Drugs

1. For drugs infused in doses of µg/kg/min (or multiples):
   a. Multiply weight (in kg) by 6; place this number of milligrams of drug in solution *totaling* 100 ml.
   b. Then 1 ml/hr delivers 1 µg/kg/min.
2. For drugs infused in doses of 0.1 µg/kg/min (or multiples):
   a. Multiply weight (in kg) by 0.6; place this number of milligrams of drug in solution *totaling* 100 ml.
   b. Then 1 ml/hr delivers 0.1 µg/kg/min.
3. For any concentration of a drug:

$$\text{Rate (ml/hr)} = \frac{\text{Weight (kg)} \times \text{Dose (µg/kg/min)} \times 60 \text{ min/hr}}{\text{Concentration (µg/ml)}}$$

From Hazinski MF: *Nursing care of the critically ill child,* ed 2, St Louis, 1992, Mosby.

of the drug mixed for each patient will vary; so errors may occur. In addition, if large doses of the drug are administered, large volumes of fluid will be required unless the concentration of the drug is increased.

Most IV pumps (with the exception of syringe pumps) provide *intermittent* rather than continuous fluid administration when the infusion rate is reduced below 3 ml/hr. At these slow infusion rates, fluid delivery is provided in small bursts. If the vasoactive drug is prepared in a high concentration and is administered at a rate <3 ml/kg/hr, the patient may actually receive the drug in several "bursts" over the course of an hour. Such intermittent infusion can lead to heart rate and blood pressure instability, particularly if a concentrated drug solution is used. The drugs should be prepared in a concentration that will enable infusion at a minimum rate of 3 to 5 ml/hr if at all possible.

All vasoactive drugs must be carefully titrated to ensure maximal therapeutic effects with minimal side or toxic effects. The correct dose of any vasoactive drug can only be determined at the bedside with careful evaluation of patient response to therapy. Patient blood levels and responses to these drugs will vary tremendously.

Sympathomimetic drugs are provided to selectively stimulate adrenergic receptors. The receptors targeted will include those to stimulate coronary artery, mesenteric, or renal blood flow; those producing an increase in heart rate and an increase in ventricular contractility; and those increasing SVR (Box 5-15). General reported effects of these administered drugs are summarized in Table 5-13.

Often a combination of vasoactive agents is used to redistribute, as well as increase, cardiac output. When titrating any vasoactive drug dose, change only one drug at a time to enable evaluation of the effect of the change on systemic perfusion.

When infusions are begun or the infusion rate is changed, consider the "dead space" in the tubing. It may be necessary to temporarily increase the infusion rate to ensure timely delivery of the drug. To "mark" the entry of the new drug or drug concentration into the patient, the nurse can aspirate blood back to the infusion port, where the vasoactive drug will enter the tubing. Then the drug infusion is begun, with the infusion rate increased until the blood is cleared to the skin entrance site.

Sympathomimetic drugs are inactivated at an alkaline pH; thus they should not be infused in tubing containing buffers (e.g., sodium bicarbonate). Extravasation of any of the sympathomimetic drugs may produce a chemical burn, which can result in tissue necrosis and tissue sloughing. If the extravasation is detected immediately, injection of *phentolamine* into the area of extravasation may minimize the burn. Hyaluronidase should *not* be used to treat these burns; it may actually worsen the tissue injury.

Dopamine Dopamine can be titrated to produce a wide variety of effects. These effects include alpha- and beta-adrenergic, as well as direct dopaminergic, effects. As a norepinephrine precursor, dopamine produces release of norepinephrine, which may produce as much as 50% of dopamine's actions. However, if the patient receives dopamine for a prolonged period, norepinephrine stores may be depleted, and effects will then become more solely dopaminergic.

Theoretically, at low doses (approximately 1 to 5 μg/kg/min), dopamine produces dopaminergic

---

Box 5-15

Clinical Effects of Adrenergic Receptor Activation

Dopaminergic Receptor Activation

Dilates renal, mesenteric, coronary, and cerebrovascular beds.
Look for an increase in urine volume.

Beta-1 Receptor Activation

Increases heart rate, cardiac contractility, and atrioventricular conduction velocity.
Look for an increase in heart rate and cardiac output.

Beta-2 Receptor Activation

Causes peripheral vasodilation and bronchodilation.
Look for improved skin perfusion, decrease in blood pressure, and decrease in wheezing.

Alpha Receptor Activation

Constricts arteries and veins
Look for increase in blood pressure and decrease in skin perfusion and urine output.

Table 5-13
Pediatric Sympathomimetic and Other Inotropic Drugs*

Drug	Dose	Effects	Cautions
Sympathomimetics			
Dobutamine	2-20 µg/kg/min	Selective beta-adrenergic effects; increases cardiac contractility and also increases heart rate (this latter effect is variable). Beta-2 effects produce peripheral vasodilatation. No dopaminergic or alpha-adrenergic effects.	Extreme tachyarrhythmias have been reported (particularly in infants); hypotension may develop; may produce pulmonary venoconstriction.
Dopamine	1-5 µg/kg/min	Dopaminergic effects predominate (including increase in glomerular filtration rate and urine volume).	Can produce extreme tachyarrhythmias; can result in increase in pulmonary artery pressure; inhibits thyroid stimulating hormone (TSH) and aldosterone secretion.
	2-10 µg/kg/min	Dopaminergic effects persist and beta-1 effects are seen (especially an increase in heart rate).	
	8-20 µg/kg/min	Alpha-adrenergic effects dominate.	
Epinephrine	0.05-0.15 µg/kg/min	Endogenous catecholamine which produces alpha, beta-1 and beta-2 adrenergic effects; at low doses, beta-1 effects dominate.	Will increase myocardial work and oxygen consumption at any dose; splanchnic constriction will occur at even low doses.
	0.2-0.3 µg/kg/min	Alpha-adrenergic effects dominate.	
Isoproterenol	0.05-0.1 µg/kg/min	Beta-adrenergic effects; beta-1 effects may result in rapid increase in heart rate; beta-2 effects may produce peripheral vasodilatation and also may effectively treat bronchoconstriction.	Monitor for tachyarrhythmias, hypotension. Will increase myocardial oxygen consumption.
Norepinephrine	0.05-1.0 µg/kg/min	Endogenous catecholamine with alpha- and beta-adrenergic effects; produces potent peripheral and renal vasoconstriction; can increase blood pressure.	May produce tachyarrhythmias, increased myocardial work, and increased oxygen consumption; may result in hepatic and mesenteric ischemia
Phosphodiesterase Inhibitors			
Amrinone	0.75-5 mg/kg IV (loading dose—slowly) 5-10 µg/kg/min	Nonadrenergic inotropic agents that produce phosphodiesterase inhibition and increase in intracellular cyclic-AMP; intracellular calcium uptake also is delayed. These effects result in improved cardiac contractility and vasodilatation, without increasing myocardial oxygen consumption. May improve both systolic and diastolic ventricular function.	Monitor for arrhythmias (especially accelerated junctional rhythm, junctional tachycardia, and ventricular ectopy); may produce hypotension (especially if patient is hypovolemic), liver and gastrointestinal dysfunction, thrombocytopenia, and abdominal pain.
Milrinone	0.05-0.075 mg/kg (50-75 µg/kg) IV (loading dose—slowly) 0.5-0.75 µg/kg/min infusion		

Modified from Hazinski MF: Shock in the pediatric patient, *Crit Care Nurs Clin North Am* 2:309, 1990.

*Infusion rate (mL/hr) = $\dfrac{\text{wt (kg)} \times \text{Dose (µg/kg/min)} \times \text{60 min/hr}}{\text{Concentration (µg/mL)}}$

effects (renal, coronary artery, mesenteric, and cerebral vasodilation); this can improve renal, mesenteric, and coronary artery perfusion and result in an increase in urine output and cardiac output. Dopamine can be an ideal drug alone for patients following renal or liver transplantation or to mitigate potential renal vasoconstrictive effects of drugs such as epinephrine or norepinephrine.

At moderate doses (approximately 2 to 10 μg/kg/min), dopaminergic effects continue, and beta-adrenergic effects may also be observed. At these doses, urine output should be maintained, and heart rate and ventricular contractility should increase. Dopamine will not affect pulmonary arterial tone directly, but it may augment the pulmonary vascular constrictive response to hypoxia and may produce pulmonary venoconstriction.

At high doses (>8 to 20 μg/kg/min), dopaminergic and beta-adrenergic effects may be reduced, and alpha-adrenergic effects begin to dominate. However, the dose at which this occurs is extremely variable and will be affected by the patient's renal and hepatic function, the underlying condition, and the duration of drug therapy. Monitor urine output closely, since it will fall when renal blood flow is reduced by vasoconstriction.

Dopamine inhibits thyroid-stimulating hormone (TSH) and prolactin release and blunts the TSH response to thyrotropin-releasing hormone (TRH); thus it will affect thyroid function studies. Dopamine also inhibits aldosterone secretion and can reduce insulin secretion.

Dobutamine Dobutamine is a synthetic sympathetic amine that produces pure beta-adrenergic effects, with neither dopaminergic nor alpha-adrenergic effects. Its beta-1 adrenergic effects increase heart rate and ventricular contractility, but beta-2 effects produce systemic vasodilation. Dobutamine may be the preferred drug for the treatment of CHF or cardiogenic shock associated with systemic vasoconstriction, since dobutamine can improve heart rate and ventricular contractility and reduce SVR. Dobutamine also increases gastrointestinal mucosal blood flow; thus it may be useful in patients with a compromise in mesenteric perfusion.

Doses of 2 to 20 μg/kg/min improve stroke volume and cardiac output, as a selective inotrope. Dobutamine can produce significant vasodilation; thus it may cause a fall in blood pressure. Dobutamine produces variable effects on heart rate in children and does not affect PVR directly.

Dobutamine can produce long-term improvement in ventricular contractility when administered to children with severe heart failure. Its effect seems to be related to improvement in the myocardial oxygen supply-demand ratio.

Epinephrine Epinephrine is an endogenous hormone released from the adrenal medulla in response to stress. Epinephrine is the drug of choice for resuscitation of children, for treatment of bradyarrhythmias unresponsive to oxygenation and ventilation, and for treatment of hypotension. It can be the ideal drug for the treatment of shock associated with hypotension, particularly septic shock.

Epinephrine can exert both beta-adrenergic effects and alpha-adrenergic effects that are somewhat dose related. Alpha-adrenergic effects, including significant peripheral vasoconstriction, are generally observed at doses exceeding approximately 0.3 μg/kg/min. Undesirable effects of epinephrine include tachyarrhythmias, increased myocardial oxygen consumption, and a compromise in renal and mesenteric blood flow. The reduction in renal blood flow associated with epinephrine may be partially mitigated by administration of low-dose dopamine.

Norepinephrine Norepinephrine is an endogenous catecholamine that functions as a sympathetic neurotransmitter. This drug is often used for the treatment of shock associated with hypotension, particularly septic shock.

Norepinephrine provides both beta- and alpha-adrenergic effects at doses ranging from 0.05 to 1 μg/kg/min. It typically produces an increase in heart rate, stroke volume, and blood pressure. Its undesirable effects include an increase in myocardial oxygen consumption, an increase in heart rate, and a decrease in renal and mesenteric blood flow. The reduction in renal and mesenteric blood flow may be mitigated, in part, through concurrent administration of low-dose dopamine.

Phenylephrine Hydrochloride (NeoSynephrine) Phenylephrine is an alpha-adrenergic drug that exerts direct effects and also stimulates norepinephrine release from storage sites. The net result of IV administration is intense vasoconstriction. This drug may be used for treatment of refractory hypotension, such as that associated with severe septic shock, spinal shock, or anaphylactic reaction. Since this drug will increase myocardial oxygen demand, it is not the drug of choice for treatment of shock associated with myocardial hypoxia or ischemia. It may also produce extreme tachycardia; thus it should be used with caution.

This drug is occasionally used for the treatment of paroxysmal SVT and intractable hypoxic spells in children with tetralogy of Fallot (for further information see Arrhythmias and Hypoxemia Caused by Cyanotic Heart Disease).

Metaraminol Bitartrate (Aramine) Metaraminol bitartrate produces predominantly alpha-adrenergic effects with milder beta-1 adrenergic effects. The alpha-adrenergic actions produce intense vasoconstriction, useful for the treatment of hypotension associated with septic or spinal shock or anaphylaxis. The beta-1 effects produce an increase in heart rate and ventricular contractility.

Metaraminol increases myocardial oxygen consumption and myocardial oxygen demand. It may produce tachyarrhythmias and reflex bradycardia. Propranolol can be used to treat these arrhythmias, and atropine will correct reflex bradycardia.

Isoproterenol Isoproterenol is a pure beta-adrenergic agonist that exerts both beta-1 and beta-2 adrenergic effects. This drug may be useful for the treatment of bradycardia unresponsive to oxygen and ventilation, particularly bradycardia associated with heart block, because it is capable of stimulating the ventricles. Isoproterenol also produces vasodilation and bronchodilation; thus it is occasionally useful for the treatment of the child with poor perfusion accompanied by bronchoconstriction. However, its usefulness is often limited by the extreme tachycardia it produces, as well as by the increase in myocardial oxygen demand associated with its administration.

Amrinone/Milrinone Amrinone and milrinone are not sympathomimetic drugs; thus they do not stimulate adrenergic receptors. Instead, amrinone and milrinone are phosphodiesterase inhibitors. Cyclic adenosine monophosphate (cAMP) is the intracellular messenger triggered by stimulation of adrenergic receptors. Phosphodiesterase is the enzyme that breaks down cAMP; thus phosphodiesterase inhibition prolongs the activity of cAMP and prolongs sympathomimetic effects. In addition, these drugs produce inotropic effects by increasing intracellular calcium concentration and delaying calcium uptake. Amrinone and milrinone are particularly useful for the treatment of severe CHF or low cardiac output.

Infusion of either of these drugs should begin with administration of a loading dose followed by a continuous infusion. Bolus doses should be administered whenever drug therapy is initiated or when an increase in dose is required. Milrinone is the more potent form of the drug.

Amrinone and milrinone will produce vasodilation; thus intravascular volume should be assessed before initiation of therapy, and fluid administration may be required. Volume expanders should be readily available during therapy. Potential complications of these drugs include thrombocytopenia, gastrointestinal dysfunction, arrhythmias, and hypotension. Milrinone may produce fewer complications.

Vasodilators Vasodilators are frequently administered to the patient in shock, to reduce ventricular afterload. Vasodilators also increase ventricular compliance; thus they enable the ventricle to accept greater end-diastolic volume without an increase in end-diastolic pressure. The result can be an increase in stroke volume without an increase in end-diastolic pressure.

The effects of vasodilators on cardiac output can be variable and are determined by the relative effects on cardiac preload and afterload, and ventricular compliance. Typically, the greatest improvement in cardiac output occurs when simultaneous volume therapy is provided to maintain right or left ventricular end-diastolic pressure (VEDP) at approximately 10 to 12 mm Hg.

Because most vasodilators dilate both arteries and veins, they may produce venous pooling and hypotension. Therefore the patient's volume status should be evaluated before and during therapy, and volume expanders should be readily available throughout therapy. If severe hypotension develops during continuous infusion therapy, the infusion should be discontinued and volume expanders administered as needed.

The vasodilators administered most often to the child in shock include amrinone, milrinone, sodium nitroprusside, and nitroglycerin. A more complete listing of vasodilators is included in Table 5-14.

Table 5-14
Pediatric Vasodilator and Antihypertensive Therapy

Drug	Dose	Effect	Caution
Amrinone (Inocor)	Loading: 0.75-5.0 mg/kg Infusion: 5-10 µg/kg/min	Nonadrenergic inotropic agent; phosphodiesterase inhibition ↑ intracellular cyclic adenosine monophosphate. Also delays intracellular calcium uptake. Overall effects result in increased cardiac contractility and arterial and venous dilation.	Can produce profound hypotension, especially if patient is hypovolemic. Can produce hepatic and gastrointestinal dysfunction, abdominal pain, and thrombocytopenia. Monitor for arrhythmias, including junctional tachycardia and ventricular ectopy.
Atenolol (Tenormin)	1-2 mg/kg/day (maximum: 4 mg/kg), given every day	Beta-1 adrenergic blocker.	Will decrease heart rate and may decrease cardiac output and renin release.
Captopril (Capoten)	Neonates and children: begin at 0.3 mg/kg/dose PO q8h, then titrate to effect Older children and adolescents: 12.5-25 mg/dose q8h	Inhibits angiotensin-converting enzyme; results in increased sodium excretion and mixed arterial and venous dilation (reduces both afterload and preload).	May cause hypotension, proteinuria, neutropenia, hyperkalemia.
Diazoxide (Hyperstat)	IV: 2.5 mg/kg/dose (maximum: 10 mg/kg/dose); may give PO	Nondiuretic cogener of thiazide diuretics. Relaxes arterial smooth muscle, causing vasodilation.	Increases blood glucose. Contraindicated if hypersensitivity to thiazides. May affect phenytoin metabolism and protein-bound substances. May produce nausea, vomiting, flushing. Monitor blood pressure.
Enalapril (Vasotec)	IV or PO: 0.01-0.025 mg/kg q6h	Inhibits angiotensin-converting enzyme; results in increased sodium excretion and vasodilation.	May produce hypotension. Pediatric experience limited.
Esmolol (Brevibloc)	IV infusion: 1-300µg/kg/min (begin at 50 or 100 µg/kg/min and titrate)	Beta-1 adrenergic blocker with selective cardiac effects.	May produce hypotension, bradycardia. Effects *will not be apparent for 30 min after infusion begins*, so titrate carefully (half-life: 9 min). May compromise myocardial function. Do not mix with other drugs. Pediatric experience limited.

From Johns Hopkins Hospital Department of Pediatrics: *The Harriet Lane handbook*, ed 14, edited by Barone M, St Louis, 1996, Mosby; Ellsworth AJ et al, editors: *Mosby's 1998 medical drug reference*, St Louis, 1998, Mosby; Hackman AM, Bricker JT: Preventative cardiology, hypertension, and diplipedemia. In Garson A, Jr et al, editors: *The science and practice of pediatric cardiology*, ed 2, Baltimore, 1998, Williams & Wilkins; Hazinski MF: *Nursing care of the critically ill child*, ed 2, St Louis, 1992, Mosby.
Continued

Table 5-14
Pediatric Vasodilator and Antihypertensive Therapy—cont'd

Drug	Dose	Effect	Caution
Hydralazine (Apresoline)	PO: 0.1-0.3 mg/kg q4-6h IV/IM: 0.1-0.5 mg/kg/dose q6-8h	True arterial dilator.	Monitor for hypotension, reflex tachycardia, lupuslike syndrome, positive antinuclear antibody.
Isoproterenol (Isoprel)	IV infusion: 0.05-0.1 µg/kg/min	Beta-1 and beta-2 adrenergic effects—beta-2 effects produce systemic vasodilation.	May cause extreme tachycardia and increased myocardial oxygen consumption (possible myocardial ischemia).
Labetalol (Normodyne, Transdate)	IV: 0.25 mg/kg, may increase dose to maximum of 1-3 mg/kg dose (maximum total: 4 mg/kg) IV infusion: 5-20 µg/kg/min or 2 mg/min	Alpha-1 and beta-1 adrenergic blocker; produces fall in blood pressure.	Monitor for hypotension, bradycardia, ventricular arrhythmias. Dilute per manufacturer's instructions. Pediatric experience limited.
Metroprolol	PO: 1-2 mg/kg/day (maximum: 5 mg/kg/day)	Selective beta-1 adrenergic blocker.	Monitor for fatigue, dizziness, headache, bronchospasm.
Milrinone	Load: 50 µg/kg over 10-15 min Infusion: 0.35-0.75 µg/kg/min	Phosphodiesterase inhibitor (more potent form of amrinone (see amrinone)	See amrinone precautions, but less likely to produce thrombocytopenia.
Minoxidil (Loniten, Minoxidil)	PO: 0.1-0.2 mg/kg/day (maximum: 1 mg/kg/day), may be given in single dose	Direct peripheral vasodilation.	May cause severe edema and is associated with hypertrichosis (may be undesirable for use in girls). Pediatric experience limited.
Nifedipine (Adalat, Procardia)	PO/sublingual: 0.25-0.5 mg/kg	Calcium channel blocker.	Monitor for hypotension, signs of decreased myocardial function, flushing, nausea, headaches.
Nitroglycerin	IV: 0.1-10+ µg/kg/min Ointment: 0.5 cm changed q2-6h (to increase effective dose, change more frequently)	Systemic and pulmonary vasodilator and venodilator, so will reduce afterload and preload.	Can produce hypotension, particularly if patient is hypovolemic. May produce headaches. Drug is adsorbed by polyvinyl chloride tubing, so a change in tubing may decrease effective dose of drug. May produce methemoglobinemia.

Drug	Dose	Action	Comments
Nitric oxide (inhaled)	Delivered mixed in inspired gas at 10-80 ppm (10-20 ppm most frequently effective) under research protocol	Selective pulmonary vasodilator (endothelial-derived relaxing factor). Has no systemic vascular effects, because will be metabolized/inactivated within hemoglobin when it enters vascular space.	Can produce methemoglobinemia (monitor levels). Can produce significant pulmonary vasodilation and result in increased pulmonary blood flow if child has intracardiac shunt.
Nitroprusside (Nipride, Nitropress)	IV: 0.5-8.0 µg/kg/min	Systemic and pulmonary artery and venodilator, so will reduce both afterload and preload.	Monitor for hypotension (particularly if patient is hypovolemic) and thrombocytopenia. Metabolites include thiocyanate and cyanide (monitor levels if therapy required >48 hr). Light sensitive.
Phentolamine (Regitine)	IV: 0.1-2.0 µg/kg/min	Alpha-adrenergic blocker with direct effects on vascular smooth muscle, so vasodilation results.	Monitor for hypotension; tolerance can develop rapidly, so short-term use is advised. Gastrointestinal dysfunction may develop.
Propranolol (Inderal)	IV: 0.15-0.25 mg/kg PO: 0.5 mg/kg/day	Beta-blocker primarily administered to children with cyanotic heart disease to prevent hypercyanotic spells.	Monitor for hypotension, decreased heart rate, cardiac output.
Reserpine (Sandril, Serpasil)	PO: 0.02 mg/kg/day	Alpha-adrenergic blocker (produces vasodilation). Most frequently used in treatment of hypertension following correction of coarctation of aorta.	Rarely used in children in shock. Monitor for hypotension, sedative effects, nausea, vomiting.
Tolazoline (Priscoline)	IV: 1-2 µg/kg/min	Alpha-adrenergic blocker that may act at histamine receptors.	Monitor for hypotension, thrombocytopenia, gastrointestinal bleeding.

From Johns Hopkins Hospital Department of Pediatrics: *The Harriet Lane handbook*, ed 14, edited by Barone M, St Louis, 1996, Mosby; Ellsworth AJ et al, editors: *Mosby's 1998 medical drug reference*, St Louis, 1998, Mosby; Hackman AM, Bricker JT: Preventative cardiology, hypertension, and diplipedemia. In Garson A, Jr et al, editors: *The science and practice of pediatric cardiology*, ed 2, Baltimore, 1998, Williams & Wilkins; Hazinski MF: *Nursing care of the critically ill child*, ed 2, St Louis, 1992, Mosby.

Sodium Nitroprusside Sodium nitroprusside is a smooth muscle relaxant that dilates both arteries and veins. A typical infusion dose of 0.5 to 8 μg/kg/min dilates arteries to reduce impedance to ventricular ejection and increase ventricular compliance, and it increases venous capacitance vessels so that blood is displaced into those storage vessels.

This drug is light sensitive; thus it is stored in amber vials before use and must be protected from light after mixing. Special opaque tubing can be used, or regular tubing can be covered with tape or foil.

The most common complication of sodium nitroprusside administration is hypotension, which is particularly likely in the hypovolemic patient and should disappear if the infusion is slowed or terminated. Prolonged infusion can result in the formation of thiocyanate and cyanide, which are by-products of nitroprusside metabolism. This toxicity is most likely to occur during high-dose or prolonged infusions or in patients with renal or hepatic disease. Thiocyanate levels should be checked every other day during prolonged therapy; toxic levels are >10 mg/dl. Clinical signs of toxicity include confusion, hyperreflexia, weakness, skin rash, tinnitus, and fatigue. Signs of cyanide toxicity include agitation, diminished level of consciousness, tachypnea, incontinence, seizures, and cardiorespiratory arrest. Metabolic acidosis is an early sign of cyanide toxicity because cyanide inhibits aerobic metabolism. Sodium nitroprusside can also inhibit platelet function.

Nitroglycerin Nitroglycerin is also an arterial and venous dilator, but its predominant effects seem to be caused by venodilation. Venodilation increases venous capacitance and ventricular compliance and reduces ventricular preload. IV infusion dose typically ranges from 0.1 μg/kg/min to as high as 25 μg/kg/min.

Polyvinyl chloride tubing will adsorb nitroglycerin, particularly when the tubing is new or the administration rate is slow. When adsorption occurs, the patient receives unpredictable levels of the drug. Therefore, whenever possible, nitroglycerin should be administered through an infusion pump with polypropylene or polyethylene tubing. This system will minimize the adsorption surface for nitroglycerin and ensure more predictable drug delivery. The tubing should not be changed frequently.

Topical nitroglycerin ointment also may be applied to the chest. A dose of approximately 1 to 1.5 cm may produce effects for 0.5 to 6 hours. The dose may be increased by more frequent reapplication of the drug. Long-acting nitroglycerin paste disks are also available, but dosing choices are limited.

Side effects of nitroglycerin therapy include hypotension and headache. Hypotension is also possible, particularly if the patient is hypovolemic, but may be corrected with volume administration or interruption of drug delivery.

Treatment of Pulmonary Hypertension Pulmonary hypertension can produce low cardiac output and complicate the management of the child with CHD, the newborn with persistent pulmonary hypertension of the newborn, or the child with respiratory failure. Alveolar hypoxia promotes pulmonary vasoconstriction, and hypoxic pulmonary vasoconstriction can exacerbate pulmonary hypertension, particularly during the postoperative period or during other times of cardiorespiratory instability.

General Management Throughout management of the child with pulmonary hypertension, factors known to stimulate pulmonary vasoconstriction must be avoided. These *pulmonary vasoconstrictors* include the four *H*s:

- Alveolar hypoxia
- Hydrogen ion (acidotic pH)
- Alveolar hyperinflation
- Hypothermia

Whenever possible, factors known to promote pulmonary vasodilation should be promoted or maintained. These *pulmonary vasodilators* include the 4 *A*s:

- Alveolar ventilation
- Alkalosis (pH approximately 7.5—ensure adequate ionized calcium concentration)
- Analgesia and sedation (anesthesia may be required)
- Avoidance of stimulation

The infant or child with reactive pulmonary hypertension should be kept well ventilated and well oxygenated. In addition, analgesics and sedatives should be provided as needed. Anesthetics may be required. A metabolic alkalosis (pH 7.5) may be maintained through hyperventilation or administration of sodium bicarbonate (which generates some carbon dioxide, necessitating an increase in ventilation).

For the infant with severe pulmonary hypertension with periodic hypertensive "crises" that produce a sudden decrease in cardiac output, meticulous prevention of pulmonary vasoconstriction is required. Alveolar oxygenation is maintained through controlled mechanical ventilatory support and administration of supplementary inspired oxygen, and a mild alkalosis is maintained. Sedatives, neuromuscular blockade, and analgesics or anesthetics are provided to prevent or treat any pain (see Chapter 3), and stimulation is minimized.

Two skilled health care providers are needed every time endotracheal suctioning is performed. The first person suctions the tube quickly and gently, maintaining sterile technique. The second person provides hand ventilation while monitoring the infant's heart rate, color, and systemic arterial oxygenation (via pulse oximetry). If the infant deteriorates during suctioning, the suctioning is interrupted and hand ventilation with increased inspired oxygen concentration is provided until the child's heart rate, color, and cardiovascular function are stable. Weaning from mechanical ventilatory support is accomplished gradually.

Vasodilator Therapy   Vasodilators may be prescribed to treat pulmonary hypertension. However, any parenteral or oral vasodilator will dilate both arteries and veins; thus this therapy may produce complications such as hypotension.

Nitric Oxide   Nitric oxide is chemically identical to endothelium-derived relaxing factor (EDRF), a vasodilator. Nitric oxide increases calcium efflux from smooth muscle and dephosphorylates myosin; thus smooth muscle contraction is reduced, producing vasodilation. Nitric oxide quickly binds with hemoglobin. When it is inhaled, it can produce selective dilation of the pulmonary vascular bed, because it is inactivated within hemoglobin before it affects SVR.

In many cardiovascular centers, inhaled nitric oxide is provided under research protocol to promote pulmonary vasodilation. It is titrated in concentrations of 10 to 80 parts per million (ppm), although it is generally effective at concentrations of 10 to 20 ppm. Methemoglobinemia may develop as a complication of nitric oxide inhalation; thus the methemoglobin concentration is evaluated on a regular basis and should be kept below 2 g/dl. Vasodilators and phosphodiesterase inhibitors may also be administered to promote pulmonary vasodilation.

For further information regarding manipulation of pulmonary vascular resistance, see Postoperative Care of the Pediatric Cardiopulmonary Surgical Patient.

Specific Guidelines for Management of Hypovolemic Shock   Volume administration is provided until systemic perfusion is adequate or evidence of systemic and pulmonary venous congestion and myocardial dysfunction are observed. Avoid hypotonic fluid, because the portion of the hypotonic fluid that is water will be distributed throughout total body water, leaving little in the vascular space. Patients may require administration of more fluid than was originally lost, since only approximately 25% of administered isotonic colloids or crystalloids will remain in the vascular space.

Evaluate the child's airway, oxygenation (with pulse oximetry), and ventilation, and support as needed. During volume resuscitation, monitor the child's systemic perfusion, urine output, and level of consciousness; all should improve with successful volume resuscitation.

Keep track of all sources of fluid administration. In addition, total all sources of ongoing fluid loss, since these may cause persistent hypovolemia. Fluid and electrolyte balance should also be monitored and maintained.

Specific Guidelines for Management of Cardiogenic Shock   Management of cardiogenic shock requires optimization of ventricular preload through careful manipulation of intravascular fluid volume. This is accomplished with diuretics or fluid administration with isotonic crystalloids or colloids. Attempt to determine the ideal filling pressures for the right and left ventricles.

Cardiac function is optimized through administration of inotropic and vasoactive agents, selected to support ventricular function and redistribute blood flow. Dopamine may be the drug of choice if renal blood flow is compromised, whereas dobutamine may be ideal if the cardiogenic shock is associated with systemic vasoconstriction. Vasodilator therapy may be indicated to reduce impedance to left ventricular ejection or to improve ventricular compliance.

Assess and support the child's airway, oxygenation (via pulse oximetry), and ventilation. Oxygen delivery is maximized through support of hemoglobin concentration, oxygenation, and cardiac output. Oxygen demand is minimized through treatment of pain and fever and maintenance of a warm environment for young infants. Maintain acid-base and electrolyte balance.

Specific Guidelines for Management of Septic Shock

Treatment of septic shock requires prevention and early detection. Any existing source of infection must be eradicated with appropriate antimicrobial agents, administered on time. The goals of cardiorespiratory support are to maximize oxygen delivery and minimize oxygen demand.

The septic patient has hypovolemia relative to the vascular space, caused by both vasodilation and capillary leak. Treatment includes volume administration with isotonic crystalloids and colloids. During volume resuscitation, pulmonary edema is likely to develop, since capillary leak is present. Therefore closely monitor pulmonary function and oxygenation and provide supplementary oxygen, intubation, and ventilatory assistance with PEEP as needed.

Heart rate and ventricular function are supported through administration of beta-adrenergic agents. Vascular tone is supported, as needed to maintain blood pressure, through administration of alpha-adrenergic agents. Combination drugs, such as epinephrine or norepinephrine in combination with low-dose dopamine, may be ideal to prevent excessive reduction in renal blood flow and urine output. Dobutamine may be useful if hypotension is not severe.

Mediator-specific therapy has thus far been ineffective in altering the clinical course of adult patients with sepsis. However, if any of these agents is shown to be effective, they should be administered during the care of the septic patient.

Mechanical Support of Cardiovascular Function

Mechanical support of cardiovascular function may be provided if conventional medical therapy fails to support effective systemic perfusion. Mechanical support can be provided through use of extracorporeal membrane oxygenation (ECMO), an intraaortic balloon pump (IABP), or a left ventricular assist device (LVAD).

Signs of successful mechanical support include elimination of metabolic acidosis, increased urine output, and improved systemic perfusion. The patient will be more responsive (unless sedated), the skin will be warm with brisk capillary refill and strong peripheral pulses, and organ function will improve. As the patient's systemic perfusion improves, mechanical support may be weaned. During weaning, systemic perfusion is closely monitored to ensure tolerance of the weaning. It may be necessary to adjust vasoactive support at this time.

Extracorporeal Membrane Oxygenation ECMO therapy can support cardiac or pulmonary function through use of cardiopulmonary bypass with a membrane oxygenator. This device is most commonly used to treat severe respiratory failure in newborns, but it may also be used to treat acute respiratory failure or cardiac failure in older infants and children. ECMO should be considered for the treatment of acute, reversible cardiac or respiratory failure unresponsive to conventional medical management.

During ECMO therapy, both a nurse and an ECMO technician (who may or may not be a nurse) are present at the bedside at all times. The ECMO technician is responsible for the function of the membrane oxygenator. The bedside nurse works closely with the ECMO technician, keeping the technician apprised of the patient's condition, including systemic perfusion and organ system function. The ECMO technician also keeps the bedside nurse informed regarding the amount of support provided by the oxygenator. Together, the bedside nurse and the ECMO technician make decisions regarding blood sampling and administration, drug administration and titration, and tolerance of any weaning of ECMO support. Mechanical ventilatory support is provided during ECMO therapy to maintain alveolar expansion and some oxygenation via the lungs. Ventilatory support becomes particularly crucial as ECMO support is weaned or if a mechanical failure develops.

ECMO support may be accomplished in several ways. All forms require removal of venous blood from the body, oxygenation and warming of the blood in the oxygenator, and return of the blood to the body. The blood must be anticoagulated to prevent clotting in the circuit. Although heparin-impregnated tubing is available, anticoagulation with heparin is the preferred method of anticoagulation during ECMO.

Venovenous ECMO diverts the patient's venous blood to the oxygenator and then returns the oxygenated blood to the patient's right atrium (or a large vein). This form of ECMO support requires good cardiac function; thus it is generally not used for the treatment of myocardial failure. Although oxygenation is provided by ECMO, all blood flow passes through the heart, and cardiac output is determined by the heart.

Venoarterial ECMO diverts venous blood to the oxygenator and returns the blood to the patient's arterial circulation. This form of ECMO may require little or no cardiac output, but blood delivered to the aorta or a large artery is often nonpulsatile. Therefore pulses are not apparent on the display of arterial waveform. Pulse oximetry may fail to function in the absence of pulses. A pulse generator can be attached to the ECMO circuit, but this is rarely done.

Once cardiac function recovers, ECMO support can be weaned to enable the heart to take over more and more responsibility for cardiac output. As ECMO support is weaned, pulsatile flow should be generated by intrinsic cardiac output.

Anticoagulation therapy during ECMO therapy is accomplished through administration of heparin into the circuit, titrated to maintain the activated clotting time (ACT) at approximately 230 to 260 seconds (normal is approximately 80 to 130 seconds). During ECMO therapy the nurse should monitor the patient closely for evidence of bleeding and monitor neurologic function for evidence of deterioration. These should be reported to a physician immediately.

During ECMO therapy for *children,* mortality is approximately 50%. The vast majority of children who die during ECMO support do so following termination of ECMO when the patient's condition is deemed to be futile. Approximately one third of deaths during ECMO therapy are the result of multiple organ failure, including brain death. A small but significant number of deaths are due to mechanical complications of ECMO, including bleeding and cannula dislodgment; thus the nurse should be prepared to respond to these emergencies.

Left Ventricular Assist Devices Although a variety of LVADs are available for use in adult patients, most are unsuitable for pediatric use because they require displacement of excessive blood volume to fill the device reservoir. Centrifugal LVADs may be used in children; they are relatively simple and inexpensive, and they do not require any filling volume. The centrifugal LVAD uses a conical head that rotates and forces blood centrifugally into the outflow tubing. This LVAD provides nonpulsatile blood flow; thus a constant mean arterial pressure is achieved.

In general, LVADs are inserted through a median sternotomy incision. Standard bypass tubing can be used in cannulation of the centrifugal LVAD. One cannula diverts blood from the apex of the left ventricle through the chest wall and into the pump while the other returns blood into the aorta.

As with ECMO circuits, anticoagulation is required during LVAD therapy, to reduce the risk of thromboembolic complications. As a result, the nurse must monitor the patient closely for signs of bleeding and for signs of systemic emboli, including emboli to the brain, kidneys, or peripheral circulation.

Potential complications of LVAD therapy are similar to those encountered during ECMO therapy and include bleeding, thromboembolic complications, infection, and mechanical failure. Thromboembolic complications and organ system effects of nonpulsatile blood flow limit the use of centrifugal LVADs to short periods. Experience with LVADs in children is extremely limited.

Intraaortic Balloon Pump The IABP is another mechanical circulatory assist device that is frequently used in adult patients with myocardial failure but has been used infrequently in children. The IABP uses an elongated balloon that is usually threaded in a retrograde fashion into the thoracic aorta, just distal to the left subclavian artery branch from the aorta.

Balloon inflation and deflation are timed with the patient's ECG to provide diastolic augmentation of blood flow. Since the child's heart rate is typically very rapid, the pump must be outfitted with a special pediatric cassette, pediatric balloon, and helium inflation cartridge for use in children.

The balloon inflates during ventricular and aortic diastole, to augment diastolic flow. This increases mean arterial pressure and coronary artery blood flow but may result in reversal of the normal systolic-diastolic relationships. The diastolic curve may actually be higher than the systolic curve on the arterial waveform display. The balloon deflates just before ventricular ejection, to facilitate ventricular ejection.

Potential complications of IABP therapy in children include bleeding, thromboembolic events, infection, leg ischemia, aortic dissection, and decreased mesenteric and renal artery perfusion. Mesenteric ischemia may produce abdominal distension and guaiac-positive stools.

Anticoagulation may be required during therapy, to prevent formation of thromboses around the balloon and catheter. Thrombocytopenia also develops as platelets coat the balloon and catheter. The nurse must monitor the patient closely for evidence of bleeding and must ensure that the balloon is cycling appropriately (either 1:1, 1:2, or 1:3 augmentation with patient's heart rate). The augmentation is usually apparent when the arterial waveform is monitored. IABP therapy has been used for a limited number of pediatric patients, with limited success.

Psychosocial Support of the Child and Family
The child in shock requires excellent medical and nursing management. Health care personnel are constantly surrounding the bedside to evaluate or treat the child. The gravity of the child's condition and the complexity of care can be overwhelming for the staff and even more threatening for the child and family.

Provide the parents with essential information without overwhelming them with details. Assume that the child can hear everything said at the bedside, even if the child is receiving sedatives. Address the child by name and always prepare the child before any touch, and certainly before any painful procedure. Provide adequate sedation and analgesia.

Parents will require frequent briefings on the status of the child, particularly when the child's condition is unstable. It is helpful to record specific terms used with the parents in the nursing Kardex to enable use of consistent terminology.

Encourage the parents to visit as much as possible and to touch the child. The nurses and physicians should touch the child frequently and gently, since this will comfort the child and the parents.

Cardiopulmonary Arrest and Cardiopulmonary Resuscitation

Etiology

Cardiopulmonary arrest in children often represents the end point of progressive deterioration in respiratory or cardiovascular function. In *adults* cardiac arrest may be a *sudden* event, resulting from a myocardial infarction and sudden arrhythmia. In *children* cardiac arrest is often a *secondary* event, the consequence of progressive shock, respiratory failure, or cardiorespiratory failure.

Cardiopulmonary arrest can be precipitated by respiratory arrest, with secondary development of hypoxic bradycardia. If the child with respiratory arrest receives prompt and skilled support of oxygenation and ventilation, cardiac arrest may actually be prevented.

A common cause of out-of-hospital cardiac arrest during the first year of life is sudden infant death syndrome. The most common cause of out-of-hospital cardiac arrest beyond infancy is trauma, including near-drowning. Many of these childhood injury deaths can be prevented with relatively simple injury prevention strategies.

Most episodes of cardiopulmonary arrest in children occur in or around the home. For this reason, parents and those responsible for the care of children (e.g., child care workers) should learn cardiopulmonary resuscitation (CPR) and injury prevention.

Unexpected cardiac arrest should be rare in the hospital. If respiratory deterioration and cardiovascular deterioration are detected and support is provided, many cardiac arrests will be avoided. In the critical care unit, oxygenation and ventilation should be supported; thus hypoxic respiratory arrest should be uncommon. As a result, cardiac arrest may be the most common form of arrest seen in the ICU.

Sudden cardiac arrhythmias may cause cardiopulmonary arrest. These arrhythmias are most commonly observed in children with CHD, myocarditis, cardiomyopathy, drug toxicity, or electrolyte imbalances.

Cardiopulmonary *arrest* will be observed in every patient who dies. Cardiopulmonary *resuscitation,* the attempt to reverse death and restore life, should *not* be attempted for every child who dies in the hospital. It is extremely important to evaluate each patient at risk for cardiopulmonary arrest. Potential limitation or prevention of resuscitative efforts should be discussed among members of the health care team, with the child (if age appropriate), and with the parents.

Pathophysiology

In *adults,* when sudden cardiac arrest occurs, sinus rhythm converts to sudden ventricular tachycardia and, ultimately, ventricular fibrillation. Thus, up until the moment of arrest, all organs, including the brain, are well perfused. If bystander CPR and (most important) early defibrillation are provided, adult survival from prehospital cardiac arrest may be 50% or higher.

Cardiopulmonary arrest in *children* is often gradual, rather than sudden, and is associated with hypoxia and hypercarbia. When terminal cardiac rhythm is documented in children, the terminal cardiac rhythm is most often bradycardia, which progresses to asystole. Thus, even before arrest develops, most organs have suffered a hypoxic insult. Even if skilled resuscitation is provided following pulseless cardiac arrest, survival averages 10% or less, and most survivors are neurologically devastated.

Only approximately 7% to 15% of children who experience prehospital cardiac arrest demonstrate ventricular tachycardia or ventricular fibrillation on initial evaluation. In some studies survival is higher in these children than in those presenting

with asystole. However, since these patients constitute only a small percentage of children who experience out-of-hospital cardiac arrest, it can be difficult to identify these patients. If automated external defibrillators (AEDs) prove to be accurate in interpreting pediatric rhythms, they may provide a helpful adjunct to the assessment and treatment of children in prehospital cardiac arrest.

Arrhythmias that may portend the development of cardiac arrest include malignant ventricular arrhythmias, including ventricular tachycardia, frequent or multiform premature ventricular contractions, complete heart block, or progressive bradycardia (including a relative bradycardia—a heart rate inappropriately low for the patient's clinical condition).

Clinical Presentation

The prearrest conditions of the child may include shock or respiratory failure. As a result, these must be recognized and treated. Airway, breathing, and circulation must be assessed in sequence when initially encountering the child at risk for cardiorespiratory deterioration and arrest (Figure 5-9)

Airway   Assess airway patency. In addition, determine if the child is capable of sustaining airway patency without assistance. If the child's ability to maintain an airway is in doubt, consider intubation.

Potential causes of airway obstruction include obstruction of the pharynx with the tongue, development of upper airway edema, or obstruction of the airway with secretions. Neurologic deterioration, anesthesia, or head injury depresses respiratory drive and compromises airway protective mechanisms such as cough and gag. Finally, injuries or conditions likely to produce progressive airway edema (e.g., smoke inhalation) may require intervention even if airway obstruction is not currently present.

When evaluating airway patency, the child's respiratory effort should be evaluated. Intubation should be provided well before oxygenation is compromised, based on evaluation of the child's respiratory effort.

Breathing   The effectiveness of the child's ventilation must be assessed. Signs of *potential* respira-

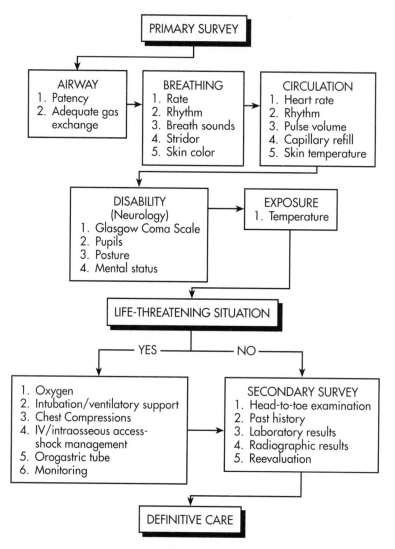

Figure 5-9 Initial evaluation of the child. (From Nichols DG et al: *Golden hour: the handbook of advanced pediatric life support,* ed 2, St Louis, 1996, Mosby.)

tory failure should be recognized and support provided before any arterial blood gas analysis is completed. If the child fails to respond to initial therapy or if the child deteriorates further despite intervention, a diagnosis of *actual* respiratory failure is made. The diagnosis of actual respiratory failure usually includes arterial blood gas analysis.

Potential respiratory failure is characterized by inappropriate respiratory effort (either excessive or inadequate) for clinical condition, altered level of consciousness, reduced air movement, or hypoxemia per pulse oximetry. If the child with potential respiratory failure fails to improve with initial supportive measures or deteriorates further, actual respiratory failure is present.

Actual respiratory failure is present when the child demonstrates hypoxemia despite oxygen administration, hypercarbia with acidosis, evidence

---

Box 5-16

Clinical Signs of Potential and Actual Respiratory Failure

Signs of Potential Respiratory Failure

Tachypnea
Increased respiratory effort
   Severe retractions
   Nasal flaring
   Stridor or wheezing
   Head bobbing in infant
   Grunting
Depressed level of consciousness
   Decreased responsiveness (including decreased response to painful stimulus)
   Irritability
   Lethargy
Inadequate air movement
   Weak cry
   Decreased chest expansion or breath sounds
Hypoxemia per pulse oximetry

Signs of Actual Respiratory Failure

Apnea or gasping
Bradycardia, poor systemic perfusion
Hypoxemia despite supplemental oxygen therapy
Hypercarbia with acidosis
Increasing intrapulmonary shunt
   Rising alveolar-arterial oxygen gradient (>25-50 mm Hg)
   Falling Pao_2/Fio_2 ratio (<180-240 mm Hg)
   Rising oxygenation index (>10)
Decreased air movement, weak cry

---

of a significant intrapulmonary shunt, and evidence of excessive respiratory effort with fatigue or inadequate respiratory effort (Box 5-16).

Circulation Cardiac arrest is present when asystole or collapse rhythms develop and central arterial pulses are not palpable. This is *not* the same as hypotension or bradycardia, which are *prearrest* conditions.

One of the prearrest circulatory conditions is shock. Signs of shock include tachycardia, poor peripheral perfusion (including delayed capillary refill despite a warm ambient temperature, diminished peripheral pulses, and oliguria), irritability or lethargy, and metabolic acidosis. The child's skin may be mottled, pale, or gray. Note that hypotension may be only a very *late* sign of decompensated shock in children and may not be present until cardiovascular arrest is imminent. For more complete information regarding recognition and management of shock in children, see Shock.

Management

An essential element in the management of all critically ill children is the anticipation of deterioration and preparation for necessary support. As part of morning and evening rounds, the critical care team should discuss potential causes and signs of deterioration in every patient and review plans for each potential problem. If and when the child deteriorates, the team should be prepared to respond quickly and skillfully.

The goals of resuscitation are to ensure an effective airway, oxygenation, and ventilation, and to restore adequate heart rate and systemic perfusion. These fundamental aspects of therapy provide the framework for resuscitative efforts. Assessment must be performed constantly, and reassessment must be performed after each intervention, to evaluate patient response (see Figure 5-9). Throughout resuscitation of infants and children, 100% oxygen is provided.

Emergency equipment should always be readily available; a hand ventilator bag and mask and an oxygen source (with necessary flowmeter and tubing) should be present at every bedside. When cardiorespiratory distress is present or arrest is suspected to be imminent, oxygen should be administered immediately. The child's airway, breathing, and circulation should then be assessed and supported.

Resuscitation efforts for the child in pulseless cardiac arrest should not continue indefinitely. If the child fails to respond to conventional resuscitation techniques within approximately 10 minutes (and two doses of epinephrine), unusual causes are sought and eliminated if found, and consideration should be given to termination of efforts. Occasionally prolonged resuscitation is indicated for the child with electrolyte imbalance or unusual drug interaction; most often these conditions produce an arrhythmic arrest. However, asystolic cardiac arrest is typically hypoxemic and hypercarbic, and the likelihood of survival diminishes dramatically if the normothermic child fails to respond to 10 minutes of resuscitation and two doses of epinephrine. Resuscitation is unlikely to be successful for near-drowning victims if there is no response despite normothermia and total resuscitation efforts of 25 minutes or longer.

Sequence of Resuscitation Resuscitation should proceed in an orderly fashion. A team leader should immediately take charge and ensure performance of critical interventions according to priority. Ideally, two to three nurses and two to three physicians are involved in the resuscitation, and several tasks are performed simultaneously (Box 5-17). The team leader should not perform the tasks but should delegate responsibility for the tasks and ensure that they are performed.

Once pulseless cardiac arrest has occurred, resuscitation focuses on establishment of oxygenation and ventilation, chest compressions, and restoration of an effective heart rate and rhythm and systemic perfusion. Guidelines for the sequence of resuscitation from pulseless arrest have been published by the American Heart Association (Figure 5-10).

Oxygen Administration and Assessment of Effort
If the child's spontaneous respiratory effort is adequate but hypoxemia is present (as indicated by

---

Box 5-17

Suggested Responsibilities of Team Members During Resuscitation

Nurse 1

Begins cardiopulmonary resuscitation (CPR); continues unless/until relieved. Directs other team members regarding tasks until relived by Physician 1. When relieved of CPR duties, remains at head of bed to assess patient and assist with intubation, medication administration.

Nurse 2

Summons help and brings cart into room. Begins to assemble initial resuscitation equipment and medications (e.g., provides bag-valve-mask to Nurse 1 if none at bedside; prepares equipment to establish IV access or intubate; begins to draw up epinephrine, atropine).

Nurse 3

Scribe. Must determine single clock to use to time and record all "code" events. Reminds Physician 1 of timing and intervals since last "round" of medications.

Potential Nurse 4

"Runner" for supplies, calls to laboratory or radiology. May also be designated communicator with parents (negotiated with Nurse 1 and Physician 1).

Physician 1

Directs code. Directs team members and monitors actions. Assesses patient. Responsible for ventilation and intubation or may direct others. Determines selection, timing of drug administration. Communicates with family. "Calls" the code if needed.

Physician 2

If ventilation and intubation are performed by others, will establish IV or intraosseous access. Also provides backup for determination of cause of arrest or reasons resuscitation was ineffective.

Respiratory Therapist

Often assumes responsibility for bag-valve-mask ventilation on arrival. Assists with establishment and monitoring of ventilation and intubation. May establish noninvasive monitoring (e.g., end-tidal carbon dioxide), or draw blood gases.

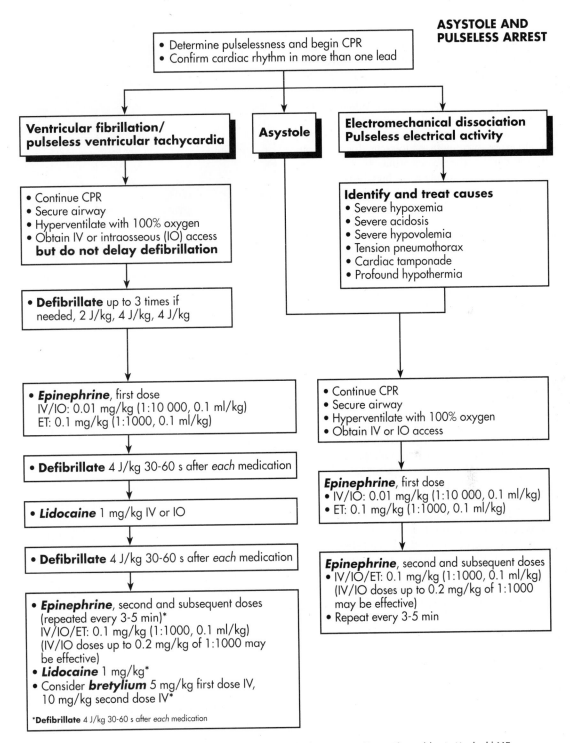

Figure 5-10 Decision tree for asystole and pulseless arrest. (From Chameides L, Hazinski MF, editors: *Pediatric advanced life support*, Dallas, 1997, American Heart Association.)

pulse oximetry), oxygen administration may succeed in correcting the hypoxemia. However, the child's airway and respiratory effort must be carefully evaluated, and intubation with mechanical ventilation must be provided if either is inadequate. If hypercarbia is associated with acidosis, mechanical ventilation is required, and oxygen administration alone or even with endotracheal intubation will not correct the hypercarbia. If respiratory fatigue is present or spontaneous breathing effort is inadequate, bag-valve-mask ventilation with 100% oxygen must be provided.

Airway   If the child is in a prearrest condition, positioning may be used to open the airway. If the airway is obstructed with secretions, suctioning is indicated. A nasopharyngeal airway is a soft plastic tube that can be inserted to facilitate suctioning of the nasopharynx. These airways can help to maintain airway patency, but they can become obstructed with secretions or can kink.

If the child is unconscious but breathing with some signs of airway obstruction, an oropharyngeal airway can be inserted to maintain an airway. These airways should *not* be inserted if the child is conscious, because they can induce gagging and vomiting. The proper size of an oropharyngeal airway is selected by placing the airway next to the face with the flange next to the corner of the mouth. An airway of proper length will reach the angle of the jaw.

If respiratory arrest has occurred, ventilation is provided with a bag-valve-mask device, using 100% oxygen. If the child demonstrates any spontaneous respiratory effort, the ventilation with bag and mask should be synchronized with the child's respiratory efforts. All nurses, respiratory therapists, and physicians involved in the care of critically ill children should be proficient in provision of bag-valve-mask ventilation (Figure 5-11). Ventilation should be provided to ensure bilateral chest expansion and good breath sounds.

Gastric distension may develop during bag-valve-mask ventilation. This distension may compromise diaphragm movement and may result in regurgitation and aspiration. If the child is unconscious, application of pressure over the cricoid cartilage (the Sellick maneuver) can prevent air entry into the esophagus and stomach during ventilation. A nasogastric tube should be inserted to decompress the stomach.

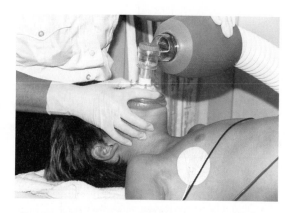

Figure 5-11   Bag-valve-mask ventilation. The chin/jaw is lifted as ventilation is provided to ensure that the airway remains open and that a good seal is made by the mask around the patient's nose and mouth. If this form of ventilation is effective, the chest should rise bilaterally during every inspiration. (From Hazinski MF: *Nursing care of the critically ill child,* ed 2, St Louis, 1992, Mosby.)

Intubation   In the hospital setting or during prehospital care by skilled providers, intubation with an endotracheal tube is the method of choice for establishment and maintenance of an airway. Intubation should be strongly considered for the following conditions:

- Respiratory arrest or apnea
- Significant functional or anatomic airway obstruction with increased work of breathing
- Inability to maintain airway (including actual or anticipated obstruction due to secretions or inflammation)
- Neurologic deterioration associated with decreased responsiveness
- Increased intracranial pressure
- Need for mechanical ventilatory support
- Need for prolonged transport or diagnostic studies in unstable patient

Whenever possible, intubation should be accomplished as an *elective* procedure with the most skilled personnel at the bedside. All necessary equipment and drugs should be assembled at the bedside before the intubation attempt (Box 5-18). The child's heart rate and pulse oximetry

Box 5-18

Equipment Required for Intubation

Cardiac monitor with audible QRS tone

Bag, mask, and oxygen source

Endotracheal (ET) tube (estimated size for body length and age and tubes 0.5 mm larger and smaller)

Laryngoscope blade and handle (and extra bulbs)

Infant: 0-1 straight blade
Small child: 1 straight blade
Child (12-22 kg): 2 straight or curved blade
Large child (24-30 kg): 2-3 straight or curved blade
Adolescent (32-34 kg): 3 straight or curved blade

Stylet

Children 3-17 kg: 6 French
Children >17 kg: 14 French

Suction equipment

Wall or portable suction
Appropriate catheter to pass easily through ET tube (usually the next French size above twice the ET tube size in millimeters should pass readily into an ET tube >3 mm)
Tonsillar suction or 12-14 French suction catheter

Nasogastric tube

Tape, benzoin, water-soluble lubricant

Gloves and goggles

Paralyzing agents, sedatives, vagolytics, lidocaine

Magill forceps for nasotracheal intubation

Modified from Hazinski MF: *Nursing care of the critically ill child*, ed 2, St Louis, 1992, Mosby.

Endotracheal tube size can be estimated from the child's age (beyond 1 year of age) using the following formula:

$$\text{mm ET tube size} = \frac{Age\ (years)}{4} + 4$$

A length-based resuscitation tape such as the Broselow tape (marketed by Armstrong) may also be used to determine proper endotracheal tube size.

A large suction catheter should be available during intubation to suction at the level of the vocal cords. In addition, a suction catheter that will fit into the endotracheal tube should also be available. This French suction catheter size can be estimated by doubling the endotracheal millimeter tube size and selecting the next largest French catheter (catheter sizes can also be estimated using a length-based resuscitation tape such as the Broselow tape).

During intubation the child's heart rate is monitored continuously with a bedside monitor, preferably with audible QRS tone so that the child's heart rate is "heard." The child's hemoglobin saturation is monitored by pulse oximetry, and color is observed throughout the intubation attempt. The child is well oxygenated and ventilated before any attempt, and the attempt should be interrupted to provide additional oxygenation and ventilation if the child's heart rate or hemoglobin saturation falls significantly or if the child's color deteriorates.

Once the tube is inserted, tube position should be immediately verified by clinical examination. Breath sounds and chest expansion should be equal bilaterally. Appropriate depth of insertion of the endotracheal tube is estimated by the following formula:

mm ET tube size $\times$ 3
$\qquad$ = Approximate cm insertion depth of tube

A chest x-ray film is obtained when possible to verify proper tube position (see Chapter 7). The tube should be at the level of the third rib, or approximately 1 to 2 cm above the carina. Once the proper position is verified, the tube should be marked with an indelible marker at the patient's lip, the centimeter marking at the lip should be noted on the nursing Kardex, and the tube should be taped in place.

hemoglobin saturation are monitored continuously. Some sedation and neuromuscular blockade is generally used, and rapid-sequence intubation is used if the child has a full stomach (see Chapter 3).

Insertion of the endotracheal tube establishes a patent airway unless small airway obstruction is present. Following intubation, oxygenation and ventilation must also be established, and location and patency of the airway must be reassessed frequently. Causes of acute deterioration in the intubated child include tube displacement or obstruction, pneumothorax, or equipment failure.

Breathing/Ventilation   Ventilation is provided during resuscitation, initially with a bag-valve-mask device and then through an endotracheal tube. Hand ventilation should provide sufficient volume to produce visible chest expansion; this should enable effective elimination of carbon dioxide. However, when cardiac arrest occurs, pulmonary blood flow is dramatically curtailed; thus the amount of exhaled carbon dioxide eliminated by the lungs may be minimal, and an end-tidal CO_2 monitor may register very low $ETCO_2$.

Hand ventilation is provided during resuscitation. If the child is successfully stabilized, ventilation can be accomplished mechanically. At that time, arterial blood gas analysis is used to guide ventilator settings and adjustments.

Circulation   Cardiac compressions are indicated for cardiopulmonary arrest, severe hypotension, or extreme bradycardia associated with signs of poor systemic perfusion unresponsive to oxygenation and ventilation. For infants, compressions are provided at a rate greater than 100/min, approximately 1 finger-breath below the nipple line. For children, compressions are provided at a rate of approximately 100/min over the lower half of the sternum. The xiphoid process should be avoided.

The optimal depth of compression for infants and children is unknown. In general, the chest is compressed approximately one half to two thirds the depth of the chest. Pulses should be palpable during chest compressions, but arterial pulsations may be impossible to distinguish from venous pulsations. If an arterial line is in place, effectiveness of chest compressions may be verified by the intraarterial pressure and pressure waveform.

Cardiac compressions produce only a small percentage of normal cardiac output. If resuscitation of the normothermic patient is not successful within 10 to 20 minutes and after two or more doses of epinephrine, the outcome is likely to be poor unless unusual extenuating circumstances are present (e.g., electrolyte imbalance).

Support of Heart Rate   Symptomatic *bradycardia* is a heart rate that is too low for age and clinical condition and is associated with a compromise in systemic perfusion. Since hypoxia is the most common cause of symptomatic bradycardia in infants and children, it should be ruled out. Chest compressions are indicated for a heart rate <60/min associated with poor systemic perfusion. If bradycardia continues despite effective support of oxygenation and ventilation, pharmacologic therapy with epinephrine or atropine is required. The cause of the bradycardia should be determined and eliminated, and pacing may be needed (Figure 5-12).

Extreme *tachycardia* can also compromise systemic perfusion. If tachycardia results in a loss of pulses, it should be treated as pulseless arrest (see Figure 5-10). However, if pulses are maintained, then the treatment is determined by the type of tachycardia that is present. The QRS width is used to distinguish narrow-complex from wide-complex tachycardia in an attempt to differentiate between supraventricular and ventricular tachycardia (Figure 5-13). Narrow-complex tachycardia can be either sinus tachycardia or SVT. Sinus tachycardia requires no treatment, since it is a symptom of a problem rather than the cause, but the cause should be identified and treated. SVT associated with poor perfusion is treated with adenosine (if IV access is available or can be established quickly) or cardioversion. Adenosine must be delivered by rapid IV push at the IV port closest to the patient, and followed by a flush. Ventricular tachycardia with pulses is treated with cardioversion (see Defibrillation and Cardioversion).

Vascular Access   If oxygenation and ventilation are supported and chest compressions are provided, vascular access should be established as quickly as possible to provide a route for IV drug administration. Vascular access should be achieved in the largest vein possible as quickly as possible. Ideally, this will be a central vein above the level of the diaphragm, since this route of administration provides the most rapid delivery of drugs to the heart.

If IV access cannot be achieved quickly in the child up to 6 years of age, an intraosseous needle should be inserted in the anterior medial aspect of

BRADYCARDIA

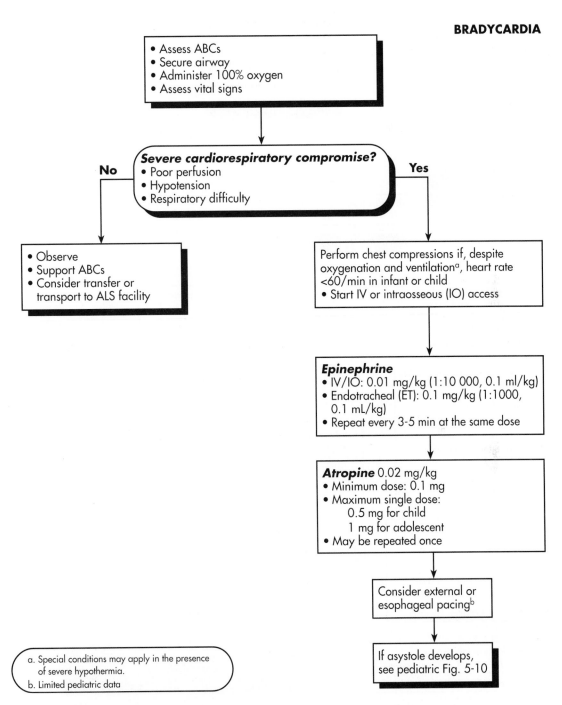

Figure 5-12 American Heart Association decision tree for treatment of symptomatic bradycardia in children. Treatment focuses on support of oxygenation and ventilation, with drug therapy and chest compressions provided as needed. (From Chameides L, Hazinski MF, editors: *Textbook of pediatric advanced life support,* Dallas, 1997, American Heart Association, p 7-8.)

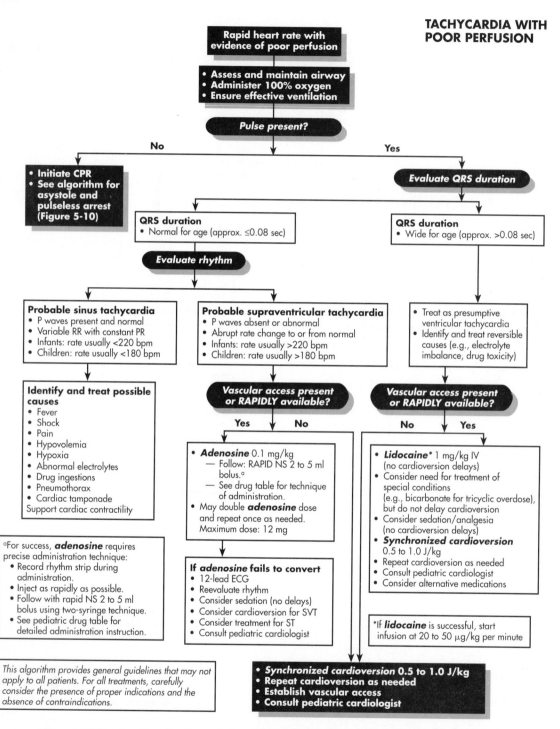

Figure 5-13 American Heart Association algorithm for treatment of tachycardia associated with poor systemic perfusion in children. (From Hazinski MF, Cummins RO: *1997-1999 handbook of emergency cardiovascular care,* Dallas, 1997, American Heart Association, p 45-46.)

the tibia. The intraosseous route provides access to a noncollapsible venous plexus during resuscitation and provides delivery of drugs to the heart in a time equivalent to central venous administration.

Each resuscitation team should follow a protocol for establishment of vascular access. If vascular access is not achieved within 90 seconds or three attempts at insertion (whichever comes first), intraosseous access is attempted if the child is 6 years old or younger, and central venous access or saphenous vein cutdown is attempted if the child is older than 6 years.

Endotracheal Drug Administration The IV route is preferred for all drugs other than oxygen. However, until IV access is achieved, some drugs can be administered by endotracheal route, specifically epinephrine, atropine, naloxone, and lidocaine (the first letters of these drugs can form the word *lean,* although this word does not indicate proper sequence of administration).

The correct endotracheal resuscitation doses of epinephrine, atropine, naloxone, and lidocaine have not yet been established. A "high" dose of epinephrine (0.1 ml of 1:1000 dilution, for a dose of 0.1 mg/kg) is currently recommended by the American Heart Association for delivery by the endotracheal route. This recommendation was made after a single adult human resuscitation study documented low serum epinephrine levels when standard IV doses were administered.

The American Heart Association currently recommends that the IV dose of other resuscitation drugs administered by the endotracheal route be considered the minimum dose of the drug by the endotracheal route. It may be necessary to increase dosage by two to three times when the drug is administered by the endotracheal route.

When drugs are administered by the endotracheal route, they should be diluted to a minimum volume of 3 to 5 ml and then instilled into the tube. After drug instillation, several breaths with a hand ventilator should be provided to encourage distribution of the drug into the tracheobronchial tree.

Intravenous/Intraosseous Drug Administration Oxygen is the first drug administered during resuscitation. Epinephrine should be the second drug and the first IV drug administered during resuscitation. Epinephrine is the most important IV drug during resuscitation, and it should be administered every 3 to 5 minutes during resuscitation of pulseless cardiac arrest.

Epinephrine is the ideal drug for use in resuscitation, because it provides both alpha- and beta-adrenergic effects. It increases SVR and can improve systolic, diastolic and coronary artery perfusion pressure, increasing blood flow to the heart and brain. Beta-adrenergic effects increase cardiac automaticity, heart rate, ventricular contractility, SVR, and blood pressure. It is thus the drug of choice for the treatment of symptomatic bradycardia, pulseless arrest, and severe hypotension.

Epinephrine should be administered by the IV route. Because the outcome of pulseless cardiac arrest in children has been so dismal, since 1992 the American Heart Association has suggested use of a "high" dose of epinephrine (0.1 mg/kg or 0.1 ml/kg of 1:1000 solution) if the initial "standard" dose of IV epinephrine (0.01 mg/kg or 0.1 ml/kg of 1:10,000 solution) is ineffective. The first IV dose administered is the "standard" dose, and second and subsequent doses may be "high" doses. If initial dose(s) of the drug are administered by the endotracheal route, the first IV dose provided is the "standard" dose.

A continuous epinephrine infusion may be administered at a dose of 0.1 to 1 μg/kg/min. This infusion may produce both chronotropic and inotropic effects if spontaneous perfusion is restored.

Atropine administration may be considered in the treatment of pulseless arrest, although there are no data that it is effective. Atropine is a vagolytic agent, and it also may be used in conjunction with epinephrine for the treatment of symptomatic bradycardia unresponsive to oxygenation and ventilation, particularly if vagal stimulation (e.g., following suctioning) was thought to contribute to the bradycardia.

The dose of atropine is 0.02 mg/kg. However, a minimum dose of 0.1 mg is recommended, since rebound bradycardia may result from extremely small doses. The maximum dose is 0.5 mg for a child and 1 mg for an adolescent. The dose may be repeated in 5 minutes for a maximum total dose of 1 mg for a child and 2 mg for an adolescent.

Glucose and calcium administration may be considered during resuscitation for *documented* deficiencies in these electrolytes. Routine administration of these electrolytes is not recommended during resuscitation.

Sodium bicarbonate or other buffers are not first-line resuscitation drugs but may be administered as part of prolonged resuscitation or to treat metabolic acidosis encountered during prearrest conditions. However, these drugs are not routinely used during resuscitation. Restoration of oxygenation, ventilation, and effective systemic perfusion will correct metabolic acidosis more efficiently than buffering agents. In addition, the buffering action of sodium bicarbonate can actually contribute to worsening of respiratory acidosis and may depress myocardial function. Bicarbonate may be indicated for hyperkalemia or tricyclic overdose.

Defibrillation and Cardioversion *Defibrillation* is required for the treatment of pulseless ventricular tachycardia or ventricular fibrillation. This defibrillation may be provided through a manual defibrillator or, in children beyond 8 years of age, through use of an AED. When manual defibrillators are used, the health care provider applies the pad/electrodes, assesses the rhythm, and selects and delivers the defibrillation "dose" (2 J/kg for the first shock, then 4 J/kg if second or subsequent shocks are required). If an AED is used for children 8 years of age or older, the health care provider applies the electrodes, and the microprocessor in the AED analyzes the rhythm, determines if a shock is indicated, charges, and waits for a signal from the operator to deliver the shock.

When pulseless ventricular tachycardia or ventricular fibrillation is present, up to three shocks are delivered in succession if the arrhythmia persists (see Figure 5-10). If the three shocks are ineffective, then chest compressions are resumed and epinephrine is provided, followed within 30 to 60 seconds by defibrillation. If that is ineffective, lidocaine (1 mg/kg IV) is administered, followed within 30 to 60 seconds by defibrillation. This regimen of alternating drugs and shocks continues, and bretylium (5 mg/kg IV, then 10 mg/kg IV) may be considered.

The paddles used for defibrillation should be the largest that can be placed on the chest without touching each other. All parts of the electrode or pad should be in complete contact with the chest. In general, infant electrodes are used for infants up to 10 kg or 1 year of age, and "adult" paddles are used for children >10 kg or 1 year of age.

Synchronized cardioversion is used for the treatment of symptomatic SVT (particularly if the SVT is unresponsive to adenosine) and ventricular tachycardia *with* pulses. In synchronized cardioversion the shock provided is timed to coincide with the patient's own QRS complex. The energy dose for synchronized cardioversion is 0.5 J/kg. To synchronize the shock, a "synchronize" button must be triggered on the defibrillator, and either external paddles that "read" the ECG are used or the defibrillator is linked by ECG cable to the bedside monitor or ECG chest electrodes.

Treatment of Electromechanical Dissociation/ Pulseless Electrical Activity Electromechanical dissociation (EMD) is a form of pulseless electrical activity (PEA), characterized by narrow QRS complexes and no pulse. The most common causes of EMD include severe hypoxemia, severe acidosis, severe hypovolemia, tension pneumothorax, cardiac tamponade, profound hypothermia, and electrolyte imbalances. Treatment of EMD requires resuscitation and elimination of the cause.

Postresuscitation Stabilization If the child responds to resuscitative efforts, postresuscitation monitoring is required. Continuous cardiorespiratory monitoring is required, including pulse oximetry and continuous ECG monitoring. Serial assessments of systemic perfusion and neurologic function should be performed until the child is definitely stable/awake. If the child's blood pressure is unstable, continuous arterial pressure monitoring is indicated. Noninvasive oscillometric blood pressure monitoring may *not* be a reliable method of blood pressure monitoring and may overestimate arterial pressure in the hypotensive patient; thus it should not be considered to be reliable when the child is unstable. At the very least, noninvasive monitoring results should be verified using sphygmomanometry, and institution of intraarterial monitoring should be considered. Monitor temperature frequently and use warming devices as needed. Temperature instability should be anticipated in small infants and following near-drowning or neurologic insult.

Humidified oxygen is provided if the child is breathing effectively spontaneously, and mechanical ventilation is required if oxygenation or ventilation is inadequate. Respiratory failure and shock should be treated if they are present. Acute respiratory distress syndrome may develop following cardiopulmonary arrest and resuscitation; thus its development should be anticipated and appropriate treatment instituted as needed (see Chapter 6). Organ systems should be assessed and supported if organ system failure develops.

Two large-bore functioning IV catheters should be inserted. An arterial catheter should be inserted if continuous arterial pressure monitoring is required. A nasogastric tube is inserted and the child should receive nothing by mouth for several hours until the child's condition can be thoroughly assessed.

Laboratory evaluation should include measurement of arterial blood gases (with appropriate adjustment in ventilatory support), serum electrolytes, calcium, glucose, and hematocrit.

The cause of the cardiorespiratory arrest should be determined and corrected to reduce the risk of subsequent arrests. Transportation to a PICU should be considered, particularly if organ system failure is present or the child is unstable.

Support of the Parents and Family The parents should be notified when CPR is necessary. If at all possible, one member of the health care team should be responsible for communication with the family at regular intervals during the resuscitation efforts. It is also essential that the number of health care members communicating with the family be limited so that consistent messages can be provided to the family.

Regular communication from the team can help prepare the family if efforts are unsuccessful. For example, the family may initially be told that the child's heart stopped but that the physicians and nurses are providing oxygen and chest compression. If resuscitation is unsuccessful, the family may be told that the physicians and nurses have provided all of the most common drugs known to be effective and the heart still has not responded. At this point, it may be helpful to express to the family concern about the effects of the arrest on the brain and brain function. If the resuscitation efforts continue to be unsuccessful, the family may be told that the child's heart has failed to respond to any of the drugs available to the physicians and the nurses. At this point, the family is somewhat prepared to hear that resuscitation efforts have been terminated.

In any discussion, refer to the child by name. Allow the family to ask questions and to make suggestions during the resuscitation. Family members may wish to be present during part of resuscitation, or they may wish to hold the child after resuscitation efforts have ceased (see Chapter 4).

If resuscitation efforts are unsuccessful, the child and bed space should be made as clean as possible for the parents' last visit with the child. If tubes must remain in place (e.g., for postmortem examination), the family should be prepared for the sight of the tubes. Family members should be allowed a private time with the child after death.

If the resuscitation is successful, the family should be allowed to spend as much time as possible with the child after the resuscitation to reassure themselves that the child is alive. The cause of the arrest and treatment plan should be explained in simple terms, and this information should be reinforced by all members of the health care team. If the child's prognosis is guarded, this should be carefully and consistently explained to the parents.

Arrhythmias

Etiology

Arrhythmias can result from CHD or its surgical correction, hypoxia, electrolyte or acid-base imbalances, drug toxicity, or myocardial injury. Arrhythmias can be symptomatic or asymptomatic; they may require urgent treatment or produce symptoms or have the potential to deteriorate into symptomatic arrhythmias.

The three most common types of clinically significant pediatric arrhythmias are bradyarrhythmias, tachyarrhythmias, and those producing collapse (loss of pulses). Hypoxia and heart block are the most common causes of bradyarrhythmias. SVT with aberrant/accessory intraatrial conduction pathways is probably the most common cause of pediatric tachyarrhythmias. Sinus tachycardia is another form of tachycardia that is not an arrhythmia but an indication that a high heart rate and cardiac output are needed. Collapse rhythms include ventricular tachycardia and ventricular fibrillation. These rhythms may indicate ventricular irritability secondary to hypoxia, acidosis, significant hyperkalemia or hypokalemia, anomalous atrioventricular (AV) conduction pathways, myocarditis, cardiomyopathy, or creation of an irritable focus during cardiovascular surgery.

Complete heart block may be congenital in origin (it may be observed in children with L-transposition), or it may result from infectious or inflammatory disease of the heart. Heart block following cardiovascular surgery can result from direct trauma to the conduction system (e.g., during placement of a ventricular septal patch or replacement of a valve) or from edema or other inflammatory reactions near the sutures. Heart block in nonsurgical patients can result from electrolyte imbalance, myocarditis, or cardiomyopathy. Some forms of heart block are congenital in origin.

Pathophysiology

Arrhythmias resulting from hypoxia typically are bradyarrhythmias, although premature ventricular contractions and ventricular tachycardia may develop if the myocardium is ischemic. Hypoxia/ischemia impairs function of the sodium-potassium pump, results in a decrease in the magnitude of the transmembrane potential, and slows myocardial conduction time. These changes may contribute to a slowing of the heart rate, as well as an increased potential for ectopy.

Acidosis reduces the rate of spontaneous pacemaker firing and the rate of diastolic depolarization. Severe hypercapnia may also increase ectopy.

Arrhythmias associated with drug toxicity or electrolyte imbalances result from alteration in the transmembrane electrolyte concentration difference. A change in serum potassium will alter the magnitude of the transmembrane potential itself. A change in serum sodium or calcium concentration can change the magnitude or duration of the action potential. Calcium imbalances can change contractility by affecting intramyocardial calcium movement.

Bradyarrhythmias   Bradycardia is a heart rate <100 beats/min in the infant and <60 beats/min in the child. If a heart rate that is normal for age occurs in a child with poor systemic perfusion, it constitutes a relative bradycardia. *The heart rate should always be evaluated in light of the child's age and clinical condition.*

Bradycardia can compromise systemic perfusion because it slows the ventricular rate; unless

stroke volume increases commensurate with the decrease in heart rate, cardiac output will fall. Bradycardia is often associated with a proportional fall in cardiac output. An additional consequence of a fall in heart rate is that more time is available for ectopic foci (e.g., an irritable ventricular focus) to take control of the cardiac rhythm. Bradyarrhythmias result most commonly from hypoxia, vagal stimulation (e.g., during suctioning), dysfunction of the sinus node, or heart block.

Tachyarrhythmias   Tachycardia is defined as a heart rate >200 to 250 beats/min in the infant and >160 beats/min in the child over 5 years of age. Although the heart rate can increase transiently during fever or episodes of crying, the term *tachycardia* is reserved for significant and persistent increases in heart rate.

Tachycardia can be a normal response to stress (e.g., pain) or to increased oxygen requirements, as in the case of sinus tachycardia. Sinus tachycardia may also be a normal response to a compromise in cardiovascular function, such as CHF. Although tachycardia can be normal and compensatory, extremely high heart rates can be associated with a fall in stroke volume and cardiac output.

Tachycardias can compromise perfusion because they reduce ventricular diastolic filling time. In addition, since the left coronary artery perfuses the left ventricle almost exclusively during diastole, a rapid heart rate will reduce coronary artery perfusion time. If the tachycardia develops from below the AV node (junctional tissue), the ventricles may be depolarized without receiving the final 25% to 30% of ventricular filling produced by atrial systole. This may be associated with a significant fall in stroke volume.

SVT is not a normal response to stress and can produce a ventricular rate that is so rapid that cardiac output falls. Ventricular tachycardia compromises ventricular diastolic filling time and stroke volume, and it eliminates synchrony between atrial and ventricular depolarization (and contraction); thus stroke volume falls dramatically. Tachyarrhythmias result from reentrant pathways (such as those responsible for some episodes of SVT) or from areas of increased automaticity.

Heart Block   Heart block is present when there is a delay or prevention of the conduction of electrical impulses through the intracardiac conduction tissue. When this occurs, the impulse must bypass the area of block; thus conduction intervals are prolonged. Heart block can be characterized as first-degree, second-degree, or third-degree heart block based on the magnitude of delay in the conduction of impulses.

Heart block can result in slowing of the ventricular rate, and complete heart block results in loss of synchrony between atrial and ventricular depolarization. Each form of heart block is presented briefly under Clinical Presentation.

Clinical Presentation

Arrhythmias may result from a wide variety of clinical insults and can produce a wide variety of ECG patterns and clinical sequelae (Table 5-15). *Whenever any arrhythmia is detected, its effect on systemic perfusion must be determined.* Arrhythmias that compromise systemic perfusion or that may deteriorate into malignant arrhythmias must be treated immediately, whereas those that do not compromise systemic perfusion can be evaluated on more of an elective basis.

Principles of Assessment Assessment of the child with an arrhythmia requires a logical approach with emphasis on evaluating the effects of the rhythm on systemic perfusion. The following principles are essential:

- Determine the effects of the arrhythmia on systemic perfusion.
- Support systemic perfusion as needed.
- Remember that patients with underlying heart disease will be less tolerant of arrhythmias than patients with normal cardiovascular structure and function.
- Obtain a long rhythm strip to document the arrhythmia, and a three-lead ECG when possible.
- Attempt to determine precipitating and alleviating factors (e.g., check electrolytes and arterial blood gases, eliminate vagal stimulation).

Assessment of Systemic Perfusion Appropriate assessment includes the following:

- Evaluation of vital signs, including pulses and blood pressure (Compare apical and

ECG pulse rates with peripheral pulses; if pulses are lost during the arrhythmia, begin cardiac compressions.)
- Evaluation of warmth of extremities and capillary refill
- Evaluation of level of consciousness
- Evaluation of urine output

Evaluation of Heart Rate Intervals and rates can be measured on ECG paper. Conventional ECG recordings include the following:

- Conventional paper speed is 25 mm/sec.
- The smallest interval represented on ECG paper is the small square. Movement across one small square or box requires 0.04 second.
- Movement across five of these small boxes requires 0.2 second (0.04 second × 5). A 0.2-second interval is indicated by a heavy black vertical line.
- A 1-second interval is represented by five heavy vertical lines.

The heart rate can be estimated two ways. The number of QRS complexes appearing in a 3-second strip (15 heavy vertical lines) is counted and multiplied by 20 for the heart rate per minute. If the RR interval is extremely irregular, a 6-second strip should be used; the number of QRS complexes occurring in that 6-second strip (30 heavy vertical lines) multiplied by 10 yields the heart rate per minute. If the heart rate is fairly regular, the heart rate can be estimated from the interval between two QRS complexes (Figure 5-14).

Rhythm Identification Characteristics of specific arrhythmias are provided in Table 5-16 with illustrations of the most common arrhythmias. If the specific identity of the rhythm is in doubt, document the rhythm with a long rhythm strip in the chart. If systemic perfusion is compromised, the arrhythmia is treated according to general classification (bradyarrhythmia or tachyarrhythmia—see Management).

Evaluation of Precipitating or Alleviating Factors
Attempt to determine if the arrhythmia was precipitated by stimulation (e.g., suctioning), hypoxia, or electrolyte imbalance. Document hemoglobin satu-

Table 5-15
Effects of Electrolyte Imbalances, Drugs, and Clinical Condition on the Pediatric Electrocardiogram

	Short QT	Long QT-U	Prolonged QRS	ST-T Changes	Sinus Tach	Sinus Brady	AV Block	V Tach	Miscellaneous
Chemistry									
Hyperkalemia			X	X			X	X	Low-voltage Ps; peaked Ts
Hypokalemia		X	X	X					
Hypercalcemia	X								
Hypocalcemia		X			X		X	X	
Hypermagnesemia						X	X		
Hypomagnesemia		X					X		
Drugs									
Digitalis	X			X		T	X	T	
Phenothiazines		T						T	
Phenytoin	X								
Propranolol	X					X			
Quinidine		X	X	X		T	T	T	
Tricyclics		T	T	T			T	T	
Verapamil						X	X		
Imipramine					T		T	T	Atrial flutter
Miscellaneous									
CNS injury		X		X	X	X	X		
Freidreich's ataxia				X	X				Atrial flutter
Duchenne's disease				X	X				Atrial flutter
Myotonic dystrophy			X	X	X		X		
Collagen disease				X			X	X	
Hypothyroidism						X			Low voltage
Hyperthyroidism					X				
Other diseases		Romano-Ward	Lyme disease				Holt-Oram, maternal lupus		

From Johns Hopkins Hospital Department of Pediatrics: *The Harriet Lane handbook,* ed 14, edited by Barone M, St Louis, 1996, Mosby. Modified from Garson A Jr: *The electrocardiogram in infants and children: a systematic approach,* Philadelphia, 1983, Lea & Febiger; and Walsh EP: Electrocardiography and introduction to electrophysiologic techniques. In Fyler DC, Nadas A, editors: *Pediatric cardiology,* Philadelphia, 1992, Hanley & Belfus.
X, Present; T, present only with drug toxicity.

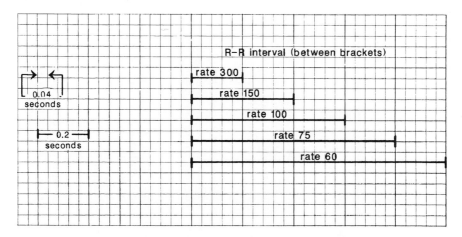

Figure 5-14   ECG time intervals and estimation of heart rate from ECG R-R interval. (From Berman w Jr: *Handbook of pediatric ECG interpretation,* St Louis, 1991, Mosby.)

ration by pulse oximetry, arterial blood gases, and serum electrolyte concentration. Note if any drugs were administered immediately before the arrhythmia, or if any drugs are currently being administered (e.g., digoxin or catecholamines) that may predispose the patient to arrhythmia. Document any factors that are associated with elimination of the arrhythmia (e.g., bag-valve-mask ventilation, vagal stimulation).

Management

General Principles   An arrhythmia that compromises systemic perfusion should be treated as an emergency. Cardiac compressions and drugs or defibrillation are required for pulseless arrest (see Figure 5-10). Bradyarrhythmias and tachyarrhythmias that compromise systemic perfusion are treated urgently (see Figures 5-12 and 5-13).

General principles of care require a focus on the patient rather than the ECG and include the following:

- Assess and support systemic perfusion at all times.
- Treat the patient, not the ECG.
- Treat symptomatic arrhythmias and those capable of deteriorating into symptomatic arrhythmias. Note that many "arrhythmias" do not require treatment.
- Treat the cause of the arrhythmia, if possible.

- Do not make the patient sicker from the therapy than from the arrhythmia.
- Note that most antiarrhythmic drugs will depress myocardial contractility; therefore monitor systemic perfusion closely.

Bradycardia   Ensure that oxygenation and ventilation are adequate. Epinephrine is an excellent chronotropic agent, and atropine may be used if vagal stimulation is thought to be contributing to the bradycardia. Esophageal pacing stimulates the atria but will not increase the heart rate if heart block is present. Ventricular pacing may be required.

Tachycardia   Tachyarrhythmias must be distinguished from sinus tachycardia. Sinus tachycardia is not treated, although the cause is identified and treated. Tachyarrhythmias are treated with defibrillation, cardioversion, or antiarrhythmics.

Heart Block   If heart block is present, isoproterenol may increase the ventricular rate. External or IV pacing may also be performed.

Antiarrhythmic Therapy   Antiarrhythmic drugs alter action potential (depolarization) or refractory periods (including repolarization), or they block beta-adrenergic stimulation (Table 5-17). Virtually all antiarrhythmic drugs will depress myocardial function; thus cardiac output and systemic perfusion must

Text continued on p. 185

Table 5-16
Characteristics of Pediatric Arrhythmias

Rhythm	Description
Bradyarrhythmias—Heart Rate Too Slow for Clinical Condition	
QRS Duration Normal (approximately, <0.08 sec)	
Sinus bradycardia 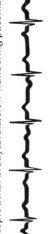	Heart rate is lower than "normal" for age or lower than appropriate for clinical condition. One P wave precedes each QRS, and one QRS follows each P wave. QRS morphology is normal (narrow, <0.08 sec); P wave axis and morphology are normal. May be caused by hypoxemia, hypotension, acidosis, hypothermia, vagal stimulation, or beta-blocking agents.
Ectopic atrial bradycardia/slow wandering pacemaker 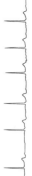	One P wave precedes each QRS, and one QRS follows each P wave. Although QRS morphology is normal, P wave is abnormal in axis and appearance. Rhythm develops when an accessory pacemaker takes over rhythm and is more rapid than (slowed) sinus rate.
Junctional rhythm	Normal sinus pacemaker is slowed and no longer driving ventricular depolarization (heart rate), so junctional tissue initiates rhythm. P wave may be absent or slower than QRS, retrograde, or present with rate faster than QRS but with dissociation between P and QRS. QRS morphology is normal, indicating normal conduction from junctional tissue through ventricles.
Heart block—first-degree 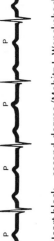	Each P is followed by a QRS, and each QRS is preceded by a P. However, PR interval is longer than normal for age and heart rate (generally >0.12-0.14 + sec). May be caused by digoxin therapy, may be associated with some congenital heart disease (atrioventricular canal), or may follow cardiovascular surgery.
Heart block—second-degree (Mobitz I—Wenckebach rhythm is illustrated here) 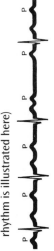	*Variable block (Mobitz I—Wenckebach rhythm):* PR interval lengthens progressively from complex to complex (and RR interval shortens) until one P wave is not followed by a QRS. Often follows cardiovascular surgery; not likely to progress. *Fixed block (Mobitz II):* A consistent proportion (e.g., 1 or 3 or 4) of P waves are not followed by a QRS, but PR interval is constant. Rhythm is uncommon in children but worrisome because it may progress to complete heart block.

Heart block—third degree

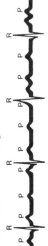

There is no temporal relationship between P and QRS. P waves are usually regular, with rate > QRS rate. May be congenital or may follow cardiovascular surgery or inflammatory diseases of the heart.

QRS Duration Prolonged (approximately >0.08 sec)
Supraventricular rhythm with block and aberrant conduction through ventricles

P waves may be difficult to see but are present. Supraventricular rhythm is frequently blocked (typically in a fixed ratio), so P waves are much more common than QRS. QRS is widened and notched as a result of abnormal conduction through ventricle.

Idioventricular rhythm

An escape rhythm (atrial and junctional tissue fail to generate impulses at a rate faster than ventricular pacer rate, so ventricular depolarization takes over rhythm). Typically QRS is wide because impulse begins outside of normal conduction pathway. Will result in decreased cardiac output because rhythm is slow and stroke volume often inadequate. *Rhythm will deteriorate and requires CPR.*

Slow rate with intraventricular conduction (e.g., right bundle branch) block

Whether rhythm generated from atrial or junctional tissue, QRS complexes are wide because right bundle branch or other ventricular conduction block slows impulse (right bundle branch block is expected postoperatively if right ventriculotomy is performed). *Rhythm may deteriorate.*

Tachyarrhythmias—Heart Rate Too Fast for Clinical Condition
QRS Duration Normal (approximately <0.08 sec)

Sinus tachycardia

One P precedes each QRS, and one QRS follows each P. P-wave morphology and appearance are normal, and rate <230/min (varies with sleep-wake cycles and activity). May be caused by fever, pain, hemorrhage, other stress, adrenergic drugs, or vagolytic agents (search for cause).

Continued

Data from Hazinski MF: Cardiovascular disorders. In Hazinski MF, editor: *Nursing care of the critically ill child*, ed 2, St Louis, 1992, Mosby; Nichols DG et al, editors: *Critical heart disease in infants and children*, St Louis, 1995, Mosby; Garson A et al, editors: *The science and practice of pediatric cardiology*, ed 2, Baltimore, 1998, Williams & Wilkins.

Table 5-16
Characteristics of Pediatric Arrhythmias—cont'd

Rhythm	Description
Tachyarrhythmias—Heart Rate Too Fast for Clinical Condition—cont'd *QRS Duration Normal* (approximately <0.10 sec)—cont'd	
Supraventricular tachycardia 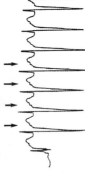	May be paroxysmal. Rapid, regular, and fixed rate. Patient maintains pulses but may develop congestive heart failure, shock. Most SVT due to reentry of depolarizing impulse from ventricles to atria (reentry or reciprocating tachycardia), so retrograde P may be present.
Supraventricular tachycardia—Wolff-Parkinson-White syndrome 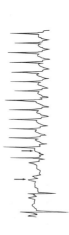	Characterized by anomalous AV conduction pathway and retrograde conduction from ventricles to atria. A delta wave (negative or positive) can be identified at beginning of QRS (arrows), which initiates tachycardia.
Junctional ectopic tachycardia (JET)	Ectopic focus initiates rhythm from junctional tissue at extremely rapid rate (110-250/min). Most commonly observed postoperatively. Stroke volume, cardiac output, and systemic perfusion typically deteriorate. P waves not visible; QRS complexes narrow.
Atrial flutter (irregular block, with irregular P-QRS ratio is shown here)	Atrial rate is approximately 300/min (range: 280-450/min), and atrial depolarization is characterized by "sawtoothed" waves. Typically, some block of atrial impulses occurs at AV node, so number of "sawtoothed" waves > number of QRS complexes. Usually one P wave is "hidden" in QRS complex.
Atrial fibrillation—rapid ventricular response 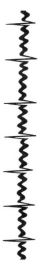	Chaotic atrial activity prevents organized atrial depolarization (and contraction). ECG baseline appears to wander (caused by fine atrial fibrillation), and QRS response is irregular, so heart rate is irregular.

Supraventricular tachycardia with aberrant ventricular conduction

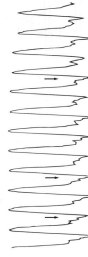

P waves may be difficult to see in all leads, but they do precede QRS complexes (*arrows*); PR interval is constant. Aberrant ventricular conduction causes wide QRS. Difficult to distinguish from ventricular tachycardia. Treat as ventricular tachycardia if patient is pulseless.

Ventricular tachycardia

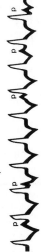

Rapid (typically >120-150/min), regular heart rate often with loss of pulses (pulseless arrest). QRS complex is wide because impulse is generated outside of normal ventricular conduction system. QRS is not related to P. With rate <150/min, pulses may be present. *Emergent rhythm.*

Collapse Rhythms—Require Immediate CPR
Electromechanical dissociation/Pulseless electrical activity

Results in loss of effective ventricular contraction, so pulses disappear and systemic perfusion is inadequate (pulseless arrest). Reversible causes include hypoxia, severe acidosis, tension pneumothorax, cardiac tamponade, hypovolemia. Treated as pulseless arrest, although reversible causes must be sought and eliminated.

Ventricular tachycardia (see strip above)

Rapid wide QRS complexes (rate usually >120-150/min) with loss of pulses. Results in inadequate ventricular filling and drastic reduction in stroke volume. Treated as pulseless arrest.

Ventricular fibrillation

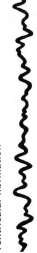

Chaotic ventricular electrical activity results in absence of complexes. Coarse or fine oscillations in ECG baseline. Lack of organized ventricular depolarization prevents organized contraction, so pulses are not present. Resuscitation is required with urgent defibrillation.

Asystole

"Straight line" ECG indicating absence of electrical activity, pulseless arrest, and poor likelihood of resuscitation.

Data from Hazinski MF: Cardiovascular disorders. In Hazinski MF, editor: *Nursing care of the critically ill child*, ed 2, St Louis, 1992, Mosby; Nichols DG et al, editors: *Critical heart disease in infants and children*, St Louis, 1995, Mosby; Garson A et al, editors: *The science and practice of pediatric cardiology*, ed 2, Baltimore, 1998, Williams & Wilkins.

Table 5-17
Pediatric Antiarrhythmic Therapy

Drug	Dose	Effect	Caution/Excretion
Adenosine (Adenocard)	IV: 0.05 mg/kg, then can increase dose by 0.05 mg/kg to 0.1-0.3 mg/kg maximum	Slows conduction through atrioventricular (AV) node and can interrupt reentrant pathways, so is ideal for treatment of supraventricular tachycardia (SVT) Of particular benefit is its short half-life (approximately 10 secs) Must administer rapid push (3.5 sec)	Use with caution in children with evidence of underlying conduction or AV node dysfunction; may cause bradycardia or hypotension Metabolized in body pool, so is unaffected by changes in hepatic or renal function
Amiodarone (Cordarone)	IV: 3-6 mg/kg PO: 10-15 mg/kg/day for 1 wk, then 2-5 mg/kg/day	Inhibits alpha- and beta-adrenergic receptors; also functions as smooth muscle relaxant Prolongs action potential and refractory period of myocardial cells	Long half-life, and often delay occurs before effects are seen May produce hypotension, heart block, bradycardia May contribute to thyroid dysfunction (monitor T_3, T_4) and keratopathy Metabolized primarily by liver
Atenolol	PO: 1-2 mg/kg/day, given bid	Sympathetic inhibition	Do not give in presence of bronchospasm
Atropine	IV/SQ: 0.02 mg/kg (minimum: 0.1 mg, maximum: 1.0 mg); also absorbed in tracheobronchial tree (may be administered via endotracheal tube)	Vagolytic (anticholinergic) agent that increases heart rate and AV conduction (it blocks acetylcholine effects at sinoatrial [SA] and AV nodes) and increases SA automaticity	Monitor for tachycardia; low doses may cause paradoxical bradycardia in infants Metabolized in liver and excreted through kidneys
Bretylium tosylate (Bretylol)	IV: 5 mg/kg bolus (over 5 min), and 5 mg/kg q6h	Increases action potential duration and effective refractory period; increases effective ventricular fibrillation threshold Inhibits norepinephrine release	May produce hypotension Aggravates digitalis toxicity 80% excreted unchanged in urine
Digoxin (Lanoxin)	See Table 5-6	Decreases SA node rate; decreases atrial automaticity Increases AV node conduction time Improves myocardial function and decreases oxygen consumption	Monitor for arrhythmias (especially high in premature neonates) Hypokalemia may potentiate toxicity 60% excreted in urine
Disopyramide (Norpace, Napamide)	IV: 1.5-2.5 mg/kg slowly as bolus PO: 2-6 mg/kg/day in 4 divided doses	Exerts quinidine-like action on myocardium (see quinidine) Sodium channel blocker with anticholinergic effects Effective in treatment of ventricular ectopy	May contribute to development of heart failure; depresses myocardial function to greater extent than quinidine Monitor for hypotension, rash, and anticholinergic effects (dry mucous membranes, GI symptoms)

Modified from Hazinski MF: *Nursing care of the critically ill child,* ed 2, St Louis, 1992, Mosby. Data from Adams FH, Emmanouilides GC, Riemenschneider TA: *Moss' heart disease in infants, children, and adolescents,* ed 4, Baltimore, 1989, Williams & Wilkins; Garson A et al: Amiodarone treatment of critical arrhythmias in children and young adults, *J Am Coll Cardiol* 4:749, 1984; Moak JP, Smith RT, Garson A: Mexiletine: an effective antiarrhythmic drug for treatment of ventricular arrhythmias in congenital heart disease, *J Am Coll Cardiol* 10:824, 1987; Moreau G: Personal communication, Vanderbilt University Medical Center, Nashville, 1991; Nestico PF, Morganroth J, Horowitz LN: New antiarrhythmic drugs, *Drugs* 35:286, 1988; Perry JC et al: Flecainide acetate for resistant arrhythmias in the young: efficacy and pharmacokinetics, *J Am Coll Cardiol* 14:185, 1989; Scott WA: Cardiac arrhythmias. In Levin DL, Morriss FC, editors: *Essentials of pediatric intensive care,* St Louis, 1997, Quality Medical; Till J et al: Efficacy and safety of adenosine in the treatment of supraventricular tachycardia in infants and children, *Br Heart J* 62:204, 1989.

Table 5-17
Pediatric Antiarrhythmic Therapy—cont'd

Drug	Dose	Effect	Caution/Excretion
Disopyramide cont'd			Metabolized in liver and 40% to 60% excreted unchanged in urine
Edrophonium (Tensilon)	IV: 0.1-0.2 mg/kg/ dose (Maximum: 10 mg/dose)	Cholinesterase inhibitor; prevents acetylcholine destruction, so prolongs cholinergic effects	May produce bradycardia, hypotension, increased bronchial secretions Metabolism unknown; IV effects last 5 min
Encainide (Enkaid)	IV: 0.5-1 mg/kg/dose PO: 2-5 mg/kg/day in 4 divided doses	Lengthens refractory period in atria and ventricles Prolongs His-Purkinje system conduction Sodium channel blocker, useful for treatment of ventricular arrhythmias and possibly SVT	May produce bradycardia, arrhythmias, hypotension Metabolized in liver and metabolites are excreted by kidneys
Ethmozine	PO: 65-200 mg/m^2 q8h	Decreases automaticity	May cause headache, vertigo, parasthesias
Flecainide (Tambocor)	IV: 1-2 mg/kg over 5-10 min	Sodium channel blocker that slows conduction through AV node and accessory AV pathways, so can be effective in treatment of SVT, including Wolff-Parkinson-White (WPW) syndrome Also slows conduction through His-Purkinje system, so can be effective in treatment of ventricular arrhythmias	May produce myocardial depression, arrhythmias, heart block, blurred vision Monitor hepatic function (may compromise function) 17% to 24% excreted unchanged in urine
Isoproterenol (Isuprel)	IV: 0.05-0.1 μg/kg/min	Beta-1 and beta-2 adrenergic agonist; increases heart rate Especially effective in treatment of bradycardias associated with heart block, since it will shorten AV conduction time	May produce tachyarrhythmias Will increase myocardial oxygen consumption Distributed throughout body; metabolized by conjugation in GI tract and enzymatic reduction in liver, lungs, and a variety of other tissues
Lidocaine (Xylocaine)	IV: 1-2 mg/kg/dose Infusion: 10-20 μg/kg/min	Sodium channel blocker depresses spontaneous ventricular depolarization but does not affect SA or AV node depolarization Especially useful in treatment of ventricular ectopy	May produce seizures in toxic doses Cimetadine and beta-blockers will reduce hepatic clearance of this drug May exacerbate SVT Metabolized (90%) in liver
Mexiletine (Mexitil)	IV: 2-5 mg/kg PO: 3-12 mg/kg/day in 3 divided doses	Sodium channel blocker; similar in effects to lidocaine Most effective in treatment of ventricular arrhythmias in children with structural heart disease	May produce nausea (administer with meals), vertigo, tremors, and paresthesias Monitor for hypotension and arrhythmias Significant renal clearance

Continued

Table 5-17
Pediatric Antiarrhythmic Therapy—cont'd

Drug	Dose	Effect	Caution/Excretion
Moricizine (Esmolol)	IV: load with 500-600 μg/kg over 2-4 min, then 200 μg/kg/min (maximum: 1000 μg/kg/min)	Decreases sympathetic input	
Phenytoin (Dilantin)	IV: 2-4 mg/kg/dose (over 5 min) PO: 2-8 mg/kg/day	Increases spontaneous depolarization of atria and ventricles Previously used in treatment of digitalis-induced arrhythmias but replaced by treatment with Fab binding fragments	May produce bradycardia, decreased myocardial contractility, hypotension, ventricular arrhythmias Hepatic metabolism
Procainamide (Pronestyl)	IV load: <1 yr: 7 mg/kg over 30 min >1 yr: 10-15 mg/kg over 30 min (Maximum dose: 500 mg) IV infusion: 20-80 μg/kg/min PO: 15-50 mg/kg/day in divided doses (5-10 mg/kg q4h)	Sodium channel blocker; suppresses automaticity in atria and ventricles and prolongs AV nodal conduction Useful in treatment of atrial fibrillation and flutter and ventricular ectopy Has anticholinergic properties so may enhance ventricular response to SVT	May depress myocardial contractility, and may produce bradycardia and hypotension Monitor for blood dyscrasias and lupuslike syndrome Acetylated in liver
Propafenone	IV: 0.1-0.2 mg/kg Loading dose then q10 min (maximum: 1 mg/kg) IV infusion: 4-8 μg/kg/min PO: 3 mg/kg tid	Sodium channel blocker; slows conduction through atria, AV node, ventricles Useful in treatment of SVT, particularly junctional ectopic tachycardia (JET)	Monitor for hypotension, arrhythmias, nausea, paresthesia, tremors May produce restlessness, sleep disturbances May increase serum digoxin concentrations Hepatic metabolism
Propranolol (Inderal)	IV: 0.01-0.15 mg/kg (over 10 min) PO: 0.2-8 mg/kg/day	Decreases heart rate, AV conduction, and ventricular contractility beta-adrenergic blockade	May augment AV block Monitor for bradycardia, decreased myocardial function Hepatic metabolism (90+%)

Modified from Hazinski MF: *Nursing care of the critically ill child,* ed 2, St Louis, 1992, Mosby. Data from Adams FH, Emmanouilides GC, Riemenschneider TA: *Moss' heart disease in infants, children, and adolescents,* ed 4, Baltimore, 1989, Williams & Wilkins; Garson A et al: Amiodarone treatment of critical arrhythmias in children and young adults, *J Am Coll Cardiol* 4:749, 1984; Moak JP, Smith RT, Garson A: Mexiletine: an effective antiarrhythmic drug for treatment of ventricular arrhythmias in congenital heart disease, *J Am Coll Cardiol* 10:824, 1987; Moreau G: Personal communication, Vanderbilt University Medical Center, Nashville, 1991; Nestico PF, Morganroth J, Horowitz LN: New antiarrhythmic drugs, *Drugs* 35:286, 1988; Perry JC et al: Flecainide acetate for resistant arrhythmias in the young: efficacy and pharmacokinetics, *J Am Coll Cardiol* 14:185, 1989; Scott WA: Cardiac arrhythmias. In Levin DL, Morriss FC, editors: *Essentials of pediatric intensive care,* St Louis, 1997, Quality Medical. Till J et al: Efficacy and safety of adenosine in the treatment of supraventricular tachycardia in infants and children, *Br Heart J* 62:204, 1989.

Table 5-17
Pediatric Antiarrhythmic Therapy—cont'd

Drug	Dose	Effect	Caution/Excretion
Quinidine gluconate	IV: 0.5 mg/kg slow drip with glucose IM: 2-10 mg/kg q3-6h prn PO: 10-30 mg/kg/day in 2 divided doses	Depresses atrial and ventricular excitability and prolongs conduction through AV node Particularly useful in treatment of atrial fibrillation or flutter and AV reentrant tachycardias (with other drugs) Has anticholinergic properties	May produce tachyarrhythmias or cardiac arrest May depress myocardial contractility Monitor for signs of blood dyscrasias Hepatic metabolism
Quinidine sulfate	PO: Begin with 3-6 mg/kg q2-3h × 5; may increase to 12 mg/kg q2-3h × 5; maintenance: 7-12 mg/kg/day in divided doses	See above	See above
Sotalol	PO: 1-4 mg/kg bid (maximum: 160 mg/24hr)	Prolongs repolarization	May cause orthostatic hypotension, torsades de pointes
Tocainide (Tonocard)	PO: 20-40 mg/kg/day in divided doses	Oral amine analog of lidocaine; suppresses ventricular arrhythmias	May produce blood dyscrasias Hepatic metabolism
Verapamil (Cordilox)	IV: 0.1-0.2 mg/kg/dose (slowly, may repeat in 30 minutes) PO: 3-6 mg/kg/day in 3 divided doses	Calcium channel blocker which blocks slow calcium inward channel; particularly slows sinus node and AV conduction Useful in treatment of supraventricular arrhythmias in older children	Contraindicated in infants since may produce cardiovascular collapse Monitor for hypotension, heart failure, atrial fibrillation Keep CaCl ready and administer in event of collapse 80% hepatic

be closely monitored. Antiarrhythmics require establishment of a therapeutic level and may have a very narrow therapeutic range before signs of toxicity develop. If a new arrhythmia develops when the antiarrhythmic therapy is initiated, consider the new antiarrhythmic as the cause. If the child receiving digoxin therapy develops a new arrhythmia, the digoxin must be considered as a potential cause of the arrhythmia.

Many antiarrhythmic drugs interact with other drugs commonly prescribed for critically ill children. Therefore the nurse must keep tract of potential drug interactions, as well as the child's electrolyte balance and response to the drugs.

Pacemaker Therapy   Pacemaker therapy is indicated for bradycardia unresponsive to oxygen administration, ventilation, epinephrine, and atropine.

It is also indicated for heart block with clinically significant bradycardia, or for the potential for sudden development of bradycardia or heart block (e.g., following cardiovascular surgery).

Several forms of pacemakers are used in pediatric critical care; with any form of pacemaker therapy, the child's ventricular rate should never fall below the set "demand" rate of the pacemaker. In addition, pacemaker function can only affect the *depolarization* sequence within the heart; it cannot ensure that ventricular *function* or myocardial *contractility* is effective. Therefore the nurse must monitor the child's systemic perfusion, as well as pacemaker function, closely.

Classification of Pacemakers   Pacemakers are classified according to a three-letter coding system designed to indicate the chamber(s) paced by the pacemaker, the chamber(s) sensed by the pacemaker, and the mode of pacemaker response if intrinsic chamber depolarization is detected. The code is summarized in Box 5-19.

Esophageal Pacing Esophageal pacing is a form of atrial pacing (AAI pacing) that is useful when emergency demand or overdrive pacing must be established quickly in the patient without heart block. A small electrode is inserted into the esophagus, positioned directly behind the left atrium. The proper position is confirmed when delivery of an electrical impulse stimulates atrial depolarization (which should be followed by ventricular depolarization). Consistent "capture" of the atrium can be achieved with lower mA pacer output if a 5- to 10-mA pulse width is provided.

Box 5-19

Classification of Pacemakers

First letter—chamber paced
  V = Ventricle
  A = Atrium
  D = Atrium and ventricle

Second letter—chamber sensed
  V = Ventricle
  A = Atrium
  D = Atrium and ventricle
  0 = None

Third letter—mode of response
  I = Inhibited
  T = Triggered
  D = Atrial triggered, ventricular inhibited
  0 = None

Optional Additional Letters
Fourth letter—programmable functions
  P = Programmable (rate and/or output)
  M = Multiprogrammable
  0 = None

Fifth letter—special tachyarrhythmia functions
  B = Bursts
  N = Normal rate competition
  S = Scanning
  E = External
  0 = None

From Intersociety Commission for Heart Disease Resources (ICHD).

This procedure is typically reserved for urgent situations. The patient is sedated and analgesics are administered before initiation of esophageal pacing, since the passage of current through the esophagus is painful.

Noninvasive (Temporary Transcutaneous or Transdermal) Pacing Noninvasive pacing through the chest wall can be used for emergency treatment of bradycardia. Although experience with pediatric patients is limited, it is clear that this form of pacemaker therapy can be extremely useful for a few hours, until more conventional methods of pacing (e.g., transvenous or implanted) can be established.

Noninvasive pacing uses two adhesive-backed electrodes that are placed in an anteroposterior relationship—one on the back of the chest (behind the heart) and one on the front of the chest (over the apex). If posterior placement is impossible, the posterior pad may be placed over the right side of the patient's chest, just under the clavicle. Precise placement of the pads is not essential, as long as the apical pad is the negative one. Three sizes of pads are generally available. In general, the smallest pads are reserved for neonates and small infants. The medium pads are used for infants 5 to 10 kg or up to 6 to 12 months of age. The large (adult) pads are used for children >10 kg, provided that the pads do not touch each other in any way. The pads selected should be the largest that will easily fit on the child without touching one another. Larger pads require larger pacemaker unit current output to capture the ventricles, but they actually deliver lower current density; thus they produce less discomfort than pacing through the smaller pads.

The adhesive pads are joined by cable to a commercially available external pacing unit. Either ventricular demand (VVI) pacing or asynchronous (fixed-rate, or VVO) pacing is provided. Regardless of the mode selected, the pacer must be able to "capture" the ventricle; thus every pacer spike should be followed by a QRS response, indicating that the pacemaker has succeeded in depolarizing the ventricle (Figure 5-15). Once effective pacing (and, if appropriate, sensing) of the ventricle is established, pacemaker settings should be recorded on the bedside flow sheet and nursing Kardex.

If the pacer fails to capture the ventricle, the output of the pacemaker unit should be increased

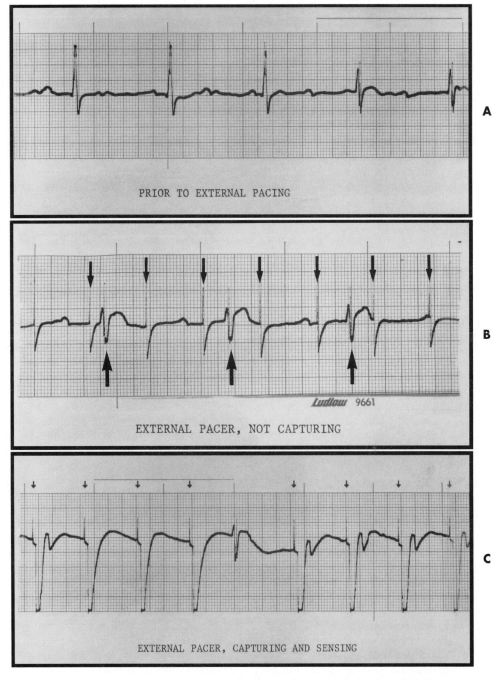

Figure 5-15 External pacing. **A,** Complete heart block with ventricular rate of approximately 43 beats/min (atrial rate is only approximately 80 beats/min). **B,** When noninvasive pacing was initiated at a rate of 76 beats/min, the pacemaker initially failed to capture the ventricle *(small arrows);* thus the intrinsic ventricular rhythm continues *(larger arrows)* at a rate of approximately 35 beats/min. **C,** Noninvasive pacing with appropriate capture of the ventricle; every pacer spike *(arrow)* is followed by ventricular depolarization. The patient's single intrinsic ventricular depolarization is appropriately sensed by the pacer, and the pacemaker is briefly inhibited. (Courtesy Carla Hansen, RN, MSN. From Hazinski MF: *Nursing care of the critically ill child,* ed 2, St Louis, 1992, Mosby.)

until capture is achieved. If the pacer has been operating satisfactorily and fails to sense or capture the ventricles appropriately after several hours of use, and the pacer settings are correct, the nurse should change the adhesive pads.

Temporary External Pacing Through Epicardial or Transvenous Leads Pediatric temporary external pacing is most frequently accomplished using pacing leads that have been placed on the epicardium in the operating room at the conclusion of cardiovascular surgery. It may also be accomplished under urgent conditions through transvenous leads that are introduced into a large vein and advanced into the right ventricular endocardium. Transvenous pacing is temporary and designed to give the child short-term support of heart rate following an episode of drug toxicity or other insult, until the child's intrinsic conduction system recovers or until a permanent pacer can be inserted.

Ventricular demand pacing is the most common form of temporary pacing provided in pediatric critical care. This allows the child's intrinsic cardiac rhythm to continue, provided that the patient's ventricular rate equals or exceeds the pacemaker demand rate. If the child's intrinsic rate consistently exceeds the pacemaker demand rate, the pacemaker is inhibited, and the surface ECG will show no evidence of pacemaker function. However, if the child's intrinsic rate falls below the demand rate, the pacemaker will initiate an electrical impulse (Figure 5-16).

During demand pacing, the pacemaker will be inhibited if the intrinsic depolarization rate exceeds the demand rate, *whether or not the rhythm is a normal one.* For example, a ventricular demand pacer will be inhibited if the patient develops supraventricular, junctional, or ventricular tachycardia if the ventricular rate exceeds the set demand rate (see Figure 5-16, *A*). Even atrial demand pacing will be inhibited by SVT. For this reason, the nurse must constantly assess the child's systemic perfusion, heart rate, and ECG and cannot rely on the pacemaker to maintain cardiac rhythm.

A demand pacemaker may provide an atrial impulse only (AAI pacing), a ventricular impulse only (VVI pacing), or both atrial and ventricular impulses (DDI pacing) if both atrial and ventricular wires are in place. Demand pacers can also be inhibited by atrial activity only (AAI pacing) or ventricular activity only (VVI or DDI pacing). DDD pacing can be triggered by atrial activity and inhibited by ventricular activity (DDD). Each of these major forms of pacing are summarized separately here.

When pacing is provided, every pacer spike should be followed by a chamber depolarization response; this indicates consistent "capture" of the chamber. An atrial pacing spike should be followed by an atrial depolarization response; a ventricular pacing spike should be followed by a ventricular depolarization (QRS) response. Pacemaker output should be adjusted until capture consistently occurs. The pacemaker output at which capture occurs is the "threshold." This threshold may increase over time during temporary pacing; thus it may be necessary to increase the output of the pacemaker to maintain capture.

Ventricular Demand (VVI) Pacing This is one of the most common forms of postoperative temporary pacing. With this form of pacing, pacemaker wires are only present in the ventricles, not in the atria. The ventricle can be paced, and intrinsic ventricular activity can be sensed. If the intrinsic ventricular depolarization rate exceeds the set demand rate, the pacemaker will be inhibited. Settings to be selected for VVI pacing include the demand rate, the sensitivity of the pacer to intrinsic impulses, and the output of the pacemaker (Box 5-20).

Atrioventricular (DVI) Sequential Pacing Any form of AV sequential pacing requires both atrial and ventricular pacing wires. With DVI pacing, both the atrium and the ventricle can be paced. However, with this form of pacing, only the intrinsic ventricular electrical activity can be sensed. Consequently, only a ventricular heart rate exceeding the demand rate set on the pacemaker can inhibit pacemaker firing. With this form of pacing, the ventricular demand rate (usually set in the range of 40 to 120 beats/min), the sensitivity to intrinsic ventricular activity, and ventricular and atrial outputs are set. In addition, the AV interval (in effect, the PR interval) is set.

The ventricular rate during DVI pacing is determined by the ventricular demand rate; this determines the maximal interval between ventricular depolarizations. The timing of the atrial output is determined by the demand ventricular rate and the set AV interval.

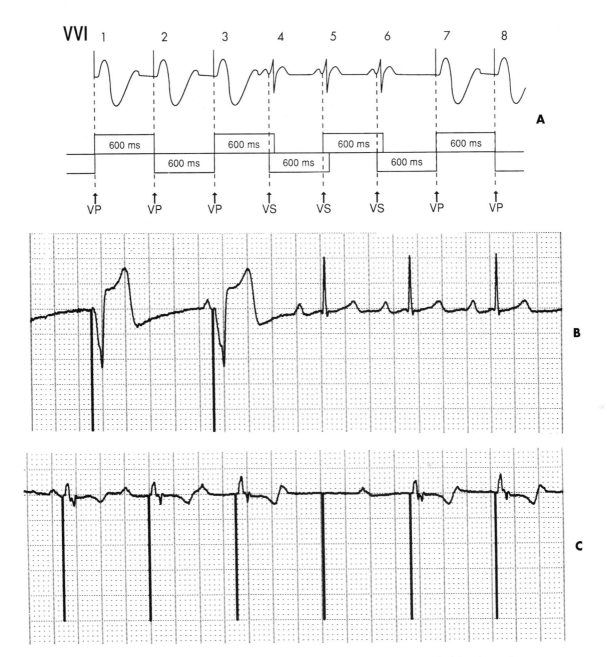

Figure 5-16   VVI pacing. **A,** Function of VVI pacer. The pacer is programmed with a demand rate of 100 (a pacing interval of 600 msec). If no intrinsic ventricular activity is sensed within 600 msec of the previous intrinsic or paced activity, a pacing stimulus is delivered *(VP)*. The fourth, fifth, and sixth complexes represent spontaneous ventricular depolarization within the 600 msec pacing interval; the pacer senses this *(VS)* and is appropriately inhibited. Note that each paced event *(VP)* occurs exactly 600 msec after the previous ventricular paced or intrinsic event. **B,** VVI pacing (inhibited). VVI demand rate is 60/min (1000-msec interval) and pacer is thus inhibited when intrinsic rate exceeds 60/min. **C,** VVI pacing with intermittent failure to capture. Pacemaker demand rate is 85/min. The fourth pacer stimulus is not followed by a QRS response. Integrity of the leads and pacemaker battery should be checked. It may be necessary to increase the pacemaker output. (From Johns JA: Pacemakers. In Kambam J: *Cardiac anesthesia for infants and children,* St Louis, 1994, Mosby.)

Box 5-20

Pacemaker Settings

Output Control (Stimulation Threshold)

This determines the amount of current delivered to the epicardium or endocardium by the pacemaker generator. The dial should be set just above the milliampere number at which the pacemaker consistently "captures" the heart by producing the depolarization of the desired chamber. The point at which the pacemaker consistently captures the chamber is called the stimulation threshold and should be verified daily, since it may increase during external cardiac pacing.

Sensitivity Control

This determines the responsiveness of the pacemaker to the patient's intrinsic cardiac electrical activity. If the control is set fully counterclockwise, the pacemaker will be *insensitive* to the patient's intrinsic cardiac activity and will fire at the set heart rate regardless of the patient's intrinsic heart rate (this may result in competition between the patient's intrinsic rhythm and the pacemaker). As the sensitivity control is turned in the clockwise direction, the pacemaker becomes more and more sensitive to patient intrinsic cardiac electrical activity. When the control is fully clockwise, the pacemaker should be inhibited consistently by the patient's intrinsic cardiac activity.

AV Interval (for AV Sequential Pacing)

This determines the interval between atrial and ventricular depolarization provided by the pacemaker. The settings are labeled in *microseconds*—the nurse utilizes milliseconds in ECG interpretation (0.04 millisecond = 40 microseconds). Therefore an AV interval of 150 microseconds is equal to an AV interval of 0.15 millisecond. Verify the AV interval on the ECG, but note that the AV interval may be shorter than the set interval if the patient's intrinsic conduction is more rapid than the interval set, but the pacemaker set interval should be the maximal interval observed.

Ventricular Rate

This is the minimal ventricular rate that should be observed. If the patient intrinsic ventricular rate falls below this rate, the pacemaker should fire and maintain the minimal rate.

Sense/Pace Lights

These will indicate whether the pacemaker is sensing patient cardiac electrical activity or pacing (the frequency of pacing should be noted on the patient vital sign record).

From Hazinski MF: *Nursing care of the critically ill child,* ed 2, St Louis, 1992, Mosby.

Case Study

Consider DVI pacing with a ventricular demand rate of 120/min and an AV interval of 125 msec. A ventricular impulse (either paced or intrinsic) should occur every half second, or every 500 msec (Figure 5-17). If no ventricular impulse is detected within 500 msec *less* the AV interval (500 msec − 125 msec = 375 msec), an atrial impulse is delivered by the pacemaker. If no ventricular impulse is detected within 125 msec after the atrial impulse, a ventricular impulse is delivered by the pacemaker. If a ventricular impulse is sensed within 375 msec after the previous ventricular impulse, or if a ventricular impulse is sensed within 125 msec of the atrial impulse, the ventricular pacer is inhibited.

DVI pacing cannot ensure that every ventricular depolarization will be preceded by an atrial depolarization. The pacemaker is inhibited by a ventricular rate exceeding the set ventricular demand rate, which may be caused by supraventricular, junctional, or ventricular tachycardia. This form of pacing is used primarily for external pacing and is not typically used for permanent pacing.

Atrioventricular DDD ("Universal") Sequential Pacing   DDD pacing provides true AV sequential pacing. Both atrial and ventricular wires are in place, and the pacemaker can pace both the atrium and the ventricle, and can sense both atrial and ventricular intrinsic activity. In addition, the pacemaker can be triggered by intrinsic atrial activity.

As in DVI pacing, a ventricular demand rate (usually between 40 and 175 beats/min) and an AV

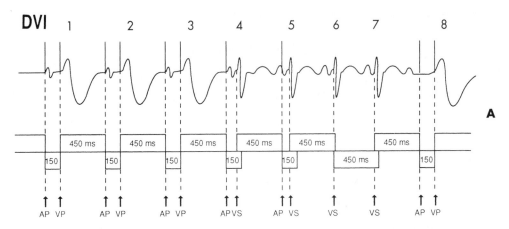

Figure 5-17 DVI pacing. **A,** This pacemaker is programmed to a demand rate of 100/min (600/msec), with an AV interval of 150 msec. This means that the VA interval (interval between intrinsic or paced ventricular activity and the need for sensed atrial activity or an atrial paced spike) is 450 msec (600 – 150 msec). *Complexes 1 to 3:* After the first atrial pacing stimulus *(AP),* the pacer waits an AV interval of 150 msec; if no intrinsic ventricular activity is sensed within that interval, a ventricular pacing stimulus *(VP)* is provided. The pacemaker VA interval is then reset, and another 450 msec passes without activity; thus an atrial pacing stimulus is again provided. This activity repeats for the first three complexes. *Complex 4:* After the fourth atrial pacing activity, spontaneous ventricular activity is sensed *(VS)* within the 150-msec AV interval; thus ventricular pacing is inhibited, and the 450-msec timing begins. *Complexes 5 and 6:* In the fifth complex, intrinsic *atrial* activity is present but not sensed by the pacer, because the DVI mode has no atrial sensors. Therefore the atrial pacing stimulus *(AP)* still follows the previous ventricular activity by 450 msec. When intrinsic ventricular activity follows the atrial stimulus within 150 msec, it is sensed *(VS)* and the pacemaker is inhibited. *Complex 7:* In this complex, intrinsic ventricular activity is sensed (VS) within the 450-msec VA interval; this inhibits both atrial and ventricular stimuli. *Complex 8:* 450 msec after the seventh ventricular complex, no ventricular activity is sensed; thus an atrial pacing stimulus *(AP)* is provided and is followed by a ventricular pacing stimulus within 150 msec when no intrinsic ventricular activity is sensed.

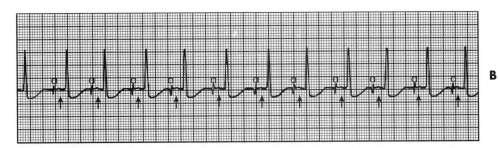

Figure 5-17, cont'd **B,** Atrial DVI pacing. The ventricular demand rate is 90/min (VV interval of 666 msec). The AV interval is 0.12 second (120 msec). Therefore the VA interval (maximum time between previous ventricular impulse and need for atrial activity) is 0.46 sec (460 msec = 666 – 120). In this strip, atrial pacing stimuli (a) are consistently delivered 460 msec after every previous ventricular impulse. Since intrinsic ventricular activity is sensed within 120 msec after each atrial stimulus, the ventricular pacer is inhibited. Note that intrinsic atrial activity is present *(arrows)* but is not sensed by the pacer and this intrinsic activity does not trigger any response (as it would during DDD pacing). *Continued*

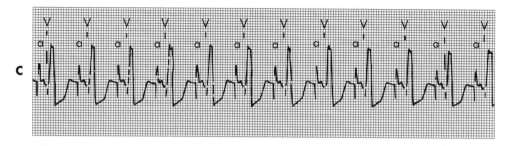

C

Figure 5-17, cont'd **C,** AV pacing with DVI pacer. The ventricular demand rate is 90/min (VV interval of 666 msec). The AV interval is 0.18 second (180 msec). The VA interval is 480 msec (666 msec − 180 msec), or 0.48 second. When no intrinsic ventricular activity is sensed within the 480-sec VA interval, an atrial pacing stimulus is delivered (a). When no intrinsic ventricular activity is sensed within 180 msec, a ventricular pacing stimulus (v) is delivered. (**A** From Johns JA: Pacemakers. In Kambam J, editor: *Cardiac anesthesia for infants and children,* St Louis, 1994, Mosby. **B** and **C** from Hazinski MF: *Nursing care of the critically ill child,* St Louis, 1992, Mosby.)

interval are set, and the atrial and ventricular outputs and sensitivities are set. As with DVI pacing, the pacemaker interval is determined by the ventricular demand rate, as well as by the AV interval.

With DDD pacing, intrinsic atrial activity *triggers* the AV interval, as well as *inhibits* the atrial pacer output. This form of pacing should ensure that each ventricular depolarization is preceded by either an intrinsic or a paced atrial depolarization, and each atrial depolarization (whether intrinsic or paced) should be followed by a ventricular depolarization within the set AV interval. Unfortunately, if the patient develops an SVT, the DDD pacer may support that rhythm by pacing the ventricle following each intrinsic atrial depolarization.

Case Study

Consider DDD pacing with a ventricular demand rate of 120/min and an AV interval of 125 msec. At a minimum, an intrinsic or paced ventricular depolarization should occur every half second, or every 500 msec. The pacemaker waits the 500 msec less the AV interval (500 msec −125 msec = 375 msec). If no activity is sensed, an atrial impulse is delivered. If intrinsic atrial activity is sensed within that 375-msec interval—although a 100-msec refractory period is protected following the last ventricular depolarization— the atrial pacemaker is inhibited but an AV interval "timer" is triggered. This explains how

DDD pacing can be atrial triggered and ventricular inhibited. If no intrinsic ventricular activity is sensed within 125 msec after the sensed atrial activity, a ventricular impulse is provided. If intrinsic ventricular activity is sensed within that 125-msec interval, the ventricular pacer is inhibited.

When DDD pacing is provided, the nurse may observe no pacer spikes, atrial pacer spikes alone, ventricular pacer spikes alone, or both atrial and ventricular pacer spikes (Figure 5-18). No pacer spikes will be observed if the patient's ventricular rate exceeds the pacemaker demand rate, and if intrinsic atrial activity occurs within an interval that triggers the AV timer; and if the patient's intrinsic AV interval is shorter than the set pacemaker AV interval. Atrial pacer spikes alone will be observed if no intrinsic atrial activity is sensed (so that an atrial impulse is provided by the pacemaker) but the patient's ventricle responds within the set AV interval. A ventricular pacing spike alone will be observed if the pacer is triggered by the patient's intrinsic atrial activity but intrinsic ventricular depolarization does not occur within the set AV interval; then the pacemaker will generate a ventricular impulse. Atrial and ventricular pacing spikes will be observed if no intrinsic atrial activity is sensed within the prescribed interval and no ventricular activity is sensed within the AV interval after the atrial impulse is provided.

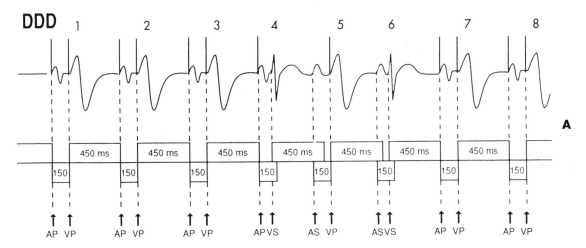

Figure 5-18 DDD pacing. **A,** The ventricular demand rate is 100/min with an AV interval of 150 msec, resulting in a VA interval of 450 msec (just as in Figure 5-17, A). The only difference between DDD pacing and DVI pacing is that the atrium is sensed in DDD pacing; and when it is sensed, that will trigger the timing of the AV interval. *Complexes 1 to 3:* No atrial or ventricular activity is sensed within the 450-msec VA interval; thus an atrial pacing stimulus *(AP)* is provided. When no intrinsic ventricular activity is sensed within the 150-msec AV interval, a ventricular pacing stimulus *(VP)* is provided. *Complex 4:* Intrinsic ventricular activity is sensed *(VS)* within the 150-msec interval following the atrial pacing stimulus; thus the ventricular pacing is inhibited, and the VA interval is reset. *Complex 5:* This complex demonstrates the difference between DVI and DDD pacing. No intrinsic ventricular activity is sensed within the 150-msec VA interval, but *atrial* activity is sensed *(AS)*. This inhibits atrial pacing and triggers the timing of the AV interval. When intrinsic ventricular activity is not sensed within the 150-msec AV interval following the atrial (sensed) activity, a ventricular pacing stimulus *(VP)* us provided. *Complex 6:* Atrial activity is again sensed *(AS)* within the 450-msec AV interval; thus atrial pacing is inhibited, and the AV interval is triggered. Intrinsic ventricular activity is sensed *(VS)* within the 450-msec AV interval; thus ventricular pacing is inhibited, and the AV interval timer is reset. *Complexes 6 and 7:* No intrinsic activity is sensed within the appropriate time intervals; thus atrial and ventricular pacing stimuli are provided.

Continued

Implantable Pacemakers Implantable pacemakers may be inserted at the time of cardiovascular surgery or whenever a child has demonstrated dependence on an external temporary pacemaker. The wires most commonly are inserted during surgery through the chest wall to the epicardium, by the transvenous route, or through percutaneous or cutdown entry to the cephalic or external jugular vein to the right ventricle. The pacemaker generator is placed under the infant's abdominal wall or in the chest under a tissue or muscle flap in the child's infraclavicular area.

A variety of pacemakers can now be implanted in infants and children. Programmable ventricular demand (VVI) or AV sequential (DVI or DDD) pacing can be provided, and the demand rate of the pacemaker can be programmed to higher rates when the child is younger and reprogrammed to lower rates as the child grows.

The most recent generation of implanted pacers are rate responsive, meaning that the demand rate of the pacemaker can be increased by sensed muscle activity or other signals, such as blood temperature, blood oxygen content, or minute ventilation. Then, after a brief period of time, the pacemaker demand rate returns to normal. The disadvantage of these pacemakers is that pacemaker battery life is reduced. However, the

CHART SPEED 25.0 mm/s **6-second strip**

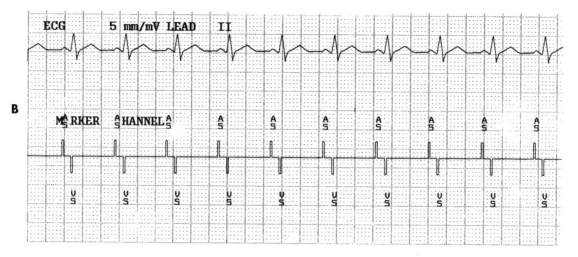

Figure 5-18, cont'd   **B,** DDD pacing (sensing only). Demand rate is 90/min, and AV interval is 130 msec. Both atrial and ventricular sensing is occurring because the patient's heart rate is 110/min and the AV interval is 0.12 or 120 msec.

CHART SPEED 25.0 mm/s **6-second strip**

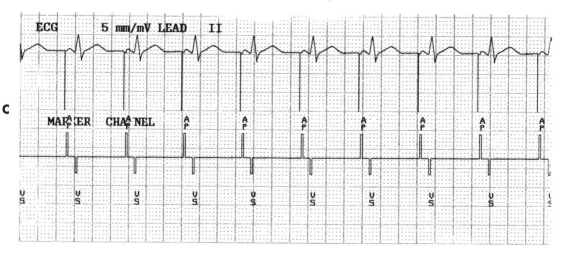

Figure 5-18, cont'd   **C,** DDD pacing with atrial pacing and ventricular sensing. Demand rate is 90/min, and AV interval is 130 msec (VA interval of 530 msec). Atrial pacing *(AP)* occurs because intrinsic activity is not sensed within the VA interval. Intrinsic ventricular activity is sensed *(VS)* within 0.10 sec (100 msec) after the atrial pacing stimulus (<130 msec); thus ventricular pacing is inhibited.

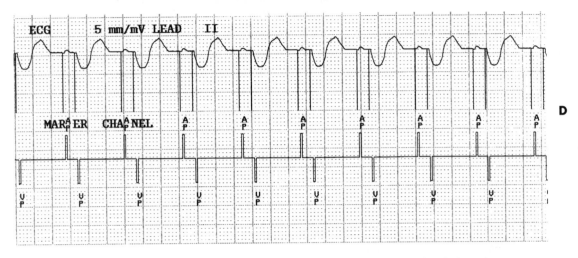

CHART SPEED 25.0 mm/s 6-second strip

Figure 5-18, cont'd   **D,** DDD pacing of atria and ventricles. Demand rate is 90/min, and AV interval is 130 msec (VA interval of 530 msec). Atrial pacing *(AP)* is provided when no intrinsic activity is sensed within the VA interval; then ventricular pacing *(VP)* is provided when no ventricular intrinsic activity is sensed within the AV interval.

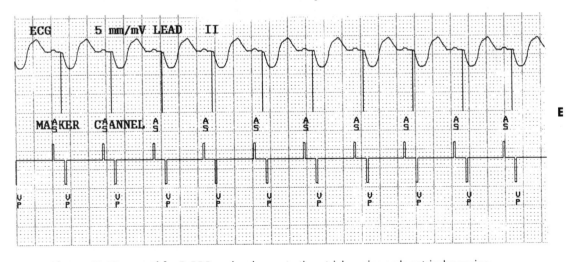

CHART SPEED 25.0 mm/s 6-second strip

Figure 5-18, cont'd   **E,** DDD pacing demonstrating atrial sensing and ventricular pacing. This strip must result from DDD rather than DVI pacing. Demand rate in 90/min, and AV interval is 130 msec (VA interval of 530 msec). Atrial activity is sensed *(AS)* within the 530-msec VA interval. This inhibits the atrial pacer and triggers the AV interval timer. When no intrinsic ventricular activity is sensed within the AV interval, ventricular pacing *(VP)* stimuli are provided. (**A** from Johns JA: Pacemakers. In Kambam J, editor: *Cardiac anesthesia for infants and children,* ed 2, St Louis, 1992, Mosby. **B** to **E** from Hazinski MF: *Nursing care of the critically ill child,* St Louis, 1992, Mosby.)

rate-responsive feature is clearly important for growing, active children.

Nursing Responsibilities During pacemaker therapy the nurse is responsible for monitoring the patient's systemic perfusion, as well as pacemaker function. The presence of a satisfactory heart rate on the cardiac monitor does not ensure effective cardiac contraction or systemic perfusion.

Regardless of the pacemaker used, the nurse must be familiar with the pacemaker parameters. These include the minimum ventricular rate that should occur with activity or programming changes. In addition, the nurse should document pacemaker activity with ECG strips preserved in the patient's chart.

At least once every shift, the nurse should verify pacemaker settings and obtain a rhythm strip to be added to the patient's chart. The nurse should note the amount of time the child's rhythm is sensed by the pacemaker vs. the frequency with which pacing occurs.

If problems arise with pacing, the integrity of the pacing system, including the unit and the wires, should be checked for loose connections, fractures, and function. The pacemaker battery should be replaced at regular intervals (typically check every 48 hours—check manufacturer's specifications and note that AV sequential pacing exhausts a battery much more quickly than ventricular demand pacing alone), and a spare battery should be taped to the pacemaker unit. A notation should be made of the date and time of the battery change and taped to the pacemaker unit.

External pacemaker wires should be kept dry and covered. The pacemaker controls should always be protected with a cover.

If the pacemaker *fails to capture* consistently, edema or inflammation may have developed at the end of the temporary electrode, and higher pacemaker output may be required to capture the ventricle. If the unit *fails to sense* properly and is competing with the patient's intrinsic rhythm, the sensitivity of the pacemaker unit may be set too low.

The child's epicardial or endocardial threshold (the minimum pacemaker output required to capture the designated chamber consistently) should be checked on a daily basis. Usually the threshold increases daily during temporary pacing—if the

threshold is near the maximum output of the pacemaker unit, consideration should be given to insertion of new electrodes or a more permanent pacing system.

Tamponade has been reported following removal of epicardial pacing wires. For this reason, these wires often are removed while the mediastinal chest tubes are still in place following cardiovascular surgery.

If the child is discharged with an implantable pacemaker, regular monitoring of pacemaker function must be performed on an outpatient basis. The child is discharged with a telephone transmitter so that the child's ECG can be transmitted by telephone to the physician's office.

A magnet is provided with some pacemakers, since the magnet can stimulate firing of the pacemaker at a fixed rate (usually approximately 100 beats/min). It may be necessary for the parents to place the magnet over the pacemaker (only if instructed by the physician or nurse) during telephone ECG transmission, to demonstrate pacemaker firing and ability to capture the chamber paced. Parents should be taught to consult a physician if the child's behavior or activity changes. Parents (and the child, if age appropriate) are usually taught to count the child's pulse daily and notify a physician if the pulse rate falls below the pacer demand rate.

Hypoxemia Caused by Cyanotic Heart Disease

Etiology

Definition Cyanosis is the blue color that may be observed in the mucous membranes, skin, sclera, and nailbeds of the child with arterial oxygen desaturation. Cyanosis is usually not visible until there is at least 5 g of reduced hemoglobin (hemoglobin not saturated with oxygen) per deciliter of blood. This level of desaturation usually correlates with a hemoglobin saturation of 70% to 85%, although the detection of the cyanosis may vary according to the child's total hemoglobin concentration and the experience of the observer. Systemic arterial oxygen desaturation will compromise oxygen delivery unless hemoglobin concentration or cardiac output increases commensurately (see

Essential Anatomy and Physiology: Oxygen Delivery, Cardiac Output, and Oxygen Consumption earlier in this chapter). Chronic hypoxemia can cause systemic consequences that may also be detrimental. These consequences and problems are presented in this section.

Because the degree of cyanosis visible is dependent on both the total amount of hemoglobin present and its saturation, cyanosis itself is not a reliable indicator of the degree of hypoxemia present. An anemic patient may be profoundly hypoxemic before cyanosis is observed, whereas a polycythemic patient may appear extremely cyanotic at only modest levels of arterial oxygen desaturation.

The detection of cyanosis is also influenced by the experience of the observer and the ambient lighting conditions. A mildly cyanotic child may appear deeply cyanotic when surrounded by blue linen and less cyanotic when surrounded by pink linen.

Acrocyanosis or peripheral cyanosis can be a normal variation of skin color observed in the extremities and around the mouth of the newborn. It is distinguishable from central cyanosis because it does not involve the mucous membranes or nailbeds. Newborn acrocyanosis is thought to be caused by vasomotor instability and is most commonly observed when the infant cries or is cold (e.g., during a bath). Acrocyanosis can also be caused by low cardiac output, peripheral vasoconstriction, and poor perfusion of the extremities.

Causes of Hypoxemia in Children Hypoxemia that is caused by cyanotic heart disease develops because some systemic venous blood is shunted into the systemic arterial circulation, bypassing the lungs. This type of shunt is referred to as a "right-to-left" intracardiac shunt, indicating that systemic venous blood, which should normally flow through the right side of the heart, into the pulmonary artery, and to the lungs, is directed instead either into the left side of the heart or into the aorta. The most common types of cyanotic CHD include the following:

- Severe obstruction to right heart or pulmonary artery flow with shunting of the blood from the right to the left side of the heart or from the pulmonary artery to the aorta

- Mixing of arterial and venous blood within the heart, such as within a single ventricle
- Transposition of the great vessels

The specific congenital heart defects that cause cyanosis are presented under Specific Diseases.

Pathophysiology

Chronic hypoxemia may produce complications resulting from inadequate oxygen delivery, as well as complications from compensatory polycythemia. Because oxygen delivery to tissues must be maintained, polycythemia is supported, but excessive hemoconcentration must be avoided.

Oxygen Delivery Chronic hypoxemia stimulates two major compensatory responses to maintain oxygen delivery: polycythemia (an increase in the RBC count) and an increase in oxygen release to the tissues. Chronic hypoxemia causes increased erythropoietin secretion by the kidneys, with a resultant increase in RBC production (called erythropoiesis). This erythropoiesis increases the amount of hemoglobin available to carry oxygen. If only 75% of available hemoglobin can be saturated with oxygen but a lot of hemoglobin is present in the blood, polycythemia can ensure that the arterial oxygen content is normal or near-normal despite hypoxemia.

Case Study

Calculate the arterial oxygen content for two patients:

	Patient 1	Patient 2
PaO_2	100 mm Hg	50 mm Hg
Hemoglobin saturation	98%	75%
Hemoglobin concentration	8 g/dl	18 g/dl
O_2 content		

$$O_2 \text{ content} = ([\text{Hgb in g/dl} \times 1.34 \text{ ml } O_2/\text{g} \times \text{Hgb sat}]) + PaO_2 \times 0.003$$

| O_2 content = | 10.8 ml O_2/dl | 18.2 ml O_2/dl |

Patient 2's arterial oxygen content is normal because compensatory polycythemia is present. Although Patient 1's PaO_2 and hemoglobin saturation are normal, oxygen content is reduced significantly by anemia. Patient 1 will not be cyanotic, whereas Patient 2 will be cyanotic.

During chronic hypoxemia, oxygen release to the tissues is facilitated by a shift in the oxyhemoglobin dissociation curve to the right. This means that at a given arterial oxygen tension (PaO_2), the hemoglobin is less well saturated. This shift results from high production of 2,3-diphosphoglycerate by the RBCs in response to chronic hypoxemia. The shift facilitates oxygen release to the tissues so that tissue oxygenation may be maintained despite hypoxemia and makes cyanosis more readily apparent in children with cyanotic heart disease.

Although polycythemia is a compensatory mechanism for chronic hypoxemia, the increase in RBC mass can produce hemoconcentration and complications of increased blood viscosity. The hemoconcentration can result from a progressive increase in hemoglobin concentration and hematocrit or from loss of plasma volume such as occurs with dehydration. Hemoconcentration may develop if an infant is placed on "NPO" status for more than a few hours for a surgical procedure or cardiac catheterization without IV hydration. Aggressive diuretic administration to control CHF can also produce hemoconcentration. For these reasons, manipulation of intravascular fluid volume in children with CHF and uncorrected cyanotic heart disease requires a great deal of skill to control CHF, yet prevent hemoconcentration.

When the hematocrit exceeds 70%, complications of increased blood viscosity, including pulmonary hypertension, dyspnea, headache, and exercise intolerance, can occur. Symptoms of hemoconcentration often develop in adolescents with uncorrected cyanotic heart disease.

Hypercyanotic Spells   Approximately one fourth of children with uncorrected cyanotic heart disease demonstrate paroxysmal hypercyanotic episodes. These episodes develop during the first year of life and occur most often in infants with tetralogy of Fallot, although they have been reported in association with other cyanotic defects.

Hypercyanotic episodes are incompletely understood but seem to be related to an acute reduction in pulmonary blood flow or an acute increase in oxygen requirements in the presence of relatively fixed oxygen delivery (e.g., CHD with limited pulmonary blood flow). In children with tetralogy of Fallot, the episodes may also be caused by contraction of the pulmonary infundibular muscle and a dramatic reduction in pulmonary blood flow.

The episodes typically occur in the morning, when the child resumes activity after a long rest. Hyperpnea may be a contributing factor.

Blood gas analysis during hypercyanotic episodes may document arterial oxygen saturations as low as 15% to 33%, with arterial oxygen tension as low as 20 mm Hg. The spells are dangerous, because this level of hypoxia probably compromises oxygen delivery to the brain; death and cerebrovascular accidents may occur during the spells. Onset of these spells is considered an indication for urgent surgical intervention to improve systemic arterial oxygenation.

Thromboembolic Events   Polycythemia increases the viscosity of the blood, which can result in the development of thromboembolus to the brain or other organs, brain abscess, or coagulopathies. Thromboembolic events are most likely to occur when the hematocrit is ≥60% to 70% and the mean hemoglobin concentration is ≥20 to 25 g/dl. The development of a microcytic anemia (a low mean corpuscular hemoglobin concentration or mean corpuscular hemoglobin volume) makes thromboembolic events more likely because this form of anemia increases the viscosity of the blood and the likelihood of RBC aggregation. Bacteremia increases the risk of formation of septic emboli.

Air can cause a cerebral thromboembolus. This air can enter the brain via an IV infusion and cause a stroke. Under normal conditions, IV air is filtered out of the blood in the lungs. However, when uncorrected cyanotic heart disease is present, some systemic venous blood is entering the left side of the heart or systemic arterial circulation without passing through the lungs first. Therefore, when the child has uncorrected cyanotic heart disease, *absolutely no air can be allowed to enter any IV tubing system or catheter, since it may produce a stroke.*

Brain Abscesses   Children with uncorrected cyanotic heart disease can develop brain abscesses, particularly beyond the age of 2 years. Congenital heart defects most commonly associated with brain abscess are uncorrected tetralogy of Fallot or transposition of the great vessels. The pathophysiology of brain abscess is incompletely understood, but it seems to be related to an episode of bacteremia and some compromise in cerebral microcirculation. Systemic venous blood normally is filtered through an effective phagocytic system in the pulmonary capillary bed. When cyanotic heart disease is present, some systemic venous blood enters the systemic arterial system without passing through the pulmonary capillary filtration system.

Coagulopathy Children with polycythemia and chronic hypoxemia often demonstrate a coagulopathy, which may cause severe postoperative bleeding. This coagulopathy includes a decrease in the synthesis of vitamin K–dependent clotting factors by the liver, which is not corrected even with administration of vitamin K. In addition, children with cyanotic heart disease and polycythemia often demonstrate thrombocytopenia (decrease in platelet number) or thrombocytopathia (decrease in platelet function even when the number of platelets may be normal).

Pulmonary Hypertension Polycythemia increases vascular shear stresses. This may contribute to the development of pulmonary hypertension. An additional potential cause of pulmonary hypertension in children with cyanotic heart disease is the development of pulmonary microemboli, which can narrow the lumina of small pulmonary arteries. These complications are most likely when the hematocrit is 60% to 70%.

Clinical Presentation

Clinical Evaluation Arterial oxygen desaturation can be caused by either cardiac or respiratory disease. If the child presents with hypoxemia, particularly during the first days of life, it may be unclear if the cyanosis is respiratory or cardiac in origin. Some clinical observations made by the bedside nurse may help to distinguish between the two causes.

Cyanosis that *decreases* with cry is often respiratory in origin, and the increase in tidal volume during vigorous cry reduces the degree of hypoxemia. Cyanosis that *increases* with cry is often cardiac in origin because the expiratory phase of crying tends to increase resistance to pulmonary blood flow and enhance any existing right-to-left intracardiac shunt.

Oxygen Delivery When polycythemia is present, the oxygen-carrying capacity of the blood is in-creased; thus the child's arterial oxygen content (milliliters of oxygen per deciliter of blood) may be nearly normal despite the presence of hypoxemia (low PaO_2). However, polycythemia must be present, and cardiac output must be adequate. The polycythemia can then produce complications (see Management, Oxygen Delivery and Polycythemia).

Although the presence of *hypoxemia* does not mean that tissue *hypoxia* is present, the nurse should ensure that the child is stable and monitor signs of tissue hypoxia or organ dysfunction. Signs of inadequate oxygen delivery (tissue hypoxia) in the child with uncorrected cyanotic heart disease may include:

- Deterioration in systemic perfusion (development of pallor, increased respiratory distress, gasping respirations, lethargy, cool extremities, diminished peripheral pulses, and oliguria)
- Significant fall in the child's arterial oxygen tension (less than the child's normal or less than 30 to 35 mm Hg)
- Increased severity of cyanosis
- Development of metabolic acidosis ("red flag" of inadequate oxygen delivery)
- Deterioration in responsiveness, heart rate, or respiratory function

When cyanotic heart disease is present, the child's hemoglobin concentration and hematocrit must be monitored closely. A fall in these values to normal or anemic levels will reduce the oxygen-carrying capacity of the blood and will compromise oxygen delivery unless cardiac output increases commensurately. Such anemia is most likely to occur following cardiac catheterization or palliative surgery.

Hemoconcentration may develop gradually as the hemoglobin concentration and hematocrit rise, or it may develop suddenly with dehydration. Sudden development of hemoconcentration, particularly in association with a bacteremia or microcytic anemia, can increase the likelihood of thromboembolic events. A microcytic anemia is present if the mean corpuscular volume or mean corpuscular hemoglobin concentration is low.

Symptoms of hemoconcentration typically develop once the hematocrit exceeds 70%. These symptoms may be vague, including fatigue, exercise intolerance, dyspnea, and headaches. If the hematocrit rises further, it may be impossible for the patient to complete activities of daily living. This level of hemoconcentration is certainly associated with an increased risk of thromboembolic events; thus neurologic function should be carefully assessed, and efforts should be made to lower an extremely high hematocrit ($\geq 70\%$).

Hypercyanotic Spells Hypercyanotic episodes require immediate intervention. These spells are most likely to develop in infants beyond 3 to 4 months of age. They typically occur in the morning and most frequently are precipitated by crying, defecation, or feeding. The child becomes deeply cyanotic, diaphoretic, irritable, and hyperpneic immediately before or during the spell and may lose consciousness or have a seizure. Characteristics of hypercyanotic spells and their treatment are included in Box 5-21.

Thromboembolic Events Neurologic function must be assessed carefully and frequently when uncorrected cyanotic heart disease is present. The risk of thromboembolic events is particularly high if the hemoglobin is >20 g/dl and the hematocrit is $>60\%$, when a microcytic anemia is present, during episodes of bacteremia or dehydration, and following cardiac catheterization or surgery. Although thromboembolic events can occur anywhere, the most serious ones are cerebral thromboembolic events, or strokes.

Signs of stroke include sudden onset of neurologic signs and symptoms, including: excessive irritability or lethargy (or sudden failure to respond), pupil dilation with decreased response to light, signs of increased intracranial pressure, paralysis, paresthesia, altered speech, or facial droop. The development of any of these signs should be reported to a physician immediately.

Brain Abscess Signs and symptoms of brain abscess formation can be extremely nonspecific. The most common trio of signs associated with brain abscess include fever, headache, and focal neurologic abnormalities. Other signs may include nausea, vomiting, or signs of increased intracranial pressure. Health care team members must have a high index of suspicion when patients are at risk for the development of brain abscess, or these signs can be missed.

Box 5-21

Recognition and Management of Hypercyanotic Episodes

Description

Most often observed during infancy

Usually occur in morning, typically following episode of crying or vagal stimulation

Characterized by progressive irritability, diaphoresis, cyanosis, hypoxemia, hyperpnea

Child may become profoundly hypoxic and lose consciousness

Stroke, death may occur

Medical and Nursing Management

Comfort child and place in knee-chest position

Administer oxygen

Notify physician

Per physician order, administer:

Morphine sulfate (0.1 mg/kg)

Propranolol (0.15-0.25 mg/kg)

Phenylephrine (2-5 µg/kg/min infusion)

ABSOLUTELY NO AIR CAN ENTER ANY IV LINE

Administer isotonic fluid bolus (10 ml/kg)

Treat documented acidosis with sodium bicarbonate

Intubate and provide ventilatory support, if needed

Schedule surgical intervention (physician)

From Hazinski MF: *Nursing care of the critically ill child,* ed 2, St Louis, 1992, Mosby.

The computed tomography (CT) scan is diagnostic for brain abscess and should be performed *before* lumbar puncture in any child with cyanotic heart disease presenting with fever, headache, and focal neurologic findings. Lumbar puncture is performed only if the CT scan is negative. Microbiologic studies are performed but may be negative; blood cultures are frequently negative, and the white blood cell (WBC) count is normal in many children with brain abscess.

Coagulopathy   The child's coagulation profile is often abnormal when cyanotic heart disease and polycythemia are present. Concentrations of vitamin K–dependent clotting factors and fibrinogen are often decreased, and the platelet number may be decreased. Bleeding time may be prolonged, particularly if platelet function is depressed.

Pulmonary Hypertension   There are no clinical signs specific to pulmonary hypertension. Nonspecific clinical signs can include shortness of breath, decreased systemic arterial oxygenation or cardiac output, or signs of CHF.

Management

The following information focuses on supportive measures that maximize the child's arterial oxygen content and minimize the child's risk of systemic consequences of chronic hypoxemia and polycythemia. Specific management of individual defects is reviewed under Specific Diseases.

The nurse must be able to recognize changes in the child's clinical condition as soon as they occur. Signs of deterioration include increased severity of cyanosis, increased respiratory rate and effort, irritability or lethargy, poor systemic perfusion, deterioration in neurologic function or responsiveness, and the development of metabolic acidosis. Report these changes to a physician immediately.

Oxygen Delivery and Polycythemia   Oxygen delivery is maintained in the presence of hypoxemia if the hemoglobin concentration remains high (15 to 21 g/dl) and cardiac output remains adequate. If relative anemia develops in the child with uncorrected cyanotic heart disease, administration of packed RBCs should be considered to increase hemoglobin concentration and oxygen-carrying capacity.

Worsening hypoxemia or cyanosis may be caused by CHF with pulmonary edema or the development of pneumonia or other complicating pulmonary conditions. If worsening hypoxemia results from a compromise in cardiac output, treatment of shock is required (see Shock). If worsening hypoxemia and cyanosis are caused by inadequate pulmonary blood flow or inadequate mixing of systemic and pulmonary venous blood, it may be necessary to establish a shunt on an urgent basis (e.g., creation of an atrial septal defect during cardiac catheterization or surgical creation of a systemic–to–pulmonary artery shunt).

If hypoxemia increases in severity during the first days of life, it may be due to the closure of the ductus, and prostaglandin E_1 (PGE_1) administration may be required to reopen the ductus. PGE_1 produces vasodilation and smooth muscle relaxation, particularly in the walls of the ductus arteriosus. PGE_1 may succeed in opening a ductus during the first days of life. This will provide a route to enhance pulmonary blood flow and result in increased arterial oxygen tension and oxyhemoglobin saturation. Doses, effects, and side effects of PGE_1 administration are presented in Box 5-22.

When polycythemia is present, microcytic anemia must be prevented or treated with administered iron supplements to reduce the risk of thromboembolic events. Hemoconcentration should be prevented, if possible. Parents and primary caretakers should be instructed to call the child's primary care provider if vomiting or diarrhea or dehydration develops or if an infant's fluid intake is compromised for any reason. Whenever an infant or child with uncorrected cyanotic heart disease is placed on "NPO" status for a procedure or surgery, an IV catheter is inserted and IV fluids are provided.

If a rising hemoglobin concentration and hematocrit are producing symptoms in the child with uncorrectable cyanotic heart disease, reduction in the hematocrit by 10% may be accomplished with a plasmapheresis technique. Whole blood is withdrawn, and only the plasma is returned to the patient after separation of RBCs by centrifuge. Alternatively, whole blood is withdrawn and replaced with fresh frozen plasma or albumin, or with isotonic crystalloid. Throughout the procedure, accomplished in a manner similar to a partial ex-

---

Box 5-22

Prostaglandin E₁ Administration to Neonates

Initial Bolus

Initial bolus of 0.1 mg/kg may be provided

Concentration

Dilute 0.3 mg PGE₁ in solution totaling 100 ml (this yields concentration of 0.3 mg/100 ml or 3 μg/ml)

Infusion

0.025-0.1 μg/kg/min

(1 ml/kg/hr of above solution provides 0.05 μg/kg/min)

Effect

Dilation of ductus arteriosus; this should improve systemic arterial oxygenation (if pulmonary blood flow is ductal dependent) or systemic blood flow (if systemic flow is ductal dependent)

Potential Side Effects

Vasodilation, hypotension

Fever

Seizurelike activity

Respiratory depression, apnea

From Hazinski MF: *Nursing care of the critically ill child*, ed 2, St Louis, 1992, Mosby.

---

change transfusion, the child's circulating blood volume and blood pressure should be maintained.

Hypercyanotic Spells   Hypercyanotic spells indicate the need for urgent surgical intervention to provide a route of effective pulmonary blood flow. However, these spells may develop unexpectedly, or they may be present in the child admitted for cardiac catheterization and surgery; thus they may require treatment until surgery can be accomplished.

If the infant has a history of hypercyanotic spells, weight-appropriate doses of morphine and a beta-blocker (typically propranolol) are prepared and kept at the bedside. If a spell develops, the infant is placed in a knee-chest position and oxygen is administered. The knee-chest position improves systemic arterial oxygen saturation, probably by isolating a significant portion of systemic venous return in the legs and by increasing resistance to systemic arterial flow; thus pulmonary blood flow increases. Oxygen administration will lower PVR and increase arterial oxygen content.

IV morphine sulfate (0.1 mg/kg/dose) and a beta-blocker (propranolol, 0.15 to 0.25 mg/kg/dose, administered slowly) probably increase pulmonary blood flow. If contraction of pulmonary infundibular muscle is responsible for the spell, these drugs should relax that muscle. They also exert effects as vasodilators. Phenylephrine (2 to 5 μg/kg/min) may be administered to increase systemic arterial resistance, potentially inhibiting a right-to-left or pulmonary-to-systemic shunt and enhancing pulmonary blood flow. Propranolol is usually administered at regular intervals until the time of surgery.

Thromboembolic Events   Thromboembolic events may occur despite every precaution. However, some preventive measures are essential. *Absolutely no air can be allowed to enter any IV fluid administration system or catheter* when uncorrected cyanotic heart disease is present.

The child's hemoglobin concentration and hematocrit should be monitored closely. If the hemoglobin concentration is >20 to 25 g/dl or the hematocrit is 60% to 70%, in the absence of dehydration, consideration should be given to pheresis. Whole blood is withdrawn and replaced with plasma, albumin, or normal saline to reduce the hemoglobin concentration and the hematocrit. Although erythropoiesis restores the hemoglobin concentration within weeks, the pheresis may provide symptomatic relief and reduce the risk of thromboembolic events for several weeks.

Brain Abscess   Brain abscess must be recognized to be treated; this requires a high index of suspicion. Once the diagnosis of brain abscess is made by CT scan, IV antibiotic therapy is initiated immediately. A combination of penicillin and chloramphenicol or metronidazole may be administered, although the selection of antibiotics will be guided by the sensitivity of the organism and antibiotic penetration into the area. Neurosurgical debridement of the abscess is often necessary but may have to wait until liquefaction of the abscess occurs.

Mortality of brain abscess is approximately 15% to 20% and varies widely with the location of the lesion, the agent, and the promptness and effectiveness of therapy. Sequelae can include seizures and residual neurologic deficits.

Coagulopathy Coagulopathies are treated symptomatically. Postoperative or postprocedure bleeding should be anticipated and blood components prepared accordingly. Directed blood donation may be possible on the day of surgery. Every transfusion carries the risk of blood-borne infection, but blood component therapy is provided as needed.

Unrefrigerated (fresh) whole blood provides the best clotting factors and platelets and thus should be obtained through directed donation on the day of surgery, if possible. If very fresh (unrefrigerated) whole blood cannot be obtained on the day of surgery, fresh whole blood (stored less than 48 hours) should be used. Blood component therapy is provided as needed to correct significant coagulopathies (see Table 5-12).

Pulmonary Hypertension Pulmonary hypertension is better prevented than treated. Prevention is accomplished through early surgical correction of cyanotic heart disease and prevention of severe hemoconcentration. If pulmonary hypertension is present, factors contributing to pulmonary vasoconstriction (alveolar hypoxia, acidosis, hypothermia, and agitation) are avoided and factors favoring pulmonary vasodilation (alveolar oxygenation, alkalosis, analgesia, and avoidance of stimulation) are supported.

Vasodilators may be administered, although oral or IV vasodilators will dilate both arteries and veins. Inhaled nitric oxide is often used to control pulmonary hypertension postoperatively.

Postoperative Care of the Pediatric Cardiovascular Surgical Patient

General principles of postoperative care are similar for all patients following cardiovascular surgery; however, there are several aspects of postoperative care that are unique to the care of children. As a

result, pediatric expertise is required to care for pediatric patients and their families after cardiovascular surgery.

Children generally require cardiovascular surgery to palliate or correct congenital heart disease (CHD); thus the surgery often requires intracardiac reconstruction that is quite different from that performed during surgical treatment of adult coronary artery disease. The better the nurse's understanding of the child's congenital heart defect, preoperative condition, surgical procedure, and potential postoperative complications, the more able that nurse will be to anticipate, recognize, and treat postoperative complications.

A specific postoperative care plan should be developed for each child that includes an illustration of the child's heart defect and surgical procedure. Very few "classic" repairs are performed exactly as they were first designed. Most cardiovascular surgeons now use modified procedures that are tailored to the child's anatomy. Therefore use of terms such as "the Fontan procedure" to describe a child's corrective surgery can lead to confusion, because few procedures to correct tricuspid atresia are performed today as Fontan originally described them. Whenever possible, the surgical procedure should be described anatomically (e.g., cavopulmonary anastomosis) rather than referred to by a proper name.

Preoperative Preparation of the Child and Family

The child's level of cognitive and psychosocial development, as well as the child's level of anxiety and comprehension of and attitudes about the surgery, should always guide plans to prepare the child for the surgery and postoperative care. The goals of surgery should be expressed in terms intelligible to and meaningful to the child. For example, the child should not be told that the surgery will make him or her "better" if the child has no appreciable symptoms from the heart disease. However, if the child's exercise tolerance has been limited by the heart disease or the child is acutely conscious of cyanosis, the child may look forward to improved function or appearance after the surgery.

Parents should be involved in the preoperative preparation of the child, and they can guide the pace and intensity of the preparation. Whenever possible, words the parents have used in explanations should be reinforced. The parents' guilt or anxiety should be addressed separately from the child's preparation.

All preparation of the child should focus on addressing the *child's* questions and concerns and on preparing the child for things the child will see, feel, or hear, at a pace that is determined by the child's tolerance. Too much attention focused on things that will happen out of the child's awareness may increase rather than relieve anxiety. A common mistake made in preoperative preparation is to provide the child with an inflexible body of information, rather than providing the child with information the *child* wants or needs to hear.

Much information can be gained from the child and given to the child in a nonthreatening manner through play. Use of a suitcase filled with equipment (e.g., dressings, syringes, tape, tubes) and a doll as the "patient" may allow the child to enact or rehearse procedures and postoperative care. Books with pictures of equipment and children postoperatively may be useful adjuncts to the preoperative preparation session (Table 5-18).

Specific words used to describe the surgical procedure, risks, and postoperative equipment to the child and family should be recorded in the chart and on the nursing Kardex so that all health care team members can use consistent terms. These terms should be reinforced during the preparation.

The infant will not understand time intervals or plans for the surgery. Therefore the older infant will require warning immediately before painful procedures and the presence of the parents for comfort. Preparation for surgery will focus on the parents.

Preparation of the toddler is particularly challenging, because the toddler has a poor concept of time intervals, a tendency to interpret painful procedures as punishment, and a fear of separation from parents. Too much information can frighten the toddler, but inadequate preparation can result in a terrified and distrustful child. Most preparation should be accomplished immediately before a painful procedure, and parents should remain with the toddler whenever possible.

The preschooler and school-age child are at ideal ages to comprehend plans for surgery and prepare for postoperative care. These children will probably benefit most from preoperative play. At this age the child is very literal in interpretation of terms and time intervals; thus word choice should be considered carefully.

The adolescent may be reluctant to ask questions and may be very concerned about privacy and modesty postoperatively. It can be useful to discuss questions that "many kids your age" have asked to provide the information in a nonthreatening manner.

Preoperative preparation should include a visit to the postoperative unit. However, it is extremely important to control the things a child and family will see during the visit. If the visitors walk into a resuscitation or crisis, anxiety can be increased rather than decreased. Occasionally the child may misinterpret something seen or heard; thus the child's behavior and reactions must be closely monitored, with plenty of opportunity for verification and clarification of the child's thoughts and concerns.

Preoperative Assessment

The nurse caring for the child postoperatively should be aware of the child's preoperative health status, intraoperative cardiovascular function, and particular postsurgical complications associated with the surgical intervention. If at all possible, the nurse should meet the child and family preoperatively and assess the child's cardiac, respiratory, and neurologic function, to better recognize changes postoperatively. Fundamental aspects of the child's preoperative condition (e.g., hearing deficit, compromise in renal function, coagulopathy, pulmonary hypertension) and allergies should be recorded on a preoperative assessment sheet, as well as in a preoperative note.

The child's age, weight, length, and body surface area (BSA) should be noted on the preoperative note and communicated to the operating room, as well as to the postoperative unit. If possible, the child should be weighed in the postoperative unit the day before surgery; that weight is recorded as the "previous day's weight" on the flow sheet prepared for use on the postoperative day.

The nurse should record unique words used by the child to refer to parents, siblings, grandparents,

Table 5-18
Psychosocial Development

Age Group	Psychosocial Development	Cognitive Development	Play	Stressors During Critical Care	Pain
Infant	Developing sense of trust vs. mistrust (Erikson). Bonding with caregiver, and will develop stranger anxiety once object permanence is present. Will normally demonstrate good eye contact. Should not be excessively irritable or lethargic.	Sensorimotor period (Piaget). Progresses from reflexive to organized responses. Development of object permanence will coincide with stranger anxiety and preference for primary caretaker.	Transitional objects may be important once object permanence develops. Social-affective play, sense-pleasure play, and sensorimotor activity are important.	Separation from parents and disruption in routines (including sleep-wake patterns) create stress. Constant environmental stimuli can cause sleep deprivation or overstimulation. Movement restriction is stressful.	Nonspecific signs may include facial grimace, flexion of extremity, or cry. Restlessness, irritability, lethargy, or poor feeding may indicate illness or pain. Tachycardia may indicate pain or other stress.
Toddler	Developing autonomy and self-control. Balance between autonomy, and shame and doubt develops during issues such as bowel and bladder control. Dependent on primary caretakers. Is learning to choose between desirable and undesirable behaviors	Beginning to think and reason. Sensorimotor period. Expanding vocabulary. Beginning to understand causal relationships and may interpret painful procedures as punishment. Understands simple explanations.	Will play more securely when primary caretakers are present. Needs active, as well as passive, play. Large muscle exercise is important when child is recovering.	Separation from primary caretakers is stressful, as is disruption in routines (including mealtimes, bedtime rituals, schedule). Movement restriction, the supine position, and strangers are all frightening.	Usually will *not* feign discomfort or pain (take complaints seriously). Splinting, guarding, etc., will provide reliable cues to pain. May successfully use Beyer's "Oucher" or Eland Color Tool.

Continued

Table 5-18
Psychosocial Development—cont'd

Age Group	Psychosocial Development	Cognitive Development	Play	Stressors During Critical Care	Pain
Preschooler	Age of discovery, curiosity, and developing social behavior and language. Balance between initiative and guilt (Erikson). Expanding imagination can cause fear. Coping styles are established. Primary caretakers still provide valuable support, security.	Magical thinking, difficulty distinguishing between reality and fantasy. Beginning to think abstractly; good concepts of time intervals. Comprehends very simple explanations. Will often interpret words literally (be careful with homophones)	Will use imagination to play fantasy roles, but may be frightened by imaginary things. Needs large muscle exercise during recovery. Play can provide clues to child's understanding of illness and treatment.	Needs support. Because body image is still developing, ICU care by strangers can be terrifying. Wounds, punctures may lead to fears that inside of body will "leak out." Often feels guilty for illness or injury. Imagination can cause fear of ICU sights, sounds.	May not be able to express or localize pain clearly. Behavioral cues: restlessness, poor appetite, aggression, withdrawal, dependent behavior. Because child may equate stoicism with "good," encourage expression. Use Eland Color Tool, "Oucher," etc., to assess.
School-age child	Learning balance of sense of industry vs. inferiority (Erikson). Learning to meet expectations of nonfamily. Acceptance of peers and teachers is important. Better able to tolerate separation from caregivers. Needs control, independence, support.	Concrete operational thought (Piaget)—able to think in abstract, think through consequences, and understand explanations. Reality and future oriented. May still feel guilty for illness, injury.	Will often engage in productive play—will have good recall of teaching events. Needs opportunity for interaction with peers, competitive games.	Will often fear loss of emotional control and privacy. Is often uncomfortable with focus on body—particularly from strangers. Fear of mutilation may be reality or fantasy based. Requires honest but simple explanations.	Usually able to localize and quantify pain well and may reliably report effects of analgesia. Needs time to mobilize resources before painful procedures. Needs control and some choice in sequence of treatments and analgesia when possible.
Adolescent	Transition between childhood and adulthood. Balance between identity and role diffusion (Erikson). May be self-conscious, acutely aware of bodily appearance. Peer relationships and future plans are important.	Logical thought, deductive reasoning, and abstract thinking. Able to imagine consequences of illness. Some magical thinking.	Peer group extremely important. Primary caretakers may provide support. Familiar activities (music, television, video games) provide distraction, comfort.	Loss of control and privacy likely to be stressful. May have difficulty being dependent on others. May be frightened by alteration in body function, appearance. Likely to be embarrassed by physical examinations.	Can accurately locate and quantify pain. Fears may intensify expressions of pain. May also attempt to be stoic.

pain, fear, thirst, urination, and defecation so that these will be recognized postoperatively. The nurse should also make note of specific comfort objects (e.g., blanket or toy) or comfort measures (e.g., sucking of the right thumb).

Preparation of the Intensive Care Unit

The child's bed space is prepared for postoperative care while the child is in surgery. If at all possible, the child should be transported from the operating room to the unit on the bed the child will occupy during postoperative care. If the child is transported on a gurney, then the postoperative bed is prepared with appropriate linen, including a draw sheet to facilitate shifting and rolling of the patient.

All major equipment needed in the postoperative care of the child should be gathered at the bedside and turned on to ensure proper working order before the child returns from surgery. Proper "warm-up" time should be allowed if needed for the bedside monitor and transducers or monitoring equipment. The following setup is required:

- Prepare bedside monitor: enter patient variables (weight, BSA); set alarm limits for heart rate, blood pressure, and pulse oximeter.
- If possible, use the infusion pumps and transducers from the operating room (transducers must be zeroed and mechanically calibrated when transferred to the bedside monitor). If new pumps are required, these must be primed and ready.
- Prepare mechanical ventilator with selection of appropriate ventilator variables (rate, tidal volume, minute ventilation, mode of support).
- Set up manual resuscitation bag and mask and endotracheal suctioning equipment, including sterile saline and syringes for endotracheal tube irrigation.
- Prepare all tubes, labels, and requisitions for postoperative blood work, additional IV fluids, and typical postoperative medications.
- Assemble one or more hemostats to clamp chest tubes if needed.
- Set up suction systems for chest drainage (chest drainage units should come with the patient).
- Tape sign at the bedside with the child's name, length, weight, BSA, and allergies.

Admission of the Child to the Critical Care Unit

The admission of the child to the critical care unit requires organization and a calm approach. Typically, two nurses "accept" the child, with very specific responsibilities designated for each nurse (Table 5-19). If the nurses are competent and experienced and the team is organized, the admission should require few words beyond the report. The surgeon and anesthesiologist should accompany the patient to the unit and should transfer care of the child to the postoperative team (nurses, physicians, therapists) with a report as the child is admitted.

Postoperative Care

Initial Assessment

When the child returns from the operating room, initial assessment focuses on airway, breathing, and circulation. If the child is intubated and receiving hand ventilation, assessment of airway patency and position and establishment of effective mechanical ventilation are priorities. If the tube is patent and appropriately placed and if ventilation is effective, the chest should rise during positive pressure ventilation, and breath sounds should be equal and adequate bilaterally. If the child is breathing spontaneously, the child's airway patency and effectiveness of ventilation should be assessed. Oxygenation is assessed through use of pulse oximetry and verified with arterial blood gas analysis as needed.

Once the child's airway, ventilation, and oxygenation have been assessed and supported appropriately, systemic perfusion is assessed. However, throughout postoperative care, the child's airway, ventilation, and oxygenation are repeatedly verified. The most common causes of acute deterioration in the intubated child are tube *D*isplacement, tube *O*bstruction, *P*neumothorax, or *E*quipment failure ("DOPE").

Cardiovascular Function and Systemic Perfusion

The child's cardiovascular function must be closely monitored during the postoperative period. Adequate cardiac output and effective systemic perfusion require a heart rate that is appropriate for the clinical condition, sufficient cardiac preload or

Table 5-19
Nursing Responsibilities During Admission of the Pediatric Cardiovascular Surgical Patient

Nurse 1	Time Frame	Nurse 2

Assess and support:
    Airway, oxygenation, ventilation (airway, breath sounds, chest expansion)
    Heart rate and rhythm
    Systemic perfusion (strength of pulses, capillary refill)
	Immediate	Locate, label, and attach arterial and venous monitoring lines to appropriate monitoring and flush systems. Zero and calibrate systems. Identify and secure intravenous lines and regulate to appropriate infusion rate

Place child on cardiac monitor. Obtain rhythm strip. Obtain vital signs; relay them to surgeon and anesthesiologist.	Within minutes	Check function, location of pacer wires, pacemaker (as needed). Attach chest tubes to suction; be sure that water seal chamber is filled correctly; label pleural drainage systems.
Remain at head of bed for patient needs (suctioning, administration of medications). Repeat vital signs every 5 min initially, then every 15 min to a maximum interval of every hour.	After several minutes	Drain chest tubes, record drainage and notify bedside nurse and physician of excessive drainage. Administer blood products as needed.

When child is stable, ask surgeon about the following:
    Complications or problems
    Nature of surgical intervention
    Fluid and medications administered
Bring parents to see child as soon as possible.
	When child is stable	Obtain postoperative blood samples. Then remain at bedside to assist bedside nurse in obtaining supplies, medications.

intravascular volume relative to the vascular space, adequate myocardial function, and appropriate ventricular afterload or impedance to ventricular ejection. The most common postoperative cardiovascular complications include arrhythmias, shock/low cardiac output, bleeding, tamponade, and congestive heart failure (CHF).

If heart rate, cardiac preload, or myocardial function is inadequate, or if ventricular afterload is excessive, cardiac output and systemic perfusion may be poor. Signs of inadequate cardiac output (shock) include tachycardia, tachypnea (if the child is breathing spontaneously), peripheral vasoconstriction, oliguria, diminished intensity of peripheral pulses, delayed capillary refill (despite a warm ambient temperature), excessive irritability or lethargy, and possible metabolic acidosis. Decompensated shock produces hypotension with possible bradycardia; these findings indicate that cardiac arrest may be imminent.

Heart Rate and Arrhythmias   The heart rate must be *appropriate* for the clinical condition, and arrhythmias that compromise cardiac output must be treated immediately. Tachycardia is expected in the postoperative period, and a normal heart rate may be inadequate. Bradycardia may be an ominous finding, indicating hypoxia, heart block, or impending cardiac arrest.

The most common arrhythmias observed in the postoperative period include sinus bradycardia, sick sinus syndrome, heart block (particularly right bundle branch block following a ventriculotomy, and first- and second-degree heart block, including Wenckebach), supraventricular tachycardia (SVT), and junctional ectopic tachycardia. Ventricular tachycardia is an ominous rhythm that may be observed in children with left heart or aortic obstructive lesions and severe left ventricular hypertrophy with strain, or in infants with severe obstruction to right ventricular outflow (e.g., pulmonary atresia with an intact ventricular septum). Ventricular arrhythmias may also develop among children who have undergone surgical procedures involving ventriculotomy incisions or in children with postoperative low cardiac output, hypoxia, acidosis, or electrolyte imbalance. For further information about arrhythmias, see Arrhythmias under Common Clinical Conditions.

If the surgical repair involves manipulation near the intracardiac conduction system (e.g., correction of an endocardial cushion defect), temporary pacing wires are placed at the time of surgery. These wires may be used for pacing in the operating room or may be coiled and taped on the chest for use during external pacing if needed. The pacing wires are placed in pairs: a pacing wire and a ground wire are placed to enable ventricular pacing, and a pacing wire and a ground wire are placed if atrial pacing is required. The pacing wires are placed on the epicardium during surgery and then brought through the child's chest wall. The ground wires are attached to the subcutaneous tissue on the outside of the chest. The function of the pacing wires should be tested even if no pacing is required. If pacing is required, the pacemaker is adjusted to provide appropriate sensing and pacing of the desired cardiac chambers.

If permanent heart block is anticipated postoperatively, permanent pacing wires may be placed at the time of surgery, with plans to implant the pacemaker and join the implanted wires to the pacemaker at a later date if needed. The placement of the wires prevents the need for later thoracotomy.

Inadequate Intravascular Volume   Inadequate intravascular volume can result from hemorrhage, negative fluid balance (excessive fluid output or inadequate intake), or significant vasodilation. If intravascular volume is severely compromised, signs of hypovolemic shock will be present. Initial signs of hypovolemia include tachycardia, peripheral vasoconstriction, oliguria, diminished peripheral pulses, delayed capillary refill, and possible metabolic acidosis. These signs are present in the child with a central venous/right atrial pressure and a left atrial/pulmonary artery end-diastolic pressure of <5 to 10 mm Hg. The heart size is usually small if hypovolemia is present. Hypotension will not

develop until significant hemorrhage or severe volume depletion has occurred.

Volume administration is required when intravascular volume is inadequate. The fluid selected should replace that lost in quantity and content. Bolus fluid administration with isotonic crystalloids or colloids is required to treat shock, and reassessment and repeat boluses may possibly be required.

Hemorrhage   Bleeding is most likely to occur in children with cyanotic heart disease (see Hypoxemia Caused by Cyanotic Heart Disease under Common Clinical Conditions), in those who have experienced complex surgical procedures, or following reoperation. Reoperation requires dissection of scar tissue that is highly vascular and will bleed diffusely. Bleeding should be anticipated in these "high-risk" patients but may develop in any patient.

Calculate the child's circulating blood volume before the child returns from the operating room, and total and evaluate all blood lost or drawn for laboratory analysis as a percentage of that circulating blood volume. The following chest tube output quantities may be clinically significant and require replacement:

- 3 ml/kg/hr for 3 or more hours
- 5 ml/kg for any 1 hour
- Chest tube output totaling 10% to 15% of circulating blood volume during the first 3 to 5 postoperative hours

Blood replacement is indicated when significant postoperative bleeding develops, and the source of the bleeding should be determined, if possible. A coagulation panel is drawn, and any coagulopathies detected should be corrected (see Table 5-12). Excessive chest tube output despite normal clotting function usually requires reoperation.

Coagulopathies are common after correction of cyanotic heart disease. Additional causes of coagulopathies following open-heart surgery include incomplete heparin reversal and activation of cold agglutinins during hypothermic surgery or blood administration. If the patient has cold agglutinins, all blood products must be warmed before administration.

Monitor the child's hematocrit to determine the need for blood administration. Although there is no ideal hemoglobin concentration or hematocrit, the hemoglobin is typically maintained with administration of packed RBCs in the range of 12 to 15 g/dl, with a hematocrit of approximately 35% to 40%. Lower hemoglobin concentration may be tolerated if the patient's cardiac function and cardiac output are good. If the patient's parents are Jehovah's witnesses, blood products may be withheld at the parents' request unless cardiovascular function is seriously compromised; then it may be necessary to obtain a court order to enable administration of blood products.

Titration of Fluid Administration A ventricular end-diastolic pressure (VEDP) of 5 to 10 mm Hg is typically required to support effective systemic perfusion. Lower filling pressures may be acceptable if ventricular function is excellent, and slightly higher pressures may be required (in the range of 12 to 15 mm Hg) if ventricular function is poor. These pressures are maintained through administration of crystalloids (normal saline or lactated Ringer's solution) or colloids (5% albumin) and blood products as needed.

During the immediate postoperative period, bolus administration of crystalloids or colloids is often necessary to replace volume lost by osmotic diuresis in response to glucose or mannitol in the pump prime. If hypothermic cardiovascular surgery was performed, vasodilation will develop as the child warms, and it may necessitate additional volume administration.

Myocardial Dysfunction and Low Cardiac Output

Signs of low cardiac output include tachycardia, tachypnea (if the child is breathing spontaneously), peripheral vasoconstriction, oliguria, diminished intensity of peripheral pulses, delayed capillary refill (despite a warm ambient temperature), hepatomegaly, metabolic acidosis, and a right ventricular end-diastolic pressure (RVEDP; per right atrial or central venous pressure) >8 to 12 mm Hg. The left ventricular end-diastolic pressure (LVEDP; per left atrial or pulmonary artery occlusion pressure) may also be >8 to 12 mm Hg.

Cardiac contractility may be impaired as a result of hypoxia, acidosis, electrolyte imbalance, intraoperative myocardial resection, or surgical alteration of pressure, flow, and resistance relationships. Hypoxia or acidosis may impair myocardial performance significantly.

Electrolyte imbalance is a frequent complication of cardiovascular surgery, and these imbalances can depress myocardial function:

- Hypokalemia can result from diuresis, dilution, or correction of acidosis.
- Hyperkalemia can complicate renal failure.
- Hypocalcemia is common and may be caused by dilution or administration of citrate-phosphate-dextran–preserved blood (the phosphate will precipitate with calcium from the serum).
- Hypoglycemia may develop in young infants, particularly if glucose administration is inadequate.
- Hyperglycemia with an osmotic diuresis can develop if glucose-containing solutions are used to prime the bypass pump.

Management of low cardiac output requires manipulation of intravascular volume. Identify the right and left ventricular "filling pressures" associated with the best cardiac output or systemic perfusion and maintain those pressures with fluid administration. Inotropic support is also indicated (see Table 5-13). Dopamine is often the drug of choice, particularly if renal perfusion and urine output are poor. Dobutamine may be selected if poor myocardial function is associated with systemic vasoconstriction but adequate blood pressure. Drugs such as amrinone or milrinone may be useful to improve myocardial function, particularly if vasoconstriction is thought to be compromising cardiac output. Manipulation of vascular resistance may also be required to alter ventricular compliance and afterload.

Inappropriate Vascular Resistance When myocardial function is poor, the compensatory systemic vasoconstriction that develops to redistribute systemic blood flow may ultimately depress cardiac output further. Therefore vasodilator therapy may be indicated for the treatment of low cardiac output, particularly if it is associated with systemic vasoconstriction (see Table 5-14). Volume administration may be required during vasodilator therapy to maintain adequate intravascular volume relative to an expanded vascular space and to maintain adequate ventricular preload.

Sodium nitroprusside and nitroglycerin are the two most common vasodilators administered by continuous infusion postoperatively. Inhaled nitric oxide may be administered to selectively dilate the pulmonary vascular bed for patients with postoperative pulmonary hypertension (see Treatment of Pulmonary Hypertension/Manipulation of Pulmonary Vascular Resistance).

Tamponade Tamponade can cause a sudden, fatal decrease in cardiac output postoperatively, or it may develop gradually, producing progressive signs of low cardiac output. Postoperative tamponade classically develops in association with postoperative bleeding, but it may also be caused by pericardial effusion.

Signs of tamponade may be similar to those of CHF or shock and include tachycardia, narrowing of the pulse pressure, and high central venous/right atrial pressure or high left atrial pressure. Isolated right or left heart tamponade may be present, resulting in elevation of only the right atrial or left atrial pressure. Other signs of tamponade, including muffled heart tones, depression of voltage of the QRS complexes on the ECG, or friction rub, may or may not be present. A pathognomonic finding attributed to tamponade is pulsus paradoxus, or a fall in systolic blood pressure by ≥ 8 to 10 mm Hg during inspiration. However, this sign is virtually impossible to detect in the tachypneic or hypotensive child; thus it may not be appreciated.

The chest x-ray film may be normal or may reveal an apparent increase in the cardiothoracic ratio. Echocardiography is diagnostic for tamponade, and pericardiocentesis is the treatment. If continued bleeding is present, surgical exploration may be required.

Treatment of Pulmonary Hypertension/ Manipulation of Pulmonary Vascular Resistance
Mechanical ventilatory support, including support of alveolar oxygenation, is one of the most important aspects of care of the child with pulmonary hypertension. Pulmonary vasoconstrictors, including alveolar hypoxia, acidosis, hypothermia, and agitation, must be avoided. In addition, factors associated with pulmonary vasodilation, including alveolar oxygenation, alkalosis, and avoidance of stimulation, are all supported. A mild hyperventilation or administration of sodium bicarbonate may be used to maintain alkalosis (pH approximately 7.5).

If the infant has severe pulmonary hypertension with periodic hypertensive "crises" that produce a sudden decrease in cardiac output, meticulous prevention of pulmonary vasoconstriction is required, sedation should be provided, and anesthesia may be needed.

In many cardiovascular centers, inhaled nitric oxide is provided under research protocol to promote pulmonary vasodilation. It is titrated in concentrations of 10 to 80 parts per million (ppm), although it is generally effective at concentrations of 10 to 20 ppm. Methemoglobinemia may develop as a complication of nitric oxide inhalation; thus the methemoglobin concentration is evaluated several times per day and should be kept below 2 g/dl. Additional vasodilators and amrinone or milrinone may also be administered to promote pulmonary vasodilation.

Two skilled health care providers are needed every time endotracheal suctioning is performed. The first person suctions the tube quickly and gently, maintaining sterile technique. The second person provides hand ventilation while monitoring the infant's heart rate, color, and systemic arterial oxygenation (via pulse oximetry). If the infant deteriorates during suctioning, the suctioning is interrupted and hand ventilation with increased inspired oxygen concentration is provided until the child's heart rate, color, and cardiovascular function are stable. Weaning from mechanical ventilatory support is accomplished gradually.

If the patient has a defect including a single ventricle or single-ventricle physiology (e.g., tricuspid atresia or hypoplastic left ventricle), the balance between systemic and pulmonary blood flow must be carefully controlled through manipulation of pulmonary vascular resistance (PVR). Cyanotic heart disease is present (no air can be allowed to enter any IV line !), and a "balanced" shunt is generally present if systemic hemoglobin saturation is maintained at 75% to 80%, with a PaO_2 of 40 to 50 mm Hg.

Excessive pulmonary blood flow will cause high hemoglobin saturations (>80%) detected by pulse oximetry but will have the undesirable effect of causing excessive pulmonary blood flow and CHF, as well as a "steal" of blood from the systemic circulation (often causing a decrease in peripheral pulses, reduction in urine volume, and possible hypotension or cooling of extremities). *Inadequate pulmonary blood flow* will produce worsening hypoxemia (hemoglobin saturation <70%). although systemic perfusion may improve (strong peripheral pulses, warm extremities, possible rise in systemic arterial blood pressure).

In patients with single ventricle physiology, PVR is controlled to determine the balance between pulmonary and systemic blood flow. Alveolar oxygenation and ventilation, pH, and vasoactive drugs can all be manipulated to alter pulmonary vascular tone and pulmonary blood flow (Table 5-20). In general, pulmonary vasodilation is promoted using the same factors involved in the treatment of the patient with pulmonary hypertension: improvement in alveolar ventilation, alkalotic pH, and administration of nitric oxide or other vasodilators. Pulmonary vasoconstriction may be stimulated through reduction in alveolar ventilation (reduce Fio_2 and/or ventilatory support) and reduction in pH. Vasoconstrictors may also stimulate pulmonary vasoconstriction. Regardless of the therapy used, the nurse must constantly assess evidence of the child's systemic perfusion and pulmonary blood flow, since adjustments in therapy will often be required.

Evaluation of Response to Therapy   During treatment of any of these causes of inadequate cardiac output, the child's response to therapy must be assessed constantly. A positive response to therapy includes possible reduction in tachycardia (but no bradycardia), better perfusion of extremities with warming of fingers and toes, improved quality of peripheral pulses, reduction of capillary refill time, increase in urine volume, and (unless the child is sedated) more appropriate response to stimulation (less excessive irritability or lethargy). If a pulmonary artery catheter is placed to enable calculation of cardiac output and vascular resistances, these calculations will aid in the evaluation of response to therapy.

Congestive Heart Failure   CHF is often present postoperatively, particularly if it was present preoperatively or if the surgical repair required a ventriculotomy. Signs of CHF include adrenergic compensatory signs (tachycardia, peripheral vasoconstriction, oliguria), signs of systemic venous congestion (hepatomegaly, periorbital edema), and signs of pulmonary venous congestion (pulmonary edema, increased work of breathing). Treatment includes elimination of excess extravascular water (with diuretics and limitation of fluid intake) and inotropic support (e.g., with a digitalis derivative or continuous infusion of inotropic drugs). Vasodilator therapy may also be required (see Congestive

Table 5-20
Manipulation of Pulmonary Vascular Resistance

Factor	To Produce Pulmonary Constriction	To Produce Pulmonary Dilation
Alveolar oxygenation	Reduce Fio_2 May "bleed in" nitrogen (or CO_2) to inspired air circuit to reduce Fio_2 to <0.21	Increase Fio_2 Increase ventilatory support
pH	Reduce Reduce mechanical ventilator support (reduce rate, tidal volume, inspiratory pressure) May "bleed in" CO_2 into inspired air circuit to increase or maintain $Paco_2$	Increase May administer sodium bicarbonate May induce hyperventilation with mechanical ventilation
Medications	Any vasoconstrictors	Nitric oxide Prostaglandin Any drug with beta-2 adrenergic effects Miscellaneous

Heart Failure under Common Clinical Conditions and Tables 5-6 and 5-7).

Pulmonary Function

Mechanical ventilatory support is generally planned for several days following complex surgical procedures. Once the child's neurologic function is assessed and documented postoperatively, sedatives, analgesics, and neuromuscular blockade may be administered as needed to ensure that the child is comfortable during mechanical ventilation (see Chapter 3).

If the Child Is Intubated If the child is intubated and mechanically ventilated postoperatively, the following should be verified and maintained at all times:

- *Airway patency and position:* Ensure that breath sounds are adequate with hand and machine ventilation and that breath sounds and chest expansion bilaterally are equal and adequate. Verify endotracheal tube tip position on chest x-ray examination. Note and mark the tube insertion point at the lips. Unexplained hypercarbia during mechanical ventilation should be presumed to be caused by tube obstruction until this has been ruled out.
- *Effectiveness of oxygenation:* Monitor pulse oximetry and color.
- *Adequacy of ventilation:* Breath sounds and chest expansion should be equal and adequate bilaterally (observe from head or foot of bed). Monitor end-tidal carbon dioxide and arterial blood gases.
- *Color, peripheral perfusion, level of consciousness, and responsiveness.*

If the intubated child suddenly becomes restless or combative, remove from mechanical ventilation, provide hand ventilation, and evaluate the above factors immediately. Causes of acute deterioration in the intubated child include ("DOPE"):

- *Tube **D**isplacement:* Into esophagus or one main stem bronchus. Breath sounds and chest expansion will be inadequate, or unequal between the right and left sides.

- *Tube **O**bstruction:* Hand ventilation will not succeed in providing chest expansion or adequate breath sounds.
- *Pneumothorax:* Decreased breath sounds and chest expansion on involved side. Tension pneumothorax causes a shift of the mediastinum away from the pneumothorax and results in severe compromise in cardiac output and oxygenation. Pulsus paradoxus (fall in systolic blood pressure by 8 to 10 mm Hg or more during inspiration) may be observed with tension pneumothorax.
- *Equipment failure:* Oxygenation and ventilation should improve with hand ventilation.

Extubation The child should not be extubated until cardiac and pulmonary function are stable and satisfactory. Ventilatory support should be continued if shock, hemorrhage, severe CHF, pulmonary hypertension, or symptomatic arrhythmias are present, or if diaphragm paralysis is present.

Extubation should be performed electively, preferably at the beginning of the day. It may also be performed immediately after surgery. The child should be breathing effectively and should be relatively alert. The endotracheal tube is suctioned immediately before extubation, and humidified oxygen is provided immediately after extubation, in concentrations higher than those provided via the endotracheal tube. The inspired oxygen can be weaned as tolerated once it is clear that the child's respiratory rate and effort are acceptable.

If the Child Is Extubated The nurse should constantly evaluate the child's respiratory rate, effort, and effectiveness. The nurse should monitor for evidence that reintubation is required.

Tachypnea may indicate complications such as atelectasis or pneumothorax, particularly if the heart rate is increasing rather than decreasing as the postoperative period progresses. Slowing of the respiratory rate in a child who is laboring is ominous and typically indicates the need for provision of ventilatory support.

Increased respiratory effort, with retractions, nasal flaring, and grunting, may be present early after extubation, particularly if some upper airway obstruction is present. However, over time, the child should get better rather than worse. Administration of dexamethasone (0.5 g/kg, maximum 10 mg, every 6 hours for six doses) during the time of extubation may reduce postextubation stridor and upper airway obstruction. Racemic epinephrine treatments may reduce mild or moderate postoperative (postintubation) subglottic edema (0.125 to 0.5 ml of 2.25% racemic epinephrine diluted with 2 to 3 ml of water or normal saline, administered via aerosol). Heliox (helium plus oxygen) may also be provided to treat upper airway obstruction but can only be used if the child requires no more than 40% oxygen in inspired air.

Potential Postoperative Pulmonary Complications   Postoperative complications include atelectasis, pneumothorax, hemothorax, pleural effusions, and chylothorax. The nurse should monitor for signs of each of these. For x-ray appearance of these complications, see Chapter 7.

- *Atelectasis:* May result from hypoventilation or development of mucus plug. Atelectasis is characterized by decreased chest expansion and decreased or altered breath sounds on the involved side and may compromise oxygenation. Treatment is chest physical therapy, but consider the need for mechanical ventilation or continuous positive airway pressure (CPAP). Mucus plugs may be removed with bronchoscopic bronchial lavage.
- *Pneumothorax:* Characterized by decreased chest expansion and decreased or altered breath sounds over involved side. Treatment requires evacuation through needle thoracostomy or with a chest tube. If a chest tube is inserted, note how long air leak (indicated by bubbling through the water seal) continues.
- *Hemothorax:* Can result from mediastinal bleeding if there is communication between the pleural spaces and the mediastinum. Hemothorax will produce blood in the chest tube or accumulation of blood in the chest, with decreased chest expansion and decreased or altered breath sounds on the involved side. Hemothorax is evacuated by the chest tube. Significant blood loss must be replaced, and surgical exploration may be required.

- *Pleural effusions:* May develop in association with CHF or postcardiotomy syndrome. Plural effusions are characterized by accumulation of intrathoracic fluid, causing decreased lung and chest expansion on the involved side and decreased or altered breath sounds over the involved area. Treatment consists of thoracentesis or chest tube insertion and treatment of the cause. Fluid obtained may be sent for culture or analysis to rule out empyema or chylothorax.
- *Chylothorax:* Chylothorax is the accumulation of lymph fluid in the chest that results from injury to or obstruction of the thoracic duct (less common) or a large lymphatic vessel (more common). Chylothorax may also develop in children with high central venous pressure, such as following correction of tricuspid atresia, or it may be congenital in origin. Chylothorax will produce fat-colored (creamy) chest drainage once the child begins eating, since this reflects the presence of fat transported from the gut into the lymphatics and thoracic duct. Treatment requires drainage (often for weeks) or repeat thoracentesis. A medium-chain triglyceride diet or total parenteral alimentation will reduce the lymphatic drainage and should allow the chylothorax to heal. Supplementation of fat-soluble vitamins is required.

Neurologic Function

Neurologic function, including level of consciousness, ability to follow commands (if age appropriate), pupil size and response to light, spontaneous movement and posturing, and response to painful stimuli, should be evaluated as soon as the child returns from surgery and on a regular basis. Withdrawal from painful stimuli should be verified by pinching the medial aspect of all four extremities (withdrawal = abduction of extremities). Factors producing pupil dilation and constriction following cardiovascular surgery are listed in Box 5-23. If neurologic abnormalities are detected, a more thorough evaluation will be required.

If postoperative mechanical ventilation is planned and sedatives or neuromuscular blockade will be required, it is advisable to allow the child to

Box 5-23

Factors Producing Pupil Dilation and Constriction Following Pediatric Cardiovascular Surgery

Pupil Dilation

Stroke, herniation
Seizures
Large doses of vagolytic agents (atropine)
Large doses of sympathomimetic drugs
Extreme hypothermia
Mydriatic drops

Pupil Constriction

Ipsilateral Horner's syndrome (ptosis, meiosis, anhydrosis on the same side as surgical incision)
Brain stem dysfunction
Opiate, barbiturate poisoning

From Hazinski MF: *Nursing care of the critically ill child,* ed 2, St Louis, 1992, Mosby.

awaken somewhat from surgical anesthesia to enable assessment of neurologic function before administration of these drugs. Then the child is periodically allowed to awaken from these drugs to verify function during subsequent days.

Potential neurologic complications from cardiovascular surgery include stroke from thromboembolic events, hemiplegia, seizures, hypoxic encephalopathy, and Horner's syndrome.

Thromboembolic events are especially likely to occur in children with cyanotic heart disease; thus evaluation for signs of this complication should be performed frequently. Signs of stroke include sudden onset of neurologic signs and symptoms, including excessive irritability or lethargy (or sudden failure to respond), pupil dilation with decreased response to light, signs of increased intracranial pressure, paralysis, paresthesia, altered speech, or facial droop.

Paraplegia has been reported following surgical correction of coarctation of the aorta, although it is an uncommon complication. It will be apparent when the upper and lower extremity on the same side of the patient's body fail to abduct when the medial aspect of each extremity is pinched. This finding should be reported to a physician immediately.

Seizures and status epilepticus may result from perioperative neurologic insult, fever, or electrolyte imbalance. It may be impossible to clinically detect the onset of seizures in a child receiving neuromuscular blockade; thus there must be a high index of suspicion to recognize subtle signs of seizures.

Signs of seizures in patients receiving neuromuscular blockade may include only pupil dilation with sluggish response to light, nystagmus, tachycardia, and possible wide fluctuations in blood pressure. The seizures are confirmed with an electroencephalogram (EEG) and treated with anticonvulsant therapy (see Chapter 8).

Hypoxic encephalopathy may develop 48 to 72 hours after a cardiac arrest or cardiopulmonary collapse with severe hypoxia. When hypoxia is severe enough to produce signs of increased intracranial pressure, it is usually devastating in outcome.

Horner's syndrome results from damage to sympathetic nervous system fibers that course along the aorta and aortic arch. Damage to these fibers can produce ipsilateral (same side as surgery) ptosis (eyelid droop), meiosis (pupil constriction), and anhydrosis (lack of sweat). The pupil constriction on the involved side may make the contralateral pupil, by contrast, appear to be dilated. When Horner's syndrome is present, both pupils should constrict briskly in response to light. Horner's syndrome requires no therapy, and the symptoms become less obvious over time.

Fluid and Electrolyte Balance

Throughout the postoperative course, the nurse should be aware of all sources of fluid intake and all sources of fluid loss, as well as the child's fluid balance during the shift. Inadequate or excessive fluid output should be corrected.

Fluid Administration During the immediate postoperative period, particularly if shock or CHF is present, bolus fluid administration may be required to optimize cardiac preload. Once appropriate intravascular volume has been established and neither shock nor fluid volume excess is present (i.e., the child is euvolemic), the fluid administration rate is typically calculated at approximately 50% to 75% of estimated maintenance fluid requirements during the first days after surgery. This limitation of fluid intake is appropriate because antidiuretic hormone release causes most postoperative patients to retain free water.

Urine Output   All urine output should be measured and tested for the presence of blood and protein. Hematuria and proteinuria are both abnormal and should be reported to a physician.

Urine output should remain approximately 0.5 to 1 ml/kg/hr if fluid intake is adequate and cardiac output and renal perfusion are effective. Urine output less than this amount is oliguria. Inadequate urine output may be caused by prerenal or renal failure.

Prerenal failure occurs when renal perfusion is compromised secondary to inadequate systemic perfusion associated with CHF, shock, or administration of vasoconstrictive drugs. Treatment of this form of renal failure is elimination of the cause.

Occasionally children will develop hemolysis during or immediately following cardiopulmonary bypass. Signs of hemolysis include excretion of a rusty-colored urine that contains cell casts and hemoglobin. Disseminated intravascular coagulation may result from widespread damage to platelets and RBCs. If hemoglobinuria is detected, renal blood flow and urine volume must be maintained at high levels until the hemoglobin is "flushed out" of the glomeruli.

If urine output is inadequate despite the presence of adequate systemic perfusion, adequate hydration, and the administration of diuretics, renal failure should be suspected. Too often when oliguria develops, repeated fluid boluses are administered before renal failure is suspected; at this point, hypervolemia may be present.

If renal failure is suspected, fluid intake should be restricted to that required to maintain intravascular volume and replace insensible water losses and urine output. Potassium administration should also be curtailed. Serum samples should be sent for blood urea nitrogen (BUN), creatinine, and potassium. A simultaneous urine sample is obtained for creatinine to estimate creatinine clearance (see Chapter 9).

If renal failure is present, dialysis may be required to control intravascular volume or serum potassium. Drug dosing must be adjusted based on estimated renal function and the portion of each drug eliminated by the kidneys (see Chapter 9).

Electrolyte Imbalances   As noted above, the most common electrolyte imbalances observed following cardiovascular surgery are hypoglycemia or hyperglycemia, hypokalemia or hyperkalemia, and hypocalcemia. These should be treated promptly to avoid the development of arrhythmias.

Analgesia

All cardiovascular surgical patients will have postoperative pain and should receive analgesics. A discussion of sedatives, analgesics, and neuromuscular blockade is presented in Chapter 3. The nurse should become familiar with the drugs used, including their onset of action, compatibilities, and side effects.

Initially, continuous infusion or intermittent IV analgesics are provided. In addition, the surgeon may provide epidural blockade to reduce thoracotomy pain. During the postoperative period, effectiveness of analgesia should be assessed and doses titrated to ensure adequate analgesia with minimal side effects.

Nutrition

Immediately after surgery, the child receives nothing by mouth. If the child is extubated immediately after surgery and is stable, nothing is provided by mouth until it is clear that reintubation will not be necessary.

If intubation is planned for several days, parenteral alimentation is provided initially, followed by enteral feedings once cardiovascular function and systemic perfusion are stable. Maintenance caloric requirements should be provided as soon as possible following surgery, averaging approximately 100 to 150 Cal/kg/day for infants and 100 Cal/kg/day for children.

Gastrointestinal complications of surgery that may compromise nutritional support include the development of a paralytic ileus or mesenteric arteritis (also known as postcoarctectomy syndrome). Signs of a paralytic ileus include decreased bowel sounds and abdominal distension. The presence of decreased bowel sounds alone should not prevent the initiation of enteral feedings, since bowel motility often increases with feedings. Initial feedings should be elemental and dilute, and small in volume. As tolerated, the concentration and volume can be gradually increased. If abdominal distension or vomiting develops after feedings are initiated, or (in the case of nasogastric feedings) if significant gastric residuals are present, it may be necessary to decrease the concentration or volume of the feeding.

Mesenteric arteritis or postcoarctectomy syndrome can complicate correction of coarctation of the aorta or interrupted aortic arch; therefore this syndrome is discussed with postoperative complications of coarctation of the aorta under Specific Diseases.

Newborn infants, particularly those who experienced preoperative shock or other compromise in systemic perfusion, are at risk for the development of necrotizing enterocolitis. This complication results from a compromise in mesenteric perfusion that increases permeability of the gastrointestinal mucosa to gram-negative bacteria or endotoxin. The neonate may develop signs of sepsis or septic shock or may develop gastrointestinal perforation and an acute abdomen. Treatment is supportive. Urgent surgical intervention will be required if perforation develops.

Thermoregulation

The child's core body and skin temperature must be monitored closely following surgery. Hypothermia or fever may be present, and both should be treated.

Many cardiovascular patients may demonstrate peripheral vasoconstriction and cold stress on return from cardiovascular surgery. If surgery is performed under hypothermic conditions, low core body, as well as low skin temperatures may be present during the immediate postoperative period. However, low cardiac output should also be ruled out as a cause of peripheral vasoconstriction.

Neonates and young infants cannot shiver to generate heat when exposed to cold. They must break down brown fat in a process that increases oxygen consumption and calories. To prevent this energy expenditure, the neonate and infant should be kept warm. This is accomplished most efficiently in the postoperative period with an overbed warmer.

Fever may be present postoperatively and may indicate a reaction to blood product administration or infection. Low cardiac output may produce cool skin with an increase in core body temperature, because heat loss through the skin is inadequate. Fever is treated with antipyretics or a cooling blanket unless it is caused by low cardiac output. The cause of any fever must be identified and treated.

Infection

Infection can develop at the site of the incision, at the site of any invasive catheter or device (including pulmonary infections and urinary tract infections), or within the heart or bloodstream. Factors that increase the risk of infection include poor nutritional status, lengthy surgical procedure, multiple blood transfusions, reoperation for bleeding, prolonged stay in the ICU, and multiple invasive tubes and catheters. If hospital personnel do not consistently wash their hands before and after patient contact, this can contribute to the spread of infection.

Broad-spectrum staphylocidal antibiotics are administered in the operating room, preferably before the incision is made. Typically, prophylactic antibiotics are also administered for 2 to 5 days after surgery.

A low-grade fever on the night after surgery is relatively common and may indicate an inflammatory response or response to administration of blood products. If the fever is high (>38° C) or persists beyond the first postoperative night, infection should be suspected and appropriate cultures obtained. If prosthetic material is used for intracardiac or great vessel repair, infection may develop at these sites until the material is endothelialized (within approximately 3 to 6 months after surgery). Until that time, any infection must be promptly detected and aggressively treated (see Bacterial Endocarditis under Specific Diseases).

The nurse should evaluate the appearance of the child's wound and catheter insertion sites daily for any evidence of infection (e.g., erythema, drainage). Wound drainage should be cultured. Deep wound infections usually require incision and drainage and may require frequent or continuous irrigation with antibiotics. Mediastinitis can cause endocarditis, particularly in the child with a prosthetic or abnormal valve, patch, or conduit.

Signs of sepsis or significant infection can include fever or hypothermia, tachycardia, tachypnea (if the child is breathing spontaneously), and alteration in the WBC count. The child may demonstrate leukocytosis, leukopenia, or an increase in the percentage of bands (new WBCs). Thrombocytopenia may also develop, although a fall in platelet count is often observed following insertion of prosthetic patches or conduits (particularly Gore-tex) as the new surface is endothelialized. These signs should be reported to a physician immediately.

Postcardiotomy Syndrome

Postcardiotomy or postpericardiotomy syndrome is the association of fever ($>38.5°$ C), leukocytosis (WBC $>12,000/mm^3$), substernal or pericardial chest pain, pericardial friction rub, pericardial and/or pleural effusion, and serial ECG evidence of pericarditis. Pericardial pain often increases with respiration and radiates to the shoulder. Less specific and less consistent findings include malaise and arthralgia.

Causes of postcardiotomy syndrome have not been identified, although an autoimmune process has been implicated. Many patients have an elevated erythrocyte sedimentation rate (>50 mm/hr) and antiheart antibodies (AHAs), and some demonstrate a rise in viral titers.

Treatment includes administration of antiinflammatory agents, such as steroids and aspirin or nonsteroidal antiinflammatory agents. In addition, the nurse must monitor for the development of pleural or pericardial effusions, including cardiac tamponade. General supportive care, including bed rest, is also needed, and the child must be protected from exposure to secondary infections.

Psychosocial Support

Cardiovascular surgery is extremely stressful for the child and family. Every member of the health care team must be sensitive to both verbal and nonverbal cues about sources of stress and anxiety for the child and family and must provide comfort whenever possible.

The child may be extremely frightened and may feel too vulnerable to complain. Explanations should be provided at an age-appropriate level before procedures or manipulations, whether or not the child appears to be awake or responsive. For additional information about the child's psychosocial and cognitive development, see Table 5-18 and Chapter 2.

Parents may feel helpless, with a loss of control. These feelings may be assuaged by the compassionate nurse who includes the parents in the care of the child, giving the parents opportunities to nurture or comfort their child whenever possible. Parents require consistent information about the child's condition, progress, and therapies, and continuous visitation (barring medical emergencies in the unit) should be encouraged.

Many medical centers care for a large number of pediatric cardiovascular surgical patients. This large volume of patients usually results in a reduced risk of death or complications because the entire health care team develops routines, protocols, and procedures so that care is streamlined, efficient, and consistently good. However, although the child's care is "routine" for the health care team, the surgical experience is far from "routine" for the child and family. A sensitive and compassionate nurse will be able to treat every child and family as special and demonstrate unique concern and warmth for each one. Additional information regarding psychosocial support is provided in Chapter 2.

Postoperative care is summarized in Box 5-24.

Specific Diseases

In this section congenital and acquired heart diseases requiring critical care are presented. Information about the clinical presentation, medical management, surgical intervention, and most common postoperative complications is provided. Since surgical corrections requiring cardiopulmonary bypass routinely are performed through a median sternotomy incision, that fact is not repeated for each defect corrected with bypass. Following any cardiovascular surgery the nurse should monitor for the following potential complications: low cardiac output/shock, bleeding, congestive heart failure (CHF), arrhythmias, pulmonary complications, fluid and electrolyte imbalance, neurologic complications, pain, and infection. If pulmonary hypertension is significant preoperatively, postoperative manipulation of

Box 5-24

Postoperative Care of the Pediatric
Cardiovascular Surgical Patient

1. **Potential inadequate airway, oxygenation, ventilation:** Ensure that oxygenation is adequate via pulse oximetry, that chest expansion and breath sounds are equal and adequate bilaterally, and that blood gases are appropriate (see Chapter 6).

   a. *If intubated:* Check tube position and patency. Ensure that mechanical ventilation results in equal and adequate breath sounds, and appropriate oxygenation and ventilation. If the child deteriorates suddenly, rule out tube displacement, tube obstruction, pneumothorax, and equipment failure.

   b. *When patient is extubated and breathing spontaneously:* Ensure that respiratory rate and effort are adequate and appropriate, that airway and ventilation are adequate, and that oxygenation and carbon dioxide elimination are appropriate.

   c. *Potential pulmonary complications:* Airway obstruction, pneumothorax or hemothorax, pleural effusion, chylothorax, pneumonia, acute respiratory distress syndrome.

2. **Potential inadequate systemic perfusion and oxygen delivery:** Monitor systemic perfusion closely; ensure that heart rate, intravascular volume/preload (central venous pressure, right atrial pressure, pulmonary artery occlusion/wedge pressure, left atrial pressure), hematocrit, and blood pressure are appropriate. Potential causes of inadequate perfusion and oxygen delivery include:

   a. *Congestive heart failure:* Monitor for signs of systemic venous congestion (high central venous/right atrial pressure, hepatomegaly, periorbital edema), pulmonary venous congestion (high pulmonary artery occlusion pressure, pulmonary edema), and decreased urine volume. Treat by supporting cardiac function with sympathomimetics/inotropic drugs (possibly including digoxin), potential vasodilator therapy, probably diuretics, limitation of fluid intake.

   b. *Hemorrhage:* Monitor excessive chest tube output (3 ml/kg/hr for 3 or more hours, or 5 mL/kg/hr for any 1 hour), or loss of 10% to 15% of circulating blood volume acutely. Notify physician. Replace blood lost, rule out coagu-

lopathy (provide blood component therapy as needed), and consider need for surgical exploration. Remember that children with cyanotic heart disease may have decreased platelet number or function and a decrease in vitamin K–dependent clotting factors. Children with uncorrected cyanotic heart disease will require a higher hematocrit to maintain oxygen content and oxygen delivery.

   c. *Tamponade:* Tamponade can result from either hemorrhage (and ineffective drainage from mediastinal tubes) or pericardial effusion. Signs of tamponade may be indistinguishable from those of low cardiac output ("classic" signs are often absent). Suspect tamponade in any child with low cardiac output and rule it out. Treatment is immediate evacuation of fluid/blood.

   d. *Inappropriate intravascular volume:* Inadequate fluid administration or aggressive diuresis can result in inadequate intravascular volume. Congestive heart failure, renal failure, excessive volume administration, and postoperative fluid retention can all contribute to excessive intravascular volume. Either condition can compromise cardiac output, and the underlying condition must be corrected.

   e. *Low cardiac output/shock:* Can be caused by tamponade (rule out), poor myocardial function, hemorrhage, or arrhythmia. Signs include diminished peripheral pulses, decreased skin perfusion, poor color, metabolic acidosis, oliguria, and hypotension (often only a late sign). Treat through optimization of intravascular volume, support of myocardial function with use of vasoactive drugs (see Table 5-13), idealization of myocardial afterload (see Table 5-14), and support of heart rate (see Table 5-16).

   f. *Arrhythmias:* Heart rate may be inappropriate for clinical condition (too fast or too slow), or arrest rhythm may develop. Support adequate heart rate. Correct hypoxia, and acid-base and electrolyte imbalances. Be prepared to institute treatment for excessively rapid or slow heart rates or rhythms (see Table 5-16).

   g. *Inappropriate pulmonary or systemic vascular resistance:* Manipulate with vasodilators (see

Continued

Box 5-24

Postoperative Care of the Pediatric Cardiovascular Surgical Patient—cont'd

Table 5-14) or other therapies as indicated (see Table 5-20)

3. **Potential neurologic dysfunction** caused by complications of cardiopulmonary bypass, perioperative stroke (thromboembolus), hypoxia, acidosis, electrolyte imbalance, or prolonged seizure activity: Evaluate neurologic function immediately after surgery and at regular intervals. Be alert for evidence of neurologic compromise that may be caused by a perioperative thromboembolic event (children with cyanotic heart disease are at particular risk), hypoxia, compromise in spinal cord perfusion (particularly following surgery for coarctation of the aorta), or seizures (signs may be subtle, and signs may be absent if the child is receiving paralytic agents). Horner's syndrome may cause ptosis, meiosis (pupil constriction, although it still reacts to light), and anhydrosis on the side of surgery and may complicate surgery near the aortic arch.

4. **Potential fluid and electrolyte (including glucose) imbalance:** This may result from cardiopulmonary bypass, from diuretic or intravascular fluid therapy, or from the development of renal failure. Correct if present. Monitor urine volume and balance of intake and output closely, and notify physician of imbalance. Monitor for complications of imbalance, such as cardiac arrhythmias.

5. **Pain:** Note that this is not potential; it is a probable (if not certain) complication of surgery.

Assess location and severity of pain, provide adequate analgesia, and monitor effectiveness (see Chapter 3).

6. **Potential nutritional compromise:** Make plans to ensure adequate caloric, protein, and fat intake. Parenteral nutrition may be provided initially, but enteral nutrition should be accomplished as soon as possible. Following correction of coarctation of the aorta during infancy, monitor for mesenteric vasculitis, which may cause abdominal distension, guaiac-positive stools, and potential intestinal perforation.

7. **Potential infection:** Infection may develop at the site of the incision, at the site of any invasive catheter or device, or within the heart (endocarditis) or bloodstream (bacteremia, viremia, etc.). Infection is particularly worrisome if prosthetic material was used as part of the surgical repair, since this material may become infected if a bloodstream infection develops. Monitor for signs of infection or sepsis and report promptly to physician. Provide broad-spectrum antibiotics as ordered on schedule. Note that postcardiotomy syndrome may develop several days or weeks after surgery.

8. **Potential child, parent, family anxiety or knowledge deficit:** Provide needed support at all times. Provide information as the child and family request it and are ready to handle it.

pulmonary vascular resistance will be required. The child with cyanotic heart disease is at additional risk for the development of coagulopathy-associated bleeding and perioperative thromboembolism, including cerebral thromboembolism. For more detailed information about postoperative care, see Postoperative Care of the Pediatric Cardiovascular Surgical Patient earlier in this chapter. For more detailed presentation of common problems, such as CHF or hypoxemia caused by cyanotic heart defects, see Common Clinical Conditions earlier in this chapter.

Potential Complications and Consequences of Congenital Heart Disease

This section begins with information about acyanotic congenital heart defects. Table 5-21 summarizes clinical, radiographic, and ECG characteristics of these defects. Table 5-22 provides details regarding the findings on the 12-lead ECG for each of the defects. Table 5-23 provides details regarding the clinical, radiographic, and ECG characteristics of cyanotic defects.

Table 5-21
Clinical, Radiographic, and Electrocardiographic Characteristics of Acyanotic Congenital Heart Defects

Defect	Clinical	Chest X-Ray	ECG
Patent ductus arteriosus (PDA)	± Congestive heart failure (CHF) Bounding pulses (low diastolic BP) if large shunt	± Cardiomegaly (LA, LV enlargement) ↑ PA, pulmonary vascular markings	± (LVH) (combined left ventricular hypertrophy [LVH] and right ventricular hypertrophy [RVH] if pulmonary hypertension develops)
Atrial septal defect (ASD)	Often asymptomatic during childhood (CHF rare) (Adults may develop atrial arrhythmias and CHF)	Right atrium, right ventricle may be enlarged ↑ PA, pulmonary vascular markings	Mild RVH
Ventricular septal defect (VSD)	CHF present if shunt large	*Large shunt:* Cardiomegaly (RV, LA, LV enlargement) ↑ PA, pulmonary vascular markings *Pulmonary hypertension:* ↓ Peripheral pulmonary vascular markings ↑ RV, main PA	*Large shunt:* LAE, LVH Possible RVH *Pulmonary hypertension:* RAE, RVH
Endocardial cushion defect (ECD)	CHF present if shunt large	*Primum ASD* (see ASD) *Complete canal:* Cardiomegaly (all chambers) ↑ PA, pulmonary vascular markings	*Primum ASD:* Left axis deviation, RAE, RVH *Complete canal:* LAE, RAE LVH, RVH, left axis deviation
Double-outlet right ventricle (DORV)	*With subaortic VSD without PS:* CHF	*With subaortic VSD without PS:* ↑ PA, pulmonary vascular markings, cardiomegaly (RV, LV, LA enlargement)	*With subaortic VSD without PS:* RVH, LVH, LAE
Pulmonary stenosis (PS)	Asymptomatic (cyanosis, CHF may be present if PS critical in infants)	May be normal ± ↑ RV size ↑ PA (poststenotic dilatation) if vascular stenosis	RVH, ±RAE look for RV "strain" (ECG reliably reflects severity)
Coarctation of the aorta (CoA)	CHF during infancy if severe, ↓ lower extremity pulses, BP ± differential cyanosis if preductal (rarely appreciable)	LV, ascending aorta enlargement (RV, PA enlargement if preductal CoA) Aortic silhouette may resemble "E" or "3" "Rib-notching" created by intercostal arteries of CoA present in older child	±LVH, (RVH if preductal CoA) ±LAE
Aortic stenosis (AS)	May be asymptomatic; CHF if AS severe during infancy	May be normal Ascending aorta dilated (if valvular AS)	±LVH, ±LAE (ECG *not* reflective of severity)
Hypoplastic left heart syndrome (HLHS)	CHF, cyanosis, shock	Cardiomegaly (RA, RV enlargement) ↑ PA, pulmonary vascular markings	RVH, right axis

From Hazinski MF: *Nursing care of the critically ill child,* ed 2, St Louis, 1992, Mosby.

Table 5-22

Characteristic 12-Lead Electrocardiographic Patterns in Congenital Heart Disease

CHD Category/Defect	Axis	P Wave	QRS	Other
Left-to-Right Shunts				
PDA				Left precordial ST/T abnormalities
ASD	+90 to 150		rSR′ in right precordium	
VSD or DORV		LAE	LVH	With high flow
		RAE	RVH	With high pulmonary vascular resistance or PS
AV canal (endocardial cushion defect)	−20 to −150	(P and QRS as with VSD above)		Counterclockwise vector loop
Obstructive Lesions				
PS	+90 to 280	±RAE	RVH	ECG sensitive index of severity
AS		±LAE	±LVH	ECG *not* a sensitive index of severity
Aortic coarctation				
In newborn	Rt axis	±RAE	RVH	
After 6-12 mo	Lt axis	±LAE	±LVH	
Anomalous drainage of pulmonary veins with obstruction	+90 to 210	RAE	RVH	qR pattern in right precordium
Right-to-Left Shunts				
Tetralogy of Fallot	+90 to 180	RAE	RVH	Early transition from right to left precordial pattern
Tricuspid atresia	−30 to −150*	RAE	LVH	*If great vessels transposed, QRS axis may be +
Pulmonary atresia	Right	RAE	**	RV forces depend on RV size
Ebstein's anomaly of tricuspid valve	Right	RAE	Wolff-Parkinson-White (WPW) pattern common	
Transposition	Right			Normal for newborn
Truncus arteriosus	Most often normal as newborn			
Miscellaneous				
Anomalous origin of left coronary artery . . . . ischemia or myocardial infarction pattern				
Asplenia/polysplenia syndrome . . . . atrial axis anomalies +RVH				

From Berman WJ: *Pediatric electrocardiographic interpretation*, St Louis, 1991, Mosby.

Bacterial Endocarditis

With the exception of an atrial septal defect, all other congenital heart defects create a risk of bacterial endocarditis until they are corrected. Even after surgical intervention, the risk of endocarditis may persist if areas of turbulent intracardiac or great vessel blood flow remain. Therefore antibiotic prophylaxis is required before surgery or pro-

cedures, including dental procedures (see paragraphs on Bacterial Endocarditis later in this chapter). Parents should be instructed to contact the child's primary care physician if fever or signs of infection develop.

The risk of bacterial endocarditis may be as high as 1.5% per year once the child enters school. Since this risk is cumulative, the risk of endocarditis may

Table 5-23
Clinical, Radiographic, and Electrocardiographic Characteristics of Cyanotic Congenital Heart Defects

Defect	Clinical	Chest X-Ray	ECG
Tetralogy of Fallot (TOF)	Cyanosis proportional to severity of pulmonary outflow obstruction	Heart size normal ± RV enlargement may tip apex of heart upward (toe of boot) ↓ PA (and mediastinum) ↓ Pulmonary vascular markings 25% demonstrate a right aortic arch	RVH, right axis
Truncus arteriosus (TA)	Cyanosis, ± CHF (unless significant PS present)	Cardiomegaly (generalized) ↑ Mediastinum, pulmonary vascular markings (unless severe PS); 33% demonstrate a right aortic arch	Biventricular hypertrophy
Pulmonary atresia (PA) with intact ventricular septum (IVS)	Cyanosis	± Cardiomegaly (RA, LV enlargement) ↓ PA, pulmonary vascular markings	RAE Some RV forces present unless RV diminutive
Tricuspid atresia (TA)	Cyanosis ± CHF	± Slight cardiomegaly (RA, LA, LV enlargement) Pulmonary vascular markings decreased in most patients (↑ pulmonary vascular markings if TGA or large VSD present with PS)	RAE, LVH Left axis deviation (↓ RV forces
Ebstein's anomaly	Cyanosis, CHF	Cardiomegaly (RA enlargement) Pulmonary vascular markings normal, increased, or decreased	RAE Right axis Wolff-Parkinson-White (WPW) syndrome possible
Transposition of the great arteries (TGA)	Cyanosis, ± CHF	Cardiomegaly (all chambers especially RA, RV) Heart: "egg-on-side" ↑ Pulmonary vascular markings (unless PS) Narrow mediastinum	May be normal in neonatal period RVH, ± RAE in child Biventricular hypertrophy of large VSD
Total anomalous pulmonary venous connection (TAPVC)	± Cyanosis ± CHF Severe cyanosis and CHF if obstructive	± Cardiomegaly *Supracardiac:* Widened mediastinum ("snowman") *Obstructive:* ↑ pulmonary vascular markings (interstitial edema)	RAE, RVH qR pattern in R precordium

From Hazinski MF: *Nursing care of the critically ill child,* ed 2, St Louis, 1992, Mosby.

Continued

Table 5-23

Clinical, Radiographic, and Electrocardiographic Characteristics of Cyanotic Congenital Heart Defects—cont'd

Defect	Clinical	Chest X-Ray	ECG
Double-outlet right ventricle (DORV)	With *subaortic VSD with PS:* Cyanosis proportional to severity of PS With *subpulmonic VSD without PS:* cyanosis, CHF	With *subaortic VSD with PS:* ↓ PA, and pulmonary vascular markings Enlargement of both ventricles With *subpulmonic VSD without PS:* Generalized cardiomegaly ↑ PA, pulmonary vascular markings	With *subaortic VSD with PS:* RVH, LVH; superior axis; ± first degree AV block With *subpulmonic VSD without PS:* RVH ± LVH

From Hazinski MF: *Nursing care of the critically ill child,* ed 2, St Louis, 1992, Mosby.

average 7.5% over 5 years. As a result, elective correction of some asymptomatic defects (e.g., small to moderate ventricular septal defect) may be recommended to eliminate the potential for endocarditis.

Pulmonary Hypertension

Pulmonary hypertension may develop as a complication of increased pulmonary blood flow or cyanotic heart disease. Since it is difficult to predict if or when pulmonary hypertension will develop, surgical correction is scheduled to eliminate the possibility. In general, if the increased pulmonary blood flow occurs under *high* pressure, the pulmonary hypertension may develop within months or years. If the increased pulmonary blood flow occurs under *low* pressure, the pulmonary hypertension may never develop or may take decades to develop. Pulmonary hypertension may also develop as a complication of cyanotic defects.

If severe pulmonary hypertension is present preoperatively, it may create postoperative problems, and efforts must be made to avoid pulmonary vasoconstrictors (see discussions on management under Management of Pediatric Shock [under Common Clinical Conditions, Shock] and under Postoperative Care, Treatment of Pulmonary Hypertension [under Postoperative Care of the Pediatric Cardiovascular Surgical Patient]).

Patent Ductus Arteriosus

Defect

Patent ductus arteriosus (PDA) is persistence of the ductus arteriosus (a fetal structure) beyond fetal life (Figure 5-19). Normal constriction may not occur after birth, particularly in premature neonates. PDA may also persist if it is required to provide a source of pulmonary blood flow with cyanotic heart disease or systemic flow with severe obstruction to left heart or aortic blood flow.

Hemodynamics and Clinical Presentation

Simple Patent Ductus Arteriosus   Blood will shunt from the aorta into the pulmonary artery under high pressure once pulmonary vascular resistance (PVR) falls. If the PDA is large, CHF, increased pulmonary blood flow, left ventricular volume overload, and bounding pulses will be observed and pulmonary hypertension may develop. Small PDAs may be asymptomatic.

Patent Ductus Arteriosus With Ductal-Dependent Pulmonary Blood Flow   If the PDA is required to provide for pulmonary blood flow in children with cyanotic heart disease, hypoxemia will be present at birth and will worsen if the ductus begins to close after birth.

Patent Ductus Arteriosus With Ductal-Dependent Systemic Blood Flow   If the PDA is required to maintain systemic blood flow in the child with left

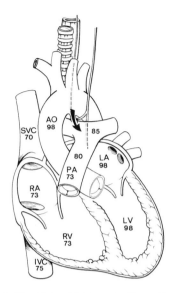

Figure 5-19 Patent ductus arteriosus. Oxygen saturations in cardiac chambers and great vessels are depicted. Positions of recurrent laryngeal nerve (adjacent to the trachea and esophagus) and vagus nerve are illustrated. (From Kambam J: Patent ductus arteriosus. In Kambam J, editor: *Cardiac anesthesia for infants and children,* St Louis, 1994, Mosby.)

heart or aortic obstruction, systemic perfusion is often poor at or soon after birth and will deteriorate quickly if the ductus begins to close after birth.

Medical and Surgical Interventions

Simple Patent Ductus Arteriosus in the Premature Neonate Ductal closure may be stimulated by administration of indomethacin, a prostaglandin synthetase inhibitor. Contraindications to the drug include renal failure, coagulopathies, hyperbilirubinemia, and thrombocytopenia. The dose is 0.1 to 0.3 mg/kg IV, which may be repeated. This drug will reduce renal blood flow; thus fluid intake should be adjusted accordingly.

Simple Patent Ductus Arteriosus Beyond the Neonatal Period The PDA may be closed with a coil during cardiac catheterization. The coil closure is most likely to be effective if the PDA is small or has a narrow waist. The PDA may be surgically divided (cut and oversewn) or ligated (tied) during

closed-heart surgery through a left thoracotomy incision, or it may be ligated during a thoracoscopy procedure.

Patent Ductus Arteriosus in the Older Adult

The ductal tissue is very friable; thus it may rupture when mobilized during surgery, resulting in massive hemorrhage. For this reason, the PDA is closed with cardiopulmonary bypass on standby.

Patent Ductus Arteriosus With Ductal-Dependent Pulmonary or Systemic Blood Flow Prostaglandin E_1 (PGE_1) administration should maintain ductal patency until palliative or corrective surgery is possible. PGE_1 is administered by continuous infusion at 0.05 to 0.1 μg/kg/min; smaller doses may be effective in maintaining ductal patency as evident by adequate hemoglobin saturation or systemic perfusion. Side effects of PGE_1 include vasodilation, hypotension, and apnea.

Postoperative Complications

Most common complications, particularly for the premature neonate, are those associated with a thoracotomy incision. Phrenic or recurrent laryngeal nerve injury may also occur. When PDA is divided in the older adult, the risk is high and hemorrhage may occur.

Aortopulmonary Window

Defect

Aortopulmonary window results from incomplete division of the aorta and pulmonary artery during fetal life. It constitutes a communication that allows shunting of blood from the aorta into the pulmonary artery once PVR falls (Figure 5-20). Shunting of blood occurs during both systole and diastole under high (aortic) pressures.

Hemodynamics and Clinical Presentation

The aortopulmonary window is usually large and unrestrictive, allowing a large shunt into the pulmonary artery. This "runoff" into the pulmonary artery may result in bounding pulses similar to those of a large PDA. Signs of CHF, increased pulmonary blood flow, and left ventricular volume overload will be present, and pulmonary hyperten-

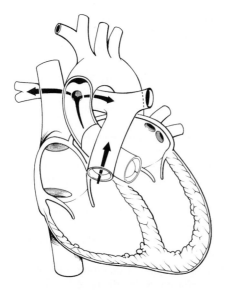

Figure 5-20 Aortopulmonary window. The defect between the aorta and pulmonary artery produces a left-to-right shunt into the pulmonary circulation that occurs during both systole and diastole. If the defect is large, the volume of the shunt will be large and under high pressure.

sion may develop rapidly. Small aortopulmonary windows may produce only a mild increase in pulmonary blood flow with minimal symptoms.

Medical and Surgical Interventions

CHF is managed medically, but surgical intervention will be required. Cardiopulmonary bypass is used to enable closure of the defect under direct visualization.

Postoperative Complications

Postoperative complications include bleeding, CHF, and shock.

Atrial Septal Defect

Defect

An atrial septal defect (ASD) is a hole in the atrial septum (Figure 5-21, *A*) that develops during fetal septal formation. The three most common types of ASDs (Figure 5-21, *B*) are:

- *Ostium secundum:* Most common, located in approximately midseptum.

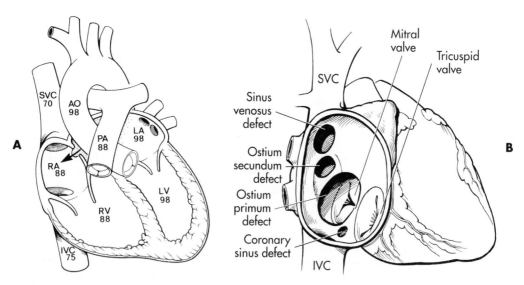

Figure 5-21 Atrial septal defect (ASD). **A,** Oxygen saturations in cardiac chambers and great vessels are depicted. **B,** Common types of ASD. (From Kambam J: Patent ductus arteriosus. In Kambam J, editor: *Cardiac anesthesia for infants and children,* St Louis, 1994, Mosby.)

- *Ostium primum:* A form of endocardial cushion defect, located low in the septum at the junction of the septum with the atrioventricular (AV) valves. It is usually associated with abnormalities of the mitral and tricuspid valves and a possible defect in ventricular septal tissue.
- *Sinus venosus defect:* Located near the junction of the superior vena cava (SVC) and right atrium. It may involve anomalous pulmonary venous return (some of the pulmonary venous return is directed into the right instead of the left atrium).

Less common forms of ASDs include Chiari network (multiple fenestrations in the atrial septum) and unroofing of the coronary sinus. When the coronary sinus in unroofed, coronary sinus blood flows into the left atrium, producing an effective right-to-left shunt of blood and hypoxemia. The unroofed coronary sinus is typically associated with a persistent left SVC.

A patent foramen ovale may serve as a channel for shunting of blood between the right and left atria. This is most commonly observed in patients with tricuspid or pulmonary atresia or in patients with transposition of the great arteries.

Hemodynamics and Clinical Presentation

Unless complex obstruction to right heart flow is present, a simple ASD produces a left-to-right shunt with right ventricular volume overload and increased pulmonary blood flow under low pressure. This defect is well tolerated and may produce no symptoms until adult years, when atrial arrhythmias, CHF, and pulmonary hypertension can develop.

If the ASD is part of an endocardial cushion defect, signs of CHF may be present (see Endocardial Cushion Defect). If an unroofed coronary sinus and persistent left SVC are present, the patient will be cyanotic, since both defects allow systemic venous blood to enter the left side of the heart.

Medical and Surgical Interventions

Most children with ASDs are asymptomatic. Surgical closure is recommended during early childhood to avoid later complications such as atrial arrhythmias and CHF. Cardiopulmonary bypass is used. A secundum ASD is closed with sutures or with a woven or pericardial patch. A primum ASD is closed with a pericardial patch; repair of the mitral valve is also undertaken at that time (see Endocardial Cushion Defect). If an ASD is present in association with tricuspid atelia or single ventricle, closure may be accomplished as a staged procedure (refer to these defects).

A sinus venosus ASD is closed with a patch to ensure that pulmonary blood flow remains on the left atrial side of the patch. The small ASDs in a Chiari network are closed with a patch.

Correction of an unroofed coronary sinus with persistent left SVC requires excision of the native atrial septum and use of a patch to isolate pulmonary venous return and the mitral valve orifice so that only pulmonary venous blood flows into the left ventricle. Alternatively, a baffle may be created to divert the left SVC blood and coronary sinus blood to the right atrium.

Some ASDs have been closed during cardiac catheterization using a "clam-shell" device passed through a catheter.

Postoperative Complications

The most common postoperative complications following closure of an ASD are arrhythmias, including sick sinus syndrome and heart block. These arrhythmias are usually transient. Approximately 2% of patients with ASDs develop postoperative CHF, most commonly related to a small left ventricle.

Ventricular Septal Defect

Defect

A ventricular septal defect (VSD) is an opening in the ventricular septum (Figure 5-22, *A*). There are five major types of VSDs (Figure 5-22, *B*):

- *Infracristal or perimembranous VSD (most common):* Located just below the crista supraventricularis.
- *Supracristal or conal VSD:* Located just above the crista supraventricularis and just below the pulmonary valve.
- *Atrioventricular (AV) canal VSD:* Located immediately under the AV valves. This VSD is part of an endocardial cushion defect.

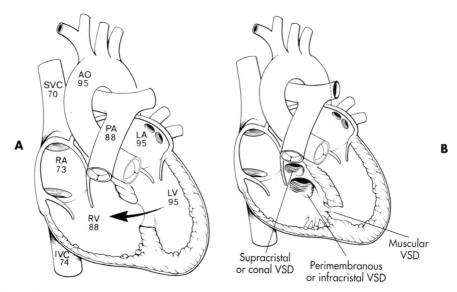

Figure 5-22 Ventricular septal defect (VSD). **A,** Oxygen saturations within the heart and great vessels are depicted. **B,** Types of VSDs. (From Kambam J: Patent ductus arteriosus. In Kambam J, editor: *Cardiac anesthesia for infants and children,* St Louis, 1994, Mosby.)

- *Muscular VSD:* May consist of a single opening low in the ventricular septum or may consist of a single opening on the left ventricular side of the septum and multiple openings on the right side of the septum.
- *Conoventricular or malalignment VSD:* Results from malalignment of the conal septum, which divides the fetal common ventricle and the truncus arteriosus during fetal life. This form of VSD is present in tetralogy of Fallot and truncus arteriosus.

Hemodynamics and Clinical Presentation

The hemodynamic consequences of a VSD depend primarily on the size of the defect and, to a lesser extent, on the location of the defect. Many VSDs (20% to 60%) close spontaneously, most often during infancy.

If the VSD is small, it allows a small shunt with few symptoms and may close spontaneously. Large defects (larger than approximately half the size of the aortic valve) produce a large amount of pulmonary blood flow; thus signs of CHF and left ventricular volume overload develop once PVR falls (typically at approximately 4 to 12 weeks of age).

The increase in pulmonary blood flow can be under high pressure if the VSD is large; thus pulmonary hypertension may develop within months.

Aortic insufficiency develops in approximately 2% to 7% of children with VSDs, most often with conal septal defects. It is caused by prolapse of the right and possibly the noncoronary cusps of the aortic valve.

Approximately 5% of children with VSDs develop secondary pulmonary infundibular stenosis. This stenosis increases resistance to right ventricular outflow and usually reduces the magnitude and pressure of the left-to-right shunt and the volume and pressure of pulmonary blood flow. If the infundibular stenosis becomes significant, it may produce signs and symptoms similar to tetralogy of Fallot.

Eisenmenger's syndrome is reversal of the direction of a shunt as a result of the development of pulmonary hypertension. Once PVR approaches or exceeds systemic vascular resistance (SVR), blood begins to shunt from right to left, and the child becomes cyanotic. The development of Eisenmenger's syndrome usually indicates that the pulmonary vascular disease is irreversible and progressive, and the defect is irreparable.

Medical and Surgical Interventions

Management of CHF is necessary when the VSD is symptomatic. Defects requiring surgical intervention include those producing severe symptoms of CHF, those producing a large amount of pulmonary blood flow, or those that contribute to a rise in pulmonary artery pressure. Surgical closure may also be recommended on an elective basis to eliminate the risk of endocarditis if the VSD persists beyond preschool years.

If the VSD is part of complex heart disease or uncorrectable heart disease, palliative rather than corrective surgery may be performed. Palliative surgery consists of *banding of the pulmonary artery* (Figure 5-23). This procedure is performed through a thoracotomy incision and does not require use of cardiopulmonary bypass. A strip of woven prosthetic material is wrapped around the main pulmonary artery and used to constrict the artery. This procedure reduces the volume and pressure of pulmonary blood flow, relieves symptoms of CHF, and should prevent the development of pulmonary hypertension.

Surgical closure of the VSD requires cardiopulmonary bypass. If at all possible, the surgeon reaches and corrects the VSD from a right atrial incision, working through the tricuspid valve to avoid the need for a ventriculotomy incision. The defect is closed with a patch. A conal septal defect can be closed through an incision in the right ventricular outflow tract or through an incision in the pulmonary artery (with retraction of the pulmonary valve). A ventriculotomy incision is occasionally necessary.

If a muscular defect is low in the ventricular septum, and if it is associated with multiple defects on the right ventricular side, the defect may be approached through an incision in the left ventricle. Unfortunately, this approach is associated with high mortality, poor left ventricular function postoperatively, apical aneurysms, and persistent VSD shunts.

Small VSDs have been closed during cardiac catheterization using a "clam shell" or umbrella passed through a catheter.

Postoperative Complications

The most common complications are CHF and arrhythmias. CHF and possible low cardiac output

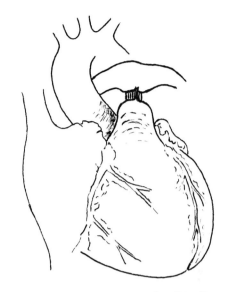

Figure 5-23   Pulmonary artery banding. (From Hazinski MF: *Nursing care of the critically ill child,* ed 2, St Louis, 1992, Mosby.)

are most likely if a ventriculotomy incision was used for the correction, if CHF was severe preoperatively, or if pulmonary hypertension is present. If CHF or low cardiac output are severe, a persistent VSD should be ruled out. Right bundle branch block virtually always results from a ventriculotomy incision, and heart block may complicate the patch insertion.

Endocardial Cushion Defect

Defect

Endocardial cushion defects (ECDs) result from malformation of the endocardial cushions during fetal life. Since the endocardial cushions participate in the formation of the lower portion of the atrial septum, the AV (tricuspid and mitral) valves, and the upper portion of the ventricular septum, an ECD can include defects in some or all of these areas of the heart (Figure 5-24).

A variety of terms have been used to classify ECDs (Table 5-24). With a complete form of AV canal, the mitral and tricuspid valve rings are *not* separate and complete; they share some bridging

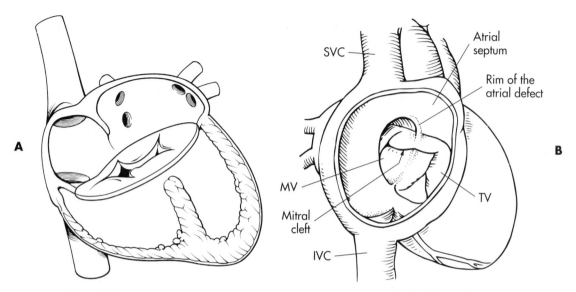

Figure 5-24   Endocardial cushion defect. **A,** Endocardial cushion defect with atrial and ventricular septal defect (ASD). Complete canal shown (note common anterior atrioventricular valve leaflet). **B,** Ostium primum atrial septal defect (ASD) form of endocardial cushion defect. Cleft in mitral valve *(MV)* can be seen through ASD. Tricuspid valve *(TV),* superior vena cava *(SVC),* and inferior vena cava *(IVC)* are also depicted. (From Fyler DC: Endocardial cushion defects. In Fyler DC, editor: *Nadas' pediatric cardiology.* Philadelphia, 1992, Hanley & Belfus.)

tissue (usually an anterior leaflet). This contributes to significant AV valvular insufficiency, increases the magnitude of left-to-right shunting that is present, and increases the complexity of surgical correction.

Hemodynamics and Clinical Presentation

The direction and magnitude of intracardiac shunting of blood is determined by the severity of inter-atrial shunting, interventricular shunting, and AV valve regurgitation, as well as by the difference between systemic and pulmonary vascular resistances. Once PVR falls, the direction of any shunting through an ASD or VSD will be left-to-right, into the pulmonary circulation. In addition, mitral and tricuspid insufficiency will be present.

Ostium Primum Atrial Septal Defect   If only an ostium primum ASD is present and AV valve function is fairly normal, symptoms may be mild, similar to those of a simple ASD. Mild mitral insufficiency may be clinically insignificant, and any blood regurgitated from the left ventricle into the

left atrium is shunted through the ASD to the right side of the heart. CHF may not be present, and the risk of pulmonary vascular disease is low.

If the ECD consists of an ostium primum ASD and significant AV valve insufficiency, severe CHF may develop once PVR falls.

Endocardial Cushion Defect With Ventricular Septal Defect   If the ECD includes a significant shunt through a VSD, particularly with a complete form of the defect, signs of CHF can be severe. The shunt is largely left-to-right once PVR falls (typically at approximately 4 to 12 weeks of age), and pulmonary blood flow is increased by a shunt through the ASD and VSD. Mitral insufficiency contributes to the left-to-right atrial shunt. The infant may occasionally become cyanotic with cry, particularly during the first weeks of life, when PVR is high. If the VSD is large, the pulmonary blood flow is under high pressure. Biventricular failure and biventricular hypertrophy are likely to be present, and pulmonary vascular disease may develop within months.

Table 5-24
Endocardial Cushion Defect

Defect	Cardiac Abnormalities
Partial (incomplete) AV Canal (or ASD-VSD)	Mitral and tricuspid valves are separate and complete. Potential defects: Ostium primum ASD with cleft in septal leaflet of mitral (and possibly tricuspid) valve(s); deficiency in ventricular septal tissue present but without shunt Isolated ostium primum Isolated cleft in mitral or tricuspid valve is rarely present alone Common atrium with cleft in mitral or tricuspid valve leaflet VSD may be present alone or in combination with AV valve deformity, with or without a primum ASD
Complete, common, or persistent common AV canal (or ASV-VSD)	One common orifice is located between atria and ventricles; mitral and tricuspid valve rings are incomplete and share some tissue.
Rastelli classification of complete AV canal	These classifications are all forms of complete AV canal; classifications are determined by anatomy of anterior AV valve leaflet. An ASD-VSD is usually present.
Type A AV canal (most common)	Anterior common leaflet is roughly divided in half into mitral and tricuspid components, with normal attachments of chordae tendineae.
Type B AV canal (least common)	Anterior common leaflet is roughly divided in half into mitral and tricuspid components, but chordae tendineae from mitral portion of valve pass through VSD to insert in right ventricular wall—these must be freed before VSD is closed.
Type C AV canal	Anterior common leaflet is not divided and has no chordal attachments; thus it floats freely.
Intermediate (transitional) form of AV canal (or ASD-VSD)	AV valve rings are incomplete. There is a deficiency in mitral valve tissue, but no true cleft. Right or left ventricular dominance may be present; right ventricular dominance suggests a small left ventricle, which may fail postoperatively.

Prepared by Michele Ilbawi, MD, The Heart Institute for Children, Oak Lawn, Ill.
AV, Atrioventricular; *ASD-VSD,* atrial septal defect-ventricular septal defect.

Associated Lesions   ECD may be associated with other congenital heart defects. In the intermediate form of AV canal, the left ventricle is small. If tetralogy of Fallot is associated with an ECD, cyanosis will be observed, and the clinical presentation will resemble that of tetralogy of Fallot. Other potential associated defects include anomalous pulmonary venous connection, PDA, VSDs, and aortic arch obstruction.

Conduction System   An ECD prevents normal development of the conduction system. The AV valve is displaced posteriorly, producing prolongation of the PR interval (first-degree heart block). The His bundle is also displaced posteriorly, and it courses along the inferior rim of the VSD; thus it may be easily injured during patch closure of a VSD.

Medical and Surgical Interventions

Preoperative CHF must be managed medically. Surgical correction will ultimately be required, but the timing will be determined by the child's anatomy and severity of symptoms. Occasionally pulmonary artery banding may be performed as a first-stage procedure to relieve symptoms of CHF and reduce the risk of pulmonary hypertension. The mitral and tricuspid valves will always be abnormal, even following surgical correction; thus antibiotic prophylaxis will be required during periods of increased risk of bacteremia.

Complete correction is the procedure of choice and is usually undertaken during infancy. Cardiopulmonary bypass is used for all procedures.

Ostium Primum Atrial Septal Defect   Correction consists of repair of clefts in the mitral valve and patch closure of the ASD. The surgery is performed through a right atrial incision. The mitral valve is repaired through the ASD, and the ASD is then closed with pericardium.

Correction of Common AV Valve Tissue With Complete AV Canal   The defect is approached through a right atrial incision. Whether or not septal defects are present, a valvuloplasty is performed on the common AV valve tissue to create two functioning AV valves (Figure 5-25). Valve chordal attachments and valve landmarks are examined to determine the best way to create separate valve rings from the

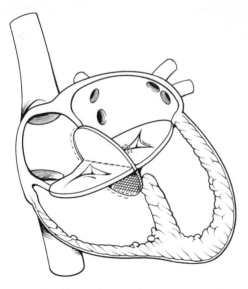

Figure 5-25 Surgical correction of endocardial cushion defect. A patch is used to close the atrial septal defect (pericardium is often used). When a complete canal is present (as shown), a second woven patch is used to close the ventricular septal defect. The patches are placed to divide common atrioventricular valve tissue, particularly the bridging anterior leaflet. Clefts in the mitral valve are sutured to prevent significant postoperative mitral insufficiency while avoiding creation of mitral stenosis.

common tissue. Clefts in the mitral valve are repaired before any septal patch is placed.

Endocardial Cushion Defect With Ventricular Septal Defect   If a complete AV canal is present, the valve tissue is repaired as described in the preceding paragraph. If an incomplete AV canal is present (i.e., the valve rings are separate and complete), then mitral valve clefts are repaired. Atrial and ventricular septal defects are then closed. Typically, a pericardial patch is used to close the ASD, and a woven patch may be used to close the VSD, although a single patch may be used to close both defects.

Postoperative Complications

Operative risk is increased by preoperative CHF, pulmonary hypertension, left ventricular hypoplasia, and severe AV valve insufficiency. Postoperative complications include low cardiac output, CHF, arrhythmias (especially heart block), respiratory failure, and hemorrhage. If CHF and mitral insufficiency are severe postoperatively, pulmonary edema and respiratory failure will be present. Pulmonary hypertension can be problematic.

Double-Outlet Right Ventricle

Defect

When double-outlet right ventricle (DORV) is present, both great vessels arise from the right ventricle. A VSD is nearly always present, but it may be located in a variety of positions relative to the pulmonary artery and aorta. Subpulmonic stenosis may also be present.

Hemodynamics and Clinical Presentation

The clinical effects of the DORV are determined by the location of the VSD relative to the great vessels, the presence and severity of subpulmonic stenosis, and the degree of mixing of systemic and pulmonary venous blood within the right ventricle (Figure 5-26).

Double-Outlet Right Ventricle With Subaortic Ventricular Septal Defect Without Pulmonary Stenosis   The location of the VSD just under the aorta results in hemodynamics very similar to those observed with a simple VSD. Once PVR falls, a

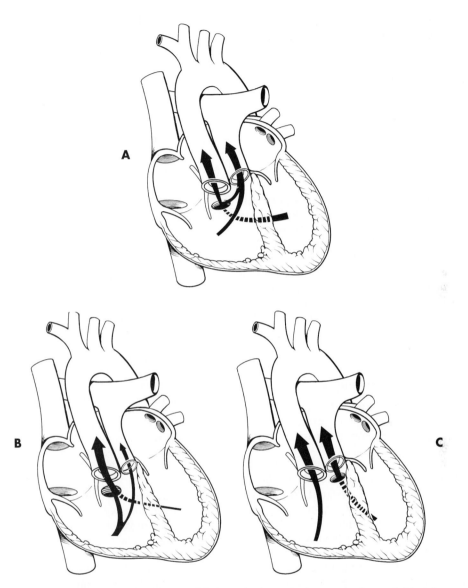

Figure 5-26 Double outlet right ventricle (DORV). There are three major forms of this defect.
A, DORV with subaortic ventricular septal defect (VSD) without pulmonary stenosis. In this form of
DORV, the VSD directs left ventricular outflow into the aorta, with some blood shunting into the
pulmonary artery. This defect produces hemodynamics similar to a simple VSD. **B,** DORV with
subaortic VSD with pulmonary stenosis. The subaortic VSD directs left ventricular outflow into the
aorta. Shunting of right ventricular outflow into the aorta (a right-to-left shunt) will occur if
pulmonary stenosis is significant. This defect produces hemodynamics similar to tetralogy of Fallot.
C, DORV with subpulmonic VSD without pulmonary stenosis. In this form of DORV, the VSD directs
left ventricular outflow into the pulmonary artery, and right ventricular outflow enters the aorta.
This produces hemodynamics similar to transposition of the great arteries.

large defect results in a large shunt, producing signs of CHF and the risk of pulmonary hypertension.

Double-Outlet Right Ventricle With Subaortic Ventricular Septal Defect and Pulmonary Stenosis This defect produces hemodynamics very similar to those resulting from tetralogy of Fallot. Cyanosis and hypoxemia are proportional to the severity of the pulmonary stenosis. Hypercyanotic spells and complications of hypoxemia and polycythemia may develop.

Double-Outlet Right Ventricle With Subpulmonic Ventricular Septal Defect Without Pulmonary Stenosis Systemic venous blood flows preferentially into the aorta, and pulmonary venous blood from the left ventricle flows through the VSD into the pulmonary artery. The hemodynamic effects of this form of DORV are very similar to those observed with transposition of the great arteries. Cyanosis is typically present from birth. Once PVR falls, pulmonary blood flow increases, and signs of CHF develop. Complications of hypoxemia and polycythemia may develop.

Medical and Surgical Interventions

CHF and/or hypoxemia must be managed (see Common Clinical Conditions earlier in this chapter). Surgical correction is illustrated in Figure 5-27.

Double-Outlet Right Ventricle With Subaortic Ventricular Septal Defect Without Pulmonary Stenosis Aggressive management of CHF is indicated, and surgical intervention is planned to prevent the development of pulmonary hypertension. Pulmonary artery banding may be performed initially, although total correction is preferred. Surgical correction is accomplished through a ventriculotomy incision and requires patch closure of the VSD in a way that diverts left ventricular output through the VSD to the aorta (a baffle).

Double-Outlet Right Ventricle With Subaortic Ventricular Septal Defect and Pulmonary Stenosis Management is similar to that provided for tetralogy of Fallot (see Tetralogy of Fallot and Pulmonary Atresia With Ventricular Septal Defect). If cyanosis and hypoxemia are severe at birth, PGE_1

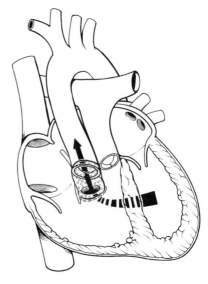

Figure 5-27 Surgical correction of double outlet right ventricle (DORV). In all forms of correction, the ventricular septal defect (VSD) is closed, and ultimately left ventricular outflow is directed into the aorta, and right ventricular outflow into the pulmonary artery. In DORV with a subaortic VSD (shown here), the VSD is patched to divert aortic blood flow through the VSD and into the aorta. DORV with subaortic VSD and pulmonary stenosis is corrected in a manner similar to tetralogy of Fallot, and DORV with subpulmonary VSD without pulmonary stenosis is corrected in a manner similar to transposition of the great arteries.

administration is required. *No air is allowed in any IV line at any time before surgical correction of the defect.* Hypercyanotic episodes may develop during the first year of life and indicate the need for urgent surgical intervention. Palliative surgery consists of creation of a systemic–to–pulmonary artery shunt. Until corrective surgery is performed, the child is at risk for the development of systemic consequences of hypoxemia and polycythemia. The infant should be kept well hydrated to avoid hemoconcentration.

Corrective surgery is performed using cardiopulmonary bypass. A ventriculotomy incision is made, and the pulmonary stenosis is excised. The VSD is then closed with a patch so that left ventricular outflow is diverted through the VSD and into the aorta. The pulmonary outflow tract may be enlarged with one or two patches. If an adequate pulmonary outflow tract cannot be created in this manner, a valved conduit may be placed between the right ventricle and the pulmonary artery.

Double-Outlet Right Ventricle With Subpulmonic Ventricular Septal Defect Without Pulmonary Stenosis

Management is very similar to that required for transposition of the great arteries but is particularly challenging because of the coexistence of the CHF and the hypoxemia. The CHF requires control of intravascular fluid volume and some diuresis, but hemoconcentration must be avoided. *No air can be allowed to enter any IV line until corrective surgery is performed.*

If cyanosis and hypoxemia are severe at birth, PGE_1 is administered until palliative or corrective surgery is performed. Palliative procedures will be aimed at improving the mixing of systemic and venous blood, such as through an atrial balloon septostomy or surgical septectomy, which should improve arterial oxygen saturation. Alternatively, pulmonary artery banding plus creation of a systemic-to-pulmonary shunt may enable control of pulmonary blood flow.

Surgical correction uses procedures described for correction of transposition of the great arteries, with simultaneous closure of the VSD. In recent years this consists of an arterial switch procedure plus VSD closure. If this procedure is not feasible, a Damus-Stansel Kaye procedure may be considered. For more information see Transposition of the Great Arteries.

Postoperative Complications

Postoperative complications will be determined by the specific type of DORV present, as well as by associated preoperative conditions such as CHF, pulmonary hypertension, or severe hypoxemia.

Double-Outlet Right Ventricle With Subaortic Ventricular Septal Defect Without Pulmonary Stenosis

Operative risk is particularly high if severe pulmonary hypertension or symptoms are present preoperatively. The ventriculotomy incision will likely contribute to some CHF and possible low cardiac output and will produce right bundle branch block. Heart block and ventricular arrhythmias may also be observed. If significant pulmonary hypertension is present, postoperative treatment will be required (see Postoperative Care of the Pediatric Cardiovascular Surgical Patient).

Double-Outlet Right Ventricle With Subaortic Ventricular Septal Defect and Pulmonary Stenosis

Surgical correction is a modification of that required for tetralogy of Fallot; thus postoperative complications will be similar. These include CHF, possible low cardiac output (may be severe if conduit insertion was required), right bundle branch block, possible heart block, and ventricular arrhythmias. The child is at risk for all potential complications of hypoxemia and polycythemia, including bleeding and perioperative thromboembolism. Use of prosthetic material increases the risk of endocarditis postoperatively and may produce a fall in platelet count as the material is endothelialized.

Double-Outlet Right Ventricle With Subpulmonic Ventricular Septal Defect Without Pulmonary Stenosis

Since surgical correction is similar to that provided for transposition of the great arteries, refer to that defect for more information. Regardless of the corrective surgery performed, potential postoperative complications include CHF, low cardiac output, and arrhythmias. The child is at risk for all potential complications of hypoxemia and polycythemia, including bleeding and perioperative thromboembolism. Use of prosthetic material increases the risk of endocarditis postoperatively and may produce a fall in platelet count as the material is endothelialized.

Pulmonary Valve Stenosis

Defect

Pulmonary valve stenosis results from improper formation of the pulmonary valve leaflets, with resultant obstruction to blood flow from the right ventricle to the pulmonary artery (Figure 5-28).

Hemodynamics and Clinical Presentation

Pulmonary valve stenosis reduces the radius of the valve orifice, increasing resistance to pulmonary blood flow. Normal right ventricular output into the pulmonary artery may be maintained if right

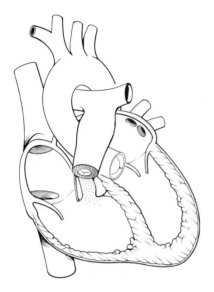

Figure 5-28 Pulmonary valve and pulmonary infundibular stenosis. Pulmonary valve stenosis is depicted as a thickening of the valve, with a narrowing of the lumen. Poststenotic dilation of the main pulmonary artery and secondary muscular infundibular stenosis are shown.

ventricular pressure can be increased sufficiently. Right ventricular output typically remains normal in the presence of *mild* (valve gradient 25 to 49 mm Hg) or even *moderate* (valve gradient 50 to 70 mm Hg) pulmonary valve stenosis. Right ventricular hypertrophy will be present, and secondary pulmonary infundibular stenosis or right ventricular fibrosis may develop. Most children with mild or moderate pulmonary stenosis are asymptomatic. However, the severity of the stenosis may increase during childhood.

When pulmonary valve stenosis is *severe* (valve gradient ≥80 mm Hg), extremely high right ventricular pressure must be generated to maintain normal right ventricular output and pulmonary blood flow. This will produce severe right ventricular hypertrophy that will ultimately contribute to the development of right ventricular fibrosis and dysfunction. Once dysfunction develops, right ventricular dilation, increased right ventricular end-diastolic pressure (RVEDP), and tricuspid insufficiency will develop. At this point, right atrial pressure is increased and signs of systemic venous congestion (including hepatomegaly) will develop. In addition, right-to-left atrial shunting may develop through a stretched foramen ovale, producing hypoxemia.

Other secondary changes may develop in the pulmonary artery and right ventricle, particularly if the pulmonary stenosis becomes progressively more severe. As right ventricular hypertrophy progresses, secondary pulmonary infundibular stenosis may develop. In addition, poststenotic dilation is present in the main pulmonary artery.

Cyanosis caused by right-to-left shunting of blood through the foramen ovale is observed in approximately one third of children with pulmonary valve stenosis under 2 years of age. It typically occurs when the stenosis is moderate or severe. Beyond 2 years of age, cyanosis is rarely observed unless severe valvular stenosis is associated with right ventricular failure.

CHF is an uncommon complication of pulmonary stenosis during childhood. When present, it is usually associated with severe pulmonic stenosis in infancy.

Occasionally severe pulmonary valve stenosis is associated with an extremely small right ventricle and tricuspid valve stenosis or atresia. This defect is known as hypoplastic right heart or critical pulmonic stenosis and will produce clinical findings similar to those of pulmonary atresia or tricuspid atresia (see Pulmonary Atresia With Intact Ventricular Septum and Tricuspid Atresia).

Medical and Surgical Interventions

The choice of therapy will be determined by the age of the child, the severity of pulmonary stenosis present, and the presence of associated lesions. Moderate and severe pulmonary stenosis are treated. Symptomatic children require urgent intervention, however, regardless of the magnitude of the valve gradient. Antibiotic prophylaxis will be required during periods of risk of endocarditis throughout the child's life, because the valve is abnormal. *Whenever cyanosis is observed, a right-to-left shunt is present, so no air an be allowed to enter any IV line.*

Mild pulmonary stenosis usually requires no treatment. The child will be monitored for signs of progression in the severity of the stenosis, including ECG evidence of severe right ventricular hypertrophy and onset of symptoms of dyspnea, fatigability, and development of CHF.

Elective balloon valvuloplasty during cardiac catheterization is recommended at 1 to 4 years of age for the treatment of moderate pulmonary stenosis even if the child is asymptomatic. Urgent balloon valvuloplasty or surgical valvotomy is required for the symptomatic child.

When pulmonary stenosis is severe in the neonatal period, PGE_1 is administered to maintain pulmonary blood flow through the ductus. Valvuloplasty is then attempted during cardiac catheterization. If the valvuloplasty results in inadequate pulmonary blood flow, creation of a systemic–to–pulmonary artery shunt may be necessary, or surgical valvotomy may be required.

Surgical valvotomy for treatment of critical pulmonary stenosis in the young infant is occasionally performed as a "blind" procedure, without use of cardiopulmonary bypass. A curved blade is inserted through a small stab incision in the pulmonary outflow tract, surrounded by purse-string sutures. A systemic-to-pulmonary shunt may be created at the same time or at a later time, if needed to ensure adequate pulmonary blood flow.

An open pulmonary valvotomy may be performed at any age and is the preferred technique of surgical intervention. This procedure requires use of cardiopulmonary bypass. The valve is approached through an incision in the main pulmonary artery, and fused leaflets are opened under direct visualization. Patch enlargement of the pulmonary artery may also be required, and the patch may include a valve cusp to prevent significant pulmonary insufficiency. If the right ventricle is small and pulmonary blood flow is still inadequate following the valvotomy, a systemic-to-pulmonary shunt may be created.

Postoperative Complications

Postoperative complications are most likely in the symptomatic neonate with severe pulmonary stenosis. Potential complications include CHF, low cardiac output, and arrhythmias. If cyanosis was present preoperatively, complications of hypoxemia and polycythemia can include postoperative bleeding and thromboembolic events.

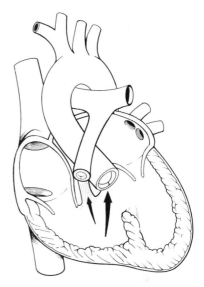

Figure 5-29 Tetralogy of Fallot. This defect consists of the association of four anomalies: a ventricular septal defect (VSD), pulmonary infundibular stenosis (often the pulmonary valve and main pulmonary artery are small), dextroposition of the aorta (the aorta shifts to the right and overrides the VSD), and right ventricular hypertrophy. Pentalogy of Fallot includes these four defects plus an atrial septal defect; this association of anomalies is often associated with a small left ventricle.

Tetralogy Of Fallot and Pulmonary Atresia With Ventricular Septal Defect

Defect

Tetralogy of Fallot is the association of four defects: VSD, pulmonary infundibular and possible valvular stenosis, rightward displacement of the aorta (so that it overrides the VSD), and right ventricular hypertrophy (Figure 5-29). If an ASD is also present, the association is referred to as pentology of Fallot. In the classic form of pentology of Fallot, the left ventricle is small, since much of pulmonary venous return is diverted to the right side of the heart through the ASD.

Occasionally the pulmonary stenosis is so severe that there is no anatomic connection between the right ventricle and the pulmonary artery. This form of severe tetralogy of Fallot may also be referred to as pulmonary atresia with VSD or pseudotruncus arteriosus (see Truncus Arteriosus).

Tetralogy of Fallot may be present with a rudimentary or absent pulmonary valve; this defect is tetralogy of Fallot with absent pulmonary valve. Tetralogy of Fallot may also be associated with AV canal defect.

Hemodynamics and Clinical Presentation

Simple Tetralogy of Fallot The consequences of this defect will be determined by the severity of the pulmonary stenosis and any associated lesions. The degree of cyanosis and hypoxemia is directly proportional to the severity of the pulmonary stenosis. If pulmonary stenosis is mild, there is little shunting of blood through the VSD, since resistance to flow through the mildly stenotic pulmonary outflow tract will be less than or equal to SVR. In fact, there may be a net left-to-right shunt through the VSD when PVR falls. This form of tetralogy is known as "pink" tetralogy. Cyanosis may be absent, although hypercyanotic spells may also develop during infancy.

With classic tetralogy, the pulmonary stenosis is moderate or severe, and cyanosis and hypoxemia will be present. The more severe the pulmonary stenosis, the more severe the hypoxemia, since more and more systemic venous blood will be shunted from the right ventricle through the VSD and into the aorta. Cyanosis may be present from birth or may develop during infancy. When pulmonary stenosis is severe during the neonatal period, hypoxemia may worsen when the ductus begins to close.

Tetralogy of Fallot With Absent Pulmonary Valve

When tetralogy of Fallot is present with absent pulmonary valve, pulmonary valvular insufficiency is present and may produce right ventricular dysfunction. In addition, aneurysmal pulmonary artery dilation compresses the tracheobronchial tree, producing airway obstruction and air trapping, and possible emphysema. Cyanosis, CHF, and respiratory distress are often present and severe.

Tetralogy of Fallot With Atrioventricular Canal

Tetralogy of Fallot may be present in association with an AV canal defect. Clinical consequences include those of tetralogy of Fallot and AV valve insufficiency. Typically, the symptoms of both the tetralogy of Fallot and the AV canal are tempered; the pulmonary stenosis prevents the development of CHF from the AV canal. However, if the pulmonary stenosis is severe, significant cyanosis and hypoxemia may be present.

Medical and Surgical Interventions

Simple Tetralogy of Fallot When cyanosis is present, the child is at risk for the development of complications of cyanosis and resultant polycythemia. *No air can be allowed to enter any IV line,* since it may shunt into the systemic arterial (and cerebral) circulation. Hypercyanotic spells may develop, indicating the need for urgent surgical intervention (management of complications of hypoxemia are presented in the discussion of hypoxemia under Common Clinical Conditions earlier in this chapter). Regardless of the type of palliative or corrective surgery, antibiotic prophylaxis will be required whenever risk of endocarditis is present.

If pulmonary stenosis is mild and no other defects are present, elective surgical correction is performed during the first years of life.

If hypoxemia is severe during the neonatal period, PGE_1 is administered to maintain ductal patency until palliative or corrective surgery can be performed. Surgical shunting procedures are described in Table 5-25 and illustrated in Figure 5-30. If the infant's subclavian artery will be used for a palliative procedure, some surgeons request that arterial punctures and cuff blood pressure measurements *not* be performed on the associated arm preoperatively or postoperatively.

Surgical correction of tetralogy uses cardiopulmonary bypass. The VSD is closed with a patch, and the pulmonary stenosis is resected. Whenever possible, closure of the VSD is accomplished with access from the right atrium through the tricuspid valve to avoid a ventriculotomy incision. The pulmonary stenosis is resected, if possible, through a pulmonary artery incision (approached through the pulmonary valve). A right ventriculotomy incision may be necessary to ensure adequate resection of the stenosis (Figure 5-31).

The pulmonary outflow tract is enlarged with one or two patches. The goal is to enlarge the pulmonary outflow tract while preserving pulmonary

Table 5-25
Palliative Shunts for Treatment of Cyanotic Heart Disease

Palliative Procedure	Resultant Anatomic Change	Circulatory Consequences
Blalock-Taussig anastomosis	Subclavian artery is separated from the arm circulation, and the distal end is sewn to the pulmonary artery.	Systemic arterial blood from the aorta flows through the subclavian artery to the pulmonary artery; this produces increased pulmonary blood flow under low pressure; this shunt is easy to take down at later surgery.
Prosthetic systemic-to-pulmonary artery shunt (modified Blalock-Taussig anastomosis or central shunt)	Prosthetic material (most commonly polytetrafluoroethylene [Gore-Tex or Impra]) is sewn between the aorta or a major systemic artery and the main, right, or left pulmonary artery; most commonly, the shunt is placed between the proximal subclavian artery and the right or left pulmonary artery (called a modified Blalock-Taussig shunt) or between the aorta and the main pulmonary artery.	Systemic arterial blood from the aorta flows through the prosthetic graft into the pulmonary artery; this produces increased pulmonary blood flow under low pressure; the shunt must be made large enough to provide adequate flow when the child grows; the flow also must be adequate to prevent thrombosis formation; this shunt is easy to take down at later surgery.
Waterston-Cooley (rarely performed)	The back of the ascending aorta is sewn to the front of the right pulmonary artery where they overlap, and an orifice is made between the back wall of the aorta and the front wall of the pulmonary artery.	Some blood from the aorta flows into the pulmonary artery; if the shunt is too large, high pulmonary blood flow under high pressure may produce congestive heart failure, and pulmonary hypertension may result; if the shunt is to small, there will be a negligible increase in pulmonary blood flow. With growth, this shunt often produces distortion of the right pulmonary artery, and may result in preferential flow of the shunted blood into the right or the left pulmonary artery; however, this is an easy shunt to construct, so it is occasionally the shunt of choice in a critically ill cyanotic baby. This shunt also can produce growth of hypoplastic pulmonary arteries; the shunt is difficult to take down, however, at later corrective surgery, and patch enlargement of the right pulmonary artery may be necessary.

From Hazinski MF: *Nursing care of the critically ill child,* ed 2, St Louis, 1992, Mosby.

Continued

valve function. If a single, transannular patch is used, pulmonary insufficiency may develop, producing right ventricular dysfunction. If a transannular patch is used, it may contain a valve cusp. Severe pulmonary stenosis may require insertion of a conduit between the right ventricle and the pulmonary artery.

Tetralogy of Fallot With Absent Pulmonary Valve
The symptomatic infant with tetralogy of Fallot with absent pulmonary valve requires treatment of CHF and support of pulmonary function. Pulmonary hygiene will be required, and bronchodilator therapy and mechanical ventilation may be required. The prone position may relieve com-

Table 5-25
Palliative Shunts for Treatment of Cyanotic Heart Disease—cont'd

Palliative Procedure	Resultant Anatomic Change	Circulatory Consequences
Glenn anastomosis	The right superior vena cava is ligated at its junction with the right atrium and is sewn to the right pulmonary artery; the right pulmonary artery may also be separated from the main pulmonary artery. NOTE: If a *left* superior vena cava is present, the same procedure may be performed with the *left* pulmonary artery.	Systemic venous blood from the head and upper extremities flows directly into the right pulmonary artery; thus superior vena caval blood no longer enters the heart; the Glenn shunt usually increases pulmonary blood flow, since approximately half of systemic venous return is flowing directly into the pulmonary circulation; the flow is under low (central venous) pressure; the shunt may also reduce cyanosis, since it reduces the quantity of systemic venous blood returning to the heart, and it increases the quantity of pulmonary venous (oxygenated) blood returning to the heart; the Glenn shunt is difficult to take down and pulmonary arteriovenous fistulas may develop.
Bidirectional Glenn anastomosis	Superior vena cava is ligated at junction of SVC and right atrium; the right pulmonary artery is not separated from remainder of pulmonary artery trunk; the SVC is then anastomosed to the right pulmonary artery.	SVC blood flows directly into right lung; this improves pulmonary blood flow and reduces volume of blood returning to the heart (so may reduce workload of single ventricle); systemic arterial oxygenation improves and signs of congestive heart failure may be relieved.
Rashkind balloon septostomy	A balloon-tipped catheter is used to tear a hole in the atrial septum during cardiac catheterization. NOTE: This procedure is performed during *cardiac catheterization,* not during surgery.	This procedure is generally only effective during the neonatal period; it creates an atrial septal defect to allow better mixing of oxygenated and venous blood within the heart; it can also allow right-to-left shunting at the atrial level; the atrial septal defect created by this procedure may contract over time.
Blalock-Hanlon septectomy	A large atrial septal defect is created. NOTE: Cardiopulmonary bypass is *not* used.	The creation of a large atrial septal defect can allow better mixing of oxygenated and venous blood within the heart (especially if the patient has transposition of the great vessels); it can also allow better flow of venous blood from the right to the left atrium; this increases pulmonary blood flow if the patient has transposition of the great vessels.
Patch enlargement of the pulmonary outflow tract	A prosthetic patch is placed across the pulmonary outflow tract. NOTE: This procedure requires use of cardiopulmonary bypass.	The patch acts as a gusset to enlarge the pulmonary outflow tract; this increases pulmonary blood flow and produces growth of the main and right and left pulmonary arteries; the patch may be left in place (or enlarged) when later correction is performed.

From Hazinski MF: *Nursing care of the critically ill child,* ed 2, St Louis, 1992, Mosby.

Table 5-25
Palliative Shunts for Treatment of Cyanotic Heart Disease—cont'd

Palliative Procedure	Resultant Anatomic Change	Circulatory Consequences
Pulmonary unifocalization procedure	Small pulmonary arteries or bronchial or collateral pulmonary vessels are joined together to fashion a common pulmonary arterial trunk of reasonable size (a patch may be used to enlarge this common arterial vessel); a shunt may provide flow from the aorta or systemic circulation to this common pulmonary artery. NOTE: This procedure may require use of cardiopulmonary bypass.	This procedure accomplishes two things: it creates a route of pulmonary blood flow of adequate size to improve oxygenation; it also fashions a common pulmonary arterial trunk which should grow in size in response to the shunt blood flow, facilitating later surgical correction (a conduit can be joined to this common pulmonary artery).

pression of the bronchi from the dilated pulmonary artery.

Palliative surgery for the *symptomatic* infant consists of ligation (tying off) of the main pulmonary artery and creation of a systemic–to–pulmonary artery shunt. This can be accomplished without cardiopulmonary bypass. Definitive correction does require cardiopulmonary bypass and requires a ventriculotomy incision for closure of the VSD and insertion of a conduit between the right ventricle and the pulmonary artery. Surgical correction for the *asymptomatic* child consists of closure of the VSD, resection of the aneurysmal pulmonary artery, and insertion of a pulmonary valve.

Tetralogy of Fallot With Atrioventricular Canal

If the infant is extremely cyanotic with limited pulmonary blood flow, creation of a systemic–to–pulmonary artery shunt may be required. When pulmonary stenosis is extremely mild, CHF may be present. Definitive correction uses cardiopulmonary bypass. An atriotomy incision is made, the atrial and ventricular septal defects are closed, and the cleft mitral valve is repaired. An incision is made in the pulmonary artery to facilitate resection of the pulmonary stenosis, and patch enlargement of the pulmonary artery may be necessary.

Postoperative Complications

Simple Tetralogy of Fallot Following *palliative* surgery, the nurse should monitor for signs of severe hypoxemia or CHF. Other postoperative

complications include those of a thoracotomy. If the child's subclavian artery was sacrificed for the shunt, arterial blood flow to that arm will be compromised postoperatively; thus arterial punctures should not be performed in that arm. It will not be possible to obtain cuff blood pressures in that arm.

Inadequate shunt blood flow may result if the shunt is too small or becomes obstructed, and hypoxemia will be worse than expected and may progress. Blood flow through a palliative shunt can be decreased by anything that increases PVR, such as atelectasis or alveolar hypoxia. These conditions should be avoided or promptly treated.

Complications of *corrective* surgery include CHF, low cardiac output, and arrhythmias. The child is at risk for all potential complications of hypoxemia and polycythemia, including bleeding and perioperative thromboembolism. CHF and right bundle branch block should be anticipated if a right ventriculotomy is performed. CHF is also more severe if residual pulmonary stenosis or pulmonary insufficiency is present postoperatively. If pentology of Fallot is present with a small left ventricle, left ventricular dysfunction and low cardiac output may be severe postoperatively.

Tetralogy of Fallot With Absent Pulmonary Valve

Postoperative complications include persistent respiratory failure, CHF, shock, and arrhythmias. The child is at risk for all potential complications of hypoxemia and polycythemia, including bleeding and perioperative thromboembolism. Pulmonary sup-

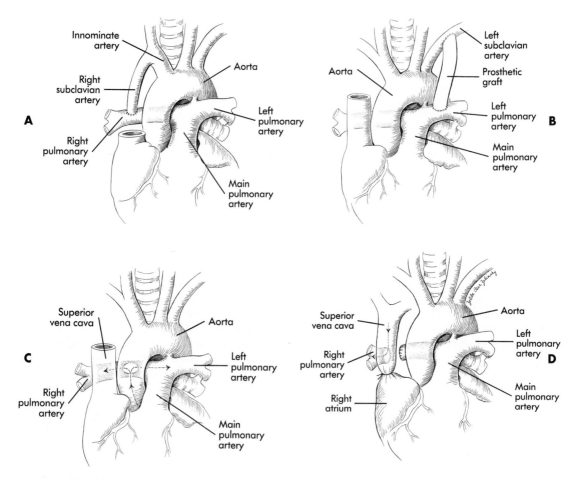

Figure 5-30   Palliative surgical procedures to increase effective pulmonary blood flow and systemic arterial oxygen saturation. **A,** Original Blalock-Taussig shunt. Patient's subclavian artery (usually the one arising from the innominate artery) is divided (tied off and cut, so it no longer provides blood flow to the arm), and the proximal end is brought down and sewn to the pulmonary artery. **B,** Modified Blalock-Taussig shunt. A prosthetic shunt, usually made of polytetrafluoroethylene (Gore-Tex or Impra) is sewn between the patient's subclavian artery and the pulmonary artery to provide a systemic-to-pulmonary artery shunt, which may be placed on either side. **C,** Waterston-Cooley shunt. This shunt is no longer performed but may occasionally be seen in older patients. A fistula is created between the back of the ascending aorta and the right pulmonary artery. This shunt was associated with complications such as pulmonary hypertension and pulmonary artery deformity. **D,** Glenn anastomosis. This shunt creates an orifice between the superior vena cava (SVC) and the right pulmonary artery. In the original Glenn procedure, the SVC is tied off at its entrance to the right atrium, so all SVC flow is directed into the right pulmonary artery. Glenn also divided the right pulmonary artery so its sole source of blood flow was the SVC. Current modifications of this shunt leave the pulmonary artery intact.

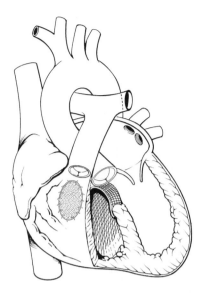

Figure 5-31 Surgical correction of tetralogy of Fallot. Pulmonary infundibular stenosis is resected, and the ventricular septal defect (VSD) is closed with a patch. The pulmonary outflow tract is enlarged with one or two patches if necessary. If possible, a right ventriculotomy incision is avoided, and this procedure is performed from the right atrium (through the tricuspid valve) and through an incision in the main pulmonary artery above the pulmonary valve. However, adequate enlargement of the pulmonary outflow tract may require a right ventriculotomy approach and patch placement at the incision site.

port will be required following correction during infancy.

Tetralogy of Fallot With Atrioventricular Canal
Potential postoperative complications include low cardiac output, CHF, and arrhythmias (particularly heart block). The child is at risk for all potential complications of hypoxemia and polycythemia, including bleeding and perioperative thromboembolism.

Truncus Arteriosus

Defect

Truncus arteriosus results from inadequate division of the common great vessel, the truncus arteriosus, during fetal cardiac development. A single, large

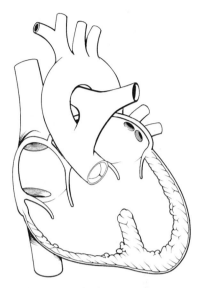

Figure 5-32 Truncus arteriosus, type I. In all forms of truncus, a large trunk arises from the ventricles, straddling a ventricular septal defect (VSD). This trunk receives the outflow from both ventricles and supplies the systemic, pulmonary, and coronary circulations. In truncus I, the main pulmonary artery branches directly from the trunk. Pulmonary stenosis may be present, although pulmonary blood flow is typically increased. The truncal valve may be stenotic or insufficient.

great vessel arises from the ventricles and gives rise to the systemic, pulmonary, and coronary circulations. Because the truncal septum contributes to closure of the conal ventricular septum, failure of truncal division also causes a large VSD. The truncus arteriosus usually has a single, large truncal valve with two to four cusps.

There are four major forms of truncus arteriosus; the types are distinguished by the origin of pulmonary arterial circulation from the large trunk (Figures 5-32 to 5-34). In truncus I, the main pulmonary artery branches off of the trunk. In truncus II and III, the right and left pulmonary arteries branch directly off of the trunk.

In truncus IV, there is no main pulmonary artery, and the pulmonary arterial circulation is supplied from the systemic arterial circulation through collateral vessels of the bronchial arteries. The distribution of the pulmonary arterial circulation is often

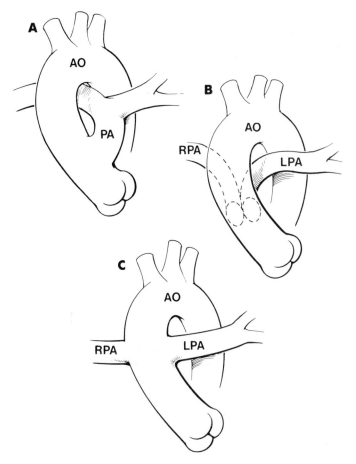

Figure 5-33 Truncus arteriosus, types I, II, and III. **A,** Type I, common trunk arising from the heart with a partial septation giving rise to the dominant aorta and main pulmonary artery. **B,** Type II has a common trunk and pulmonary arteries arising from the posterior surface of the common trunk. **C,** Type III has a common trunk and pulmonary arteries arising from the lateral walls of the common trunk. *AO,* Aorta; *PA,* pulmonary artery; *LPA,* left pulmonary artery; *RPA,* right pulmonary artery. (From Graham TP Jr, Merrill W, Kambam J: Truncus arteriosus. In Kambam J, editor: *Cardiac anesthesia for infants and children,* St Louis, 1994, Mosby.)

normal, but it originates from the aorta/systemic arterial circulation.

Hemodynamics and Clinical Presentation

The single great vessel arises from both ventricles, straddling the large VSD and receiving the output of both ventricles. The large VSD causes equalization of ventricular pressures; both ventricles share a common outflow tract, so that both right and left ventricular pressures will be high.

Both pulmonary and systemic blood flow enter the trunk, and the trunk gives rise to the systemic, pulmonary, and coronary circulations. Although there may be preferential streaming of oxygenated blood into the aortic trunk component, some systemic venous blood will enter the systemic arterial circulation; thus hypoxemia will be present. The level of systemic arterial oxygenation (or, conversely, hypoxemia) will be determined by the volume of pulmonary blood flow. The greater

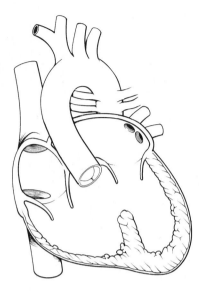

Figure 5-34 Truncus arteriosus, type IV. In all forms of truncus, a large trunk arises from the ventricles, straddling a ventricular septal defect (VSD). This trunk receives the outflow from both ventricles and supplies the systemic, pulmonary, and coronary circulations. In truncus type IV, there is no main pulmonary artery, and the pulmonary arterial circulation is supplied from the systemic arterial circulation through collateral vessels of the bronchial arteries. The distribution of the pulmonary arteries is normal, but it originates from the arterial circulation. This distribution separates truncus type IV from pulmonary atresia with VSD. In pulmonary atresia, collateral vessels from the aorta supply the pulmonary circulation, but the distribution of these vessels is not normal.

the pulmonary blood flow, the larger the proportion of pulmonary venous (oxygenated) blood entering the truncus, and the milder the hypoxemia. If pulmonary blood flow is severely compromised, little oxygenated blood will return to the left atrium and left ventricle; thus proportionately little of the truncal blood flow will be oxygenated, and hypoxemia will be severe. Whether or not cyanosis is readily apparent, the child is at risk for all complications of hypoxemia and polycythemia.

Nearly all infants with truncus arteriosus demonstrate signs of CHF or cyanosis in the first months of life. Clinical presentation of truncus ar-

teriosus is also affected by the presence of other intracardiac abnormalities. Abnormal origin of the coronary arteries is common, and interrupted aortic arch may also be present. The truncal valve may be stenotic or insufficient.

If pulmonary stenosis is absent, pulmonary blood flow will be increased, hypoxemia will be mild, but severe CHF will be present, and the risk of pulmonary hypertension will be high. If the truncal valve is also insufficient, severe CHF and cardiac decompensation can result. Cyanosis may be present during cry or exercise.

If pulmonary stenosis is mild to moderate, a balanced shunt may be present. The pulmonary stenosis may be sufficient to prevent CHF or the risk of pulmonary hypertension, while not severe enough to cause profound hypoxemia and cyanosis.

Severe pulmonary stenosis compromises pulmonary blood flow. Hypoxemia is usually severe at birth and worsens once the ductus arteriosus begins to close.

Medical and Surgical Interventions

Nonsurgical treatment of the infant with truncus arteriosus is aimed at reducing the signs and symptoms of CHF and preventing the complications of pulmonary hypertension and arterial hypoxemia and polycythemia. Since all patients with truncus arteriosus have some systemic venous blood entering the systemic arterial circulation, *no air can be allowed to enter any IV line* until corrective surgery has been performed. Antibiotic prophylaxis must be provided throughout life during periods of risk of bacteremia.

CHF must be managed aggressively, but dehydration and hemoconcentration must be avoided. Surgical intervention is scheduled to minimize the risk of pulmonary hypertension. Pulmonary artery banding may be performed to relieve symptoms of CHF unresponsive to medical management and to prevent the development of pulmonary hypertension. However, this procedure is associated with high mortality and may not prevent the development of pulmonary vascular disease. For this reason, complete correction is usually preferred to pulmonary artery banding for the symptomatic infant.

If truncus arteriosus is associated with severe obstruction to pulmonary blood flow and hypoxemia, PGE_1 should be administered at birth to

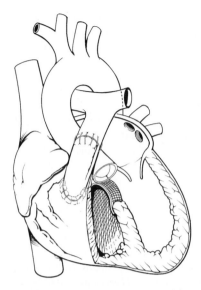

Figure 5-35   Surgical correction of truncus arteriosus, type I. Correction of all forms of truncus requires separation of the pulmonary circulation from the trunk, patch closure of the ventricular septal defect (VSD) so that left ventricular outflow is directed into the trunk, and joining of the right ventricle with the separate pulmonary circulation. A valved pulmonary artery homograft is most often used, and anticoagulation will not be required postoperatively.

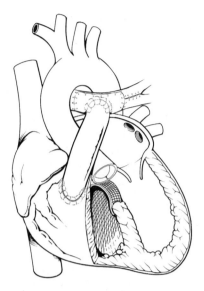

Figure 5-36   Surgical correction of truncus arteriosus, type IV, with unifocalization of the pulmonary artery supply. Correction of all forms of truncus requires separation of the pulmonary circulation from the trunk. With this form of truncus, the pulmonary arteries are separated from the descending aorta and must be joined together to form a single vessel (this is called "unifocalization"). A patch may be used to create a pulmonary artery of sufficient size. As with all forms of truncus correction, the ventricular septal defect (VSD) is closed with a patch, so that left ventricular outflow is directed into the trunk. The right ventricle is joined with new pulmonary artery (created from the pulmonary arteries removed from the trunk). A valved pulmonary artery homograft is most often used, and anticoagulation will not be required postoperatively.

maintain ductal patency until palliative or corrective surgery can be performed. A systemic–to–pulmonary artery shunt may be created to increase pulmonary blood flow and systemic oxygenation and to help the pulmonary arteries to grow. The shunt may also be performed as part of a *unifocalization* procedure, which joins right and left pulmonary arteries or pulmonary artery branches (which have been separated from the truncus or aorta) to form a single common pulmonary artery joined to the shunt. Later repair will then join this common pulmonary artery with the right ventricle.

Surgical correction is usually accomplished during infancy. This eliminates the risk of complications such as pulmonary vascular disease or thromboembolic events. Cardiopulmonary bypass is required (Figures 5-35 and 5-36).

There are three goals of surgical correction: establishment of continuity between the right ventricle and the pulmonary artery, closure of the VSD,

and correction of any associated lesions. The procedure is a modification of one developed by Rastelli. The pulmonary artery or arteries are separated from the trunk, and any remaining defects in the aorta are patched. The trunk then becomes the aorta only. If the pulmonary arteries are removed as separate vessels, they must be joined together to create a common pulmonary artery (unifocalization). If a systemic–to–pulmonary artery shunt was created, this is ligated (tied off).

A right ventriculotomy incision is made. The VSD is closed with a baffle patch so that left ventricular output is diverted into the aorta. A valved homograft conduit (usually a pulmonary artery homograft) is attached to the right ventricle and joined to the pulmonary artery. Nonvalved homograft conduits are occasionally used if PVR is low. Anticoagulation is not required postoperatively when valved homografts are used.

The conduit size selection is important; too small a conduit will produce obstruction to pulmonary flow. Too large a conduit will be compressed when the chest is closed. Occasionally, despite the selection of an ideal conduit, the sternum cannot be closed at the end of surgery. If this occurs, the skin and subcutaneous tissues can be closed but the sternum can be left separated for several days and then closed as tolerated.

Postoperative Complications

The child is at risk for complications of cyanotic heart disease, including bleeding and thromboembolism. In addition, when repair is accomplished during early infancy, crowding within the thorax due to insertion of the conduit can result in tamponade and in compression of coronary arteries (see Postoperative Complications, p. 211)

CHF (particularly right ventricular failure) and low cardiac output are common complications. Any postoperative bleeding can contribute to tamponade, since there is little room in the mediastinum. Tamponade must be ruled out whenever signs of low cardiac output develop. Right bundle branch block should be anticipated as a result of the ventriculotomy, and heart block may occur. If pulmonary hypertension is present preoperatively, postoperative pulmonary hypertensive crises should be anticipated, and pulmonary vascular resistance should be reduced through maintenance of alveolar oxygenation, alkalosis, and sedation (see p. 211).

Pulmonary Atresia With Intact Ventricular Septum

Defect

Pulmonary atresia is a failure of pulmonary valve development or failure of appropriate septation of the truncus arteriosus into both a pulmonary artery and an aorta (Figure 5-37). As a result, there is lack of anatomic continuity between the right ventricle and the pulmonary artery. The pulmonary valve annulus may be very small, and the main pulmonary artery may be absent or rudimentary. The right and left pulmonary arteries may be of normal size, or they may be extremely small.

In most patients with pulmonary atresia and an intact ventricular septum (IVS), the right ventricle is extremely small and thick walled, and the tricuspid valve is often stenotic. This form of the defect may also be called hypoplastic right heart syndrome.

Hemodynamics and Clinical Presentation

Since systemic venous blood cannot pass out of the right ventricle, it must pass through a stretched foramen ovale or a true ASD to the left side of the heart, causing cyanosis. There must be some source of pulmonary blood flow, such as a PDA, or the patient will die of progressive hypoxemia.

The lack of right ventricular outflow creates tremendous right ventricular afterload; as a result, the rudimentary right ventricle is hypertrophied. Right ventricular hypertension is extreme; Right ventricular pressures are often higher than left ventricular or systemic pressures. Endocardial fibroelastosis is typically present.

The extreme right ventricular hypertension can stimulate the formation of myocardial sinusoids between the right ventricle and the coronary arteries. These sinusoids allow *desaturated* systemic venous blood from the right ventricle to flow retrograde into the left anterior descending or right coronary artery. Forward flow of blood through the coronary arteries will be impeded. This results in ischemia of both ventricles and may contribute to the development of malignant ventricular arrhythmias.

The tricuspid valve is incompetent, and the right atrium is dilated. Some interatrial communication is always present, but it may be restrictive.

The left side of the heart receives both systemic and pulmonary venous blood; thus the left atrium and mitral valve are enlarged, and left ventricular hypertrophy is present. Left ventricular dysfunction may develop and can be exacerbated by the formation of the right ventricular sinusoids.

The neonate with pulmonary atresia and IVS is cyanotic at birth, particularly once the ductus arteriosus begins to close. The high right atrial pressure produces signs of systemic venous congestion, in-

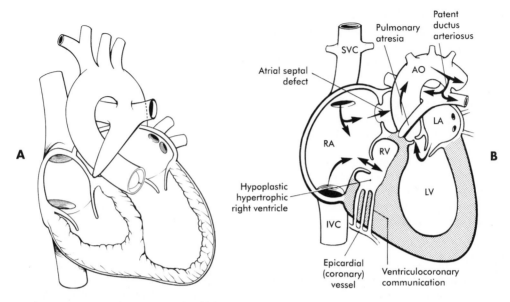

Figure 5-37 Pulmonary atresia with intact ventricular septum. **A,** There is no outflow from the right ventricle, and that ventricle is small but extremely hypertensive and hypertrophied. There must be a source of pulmonary blood flow, such as the patent ductus arteriosus *(PDA)* depicted here. **B,** Depiction of sinusoids, which may develop between the coronary arteries and the hypertensive right ventricular cavity. The blood flows from the right ventricle into the coronary arteries (particularly the left anterior descending branch), resulting in delivery of desaturated (systemic venous) blood to the tissues perfused by this system. (From Striepe V: Pulmonary atresia with intact ventricular septum. In Kambam J, editor: *Cardiac anesthesia for infants and children,* St Louis, 1994, Mosby.)

cluding hepatomegaly and periorbital edema. Signs of biventricular CHF may be present.

Medical and Surgical Interventions

PGE₁ administration is required to maintain ductal patency during the neonatal period until surgical intervention can be accomplished. The infant is at risk for the development of complications of hypoxemia and polycythemia. *No air can be allowed to enter any IV line.* Antibiotic prophylaxis will be required throughout the child's life during periods of increased risk of bacteremia.

CHF may also be present, requiring careful management of intravascular volume while avoiding hemoconcentration. Cardiac catheterization is performed during the first days of life. If the ASD or foramen ovale is restrictive, it is enlarged with a balloon (balloon septostomy) during cardiac catheterization.

The surgical approach is designed to improve pulmonary blood flow and ultimately separate pulmonary and systemic blood within the heart. If at all possible, two-ventricle cardiac function is maintained, but the surgical approach is always individualized.

Palliative surgery may be performed to provide some pulmonary blood flow without the use of cardiopulmonary bypass. A closed-heart pulmonary valvotomy (similar to that performed for critical neonatal pulmonary valve stenosis) may be performed to decompress the right ventricle. The pulmonary valve and main pulmonary artery often are too small to provide an adequate route of pulmonary blood flow after the valvotomy; thus a systemic–to–pulmonary artery shunt may also be created.

If the child with pulmonary atresia and IVS has no main pulmonary artery, a pulmonary-to-systemic shunt is created in the newborn period, with later corrective surgery similar to that performed for tricuspid atresia (later bidirectional Glenn, cardiopulmonary anastomosis, or Fontan-type surgery).

Corrective surgery uses cardiopulmonary bypass and is becoming the preferred technique to provide a route of pulmonary blood flow and attempt to preserve a two-ventricle heart. A pulmonary valvotomy is performed under direct visualization, using an incision in the pulmonary artery, just above the pulmonary valve. The valve is opened maximally, even if insufficiency is created. In addition, a patch may be placed to enlarge the pulmonary artery. This patch may be placed across the pulmonary valve and may include a valve cusp to minimize postoperative pulmonary insufficiency. The ASD is also closed.

If the right ventricle is too small to support the pulmonary circulation, blood flow from the vena cavae or right atrium may be diverted into the pulmonary artery. This form of surgery is a variant of the Fontan-type corrective procedures performed for tricuspid atresia (see Tricuspid Atresia). If at all possible, the right ventricle is incorporated into this procedure to allow some blood to flow through the right ventricle into the pulmonary artery, even when most of the pulmonary blood flow is from the vena cavae or right atrium.

Postoperative Complications

Postoperative complications include those associated with cyanotic heart disease, particularly postoperative bleeding and thromboembolism. Low cardiac output and severe CHF (including hepatomegaly, ascites, and pleural effusions) are often present. Arrhythmias, including sudden malignant ventricular arrhythmias, may be problematic. Postoperative care following Fontan-type surgical procedures is summarized under Tricuspid Atresia.

Tricuspid Atresia

Defect

Tricuspid atresia results from complete lack of formation of the tricuspid valve during fetal cardiac development (Figure 5-38). There is no blood flow between the right atrium and the right ventricle. Tricuspid atresia is associated with a very small right ventricle and some form of interatrial shunt. A VSD is often present.

There are several forms of tricuspid atresia. The defect may be associated with normally related

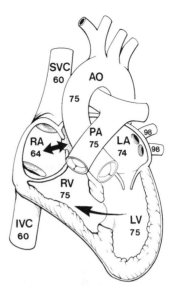

Figure 5-38 Tricuspid atresia with normally related great arteries and ventricular septal defect and pulmonary stenosis (type I, B). Typical oxygen saturations within the cardiac chambers and great vessels are depicted. This defect may also be present in association with transposition of the great arteries and without pulmonary stenosis. (From Striepe V: Tricuspid atresia. In Kambam J, editor: *Cardiac anesthesia for infants and children,* St Louis, 1994, Mosby.)

great arteries (type I) or with transposition of the great arteries (type II). The presence or absence of pulmonary stenosis is used to further subdivide the defects (Box 5-25).

Hemodynamics and Clinical Presentation

Nearly half of all infants with tricuspid atresia are diagnosed in the first day of life because of the presence of either cyanosis or a heart murmur. Tricuspid atresia is a cyanotic heart defect; thus the child is at risk for all complications of hypoxemia and polycythemia.

Because there is no communication between the right atrium and the right ventricle, the only way for blood to leave the right atrium is through an interatrial communication, such as a patent foramen ovale. Systemic venous blood enters the right atrium and passes through the interatrial communication to the left atrium. If the interatrial com-

Box 5-25

Classification of Tricuspid Atresia

Type I Tricuspid Atresia: Normally Related Great Arteries (Most Common)

I, A: No VSD, and pulmonary atresia is present

I, B: Small VSD and pulmonary stenosis (most common)

I, C: Large VSD without pulmonary stenosis

Type II Tricuspid Atresia: D-Transposition of the Great Arteries

II, A: VSD with pulmonary atresia

II, B: VSD with pulmonary stenosis

II, C: VSD without pulmonary stenosis

Type III Tricuspid Atresia: With L-Transposition of the Great Arteries

munication is restrictive, signs of severe systemic venous congestion will be present. Systemic and pulmonary venous blood mix in the left atrium and the left ventricle; thus hypoxemia is present.

In most forms of tricuspid atresia a VSD is present, although the great vessels may be normally related or transposed. If there is no restriction to pulmonary blood flow (i. e., no pulmonary stenosis or restrictive VSD with normally related great arteries), pulmonary blood flow will be increased at high pressure. The greater the volume of pulmonary blood flow, the greater the proportion of oxygenated blood returning to the left ventricle and the higher the systemic arterial oxygen saturation. However, the price of this increase in pulmonary blood flow is severe CHF and the risk of pulmonary hypertension. Increased pulmonary venous return will contribute to the development of left ventricular volume overload and left ventricular dysfunction.

Significant pulmonary stenosis will decrease pulmonary blood flow, resulting in severe cyanosis and hypoxemia whether the great vessels are normally related or transposed. If pulmonary atresia is present, cyanosis will be profound, particularly once the ductus begins to close, because the ductus arteriosus provides the only source of pulmonary blood flow. Systemic consequences of hypoxemia and polycythemia may be present, and hypercya-

notic episodes often develop. These spells indicate the need for urgent surgical intervention.

Over half of all infants with tricuspid atresia have a VSD, normally related great arteries, and pulmonary stenosis with decreased pulmonary blood flow. This typically produces significant cyanosis but no heart failure.

Medical and Surgical Interventions

The infant with tricuspid atresia is at risk for all complications of chronic hypoxemia and polycythemia. *No air can be allowed to enter any IV line.* Maintenance of optimal fluid balance may be challenging in the presence of CHF; the infant must be kept sufficiently hydrated to avoid hemoconcentration. Antibiotic prophylaxis will be required throughout the child's life during periods of increased risk of bacteremia.

If cyanosis is severe at birth, PGE_1 is administered to maintain ductal patency until diagnostic studies and surgery can be performed. Progressive hypoxemia or hypercyanotic episodes indicate the need for urgent surgical intervention.

Cardiac catheterization is performed in the first days of life. If the interatrial communication is restrictive, a balloon atrial septostomy is performed to enlarge it and reduce systemic venous congestion.

Palliative Surgery Some forms of palliative surgery are performed without cardiopulmonary bypass, whereas others require bypass. Palliative surgery can be performed to improve pulmonary blood flow and/or decompress the right atrium and the left ventricle.

Potential palliative shunts to improve pulmonary blood flow without the need for cardiopulmonary bypass include the traditional systemic–to–pulmonary artery shunts (see Figures 5-30 and 5-39) or a central shunt (aorta to pulmonary artery). Systemic venous–to–pulmonary artery shunts or right atrium–to–pulmonary artery shunts can also improve pulmonary blood flow, decompress the right atrium, and decompress the left ventricle. The left ventricle is decompressed by these procedures because diversion of systemic venous blood directly into the pulmonary circulation prevents the left ventricle from handling all of systemic and pulmonary venous return. These systemic venous–to–pulmonary artery shunts include an SVC–to–

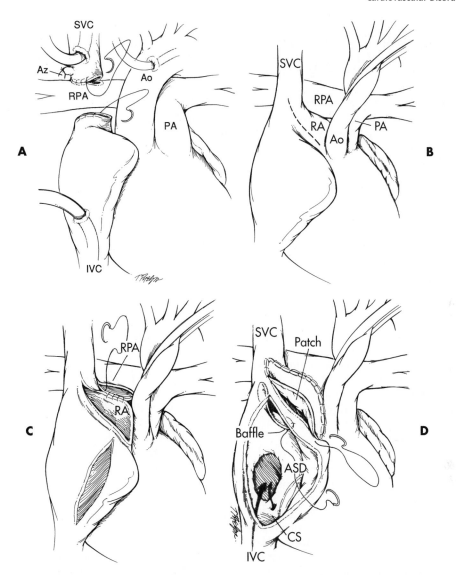

Figure 5-39 Palliative procedures for tricuspid atresia and single ventricle. **A,** Bidirectional Glenn operation. The proximal superior vena cava *(SVC)* and inferior vena cava *(IVC)* are cannulated for cardiopulmonary bypass. After transection of the SVC, the cephalad end is anastomosed to the right pulmonary artery *(RPA),* and the cardiac end of the SVC is oversewn. The azygous *(Az)* vein is ligated. IVC blood flows through the atrial septal defect (ASD) and thus contributes to left ventricular preload. *Ao,* Aorta. **B,** Hemi-Fontan operation from the surgical view showing spiral incision extending from the superior vena cava *(SVC)* onto the surface of the right atrium *(RA).* **C,** After incision of the pulmonary artery *(RPA),* a vascular confluence is created, incorporating the cardiac end of the SVC, cephalad portion of the RA, and the RPA. **D,** This confluence is roofed with a patch of polytetrafluoroethylene (PTFE). A second PTFE baffle forms the floor of this confluence and separates the inferior vena cava *(IVC)* and coronary sinus *(CS)* blood from SVC blood, thus allowing IVC and coronary blood to enter the left atrium via the atrial septal defect *(ASD).* (From Okanlami O et al: Tricuspid atresia and the Fontan operation. In Nichols DG et, editors: *Critical heart disease in infants and children,* St Louis, 1995, Mosby.)

pulmonary artery shunt (Glenn or modified Glenn, including a bidirectional Glenn) or a right atrium–to–pulmonary artery shunt, which is also called a hemi-Fontan procedure.

A Glenn procedure can be performed with or without cardiopulmonary bypass. It diverts SVC blood flow into the right pulmonary artery. The shunt is often constructed as a bidirectional Glenn so that SVC blood flow enters the right pulmonary artery but flows into both the right and left pulmonary arteries (Figure 5-39, *A*). This procedure diverts all SVC blood away from the heart and reduces the right atrial, left atrial, and left ventricular volume load. By directing a significant portion of systemic venous blood directly into the pulmonary circulation, systemic oxygenation is improved, particularly in young children.

If a Fontan-type correction is anticipated, the right atrium can be connected to the pulmonary artery in a hemi-Fontan procedure. This procedure uses cardiopulmonary bypass and creates a window at the point where the SVC, the right atrium, and the right pulmonary artery come into contact (Figure 5-39, *B*). A patch is then used to isolate the SVC blood so that it can only flow into the pulmonary artery. Inferior vena caval (IVC) and coronary sinus blood continue to flow through the ASD into the left atrium (Figure 5-39, *C* and *D*).

Corrective Surgery   Corrective surgery for tricuspid atresia separates systemic and pulmonary venous blood within the heart and diverts systemic venous blood into the pulmonary circulation. The original corrective procedure, as described by Fontan, is rarely performed. However, the Fontan name is still applied to a family of corrective procedures that divert systemic venous or right atrial blood flow into the pulmonary circulation. These procedures can be performed to correct a variety of congenital heart defects that result in single-ventricle physiology, including tricuspid atresia, single ventricle, and hypoplastic left heart syndrome.

One form of corrective procedure creates a cavopulmonary connection or tunnel to isolate SVC and IVC blood from the rest of the right atrium and divert it into the pulmonary arteries (Figure 5-40, *A*). The original Glenn procedure may remain in place. The main pulmonary artery is transected

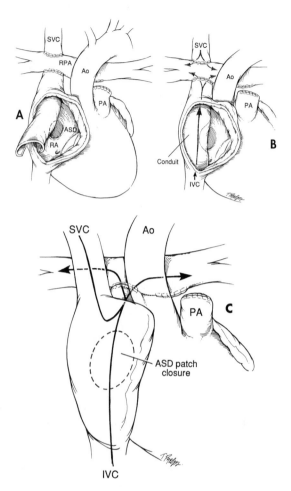

Figure 5-40   Corrective procedures for tricuspid atresia and single ventricle. **A,** Total cardiopulmonary anastomosis with previous bidirectional Glenn shunt in place. Right atrium *(RA)* is opened. Atrial septal defect *(ASD)* is enlarged by sparing the atrioventricular node. **B,** Intraatrial conduit is fashioned from Gore-Tex and positioned to convey inferior vena cava *(IVC)* blood to the SVC-RPA anastomosis. The posterolateral wall of the conduit is made up of the atrial wall. *Ao,* Aorta. **C,** Direct atriopulmonary connection: the roof of the right atrium is anastomosed to the undersurface of the right pulmonary artery. The proximal main pulmonary artery *(PA)* is oversewn. After patch closure of the atrial septal defect *(ASD),* a woven Dacron roof patch covers the atriotomy *(not shown). SVC,* Superior vena cava. (From Okanlami O et al: Tricuspid atresia and the Fontan operation. In Nichols DG et al, editors: *Critical heart disease in infants and children,* St Louis, 1995, Mosby.)

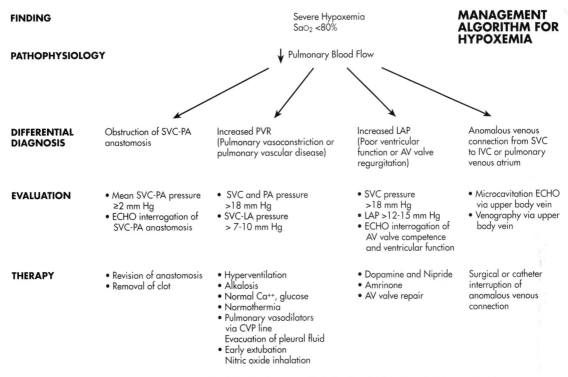

Figure 5-41 Management algorithm for hypoxemia following bidirectional Glenn or hemi-Fontan procedure. (From Okanlami O et al: Tricuspid atresia and the Fontan operation. In Nichols DG et al, editors: *Critical heart disease in infants and children,* St Louis,1995, Mosby.)

and oversewn, and any systemic–to–pulmonary artery shunt is ligated. The ASD is also closed. At the end of the procedure, all pulmonary blood flow comes from the cavopulmonary anastomosis. This cavopulmonary tunnel may also be placed on the outside of the right atrium.

An alternative corrective procedure is the atriopulmonary connection, which connects the posterior right atrium directly to the pulmonary artery. SVC and IVC blood flow into the pulmonary artery, and the ASD is closed (Figure 5-40, *C*).

Postoperative Complications

Because the child has cyanotic heart disease, bleeding or thromboembolism may complicate either palliative or corrective surgery. Until corrective surgery has completely separated systemic and pulmonary venous blood, *no air can be allowed to enter any IV line.*

Following the palliative Glenn or hemi-Fontan procedures, the patient may demonstrate persistent hypoxemia, which usually indicates the presence of increased PVR, ventricular dysfunction, or obstruction at the site of surgery. Management of persistent hypoxemia is presented in Figure 5-41.

Following the cavopulmonary anastomosis or atriopulmonary connection, low cardiac output is the most common and most severe complication. It is often caused by inadequate flow of blood into the pulmonary circulation as a result of hypovolemia, obstruction at the site of surgery, or elevated PVR. Low cardiac output may also be caused by left ventricular dysfunction. Management of low cardiac output following corrective surgery (Fontan-type correction) is summarized in Figure 5-42.

Additional postoperative complications include residual hypoxemia and systemic venous congestion. Systemic venous congestion can lead to addi-

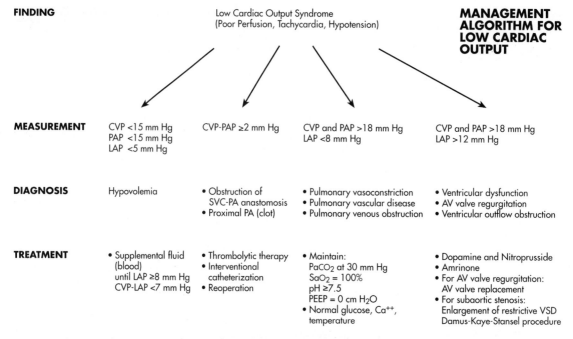

Figure 5-42   Management algorithm for low cardiac output after Fontan-type correction of tricuspid atresia or single ventricle. *CVP,* Central venous pressure; *PAP,* pulmonary artery pressure; *LAP,* left atrial pressure; *SVC,* superior vena cava; *PA,* pulmonary artery; *AV,* atrioventricular; *PEEP,* positive end-expiratory pressure; *VSD,* ventricular septal defect. (From Okanlami et al: Tricuspid atresia and the Fontan operation. In Nichols DG et al, editors: *Critical heart disease in infants and children,* St Louis,1995, Mosby.)

tional complications, including chylothorax, pleural effusion, pericardial effusion, and ascites. Chylothorax can require long-term management with chest tube insertion or insertion of a valved pulmonary-to-abdominal shunt (which can be pumped to drain lymph fluid from the chest into the abdominal cavity, where it is absorbed). Administration of a medium-chain triglyceride diet and supplementation of fat-soluble vitamins may also be required. Systemic venous hypertension will produce liver congestion and may produce liver dysfunction.

Arrhythmias, including supraventricular tachycardia (SVT), atrial flutter, junction ectopic tachycardia, and complete heart block, may also be problematic postoperatively. Neurologic complications can include thromboembolic events.

A small number of children develop protein-losing enteropathy (loss of protein via the gut) fol-

lowing Fontan-type procedures. These children exhibit systemic edema and low serum albumin and may demonstrate signs of intravascular volume depletion (particularly if diuretic therapy is aggressive). Treatment is supportive and may require albumin administration.

Single Ventricle or Univentricular Heart

Defect

The term *single ventricle* or *univentricular heart* refers to a variety of congenital heart defects that are characterized by the presence of a single, dominant ventricle that ultimately receives both systemic and pulmonary venous blood. This ventricle can be a single-inlet ventricle, as occurs with atresia of one AV valve (e.g., tricuspid atresia or mitral atresia). Alternatively, the ventricle may be a double-inlet ventricle to which both AV valves are joined.

Occasionally an extremely large VSD results in the creation of a functional single ventricle. However, if a rim of septal tissue separates two reasonably sized ventricles and if normal conduction tissue is present in that septal rim, this defect should be referred to as a common ventricle rather than a single ventricle.

The single ventricle can be described by its associated AV inlets and its morphology (structure and appearance). The most common form of single ventricle has two AV valves and left ventricular morphology and may be referred to as a double-inlet left ventricle.

Hemodynamics and Clinical Presentation

A wide spectrum of associated cardiac anomalies may be associated with a single ventricle (see Tricuspid Atresia and Hypoplastic Left Heart Syndrome). However, the ultimate result of these defects is that one ventricle receives both systemic and pulmonary venous blood and is responsible for perfusion of the systemic, pulmonary, and coronary circulations. Some systemic venous blood is entering the systemic arterial circulation; thus hypoxemia and polycythemia are present, and the child is at risk for complications of these problems.

Associated abnormalities, such as pulmonary or aortic atresia, may also complicate the child's clinical presentation and management. Intracardiac conduction may be abnormal, producing heart block or arrhythmias.

The clinical signs associated with a single ventricle will be determined by the volume of pulmonary blood flow, the mixing of pulmonary and systemic venous blood, and the presence of associated defects. Typically, the child develops signs of CHF and/or cyanosis during the first months of life.

If the single ventricle is present without significant obstruction to pulmonary blood flow, signs of CHF and the risk of pulmonary hypertension will predominate. Hypoxemia may not be severe.

If obstruction to pulmonary blood flow is present, hypoxemia will be present from birth. If pulmonary atresia is present, pulmonary blood flow may be dependent on the ductus arteriosus, and hy-

poxemia may become severe when the ductus begins to close.

Medical and Surgical Interventions

Management is determined by the child's symptoms and anatomy. Unless or until corrective surgery is performed, *no air can be allowed to enter any IV line.* Antibiotic prophylaxis will be required throughout the child's life during periods of increased risk of bacteremia.

CHF requires careful management of intravascular volume, but hemoconcentration must be avoided. Pulmonary artery banding may be performed to reduce pulmonary blood flow, relieve symptoms of CHF, and prevent the development of pulmonary hypertension (see Figure 5-23).

If obstruction to pulmonary blood flow is present, PGE_1 administration will probably be required during the first days of life to maintain ductal patency until palliative or corrective surgery can be performed. Palliative surgery usually consists of a systemic–to–pulmonary artery shunt. If pulmonary atresia is present, a pulmonary artery unifocalization procedure may be performed when the shunt is constructed to create a single common pulmonary artery from several collateral vessels (see Figure 5-36).

Correction of a single ventricle most often uses one of the modified Fontan procedures (see Figure 5-40, *A* through *C*). Septation of the single ventricle may also be attempted if two AV valves are present and the single ventricle is of the left ventricular morphology with a rudimentary right ventricle. However, the corrective procedure must also consider the presence of any associated defects; thus the particular surgical approach will be individualized. Cardiac transplantation may also be performed.

Postoperative Complications

Postoperative complications include those associated with hypoxemia and polycythemia, including bleeding and thromboembolism. Additional potential complications are largely the same as those observed following correction of tricuspid atresia and include low cardiac output, severe systemic venous congestion, and complete heart block. If pulmonary hypertension was present preoperatively, it may be problematic postoperatively. (See Treatment of Pulmonary Hypertension, pp. 156 and 211.)

Ebstein's Anomaly

Defect

Ebstein's anomaly is a congenital anomaly of the tricuspid valve (Figure 5-43). The valve leaflets are dysplastic, and two of the leaflets (the medial or septal leaflets and the posterior leaflet) are displaced inferiorly, adhering to the right ventricular wall.

The anatomy of this defect varies widely, and additional associated intracardiac abnormalities are common. Atrial or ventricular septal defects and L-transposition ("corrected transposition" or ventricular inversion) are often present. When L-transposition is present, the anomalous tricuspid valve is on the *left* side, receiving pulmonary venous return.

Hemodynamics and Clinical Presentation

Hemodynamic alterations and clinical effects resulting from Ebstein's anomaly vary widely. These alterations and effects are determined largely by the right atrial pressure, tricuspid valve function, and right ventricular size and function, as well as by any associated defects. The following information assumes that the malformed tricuspid valve is on the *right* side of the heart; if a left-sided tricuspid valve is present, signs of pulmonary edema (and other signs characteristically associated with left ventricular failure) may be present.

The inferior displacement of the tricuspid valve leaflets effectively incorporates a variable portion of the right ventricle into the right atrium; thus that portion of the ventricle is "atrialized." As a result, functional right ventricular size is compromised and the right atrium is dilated. The atrialized portion of the right ventricle may appear normal, or it may be extremely thin with little ability to contract.

The tricuspid valve may be competent or grossly insufficient and may be stenotic. If the valve is competent and not stenotic, the child may be asymptomatic during childhood or may have only occasional episodes of cyanosis. Significant tricuspid valve insufficiency or stenosis produces right atrial and systemic venous hypertension, including hepatomegaly and systemic edema.

Right atrial dilation produces atrial tachyarrhythmias, including atrial flutter or fibrillation or other SVTs. Right-to-left shunting of blood through the foramen ovale is most common during the neonatal period and will produce hypoxemia. If this shunt is large, forward flow of blood through the right ventricle will be compromised, and systemic hypoxemia may be present with low cardiac output.

Right ventricular dysplasia and dysfunction contribute to tricuspid insufficiency, CHF, right-to-left interatrial shunting of blood, and cyanosis and hypoxemia. Severe right ventricular dilation produces bulging of the ventricular septum toward the left ventricle with resultant left ventricular outflow

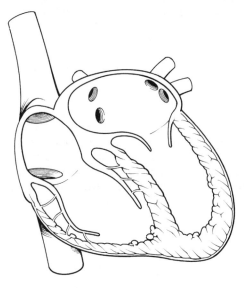

Figure 5-43   Ebstein malformation of the tricuspid valve. Ebstein's malformation consists of downward displacement of the septal and posterior leaflets of the tricuspid valve. A large portion of the right ventricle is "atrialized." This valve is pictured in normal position on the right side of the heart, where insufficiency will produce systemic venous congestion. Ebstein's anomaly may also be associated with L transposition, so that the tricuspid valve is on the left side, where insufficiency will produce pulmonary edema. (From Rao PS, Kambam J: Ebstein's malformation of the tricuspid valve. In Kambam J, editor: *Cardiac anesthesia for infants and children,* St Louis, 1994, Mosby.)

tract obstruction. The right atrial dilation may be associated with stasis of systemic venous blood and emboli to the left atrium, which may cause a stroke.

The child with Ebstein's anomaly is at risk for all of the systemic consequences of hypoxemia and polycythemia. Intracardiac conduction defects, including the presence of intraatrial conduction pathways, may also be present, and SVTs often develop. The PR interval is usually prolonged.

Medical and Surgical Interventions

Nonsurgical management of the child with Ebstein's anomaly requires treatment of CHF and management of atrial arrhythmias. Aggressive diuresis must be avoided, since it may lead to hemoconcentration. Since a right-to-left shunt is often present, *no air can be allowed to enter any IV line.* Antibiotic prophylaxis will be required throughout the child's life during periods of increased risk of bacteremia.

If pulmonary blood flow is severely compromised, administration of PGE_1 will be required during the first days of life. Indications for surgical intervention include severe cyanosis and increasing polycythemia, severe CHF refractory to medical management, tachyarrhythmias secondary to an accessory intraatrial conduction pathway, paradoxical emboli, and progressive disability.

Any surgical intervention for Ebstein's anomaly is palliative in nature. Classical palliative procedures for cyanotic heart disease generally do not result in clinical improvement. The Glenn anastomosis (SVC to pulmonary artery) may improve systemic arterial oxygen saturation and relief of symptoms of CHF. This procedure may produce only minimal or temporary relief, however.

"Corrective" surgery for Ebstein's anomaly is still being refined. The surgeon may attempt to plicate the atrialized portion of the right ventricle and repair the tricuspid valve (Figure 5-44). This plication is accomplished using cardiopulmonary bypass and an incision in the right atrium. Sutures are inserted in the area of the normal valve ring and then through the rim of the displaced valve; when the sutures are pulled together, the valve is pulled toward the normal position. This creates an isolated outpouching of the atrialized right ventricle. A valvuloplasty of the tricuspid valve is performed, and the tricuspid valve may be replaced. Any ASD or patent foramen ovale is closed.

Alternatives to plication of the right ventricle include variations of the Fontan-type procedures for tricuspid atresia. These procedures bypass the dysfunctional tricuspid valve and right ventricle. Cardiac transplantation may also be performed.

Postoperative Complications

Ebstein's anomaly is a cyanotic defect; thus the child is at risk for all of the potential complications associated with hypoxemia and polycythemia, including potential bleeding and thromboembolism. Low cardiac output and CHF may be severe postoperatively, particularly if the child was symptomatic preoperatively. Sudden malignant arrhythmias, including complete heart block and ventricular fibrillation, may develop. If pulmonary hypertension was present preoperatively, it may be problematic postoperatively.

Transposition of The Great Arteries

Defect

Transposition of the great arteries (TGA) is present when the aorta arises from the anatomic right ventricle and the pulmonary artery arises from the anatomic left ventricle (Figure 5-45). This form of transposition is referred to as D-transposition (dextro-transposition), because the aorta lies anterior and to the right of the pulmonary artery. Some form of interatrial communication is usually present, and a VSD or pulmonary stenosis may be present.

Hemodynamics and Clinical Presentation

With *simple D-TGA,* systemic venous blood enters the right atrium and then flows into the right ventricle and aorta; thus it recirculates through the system. Pulmonary venous blood enters the left atrium and flows into the left ventricle and the pulmonary artery; it is then returned to the pulmonary circulation. If there is no additional defect to allow mixing of systemic and pulmonary venous blood, the infant with TGA will die of progressive hypoxemia.

The newborn with TGA usually demonstrates signs of severe hypoxemia at birth and is usually tachypneic and hyperpneic. The severity of the hy-

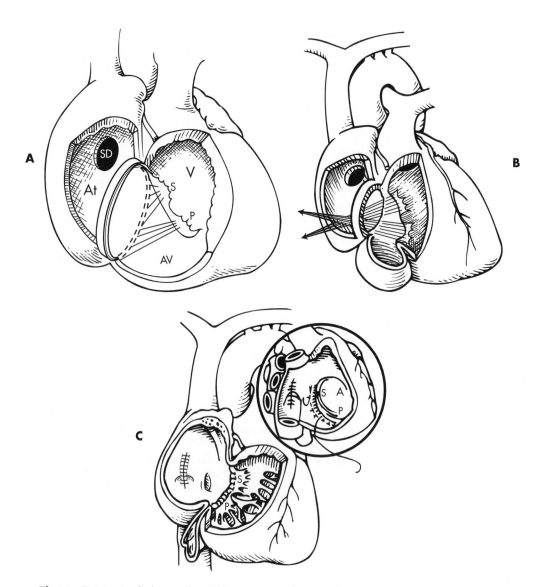

Figure 5-44 Surgical correction of Ebstein's anomaly. *At,* Atrium; *SD,* septal defect; *V,* ventricle; *S,* septal leaflet; *P,* posterior leaflet; *AV,* atrialized ventricle; *A,* anterior leaflet. **A,** Restoring the spiral line of valve attachment to an oval annulus to produce an orifice. **B** and **C,** Abnormal leaflets transposed to normal functional position, annulus reduced in size, and atrialized ventricle excluded. *Inset,* Superior view of competent eccentric valve closure is shown. (From Hardy KL et al: Ebstein's anomaly, further experience with definitive repair, *J Thorac Cardiovasc Surg* 58:556, 1969.)

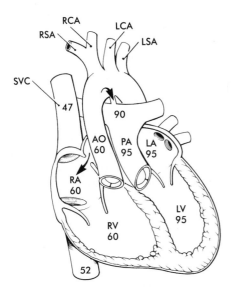

Figure 5-45 Transposition of the great arteries. Oxygen saturations in the cardiac chambers and great vessels are depicted with some shunting (mixing) of blood at the atrial level and through a patent ductus arteriosus. *RCA,* Right carotid artery; *LCA,* left carotid artery; *RSA,* right subclavian artery; *LSA,* left subclavian artery; *SVC,* superior vena cava; *AO,* aorta; *PA,* pulmonary artery; *LA,* left atrium; *LV,* left ventricle; *RV,* right ventricle. (From Kambam J: Transposition of the great arteries. In Kambam J, editor: *Cardiac anesthesia for infants and children,* St Louis, 1994, Mosby.)

poxemia is determined by the amount of mixing of systemic and pulmonary venous blood and by the amount of pulmonary blood flow. If there is little mixing, hypoxemia will be severe; if good mixing occurs, hypoxemia may be less severe. Since hypoxemia is always present, the child is at risk for the development of complications of hypoxemia and polycythemia. Pulmonary vascular disease may also develop during infancy, whether or not pulmonary blood flow is increased.

The severity of the hypoxemia is affected by the amount of effective pulmonary blood flow. This refers to the amount of systemic venous blood that enters the pulmonary circulation. Systemic arterial oxygenation will not improve if only pulmonary venous (oxygenated) blood returns to the pulmonary circulation. If no VSD is present, the neonate is dependent on mixing of blood through a

PDA and some form of interatrial communication, such as a patent foramen ovale.

The *ductus arteriosus* usually remains patent for several days after birth. Bidirectional shunting of blood occurs at this level until PVR falls. Once PVR falls, the PDA provides a systemic–to–pulmonary artery shunt, increasing effective pulmonary blood flow. If the PDA begins to close, hypoxemia will become severe.

If a *restrictive ASD or patent foramen ovale* is present, very little shunting and mixing of blood will occur at the atrial level. Profound hypoxemia (PaO₂ of 15 to 25 mm Hg) and cyanosis will be present.

If a *moderate ASD or patent foramen ovale* is present, bidirectional shunting of blood can occur at the atrial level. Right-to-left shunting of blood tends to occur during ventricular diastole and during patient inspiration, because the left ventricle and pulmonary outflow tract offer less resistance to flow than the right ventricle and systemic circulation. Left-to-right shunting of blood tends to occur during ventricular systole, because the left atrium is less distendible than the right atrium.

If a *large, unrestrictive ASD or foramen ovale* is present, bidirectional shunting can occur freely at the atrial level. This results in excellent mixing of blood and improvement in systemic arterial oxygen saturation. The arterial oxygen tension will probably average approximately 30 to 45 mm Hg.

If a *VSD* is present, the direction and magnitude of the ventricular shunting will be determined in part by the location and size of the VSD. Bidirectional shunting of blood will occur while PVR is high. When PVR falls, blood will shunt from the right ventricle through the VSD into the pulmonary circulation. If the VSD is large, the shunt into the pulmonary circulation will be large and signs of CHF will be present, but systemic arterial oxygenation will improve. The increase in pulmonary blood flow and enhanced pulmonary venous return contribute to a left-to-right shunt through any existing ASD or patent foramen ovale. Thus mixing of systemic and pulmonary venous blood is enhanced, and systemic arterial oxygenation rises. This occurs at the price of CHF and significant risk of pulmonary hypertension, however.

If a *VSD and mild or moderate pulmonary stenosis* are present, a balanced shunt may be present at the ventricular level. This combination of defects may increase systemic arterial oxygen saturation, yet the pulmonary stenosis prevents excessive pulmonary blood flow and the development of CHF and pulmonary hypertension.

If *a VSD and severe subvalvular pulmonary stenosis* are present, the total amount of pulmonary blood flow will be reduced. Profound hypoxemia and acidosis usually develop once the ductus begins to close.

Medical and Surgical Interventions

Severe hypoxemia is likely to be present at birth. Until corrective surgery is performed, *no air can be allowed to enter any IV catheter.* Antibiotic prophylaxis will be required throughout the child's life during periods of increased risk of bacteremia

PGE_1 is administered to increase pulmonary blood flow and enhance mixing of systemic and pulmonary venous blood. This should improve systemic arterial oxygen saturation. A balloon septostomy may be performed during cardiac catheterization to improve mixing of blood if hypoxemia is severe and no VSD is present.

Palliative Procedures   Possible palliative procedures for TGA include a balloon septostomy performed during cardiac catheterization, an atrial septectomy, pulmonary artery banding, or creation of a systemic–to–pulmonary artery shunt. These may be performed without cardiopulmonary bypass. However, surgical correction is now favored during early infancy.

Pulmonary artery banding may be performed for the infant with TGA and VSD to prevent the development of pulmonary hypertension or to prepare the left ventricle for an increase in afterload before the arterial switch procedure. If an arterial switch procedure is planned for the child with TGA without a VSD, but it cannot be performed in the newborn period, banding of the pulmonary artery will maintain left ventricular muscle mass. Banding is performed without use of cardiopulmonary bypass.

Corrective Procedures   A variety of surgical procedures may be performed to correct TGA. The preferred procedure for correction of simple TGA is the arterial switch procedure. However, the surgical approach is always individualized, and a variety of procedures may be used. If a VSD and subpulmonic stenosis are present, the arterial switch procedure

cannot be performed, because the subpulmonary stenosis will become subaortic stenosis.

The arterial switch procedure may be referred to as the *Jatene* procedure. It is accomplished with cardiopulmonary bypass, hypothermia, and a brief period of circulatory arrest (Figure 5-46). Any existing intracardiac defects are corrected. The great vessels are transected approximately 1 to 2 cm above the semilunar valves (the aorta is transected beyond the coronary artery ostia) and "switched." Each great vessel is sewn to the great vessel remnant ("stump") arising from the correct ventricle, so the pulmonary artery will now arise from the right ventricle and the aorta will arise from the left ventricle. The coronary arteries are removed from the original aorta and are reimplanted into the "new" aorta.

Intraatrial correction (venous switch or atrial repair) of TGA may occasionally be performed if the child's anatomy is unsuited to the arterial switch. Examples of these procedures are the *Mustard* and the *Senning* procedures. The atrial septum may be excised. Systemic and pulmonary venous blood are rerouted either within the atria or using a portion of the atrial wall to the appropriate outflow ventricle. Systemic venous blood is diverted to the mitral valve and flows into the left ventricle and then into the pulmonary artery. Pulmonary venous blood returning to the left atrium is diverted to the tricuspid valve, where it flows into the right ventricle and then into the aorta. These intraatrial or venous switch procedures require the right ventricle to function as the systemic ventricle; thus long-term results may be suboptimal.

If a VSD and pulmonary stenosis are present, corrective surgery similar to that performed to correct truncus arteriosus is used. This procedure is the *Rastelli* procedure. A right ventriculotomy incision is made. The VSD is closed so that left ventricular output is diverted through the VSD into the aorta. A pulmonary valved homograft is placed between the right ventricle and the (transposed) pulmonary artery.

The *Damus-Stansel-Kaye* procedure may be useful for correction of TGA with severe right ventricular outflow tract (aortic) obstruction or for correction of a DORV with a subpulmonic VSD. It may also be useful for the treatment of a single ventricle and severe subaortic stenosis. The pulmonary artery is transected before the bifurcation, and the main pulmonary trunk is sewn into the aorta. This enables left ventricular outflow to enter the original pul-

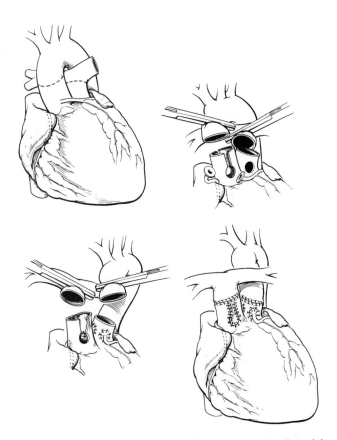

Figure 5-46 Surgical correction of transposition of the great arteries: "arterial switch" (Jantene) procedure. The aorta and pulmonary arteries are transected, and the coronary arteries are removed from the aorta. The great vessels are "switched" so that they will arise from the correct ventricles, and the coronary arteries are moved to the new aorta. (From Kambam J: Transposition of the great arteries. In Kambam J, editor: *Cardiac anesthesia for infants and children,* St Louis, 1994, Mosby.)

monary artery trunk and then the aorta. A pulmonary homograft is sewn between the right ventricle and the pulmonary artery bifurcation.

Postoperative Complications

The child is at risk for all complications of hypoxemia and polycythemia, including bleeding and thromboembolism. Postoperative complications include low cardiac output, CHF, and arrhythmias. Low cardiac output should be anticipated after any corrective procedure. CHF may be severe if a right ventriculotomy was performed. Supraventricular and junctional arrhythmias are most common following intraatrial correction of transposition, and

right bundle branch block should be anticipated if conduit insertion was performed. Heart block may complicate VSD closure.

Total Anomalous Pulmonary Venous Connection and Scimitar Syndrome

Defect

Total Anomalous Pulmonary Venous Connection
Total anomalous pulmonary venous connection (TAPVC; also known as total anomalous pulmonary venous drainage or total anomalous pul-

monary venous return) results from failure of the pulmonary veins to join normally to the left atrium during fetal cardiopulmonary development (Figure 5-47). As a result, the pulmonary veins join the systemic venous circulation, and mixed venous blood then returns to the heart. Some of the mixed venous blood then passes from the right atrium through a patent foramen ovale or ASD into the left atrium.

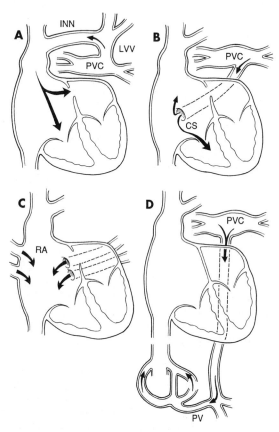

Figure 5-47 The four most common anatomic defects in total anomalous pulmonary venous connection (TAPVC). **A,** TAPVC drainage to the innominate vein *(INN)* via a left vertical vein *(LVV). PVC,* Pulmonary venous confluence. **B,** TAPVC from the common PVC to the coronary sinus *(CS).* **C,** TAPVC to the right atrium *(RA).* **D,** Infradiaphragmatic TAPVC from the common PVC to the portal vein *(PV).* (From Murphy AM, Greeley WJ: Total anomalous pulmonary venous connection. In Nichols DG et, editors: *Critical heart disease in infants and children,* St Louis, 1995, Mosby.)

TAPVC is labeled according to the site of insertion of the pulmonary veins into the systemic circulation, and the presence or absence of obstruction at the connection site.

Scimitar Syndrome Scimitar syndrome is a form of partial anomalous pulmonary venous return. In this syndrome, the right pulmonary veins join the IVC, and the lower portion of the right lung is perfused by anomalous arteries branching from the descending aorta. The anomalous pulmonary arterial supply produces right pulmonary sequestration (nonfunctional embryonic tissue perfused by anomalous systemic arteries).

Hemodynamics and Clinical Presentation

Total Anomalous Pulmonary Venous Connection
With all forms of TAPVC, pulmonary and systemic venous blood mix, and this mixed venous blood ultimately returns to the right atrium. Some mixed venous blood will enter the left atrium through a patent foramen ovale or through a true atrial septal defect. As a result, the oxygen saturation of the blood in both the right and left sides of the heart (and the systemic arterial oxygen saturation) will be equal. Approximately half of all infants with TAPVC are cyanotic in the first month of life.

In most cases of TAPVC, once PVR falls, a large portion of the mixed venous blood flows preferentially into the right ventricle and pulmonary artery. This produces increased pulmonary blood flow under low pressure, similar to that resulting from a large ASD. CHF may not be present or may develop in later infancy or childhood.

When pulmonary blood flow is large, the volume of pulmonary venous return will be large. If the pulmonary venous connection is unrestrictive, pulmonary venous blood will pass freely into the systemic venous circulation. The mixed venous blood (and hence the systemic arterial blood) will have a high oxygen saturation because a high portion of this blood is pulmonary venous blood. Cyanosis will be present but may be minimal and present only on exertion or vigorous cry.

If there is obstruction at the connection of the pulmonary veins to the systemic venous circulation, pulmonary venous pressure will rise, resulting in pulmonary interstitial edema. Cyanosis will be present and may be severe. CHF and respiratory distress will be present and may be severe. PVR is high, and the risk of pulmonary hypertension is high. Infradiaphragmatic TAPVC is usually associated with pulmonary venous obstruction.

Scimitar Syndrome   When scimitar syndrome is present, the right lung is usually hypoplastic, and abnormalities of right lung bronchial branching are also present. The vascular and bronchial anomalies result in sequestration of the right lower lobe and progressive signs and symptoms of respiratory distress. Chronic pulmonary infections and air trapping are likely to develop. The scimitar syndrome gains its name from the crescent-shaped opacification along the right heart border to the diaphragm that is created by the anomalous pulmonary vein coursing along the right heart border to the IVC.

Medical and Surgical Interventions

Total Anomalous Pulmonary Venous Connection The child is at risk for complications of hypoxemia and polycythemia. Until corrective surgery is performed, *no air can be allowed to enter any IV catheter.* Antibiotic prophylaxis will be required throughout the child's life during periods of increased risk of bacteremia.

The symptomatic infant with TAPVC requires vigorous management of CHF, as well as prevention of pulmonary vascular disease and the systemic consequences of cyanotic heart disease. If pulmonary venous obstruction is present, pulmonary support and prompt surgical intervention will be required. Urgent surgical intervention is required for any symptomatic infant or child with TAPVC.

Surgical correction is accomplished with cardiopulmonary bypass. The procedure reattaches the anomalous pulmonary veins to the left atrium and closes any interatrial communication. If a PDA is present, it is closed.

Scimitar Syndrome   Scimitar syndrome and pulmonary sequestration are corrected by lobectomy. The involved lobes of the lung are removed, and anomalous arteries and veins are ligated.

Postoperative Complications

Total Anomalous Pulmonary Venous Correction The child with TAPVC is at risk for potential com-

plications associated with cyanotic heart disease, including bleeding and thromboembolism. Postoperative complications will be most severe if preoperative obstruction to pulmonary venous return is present. The infant will require expert pulmonary support and management of pulmonary hypertension. If CHF is present preoperatively, it will likely be present postoperatively.

Scimitar Syndrome   Potential complications are most often those of a thoracotomy. Bleeding may also develop.

Coarctation of the Aorta

Defect

Coarctation of the aorta (CoA) is a discrete narrowing in the aortic arch, usually just distal to the origin of the left subclavian artery (Figure 5-48). The CoA may be present as a single lesion or in combination with other defects, such as a VSD. A bicuspid aortic valve is present in most patients with CoA.

Hemodynamics and Clinical Presentation

The aortic narrowing increases resistance to aortic flow. As a result, the left ventricle must increase pressure to maintain flow through the narrowed segment. Pressure in the aorta and major aortic branches proximal to the narrowing is high, whereas pressure in the aorta and major aortic branches distal to the narrowing is often low. If the kidneys are perfused at low pressure from the aorta, renin release will be stimulated, which will exacerbate the hypertension in the proximal aorta but will not improve pressure in the distal aorta.

CoA may be detected by evaluating blood pressure and pulses in all four extremities. Blood pressure in the extremities perfused by the aorta proximal to the coarctation will be high, and pulses will be strong, whereas the blood pressure in the extremities perfused by the aorta distal to the CoA will usually be low and associated with diminished pulses.

When the aortic obstruction is severe, signs of CHF will develop within the first weeks of life. These signs will be more severe if a VSD is present with the CoA, since the obstruction to left ventricu-

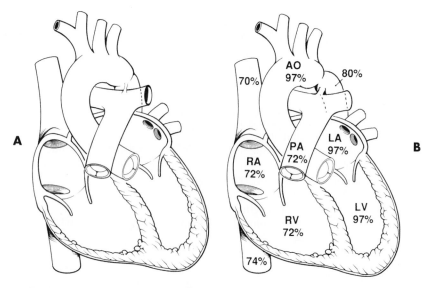

Figure 5-48   Coarctation of the aorta. Oxygen saturations in cardiac chambers and great vessels are depicted. **A,** Postductal coarctation. **B,** Preductal coarctation. While the ductus arteriosus is patent, the descending aorta is perfused by the right ventricle through the ductus. *RA,* right atrium; *RV,* right ventricle; *PA,* pulmonary artery; *AO,* aorta; *LA,* left atrium; *LV,* left ventricle.

lar outflow will increase the magnitude of the shunt into the pulmonary circulation. Many children with CoA demonstrate a prominent interatrial shunt. If CHF does not develop during the first weeks of life, the only symptoms of the CoA during childhood may be upper extremity hypertension.

Some differences in hemodynamics and clinical presentation are based on the location of the CoA in relation to the ductus arteriosus. If the CoA is located *proximal* to the ductus arteriosus, it is called a *preductal* coarctation. The descending aorta is perfused with blood flow from the right ventricle through the ductus arteriosus. This is a normal route of blood flow during fetal life; thus there may be no stimulus during fetal life for the development of collateral vessels to provide blood flow beyond the CoA. After birth, if the ductus begins to close, descending aortic blood flow will be severely compromised and signs of poor systemic perfusion will develop.

Preductal CoA results in perfusion of the ascending aorta and generally of the head and upper extremities with oxygenated blood from the left ventricle. The descending aorta, however, is perfused with systemic venous blood from the right ventricle. This results in hypoxemia in the lower extremities and tissues perfused by the descending aorta. This differential oxygenation may result in a differential cyanosis that is visible or in a difference in oxygen saturation detectable by pulse oximetry.

When the coarctation is located *beyond* the ductus arteriosus, it is known as a *postductal* coarctation. The coarctation obstructs normal aortic blood flow even during fetal life; thus the development of collateral flow pathways may be stimulated. These collateral vessels may provide a route of blood flow into the descending aorta beyond the coarctation that will provide adequate flow but at low pressure.

A *periductal* CoA may be located at the level of the ductus arteriosus. The ductus often fails to constrict, and bidirectional shunting of blood from the proximal aorta into the ductus and from the ductus into the distal aorta often occurs. Lower extremity hypoxemia may be present with periductal coarctation.

Medical and Surgical Interventions

CoA is often a chronic disease. Even if successful surgical intervention is performed, the CoA may recur, and the child may have an associated bicuspid aortic valve or other cardiovascular anomalies. As a result, antibiotic prophylaxis will be required throughout the child's life during periods of increased risk of bacteremia.

Any symptomatic infant with CoA requires treatment of CHF. If simple *postductal* coarctation is present, the infant will generally improve with medical management, and surgical intervention is planned.

If *preductal* CoA is present and descending aortic blood flow is dependent on the ductus arteriosus, the neonate may demonstrate cyanosis (and possibly differential cyanosis of the lower extremities) at birth and signs of poor systemic perfusion and shock when the ductus begins to close. PGE_1 administration should begin immediately and should be titrated to maintain effective systemic perfusion and urine output.

CoA is corrected during infancy. Unrepaired CoA can result in refractory hypertension and increased risk of cerebrovascular complications such as cerebral aneurysm.

Aortic angioplasty may be performed during cardiac catheterization to dilate the aorta and reduce the severity of aortic obstruction using a balloon-tipped catheter. This procedure may provide temporary or minor reduction in the aortic narrowing, but it may also produce intimal tears and aortic aneurysms. This technique seems to be most effective for dilating the site of recoarctation or for older infants and children. If balloon angioplasty is performed, the infant and child must be closely monitored for evidence of aortic aneurysm formation.

Surgical correction of CoA is typically accomplished without cardiopulmonary bypass, through a left thoractomy incision. If the coarctation is present with a VSD and both will be corrected simultaneously, cardiopulmonary bypass is required and a median sternotomy approach is used. The CoA itself may be corrected through an incision along the length of the aorta through the narrowed segment, with patch enlargement of the aorta. The most popular method of CoA repair uses a subclavian flap. The left subclavian artery is tied off and

cut several inches above its origin from the aorta. The artery is sliced longitudinally and opened and brought down to enlarge the aorta. If this procedure is performed, then no blood pressure will be obtainable in the left arm postoperatively, and no arterial punctures should be attempted in that arm.

A patch may also be used to repair the narrowing of the CoA in a manner that allows growth of the aorta. When repair is accomplished in older children, the narrowed segment is typically removed. The two aortic segments are then sewn together.

If a PDA is associated with the CoA, it is divided. If a VSD is present, it may be closed at the time of CoA correction. Occasionally pulmonary artery banding is performed with CoA repair, and the child returns for later VSD closure.

Postoperative Complications

Postoperative complications include those of a thoracotomy incision. If cardiopulmonary bypass is used, postoperative complications can include all potential postoperative problems. If CHF was present preoperatively, it will likely be present postoperatively. Bleeding may also occur. The surgical repair is in the area of the thoracic duct, the recurrent laryngeal nerve, the phrenic nerve, and the spinal cord artery. Injury to these structures may produce chylothorax, hoarseness, hemidiaphragm paralysis, or lower extremity paralysis, respectively. These complications should be ruled out.

If a Gore-Tex patch is used to repair the aorta, the child's platelet count may fall postoperatively as the Gore-Tex is endothelialized. Postoperative fever should be reported to a physician immediately, and blood cultures will be drawn to rule out bacteremia. Infection of the patch would be devastating. Endocarditis prophylaxis will be required during periods of increased risk of bacteremia for at least 6 months following repair (until the site endothelializes) and for the child's lifetime if additional defects, such as a bicuspid aortic valve, produce areas of turbulent intracardiac or great vessel blood flow.

Paradoxical hypertension frequently occurs postoperatively and must be managed with antihypertensive therapy, or it will increase the risk of bleeding at the surgical site and increase the risk of mesenteric arteritis. Enalapril (Vasotec, 0.01 to

0.02 mg/kg IV or PO), sodium nitroprusside (continuous infusion of 2 to 8 µg/kg/min), propranolol (0.1 to 0.25 mg/kg every 6 hours), or reserpine (Serpasil, 0.04 to 0.07 mg/kg IM every 6 hours) can be administered to control the hypertension.

Mesenteric vasculitis, also known as *postcoarctectomy syndrome,* is a form of gastrointestinal vascular dysfunction that develops after coarctation repair restores a pulsatile (and possibly a hypertensive) blood flow to the mesenteric arteries. This vasculitis has been linked with postoperative hypertension, and risks can be nearly eliminated with control of blood pressure.

Mesenteric vasculitis can cause abdominal distension, vomiting, pain, bowel ischemia, gastrointestinal bleeding, and bowel necrosis. Enteral feeding is often withheld for several days postoperatively to ensure that bowel function is adequate before feeding. All gastrointestinal output should be checked for the presence of blood, and the infant's abdominal girth should be measured frequently (once or more per shift).

Postoperative pulmonary complications can include the development of a chylothorax or leak of lymph fluid into the pleural cavity. This leak results from injury to a major lymphatic vessel and should be suspected if a cloudy or milky fluid drains from the chest tube. The drainage generally becomes more milky once the child begins feeding (especially of fat-containing food). The chylothorax is generally managed conservatively. A chest tube drains the lymph, and the child is placed on a medium-chain triglyceride diet until the drainage tapers off. Occasionally attempts are made to seal the chylothorax through instillation of concentrated antibiotics, which may fuse the pleural layers together.

Interrupted Aortic Arch

Defect

Interrupted aortic arch (IAA) is an absence of a portion of the aortic arch. There are three major types, labeled according to the aortic site of interruption:

- *Type A* (most common): The entire aortic arch is intact, and the interruption occurs just beyond the left subclavian artery.

- *Type B:* The aorta is interrupted between the left carotid and the left subclavian artery; thus the left subclavian artery arises from the descending aortic segment.
- *Type C* (least common): The aorta is interrupted between the innominate and the left carotid arteries; thus the left carotid and subclavian arteries receive blood from the right ventricle through the ductus arteriosus.

IAA is frequently associated with additional congenital heart defects, including bicuspid aortic valve, VSD, and aortic hypoplasia. Nearly half of infants with IAA have additional noncardiac anomalies. IAA is frequently associated with DiGeorge's syndrome, which includes congenital absence of the parathyroids (and possible hypocalcemia) and aplasia of the thymus (which causes decreased immune response).

Hemodynamics and Clinical Presentation

Clinical signs and symptoms of IAA are virtually identical to those produced by severe coarctation and will be influenced by the location of the interruption and the presence of any associated defects.

The interruption of the aorta provides an area of high resistance; thus the left ventricle increases pressure in an attempt to maintain blood flow through the interrupted segment. This results in hypertension in the aorta proximal to the interruption. Hypotension is often present in arteries served by the aorta distal to the interruption (unless this flow is maintained by the right ventricle through a large PDA).

Unless TGA is associated, the ascending aorta proximal to the interruption receives blood from the left ventricle, and the descending aorta and the aorta distal to the obstruction receive blood from the right ventricle through the ductus arteriosus. The right ventricle will increase pressure to maintain blood flow to the aorta distal to the obstruction; thus this blood pressure may be relatively normal when the ductus arteriosus is patent. Differential cyanosis may be observed, and differential oxygen saturation may be detectable with pulse oximetry, since the tissues perfused with systemic venous blood from the right ventricle will be hypoxemic.

Signs of poor systemic perfusion (shock) will develop when the ductus begins to close within the first days of life. The obstruction in the aorta causes signs of severe CHF.

Any associated lesions, such as VSD, will contribute to the clinical picture. Since the IAA causes severe obstruction to left heart outflow, left-to-right shunting through a VSD will be significant even in the first days of life. Signs of CHF can be severe.

Medical and Surgical Interventions

Initial treatment focuses on establishing and maintaining patency of the ductus arteriosus and treating signs of CHF and shock. Once the infant is stable, surgical intervention is required. Since the neonate is dependent on the ductus arteriosus to maintain flow to the aorta distal to the interruption, PGE_1 is administered to restore and maintain ductal patency.

Surgical correction is accomplished through a median sternotomy using cardiopulmonary bypass. The IAA and any existing lesions are corrected in the same procedure. The segments of aorta are joined, using a patch or conduit if necessary (Figure 5-49).

Postoperative Complications

Postoperative complications are identical to those following coarctation repair (see Coarctation of the Aorta), with the addition of complications of cardiopulmonary bypass and any complications associated with correction of additional cardiac lesions. The site of repair of the IAA can become a site of endocarditis if bacteremia is present, particularly if a patch or conduit was used for the repair. Endocarditis prophylaxis will be required during periods of increased risk of bacteremia for at least 6 months following repair (until the site endothelializes) and for the child's lifetime if additional defects, such as a bicuspid aortic valve, produce areas of turbulent intracardiac or great vessel blood flow.

Potential postoperative complications include CHF, low cardiac output, bleeding, chylothorax, hoarseness (from recurrent laryngeal nerve injury), hemidiaphragm paralysis, and lower extremity paralysis. If CHF was present preoperatively, it will likely be present postoperatively. If an associated VSD is present and closure requires a ventriculotomy, CHF may be severe and right bundle branch block and heart block may occur. If preop-

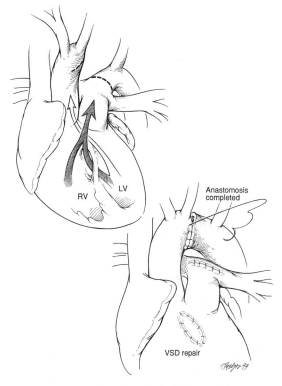

Figure 5-49   Surgical repair of interrupted aortic arch. *RV,* Right ventricle; *LV,* left ventricle; *VSD,* ventricular septal defect. (From Schwengel DA, Nichols DG, Cameron DE: Coarctation of the aorta and interrupted aortic arch. In Nichols DG et al, editors: *Critical heart disease in infants and children,* St Louis, 1995, Mosby.)

erative pulmonary hypertension was present, it may produce postoperative problems.

Management of systemic hypertension is required in most patients following correction of IAA. Enalapril (Vasotec, 0.01 to 0.02 mg/kg IV or PO), sodium nitroprusside (continuous infusion of 2 to 8 μg/kg/min), propranolol (0.1 to 0.25 mg/kg every 6 hours), or reserpine (Serpasil, 0.04 to 0.07 mg/kg IM every 6 hours) can be administered to control the hypertension.

Mesenteric vasculitis, also known as *post-coarctectomy syndrome,* is a form of gastrointestinal vascular dysfunction. It may develop after coarctation repair or repair of IAA restores a pulsatile (and possibly a hypertensive) blood flow to the mesenteric arteries. This vasculitis has been linked with postoperative hypertension, and risk can be nearly eliminated with control of blood pressure. Mesenteric vasculitis can cause abdominal distension, vomiting, pain, bowel ischemia, gastrointestinal bleeding, and bowel necrosis. Enteral feeding is often withheld for several days postoperatively to ensure that bowel function is adequate. All gastrointestinal output should be checked for the presence of blood, and the infant's abdominal girth should be measured frequently (once or more per shift).

Vascular Anomalies and Rings

Defect

Vascular rings are created by abnormal branches of the aorta and systemic arteries that encircle the trachea and esophagus. Most commonly a double aortic arch, right aortic arch with left ligamentum arteriosus (or aberrant left subclavian artery), anomalous innominate or left common carotid artery, or pulmonary artery sling is present (Table 5-26).

Hemodynamics and Clinical Presentation

The consequences of the vascular ring are determined by the location of the anomalous vessels. Significant compression of the trachea and esophagus produce upper airway obstruction and respiratory distress. Recurrent respiratory infections, wheezing, stridor, and congestion are often present. Feeding difficulties arise from dysphagia and esophageal compression of the trachea. Cyanotic episodes and apnea indicate severe obstruction, risk of respiratory arrest, and the need for urgent surgical intervention.

Medical and Surgical Interventions

The child with vascular ring and respiratory distress must be monitored closely for apnea and respiratory distress. Surgical intervention is planned during infancy before tracheal growth is compromised.

Surgery is accomplished through a thoracotomy and without use of cardiopulmonary bypass. The anomalous connections are divided to eliminate the tracheal compression. If an anomalous in-

nominate artery is present, it is pulled away from the trachea and suspended with sutures from the back of the sternum.

Postoperative Complications

Postoperative complications include those of a thoracotomy. Many of the potential complications described following repair of coarctation of the aorta may occur following repair of a vascular ring and include hoarseness from recurrent laryngeal nerve injury, hemidiaphragm paralysis from phrenic nerve injury, and chylothorax.

Aortic Stenosis

Defect

Aortic stenosis (AS) is a narrowing of the left ventricular outflow tract. AS can be characterized by the location of the obstruction in relation to the aortic valve:

- *Valvular AS* (most common): A narrowing at the valve is caused by fused commissures or a bicuspid valve.
- *Subvalvular AS/subaortic stenosis* (several forms): The obstruction can be caused by a fibrous diaphragm below the valve, muscular hypertrophy of the ventricular septum (called idiopathic hypertrophic subaortic stenosis), or fibromuscular tubular narrowing of the left ventricular outflow tract (also called tunnel subaortic stenosis).
- *Supravalvular/supraortic AS* (least common): An obstruction is caused by fibromembranous narrowing of the aorta above the aortic valve and coronary arteries. This form can be associated with Williams' (elfin facies) syndrome, which includes a characteristic facial appearance (short palpebral fissures and thick lips) and mental retardation.

Hemodynamics and Clinical Presentation

When left ventricular outflow is obstructed, the left ventricle will generate greater pressure to maintain normal flow beyond the area of resistance. Left ventricular hypertension and hypertrophy will be proportional to the severity of the obstruction. The types of symptoms resulting from the AS will be

Table 5-26
Vascular Rings

Lesion	Symptoms	Plain Film	Barium Swallow	Bronchoscopy	Angiography	Treatment
 Double arch	Stridor Respiratory distress Swallowing dysfunction Reflex apnea	AP—Wider base of heart Lateral—Narrowed trachea displaced forward at C3-C4	Bilateral indentation of esophagus	Bilateral tracheal compression—both pulsatile	Diagnostic but often unnecessary	Ligate and divide smaller arch (usually left)
 Right arch and ligamentum/ductus	Respiratory distress Swallowing dysfunction	AP—Tracheal deviation to left (right arch)	Bilateral indentation of esophagus R > L	Bilateral tracheal compression—r. pulsatile	Usually unnecessary	Ligate ligamentum or ductus

Continued

From Keith HM: Vascular rings and tracheobronchial compression in infants, *Pediatr Ann* 6(8):542-543, 1977.

Table 5-26
Vascular Rings—cont'd

Lesion	Symptoms	Plain Film	Barium Swallow	Bronchoscopy	Angiography	Treatment
Anomalous innominate	Cough Stridor Reflex apnea	AP—Normal Lat.—Anterior tracheal compression	Normal	Pulsatile anterior tracheal compression	Unnecessary	Conservative Apnea → suspend innominate artery
Aberrant right subclavian	Occasional swallowing dysfunction	Normal	AP—Oblique defect upward to right Lat.—Small defect on right posterior wall	Usually normal	Diagnostic but often unnecessary	Ligate artery
Pulmonary sling	Expiratory stridor Respiratory distress	AP—Low l. hilum, r. emphysema/atelectasis Lat.—Anterior bowing of right bronchus and trachea	± Anterior indentation above carina between esophagus and trachea	Tracheal displacement to left Compression of right main bronchus	Diagnostic	Detach and reanastomose to main pulmonary artery in front of trachea

From Keith HM: Vascular rings and tracheobronchial compression in infants, *Pediatr Ann* 6(8):542-543, 1977.

determined by the severity, as well as the location, of the AS.

Mild to Moderate Aortic Stenosis   Most children are asymptomatic, although dyspnea, exercise intolerance, or fatigability may be present. Mild left ventricular hypertrophy is present.

Severe Aortic Stenosis   Profound CHF often develops during the first weeks of life. Tachypnea, increased respiratory effort, diffuse rales, poor feeding, diaphoresis, and poor weight gain are often present. Pulmonary edema can produce respiratory insufficiency and pulmonary hypertension.

Severe AS and resulting left ventricular hypertrophy produce severe thickening of the left ventricle. Perfusion of the myocardium and endocardium requires a longer time when the ventricle is thick than when the ventricle is of normal size. Tachycardia reduces diastolic time and left main coronary artery perfusion time; thus ischemia is particularly likely to develop when the heart rate is high.

Urgent surgical intervention is required if the child develops angina (this is difficult to detect in children), syncope, or appearance of a "strain" pattern on the ECG. Abdominal pain and diaphoresis may be noted. Peripheral pulses and systemic arterial blood pressure are usually normal, although severe AS may produce CHF and may compromise cardiac output.

Coronary Artery Perfusion   When *valvular* or *subvalvular* AS is present, the area of obstruction is proximal to the coronary arteries; thus coronary artery flow cannot increase during exercise and other periods of increased oxygen requirements. Tachycardia can compromise coronary artery, myocardial, and subendocardial blood flow.

When *supravalvular* AS is present, the area of obstruction is distal to the coronary arteries; thus coronary artery perfusion is usually adequate, even during episodes of tachycardia. Because the coronary arteries receive hypertensive flow, they may become dilated and tortuous.

Idiopathic Hypertrophic Subaortic Stenosis
Idiopathic hypertrophic subaortic stenosis (IHSS) is a dynamic form of subvalvular AS that is caused by thickening of the left side of the ventricular septum.

As the left ventricle hypertrophies, the severity of the obstruction increases. This defect is associated with cardiomyopathy (see Cardiomyopathy).

Medical and Surgical Interventions

The management of AS is based on the severity and location of the obstruction; therefore management of each form of AS is presented separately in the following paragraphs. Correction of AS should generally be regarded as palliative, since the stenosis can recur. Antibiotic prophylaxis will be required throughout life, since the left ventricular outflow tract will always be a site of turbulent flow, creating increased risk of bacterial endocarditis whenever bacteremia is present.

In general, regardless of the location of the AS, surgical intervention is planned to prevent the development of severe left ventricular hypertrophy and strain. If left ventricular outflow tract obstruction is severe, the defect may be treated as a form of hypoplastic left heart syndrome, with plans made to stage surgical correction to ultimately use the right ventricle and right ventricular outflow tract to support the systemic circulation. Cardiac transplantation is also an alternative if adequate relief of left ventricular outflow tract obstruction cannot be achieved.

Once symptoms develop, particularly if symptoms of CHF or left ventricular strain are present, urgent surgical intervention is required. The risk of left ventricular ischemia and malignant ventricular arrhythmias is high; thus strict activity limitation is imposed. The infant should not be allowed to cry vigorously or for prolonged periods.

Valvular Aortic Stenosis   The goal of intervention is to relieve as much stenosis as possible without creating severe insufficiency. Valvular AS may be treated by valvuloplasty during cardiac catheterization or with surgery. If the valve annulus is critically small, however, complex surgery may be necessary to sufficiently relieve the obstruction.

The valvuloplasty is accomplished during cardiac catheterization through insertion of a catheter that contains a balloon retrograde into the aorta through the valve. The balloon is positioned at the valve and is inflated to tear or separate valve leaflets. This valvuloplasty should reduce the obstruction and relieve the symptoms.

Surgical valvotomy can be accomplished without use of cardiopulmonary bypass, using a *"blind" valvotomy* technique, with insertion of a curved blade through a puncture (surrounded by purse-string sutures to prevent bleeding) just below the aortic valve. However, this procedure may not produce optimal relief of obstruction; thus *"open" valvotomy* under direct visualization using open-heart surgery is often preferred (Figure 5-50). The aorta is entered above the valve, and the fused commissures are incised.

Valve replacement may be necessary if valvotomy has failed to relieve the AS sufficiently or if repeat valvotomy has produced significant aortic insufficiency. Unfortunately, mechanical valves will require anticoagulation postoperatively, which may be difficult to manage during childhood. To avoid this problem, the aortic valve may be replaced with a cryopreserved homograft valve, using it to replace the aortic root (with re-implantation of the coronary arteries).

Correction of severe stenosis may be accomplished during childhood and adolescence through replacement of the aortic valve and valve root with the patient's own pulmonary valve. This *pulmonary autograft procedure,* known as the *Ross procedure,* may enable the new aortic valve to grow with the patient, since the valve is one of the patient's own semilunar valves (Figure 5-51).

This pulmonary autograft procedure requires cardiopulmonary bypass. An incision is made in the main pulmonary artery (above the valve) and in the right ventricle (below the pulmonary valve), and a cuff of pulmonary artery, including the valve, is removed. This cuff is replaced with a cryopreserved homograft. The aorta is transected above and below the valve, and the coronary arteries are separated from this segment. The pulmonary autograft cuff is then used to replace the aortic valve, and the coronary arteries are reimplanted into this cuff. No anticoagulation will be required postoperatively because this valve tissue is the patient's own, and pulmonary homografts do not require anticoagulation.

Subvalvular Aortic Stenosis   Resection of subvalvular stenosis requires cardiopulmonary bypass. If subvalvular AS is discrete, it can be resected through an incision in the aorta, working through the

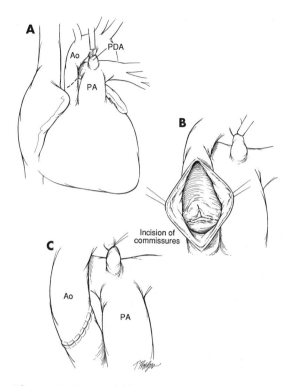

Figure 5-50   Surgical correction for critical neonatal aortic valve stenosis with open valvotomy. **A,** In neonates with critical aortic stenosis, the heart is approached through a median sternotomy. The pulmonary artery *(PA)* often appears to be tensely distended and much larger than the aorta *(Ao).* In fact, in severe cases the aorta may be only 5 to 7 mm in diameter. Valvotomy is performed on cardiopulmonary bypass (CPB) by cannulating the ascending aorta and the right atrium *(not shown).* The patent ductus arteriosus *(PDA),* which can be quite large, is controlled with a snare. **B,** An aortotomy is performed, revealing the stenotic aortic valve. The line of commissural fusion is appreciated and opened with a knife blade so that the commissurotomy extends almost to the annulus. **C,** The aortotomy is closed, and the patient is weaned from CPB. It is not necessary to provide cardioplegia. The ductus arteriosus can be tied securely at the completion of the procedure unless, in unique circumstances, it is considered prudent to leave the ductus open with the patient receiving prostaglandin E_1 for a few postoperative days. (From Ungerleider RM: Congenital aortic stenosis. In Nichols DG et al, editors: *Critical heart disease in infants and children,* St Louis, 1995, Mosby.)

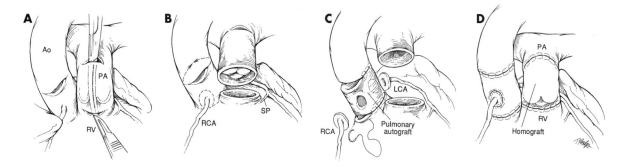

Figure 5-51 Surgical correction of critical aortic stenosis with pulmonary autograft: Ross procedure. **A,** The pulmonary autograft procedure is performed by making a small incision in the aorta *(Ao)* after the patient has been placed on cardiopulmonary bypass and the heart has been protected with cardioplegia solution. After it has been determined that the aortic valve will indeed need to be replaced, an incision is made in the main pulmonary artery *(PA)* adjacent to the origin of the right pulmonary artery, and a right-angle clamp is placed across the pulmonary artery and used to identify the right ventricular surface proximal to the pulmonary valve. An incision is then made in the right ventricle *(RV)*, and **B,** the proximal pulmonary valve is removed with a cuff of muscle tissue. The posterior division of the valve from the right ventricle should follow a horizontal plane to prevent injury to the first septal perforator *(SP)* of the left anterior descending coronary artery. After the proximal portion of the pulmonary valve has been removed, the pulmonary artery is transected at the level of the bifurcation through the initial incision made in the pulmonary artery. **C,** With the autograft removed, the previously performed incision in the aorta is extended so that the aorta is transected above the level of the valve. The coronary arteries are then removed with large buttons of surrounding sinus tissue, and all remaining aortic tissue, as well as the aortic valve, is removed from the base of the heart. The pulmonary autograft is then sewn to the base of the heart. The left coronary artery *(LCA)* and the right coronary artery *(RCA)* are implanted into the autograft. **D,** The procedure is completed by placing a cryopreserved homograft in the right ventricular outflow tract to reestablish right ventricle–to–pulmonary artery continuity. (From Ungerleider RJ: Congenital aortic stenosis. In Nichols DG et al, editors: *Critical heart disease in infants and children,* St Louis, 1995, Mosby.)

valve. If the AS is muscular, resection of the muscle may also be accomplished through an aortic approach. If tunnel narrowing of the outflow tract is associated with a small aortic valve annulus, an incision may be made in the left ventricular outflow tract and across the valve to allow insertion of a patch and an aortic valve. This procedure is known as the *Konno procedure* (Figure 5-52). The Konno procedure uses an incision in the aorta, as well as a right ventriculotomy, to gain access to the left ventricular outflow tract from the side of the ventricular septum. An incision is made through the aortic valve and into the septum from the right ventricular side, and a patch is placed to enlarge this area. The right ventriculotomy is then closed with a patch to enlarge the right ventricular outflow tract and prevent compression from the enlarged left ventricular outflow tract.

Occasionally subaortic stenosis is so severe that it cannot be relieved by patch insertion or resection. Rarely, a valved conduit may be inserted between the left ventricle and the descending aorta. Cardiac transplantation may also be considered.

Supravalvular Aortic Stenosis   Supravalvular AS is corrected using cardiopulmonary bypass. An incision is made in the aorta above the aortic valve. Any discrete membrane is excised, and if the area of narrowing is extensive, a patch is placed to enlarge the aorta.

Postoperative Complications

Postoperative complications include bleeding, low cardiac output, CHF, and malignant ventricular arrhythmias. Low cardiac output can be particularly

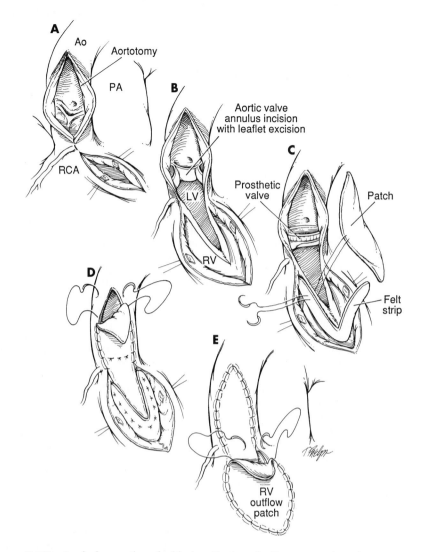

Figure 5-52 Surgical correction of critical aortic stenosis: Konno procedure. An aortoventriculoplasty is performed with the patient on cardiopulmonary bypass, the aorta cross-clamped, and the heart protected with cardioplegia solution. **A,** A vertical aortotomy is extended toward the left of the right coronary artery *(RCA)* and connected to a right ventriculotomy, which is performed below the pulmonary valve, and also extended toward the left of the right coronary artery, as shown by the dashed line. Once this incision has been performed, a second incision can be made across the aortic valve annulus **(B)** and into the interventricular septum, as shown. The aortic valve leaflets are removed. A prosthetic valve can then be placed into the annular position, using interrupted (or continuous) sutures for the posterior portion of the valve ring. **C,** A prosthetic patch is placed as shown so that the sutures are brought through the patch, then through the interventricular septum, and then through a Teflon felt strip. This reconstructs and enlarges the left ventricular *(LV)* outflow tract and places the patch on the LV surface so that the LV pressure will help to hold the patch in place. This patch is then secured **(D)** to the anterior portion of the prosthetic valve ring, and the suture line for the patch is continued around the aortotomy. **E,** Finally, the right ventricular *(RV)* outflow tract is repaired with an additional patch of either Gore-Tex or pericardium. *Ao,* aorta; *PA,* pulmonary artery. (From Ungerleider RM: Congenital aortic stenosis. In Nichols DG et al, editors: *Critical heart disease in infants and children,* St Louis, 1995, Mosby.)

problematic following correction of critical AS. Inotropic support and afterload reduction will probably be required postoperatively and should be weaned carefully. If resection of subvalvular AS is performed, heart block (especially third-degree heart block) may be present. If CHF was severe preoperatively, it will probably be present postoperatively. If pulmonary hypertension is present with pulmonary edema preoperatively, pulmonary support must be skilled and treatment of pulmonary hypertension will be required.

Hypoplastic Left Heart Syndrome

Defect

Hypoplastic left heart syndrome is an association of anomalies consisting of a diminutive left ventricle, aortic and/or mitral valve stenosis or atresia, normally related great vessels, and an intact ventricular septum (Figure 5-53). The entire left side of the heart is too small to support the systemic and coronary circulations.

Hemodynamics and Clinical Presentation

The small left ventricle and aorta do not provide sufficient flow to support the systemic and coronary circulations. As a result, the neonate is dependent on flow from the right ventricle through the ductus arteriosus to perfuse the ascending aorta and coronary arteries in a retrograde fashion, and the descending aorta with antegrade flow.

At birth, the neonate may appear to be normal, but the infant will demonstrate poor systemic perfusion once the ductus begins to close. Signs of shock, CHF, cyanosis, and pulmonary edema may develop and progress rapidly. Right ventricular hypertrophy will be present, since the right ventricle supports all circulations.

Medical and Surgical Interventions

If the hypoplastic left heart syndrome is to be managed aggressively, PGE$_1$ infusion is required to maintain ductal patency. Since all circulations are perfused by the right ventricle, until complete correction and separation of systemic and pulmonary blood flow is accomplished surgically, *no air can be allowed to enter any IV line.* The infant is at risk for all complications associated with hypoxemia

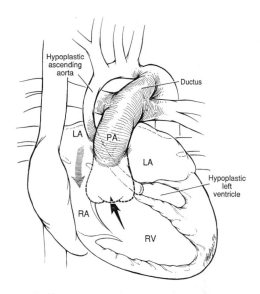

Figure 5-53 Hypoplastic left heart syndrome: native anatomy. Note the hypoplastic left ventricle, aortic valve atresia, and diminutive ascending aorta. Systemic blood flow is propelled by the right ventricle via the pulmonary artery *(PA)* and ductus arteriosus. Pulmonary venous return enters the right side of the heart through the foramen ovale or an atrial septal defect. *LA,* Left atrium; *RA,* right atrium; *RV,* right ventricle. (From Nichols SC, Steven JM, Jobes AB: Hypoplastic left heart syndrome. In Nichols GD et al, editors: *Critical heart disease in infants and children,* St Louis, 1995, Mosby.)

and polycythemia until that time. Lifelong antibiotic prophylaxis will be required during periods of increased risk of bacteremia.

Pulmonary support is provided preoperatively, if needed, but high levels of inspired oxygen must be avoided. Alveolar oxygenation can stimulate pulmonary vasodilation and result in excessive pulmonary blood flow and "stealing" of blood flow from the systemic circulation. As a result, mild alveolar hypoxia and mild acidosis are maintained preoperatively to improve systemic circulation.

There are three options for the treatment of hypoplastic left heart syndrome:

- Provision of comfort measures only, with no surgical intervention provided (The lesion will be fatal.)

- Surgical palliation with a Norwood-type procedure, which manages the defect as a variant of a single (right) ventricle
- Cardiac transplantation

Comfort Measures If comfort measures only are provided, the parents are helped to cope with the newborn's impending death. For further information, see Chapter 4

Norwood Procedures The Norwood procedures are accomplished in at least two stages over the first months of life. All require cardiopumonary bypass.

Norwood Stage I The goals of the first stage are to establish unobstructed systemic blood flow, to normalize pulmonary blood flow and pressure, and to eliminate obstruction to pulmonary venous return by providing adequate interatrial communication (Figure 5-54). The main pulmonary artery is transected, and the proximal pulmonary artery is sewn to the ascending aorta, using an adult pulmonary artery homograft to enlarge the aorta. This creates a truncus that receives blood flow predominantly from the right ventricle with little effective left ventricular ejection. A systemic-to-pulmonary shunt is created, and the existing ASD or patent foramen ovale is enlarged to ensure that there is unrestricted flow from the left to the right atrium.

At the end of this procedure, the right ventricle receives both systemic and pulmonary venous blood and ejects that blood into the new aorta that was fashioned from the aorta and pulmonary artery. Blood flow into the pulmonary artery occurs through the systemic–to–pulmonary artery shunt.

Norwood Stages II and III Final correction of hypoplastic left heart syndrome uses a version of the Fontan-type procedures to divert systemic venous blood away from the right ventricle and into the pulmonary circulation. A bidirectional Glenn (SVC to pulmonary artery) may be performed during early infancy, followed by a cavopulmonary anastomosis a few months later. The right ventricle will then function as the systemic ventricle (see Tricuspid Atresia, Medical and Surgical Interventions).

Cardiac Transplantation If cardiac transplantation is planned, PGE_1 administration continues.

If at all possible, the child should be allowed to breathe spontaneously, and a mild hypoxemia and acidosis are maintained to prevent excessive pulmonary blood flow. CHF is treated, but hemoconcentration must be avoided. The wait for a heart for transplantation is often weeks or months. Since IV access must be maintained to provide PGE_1 infusion, the risk of infection is high. Any infection must be prevented or promptly treated. For more information, see Cardiac Transplantation.

Postoperative Complications

Postoperative complications include CHF, low cardiac output, and malignant ventricular arrhythmias. Until complete correction is performed, the infant is at risk for complications of hypoxemia and polycythemia, including bleeding and cerebral thromboembolism. *No air can be allowed to enter any IV line* until complete correction has been accomplished.

After the first stage of the Norwood corrections, oxygenation, ventilation, and support of systemic arterial circulation must be carefully managed to optimize the balance of pulmonary and systemic blood flow. The PaO_2 is generally maintained at approximately 35 to 50 mm Hg, and the oxyhemoglobin saturation at 70% to 80%. Excessive systemic oxygenation (associated with a PaO_2 >35 to 50 mm Hg or oxygen saturation >80%) indicates excessive pulmonary blood flow, which may produce pulmonary edema and "steal" of blood flow from the systemic circulation. Inadequate pulmonary blood flow (associated with a PaO_2 <35 to 50 mm Hg or oxygen saturation <70%) will result in severe hypoxemia.

Pulmonary hypertensive crises may cause sudden deterioration in the newborn; thus management of pulmonary hypertension must be skilled but cannot produce excessive pulmonary vasodilation. Sedation and analgesia are provided, and stimulation is minimized. Inotropic support and systemic vasodilation (e.g., captopril, 0.5 mg/kg/day) will enhance systemic perfusion.

Pulmonary vascular resistance is presented in detail under Postoperative Care of the Pediatric Cardiovascular Surgical Patient earlier in this chapter (see p. 211).

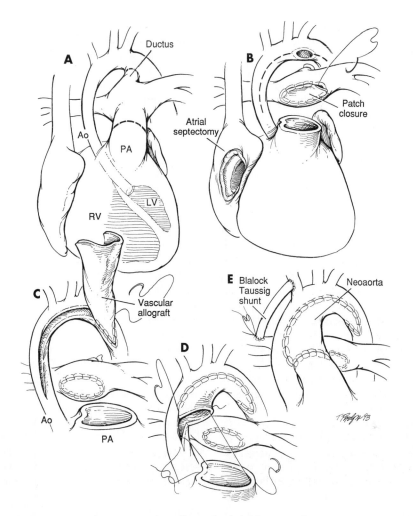

Figure 5-54   Norwood-type correction of hypoplastic left heart syndrome: stage I Norwood procedure. **A,** Transection points of the main pulmonary artery *(PA)* and ductus arteriosus. *Ao,* Right aorta; *LV,* left ventricle; *RV,* right ventricle. **B,** Atrial septectomy to avoid pulmonary venous hypertension. Patch closure of the distal main PA. Division and ligation of the ductus arteriosus. **C** and **D,** Construction of a "neoaorta" using the proximal main PA, diminutive ascending aorta, and vascular allograft. **E,** Pulmonary blood flow supplied by a right modified Blalock-Taussig shunt connecting the right subclavian artery to the right PA. (From Nichols SC, Steven JM, Jobes AB: Hypoplastic left heart syndrome. In Nichols Dg et al, editors: *Critical heart disease in infants and children,* St Louis, 1995, Mosby.)

Bacterial Endocarditis

Pathophysiology

Bacterial endocarditis is an inflammation of a valve, endocardium, or endothelium that results from a bacterial agent. Streptococcus and staphylococcus are most commonly involved. Endocarditis may also result from fungal agents (but is not addressed here). A small number of patients with endocarditis are culture negative.

Endocarditis is most likely to affect children with underlying cardiovascular disease, such as

VSD, AS, tetralogy of Fallot, CoA, PDA, and TGA. Endocarditis may also develop in children with long-dwelling intracardiac catheters.

Turbulent blood flow results in mural tissue damage with deposition of platelets and fibrin and thrombus formation. Circulating bacteria become trapped in this thrombus, becoming the focus of the endocarditis. The bacterial colonies become encased in a fibrin network, making phagocytosis or antibiotic penetration difficult.

Endocarditis may contribute to the development of valvular insufficiency. Portions of the lesions may embolize to the brain or systemic arterial circulation.

Clinical Presentation

Endocarditis often causes fever and may be associated with the development of new or changing murmurs and subtle signs of illness such as malaise, headache, or arthralgia. Signs of embolism to the systemic circulation include pain, compromise of extremity perfusion, renal dysfunction, arthralgia, and focal neurologic signs. Skin lesions, including petechiae, Osler nodes (tender red nodules), splinter hemorrhages, and Janeway lesions (painless hemorrhagic lesions on the palms or soles) may be present.

Endocarditis is confirmed by a positive blood culture, although repeated blood cultures may be required to isolate the organism. Additional non-specific laboratory tests suggestive of endocarditis include positive acute-phase reactants, and elevated erythrocyte sedimentation rate and C-reactive protein.

Medical and Surgical Interventions

Prevention of endocarditis is more desirable than therapy. The American Heart Association has published extensive recommendations regarding antibiotic prophylaxis for the prevention of endocarditis under a variety of conditions (Table 5-27).

Treatment of endocarditis requires several weeks of IV antibiotic therapy. The choice of antibiotic therapy is determined by the organism and its sensitivity to penicillin, as well as its location. Antibiotic therapy and dosages are summarized in Table 5-28.

Throughout therapy, support of cardiovascular function is required. Valvular endocarditis may

result in CHF or low cardiac output. Surgery may eventually (after a complete course of antibiotics) be required to replace an infected valve or patch.

Myocarditis

Pathophysiology

Myocarditis is an inflammatory process that involves the cardiac muscle. It may be caused by almost any pathogen, including a bacterium, virus, rickettsia, fungus, protozoa, or parasite, although most known cases in the United States are associated with a viral illness, a systemic infection, or active infective endocarditis. Noninfectious myocarditis may be caused by systemic diseases such as lupus, drug toxicity, or radiation therapy.

A pathogen invades the myocardium or an insult damages it, producing either temporary or permanent damage to the myocardial structure. It can interfere with normal myocardial cell function, resulting in necrosis of some myocardial tissue. The inflammatory response results in infiltration of the involved area with WBCs and possible formation of antigen-antibody complexes. Over time, necrotic tissue is resorbed or replaced with scar tissue. Focal hemorrhages, edema, fatty infiltration of muscle, and fibrosis may result.

Myocardial dysfunction caused by myocarditis is usually temporary. However, some patients develop progressive cardiac dilation with decreased ventricular function and AV valve insufficiency or malignant ventricular arrhythmias. Occasionally myocarditis produces a rapid and fatal decrease in myocardial function.

Clinical Presentation

Most children with myocarditis have a history of bacterial or viral illness or of systemic disease, drug toxicity, or radiation therapy known to be associated with the development of myocarditis. Potential signs of myocarditis include:

- Signs of inflammation: fever, and tachycardia disproportionate to the degree of fever
- Arrhythmias
- Signs of CHF, including systemic and pulmonary venous congestion, tachycardia, gallop rhythm, and tachypnea

Table 5-27
Antibiotic Prophylaxis for Prevention of Bacterial Endocarditis

Situation	Agent	Regimen
Prophylaxis for Dental, Oral, Respiratory Tract, or Esophageal Procedures		
Standard general prophylaxis	Amoxicillin	50 mg/kg (maximum: 2 g) PO 1 hr before procedure
Standard—unable to take oral medications	Ampicillin	50 mg/kg (maximum: 2 g) IM or IV within 30 min before procedure
Allergic to penicillin	Clindamycin	20 mg/kg (maximum: 600 mg) PO 1 hr before procedure
	OR	
	Cephalexin or cefatroxil*	50 mg/kg (maximum: 2 g) PO 1 hr before procedure
	OR	
	Azithromycin or clarithromycin	15 mg/kg (maximum: 500 mg) PO 1 hr before procedure
Allergic to penicillin, unable to take oral medications	Clindamycin	20 mg/kg (maximum: 600 mg) IV within 30 min of procedure
	OR	
	Cefazolin*	25 mg/kg (maximum: 1 g) IM or IV within 30 min of procedure
Prophylactic Regimens for Genitourinary, Gastrointestinal (Excluding Esophageal) Procedures		
High-risk patients (prosthetic valves, previous subacute bacterial endocarditis, complex cyanotic congenital heart disease [CHD], surgically constructed systemic-pulmonary shunts or conduits)	Ampicillin plus gentamicin	Ampicillin, 50 mg/kg IM or IV (not to exceed 2 g), plus gentamicin, 1.5 mg/kg, within 30 min of starting procedure; *then* 6 hr later: ampicillin, 25 mg/kg IV/IM, or amoxicillin, 25 mg/kg PO
High-risk patients allergic to ampicillin/amoxicillin	Vancomycin plus gentamicin	Vancomycin, 20 mg/kg IV (maximum: 1 g) over 1-2 hr plus gentamicin, 1.5 mg/kg IV/IM; complete injection or infusion within 30 min of starting procedure
Moderate-risk patients (most CHD other than high-risk or when no prophylaxis is required; acquired valvular dysfunction, hypertrophic cardiomyopathy, mitral valve prolapse with valvular regurgitation)	Amoxicillin or ampicillin	Amoxicillin, 50 mg/kg (maximum: 2 g) PO 1 hr before procedure, or ampicillin, 50 mg/kg IM/IV within 30 min of starting procedure
Moderate-risk patients allergic to penicillin	Vancomycin	Vancomycin, 20 mg/kg IV (maximum: 1 g) over 1-2 hr; complete injection or infusion within 30 min of starting procedure

Modified from Dajani AS et al: Prevention of bacterial endocarditis: recommendations by the American Heart Association, *JAMA* 277:1794-1801, 1997.
*NOTE: Cephalosporins should not be used for patients with immediate hypersensitivity or anaphylaxis to penicillins.

Table 5-28
Dosages, Routes, and Schedules for Antimicrobial Agents Used in Treatment of Infectious Endocarditis

Drug	Dosage and Route: Pediatric	Dosage and Route: Adult	Schedule
Amphotericin B	1 mg/kg/24 hr IV	1 mg/kg/24 hr IV	Daily
Ampicillin	300 mg/kg/24 hr IV	12 g/24 hr IV	Continuously or q4h
Cefazolin	80-100 mg/kg/24 hr IV	3 g/dose IV	q8h
Cefotaxime	100-200 mg/kg/24 hr IV	2 g/dose IV	q4-6h
Ceftazidime	100-150 mg/kg/24 hr IV	2 g/dose IV	q8h
Ceftriaxone	50-100 mg/kg/24 hr IV or IM	2 g/24 hr IV or IM	q12-24h
Cephalothin	100-150 mg/kg/24 hr IV	2 g/dose IV	q4-6h
Flucytosine	100-150 mg/kg/24 hr PO	100-150 mg/kg/24 hr	q6h
Gentamicin	2.0-2.5 mg/kg/dose IV or IM	1 mg/kg/dose IV or IM	q8h
Nafcillin	150-200 mg/kg/24 hr IV	12 g/24 hr IV	q4-6h
Oxacillin	150-200 mg/kg/24 hr IV	12 g/24 hr IV	q4-6h
Penicillin G	150,000-200,000 units/kg/24 hr IV	10-20 million units/24 hr IV	Continuously or q4h
Penicillin G, high dosage	200,000-300,000 units/kg/24 hr IV	20-30 million units/24 hr IV	Continuously or q4h
Rifampin	10 mg/kg/dose PO	300 mg/dose PO	q12h
Streptomycin	15 mg/kg/dose IM	7.5 mg/kg/dose IM	q12h
Vancomycin	40 mg/kg/24 hr IV	30 mg/kg/24 hr IV	q6-12h

From Berkowitz FE: Infective endocarditis. In Nichols DG et al, editors: *Critical heart disease in infants and children,* St Louis, 1995, Mosby.

- Lethargy, weakness, myalgia, or constant fatigue
- Chest pain
- Pericardial or pleural friction rub

Potential signs of significant myocardial dysfunction include:

- Signs of shock and poor systemic perfusion
- Tricuspid or mitral murmur signaling progressive ventricular dilation and development of AV valve insufficiency
- Pulsus alternans resulting from depressed ventricular contractility

The ECG may be normal, although it frequently reveals nonspecific ST segment changes consistent with myocardial injury. Diffuse myocarditis produces a decrease in QRS and T-wave voltage. Arrhythmias, including malignant ventricular arrhythmias and heart block, may be noted. The chest x-ray film may reveal cardiomegaly, and the echocardiogram will enable evaluation of ven-

tricular contractility and AV valve function and rule out the presence of any pericardial effusion.

Laboratory signs of myocarditis include an elevated erythrocyte sedimentation rate and rise in serum myocardial enzymes. Bacterial or viral cultures are often negative. Myocarditis must be differentiated from rheumatic fever and symptoms of systemic arteriovenous fistula.

Medical and Surgical Interventions

Treatment of myocarditis requires identification and treatment of the underlying cause, as well as support of cardiovascular function. CHF, shock, and arrhythmias are treated if they occur. The goals of therapy include maximization of oxygen delivery (support oxygenation and hemoglobin concentration, optimize heart rate and cardiac preload, maximize cardiac contractility, and reduce afterload) and minimization of oxygen demand. Fever is controlled with antipyretics, and bed rest is usually recommended. Pain is treated, and parents or primary caretakers are kept nearby to minimize anxiety. Myocardial biopsy can confirm the diagnosis and may enable identification of the cause.

Gamma globulin (2 g/kg over 24 hours) seems to improve survival and left ventricular function. Use of other antiinflammatory agents may be prescribed, but their use is controversial because they may contribute to secondary infections. Optimal agents have not been determined, but the ones used often include corticosteroids and possibly cyclosporine or azathioprine. Myocardial gallium uptake may be used to select patients most likely to benefit from immunosuppressive therapy.

Kawasaki's Disease (Mucocutaneous Lymph Node Syndrome)

Pathophysiology

Kawasaki's disease is a microvascular inflammatory disease of unknown etiology. During the first days of the disease, generalized microvasculitis is present. Myocarditis develops within 3 to 4 weeks and is associated with WBC infiltration and edema of the conduction system and myocardium. Severe valvulitis may also be present.

Coronary artery dilation develops in approximately one third to one half of involved patients and can be detected by echocardiogram approximately 12 to 24 days after the onset of symptoms. Approximately 15% to 20% of affected patients develop coronary artery aneurysms. These aneurysms seem most likely to occur in children who demonstrated extremely high fever lasting 14 or more days. The aneurysms usually affect the left main coronary artery or the proximal segments of the left anterior descending branch of the right coronary artery. Although the aneurysms ultimately calcify, extremely large aneurysms may produce coronary insufficiency and lead to myocardial ischemia, CHF, or myocardial infarction.

Clinical Presentation

The diagnosis of Kawasaki's disease is made if at least five of the major diagnostic criteria are present. These include:

- Fever (usually high, typically lasting ≥5 days)

- Skin rash/conjunctivitis
- Cervical lympadenopathy
- Mucosal inflammation (reddening of the lips and erythema of the buccal mucosa)
- Erythema of the hands and feet (they may be extremely tender and painful)
- Desquamation of the hands and feet (occurs approximately 2 to 4 weeks after onset of symptoms)
- Conjunctivitis

Symptoms of myocarditis or CHF may be apparent, and pericarditis is present in approximately one third of patients. If severe coronary artery aneurysms are present, the child is at risk for sudden myocardial infarction. Signs of myocardial infarction can be subtle in children and may include severe chest pain, vomiting, crying, abdominal pain, malignant ventricular arrhythmias, shock, and possibly cardiac arrest.

Additional conditions associated with Kawasaki's disease may include aseptic meningitis, diarrhea, jaundice, uveitis, and urethritis. Laboratory findings include nonspecific signs of an inflammatory process (including elevation in C-reactive protein and erythrocyte sedimentation rate), and evidence of thrombocytosis. The antistreptolysis is negative or low, and a sterile pyuria or proteinuria may be present.

Medical and Surgical Interventions

Treatment consists of administration of antiinflammatory agents, support of cardiovascular function, and monitoring for the development of complications such as pericarditis and coronary artery aneurysms.

Aspirin (80 to 100 mg/kg/day) and IV gamma globulin (400 mg/kg/day for 3 to 5 days) will significantly improve the outcome of Kawasaki's disease. The aspirin dose may be reduced if the patient is afebrile and asymptomatic approximately 2 weeks after the onset of symptoms, but it is continued until all signs of inflammation have disappeared and the coronary arteries are found to be normal.

Echocardiograms are performed frequently during the first days and weeks of the disease and then every 6 months after inflammation has subsided. If large coronary artery aneurysms are detected, close monitoring is essential. Serial ECGs and cardiac isoenzymes are checked on a regular basis, and tissue plasminogen activator (t-PA) is readily available for administration if signs of a myocardial infarction develop. Coronary artery bypass grafting will be required if significant coronary artery stenosis develops.

Lyme Disease and Rocky Mountain Spotted Fever

Pathophysiology

Lyme disease and Rocky Mountain Spotted Fever (RMSF) are both tick-borne diseases that can produce infection, myocarditis, and myocardial dysfunction. Lyme disease is caused by the spirochete *Borrelia burgdorferi*. RMSF is produced by the coccobacillus *Rickettsia rickettsii.*

Clinical Presentation

Lyme Disease   The clinical course is divided into three phases. Initially, cutaneous manifestations appear, including an oval erythematous patch at the site of the bite (the area of redness expands and shows a central clearing with a red rim), which may be associated with flulike signs. Additional erythematous patches may appear. Approximately 4 to 12 weeks after the skin rash, signs of cardiovascular or neurologic complications develop, including carditis and conduction abnormalities, and cranial neuropathies, meningitis, or encephalitis. Finally, signs of chronic infection develop, characterized by arthritis, which can develop months or years after the tick bite.

Rocky Mountain Spotted Fever   The incubation period for RMSF is 1 to 14 days, with clinical signs usually developing within a week. The clinical course can vary from mild to life threatening. The most common clinical findings are fever, rash, headache, and myalgia. The rash initially appears on the extremities and then is visible on the trunk. The soles and palms are often involved. The rash may begin as papular, maculopapular, or erythematous but often becomes petechial in appearance. Additional nonspecific signs include nausea, vomiting, diarrhea, abdominal pain, conjunctivitis,

lymphadenopathy, and meningoencephalitis. A diffuse vasculitis and myocarditis may develop, contributing to the development of capillary leak, CHF, and shock. Serologic tests may confirm the diagnosis; antibodies can usually be detected by day 7 to 10 of the disease.

Medical and Surgical Interventions

Treatment for both diseases consists of antibiotic therapy and supportive care. Cardiovascular function is supported as needed, and other organ systems (e.g., neurologic) are also assessed and supported. Antibiotic therapy is included here.

Lyme Disease   Doxycycline (100 mg bid PO) is the drug of choice for children older than 9 years of age, and penicillin V (50 mg/kg/24 hours, maximum 2 g/24 hours, administered tid PO) or amoxicillin (25 to 50 mg/kg/24 hours, up to 2 g/24 hours, given tid PO) is given to children 9 years of age or younger. Penicillin-sensitive patients can be treated with erythromycin (30 mg/kg/24 hours).

Rocky Mountain Spotted Fever   Tetracycline (30 to 40 mg/kg/24 hours, given every 6 hours PO, or 20 mg/kg/24 hours administered IV every 8 to 12 hours over 2 hours) is the antibiotic of choice for children older than 9 years of age. Children 9 years of age or younger are treated with chloramphenicol (50 to 75 mg/kg/24 hours given qid PO). Therapy is continued until the patient is afebrile, with a minimum course of 2 days; a typical course is 6 to 10 days.

Cardiomyopathy

Pathophysiology

Cardiomyopathy is an abnormality of the ventricular myocardium. Primary cardiomyopathy indicates that the myocardial dysfunction is not related to CHD, pulmonary or systemic venous hypertension, or coronary or valvular heart disease.

Cardiomyopathy may develop as a complication of systemic disease, viral infection, or exposure to chemicals or drugs. Some forms of CHD produce secondary ventricular dysfunction with effects similar to those of cardiomyopathy.

Three forms of cardiomyopathy are identified:

- *Dilated congestive cardiomyopathy:* Ventricles dilate and contract poorly; ejection fraction is low; ventricular end-diastolic pressure (VEDP) is high, resulting in systemic and pulmonary venous congestion. Stasis of blood may contribute to the development of intraventricular thrombi that may embolize to the systemic or pulmonary venous circulations. Biopsy reveals either hypertrophied or atrophied myocardial cells without evidence of inflammation.
- *Hypertrophic cardiomyopathy (idiopathic hypertrophic subaortic stenosis, or IHSS):* Progressive and asymmetric thickening of the myocardium, particularly in the area of the ventricular septum. This thickening obstructs left ventricular outflow and encroaches on the left ventricular cavity. Ventricular compliance and ejection fraction are decreased, and malignant ventricular arrhythmias may contribute to sudden death. Biopsy reveals an abnormal and disorganized arrangement of myocardial cells, myofibrils, and myofilaments. Coronary arteries are often thickened.
- *Restrictive/obliterative cardiomyopathy:* This form is relatively uncommon in the United States but common in equatorial countries, because it is related to repeated tropical infections

Clinical Presentation

Some children with cardiomyopathy remain asymptomatic during childhood, whereas others develop signs of severe CHF, low cardiac output, or arrhythmias, which may be fatal. Extreme lethargy with decreased exercise tolerance is often present, and the child may complain of chest pain.

Left ventricular outflow tract obstruction or dilational mitral regurgitation may produce a murmur. Chest pain and syncope are other potential signs of severe left ventricular outflow tract obstruction.

If ventricular dilation is present, cardiomegaly will be noted on chest radiographs. The ECG is usually abnormal, although there are no specific criteria diagnostic for cardiomyopathy. Evidence of left and possibly right ventricular hypertrophy is usually present, and ST segment changes consistent with myocardial injury may be noted. Additional findings may include arrhythmias, T-wave inversion, abnormal Q waves, or diminished R waves. The echocardiogram will demonstrate ventricular dilation or left ventricular outflow tract obstruction.

Medical and Surgical Interventions

Treatment of cardiomyopathy requires elimination of any causative or contributing factors and support of cardiovascular function. CHF, low cardiac output, and arrhythmias must be skillfully treated. Cardiac transplantation is the treatment of choice for most symptomatic forms of cardiomyopathy unresponsive to medical management.

Beta-adrenergic agents may be useful in the treatment of both dilated congestive and hypertrophic cardiomyopathy. Improvement may result from propranolol (2 mg/kg/day in infants and young children, and 160 to 321 mg/day in older children), because it reduces left ventricular outflow tract obstruction or reduces myocardial oxygen requirements.

Calcium channel blockers such as verapamil have been less effective in the treatment of hypertrophic cardiomyopathy, and sudden death may be associated with their use. Digoxin therapy is usually avoided in infants with hypertrophic cardiomyopathy because it may contribute to further hypertrophy. Use of vasodilators or inotropic agents must be individualized and titrated very carefully to patient response. The patient may be admitted to the critical care unit for short-term dobutamine therapy, since this may improve ejection fraction and produce symptomatic improvement.

Because sudden, malignant, and potentially fatal arrhythmias may develop at any time, the staff must maintain a high level of preparedness for resuscitation. If the cardiomyopathy is determined to be progressive, the child may be listed as a candidate for cardiac transplantation. Unfortunately, the wait for a donor heart may be long. The wishes of the child and family regarding resuscitation should be clarified before any need for resuscitation occurs, and proper written documentation should be placed in the child's chart. If the child is considered to be terminally ill, see Chapter 4.

If thromboembolism develops, anticoagulation will be required. Careful monitoring of systemic perfusion and cerebral function will be required.

Cardiac Tumors

Pathophysiology

Primary cardiac tumors are uncommon in children and are usually benign. They can, however, produce hemodynamic compromise, hemolysis, or embolism.

Rhabdomyoma is the most common cardiac tumor seen in children. It is a benign tumor that usually consists of multiple tumors within the walls of the ventricles. A fibroma, the second most common tumor seen in children, is also benign. It typically is a solid tumor that is often located in the left ventricle, growing into the left ventricular outflow tract.

Clinical Presentation

Cardiovascular effects occur when the tumor obstructs a coronary artery or valve or the outflow tract of the left ventricle. Arrhythmias may also develop.

Medical and Surgical Interventions

These tumors can be successfully removed during cardiovascular surgery, using cardiopulmonary bypass. The fibroma may not be excised completely but can be successfully debulked.

Postoperative Complications

Tumor resection typically results in elimination of all symptoms; thus postoperative complications would more likely be related to cardiopulmonary bypass or the median sternotomy incision. Arrhythmias may develop at the site of myocardial resection.

Cardiac Transplantation

Cardiac transplantation has been performed with increasing success since 1967. In recent years the greatest number of pediatric cardiac transplantations have been performed in infants and very young children.

Indications

Cardiac transplantation is considered for end-stage cardiomyopathy, endocardial fibroelastosis, inoperable CHD, ventricular failure following palliation for CHD, or retransplantation for cardiac graft failure.

Contraindications

Factors that would render a child unsuitable as a candidate for receipt of a cardiac transplant are relatively few and include active systemic infection, elevated PVR (PVR ≥6 Wood units), recent pulmonary embolism or infarction, active malignancy, other organ failure, significant extracardiac anomaly, and chromosomal abnormality that would decrease longevity. A strong social support system is also required, with the ability to ensure compliance with the medical care needed after transplantation.

Obtaining a Donor Heart

The limited pool of donor organs remains the greatest limitation to cardiac transplantation and results in many children and adults dying every year while waiting for organ transplantation. When a donor is available, the donor heart is computer matched with recipient need through the United Network of Organ Sharing (UNOS). It is matched for size, ABO blood group compatibility, and, if possible, cytomegalovirus status. Tissue matching is not possible in the time available.

Posttransplant Care

The three most common problems observed during the early postoperative period include hyperacute rejection, bleeding, and right heart failure.

Hyperacute rejection typically occurs in the operating room or within hours of the transplant and produces signs of refractory low cardiac output and inadequate systemic perfusion, indicative of failure of the transplanted heart.

Bleeding is often secondary to preoperative hepatic congestion and hepatic dysfunction. Signs of bleeding include chest tube output >3 ml/kg/hr for 3 or more hours or >5 ml/kg/hr for any 1 hour. Signs of coagulopathy include petechiae or ecchymoses. Treatment is supportive and requires blood component therapy (see Table 5-12).

Right heart failure is most frequently caused by preoperative pulmonary hypertension. Management of pulmonary hypertension includes maintenance of excellent alveolar oxygenation, alkalosis, analgesia and sedation, and possible use of nitric oxide (see Postoperative Care, pp. 156 and 211. Two people should be used to suction the intubated child with pulmonary hypertension to ensure efficient suctioning without compromise of oxygenation. Right ventricular function is also supported with judicious fluid administration (to optimize preload) and use of inotropic agents and vasodilators, if necessary.

The transplanted heart is no longer innervated by sympathetic nervous system fibers. Therefore, if sympathetic nervous system stimulation is needed, exogenous catecholamine administration will be required. Sympathomimetic drugs that stimulate alpha-2 and beta-adrenergic receptors will probably be more effective than those that stimulate alpha-1 (innervated) receptors. For this reason, dobutamine will probably produce more significant effects on heart rate and contractility than dopamine.

Renal dysfunction and failure may develop postoperatively. Causes include prerenal conditions such as low cardiac output or complications of immunosuppressive therapy.

Immunosuppression

Immunosuppressive therapy should be accomplished according to the protocol established at the transplant center, and a comprehensive review of potential therapies is beyond the scope of this chapter. Common immunosuppressive drugs and dosages are included in Table 5-29. The major drugs used are summarized briefly here:

- Cyclosporine acts on T lymphocytes, preventing their activation. If serum creatinine levels are normal preoperatively, the patient receives a preoperative dose and then receives IV cyclosporine postoperatively until oral feedings have resumed. If the creatinine is elevated, the cyclosporine dose is delayed for several hours. Once oral feedings are tolerated, cyclosporine is administered orally. Serum levels of 250 ng/ml are maintained during the immediate postoperative period. If the patient is rejection

Table 5-29
Pediatric Immunosuppressive Drugs and Dosages Following Cardiac Transplantation

Drug	Dosage
Prednisone	1 mg/kg/day then taper
Azathioprine	1-3 mg/kg/day
Cyclosporin A	10-20 mg/kg/day
Rabbit antithymocyte serum	0.2-0.5 ml/kg/dose
Monoclonal OKT-3	0.1-0.2 mg/kg/day

From Byren BJ, Kane PL, Cameron DE: Cardiac transplantation. In Nichols DG et al, editors: *Critical heart disease in infants and children,* St Louis, 1995, Mosby.

free, the dose is tapered after 6 months (to maintain a level of 150 to 200 ng/ml) and then again at 1 year (to maintain a level of 100 ng/ml). Side effects include nephrotoxicity, hypertension, and hepatotoxicity.

- Corticosteroids (methylprednisolone, then prednisone) inhibit the inflammatory response, suppressing circulating B and T lymphocytes. Methylprednisolone is administered at surgery and for 3 days (6 mg/kg/day); then oral prednisone is used (1 mg/kg/day). The prednisone dose is tapered to 0.4 mg/kg/day over 2 weeks, then to 0.2 mg/kg/day at 6 months, and finally to an alternate-day schedule by 1 year.

- Azathioprine (AZT) interferes with DNA synthesis, particularly in lymphoid cells, and it decreases granulocyte number and function. It may be administered preoperatively and is provided daily postoperatively. AZT will be held if significant leukopenia (WBC count $<5000/mm^3$) develops. Side effects include leukopenia, anemia, thrombocytopenia, and hepatic dysfunction.

Additional drugs that may be administered during rejection episodes include OKT3, a monoclonal antibody that reacts with the T3 surface antigen present on mature lymphocytes, inhibiting T-cell functions. It is typically administered only once during the posttransplant period, because subsequent doses can result in serum reactions. Antithymocyte serum or globulin (ATS) is a polyclonal antibody formed in response to human thymus injection. ATS acts against human lymphocytes and is administered during rejection. Potential side effects include sensitivity reaction and fever, urticaria, and possibly anaphylaxis.

Acute rejection may occur approximately 7 to 10 days after transplantation. Signs of acute rejection include irritability and feeding problems in the infant, behavioral changes in the child, vomiting, temperature instability, tachycardia, and tachypnea. Signs of poor systemic perfusion may be present. Serial echocardiograms document decreased myocardial contractility and failure. The diagnosis is confirmed by biopsy and is treated with a bolus of corticosteroids, with addition of antithymocyte globulin if needed.

Common Diagnostic Tests

The purpose of this section is to describe common diagnostic tests that may be performed to evaluate cardiovascular function. Preparation required for the tests and posttest care are summarized.

Echocardiography

Echocardiography is an essential noninvasive tool to diagnose congenital heart disease and evaluate myocardial function. This painless procedure transmits high-frequency pulsed-sound waves into the chest through a transducer, which then receives the sound waves reflected back from the heart. The variations in characteristics of the reflected sound can be used to generate an image of the heart, to evaluate dimensions of cardiac chambers and great vessels, to locate and evaluate motion of cardiac valves, to identify heart lesions, and to evaluate ventricular function. Doppler echocardiography reflects sound waves from RBCs; thus it can be used to evaluate blood flow, areas of intracardiac or great vessel obstruction, and peak ventricular pressures and shunts.

No preparation is required, and no complications result from the procedure.

Nuclear Cardiology

Radionuclide imaging is an extremely reliable method of evaluating ventricular function and myo-

cardial perfusion. These studies use an injected radionuclide (e.g., technetium or thallium) and monitor its movement through the cardiac chambers, vascular space, or myocardial muscle. The images derived from this process enable evaluation of myocardial perfusion, ejection fraction, myocardial contractility, and ventricular size.

The only preparation required for the procedure is injection of the radionuclide by laboratory personnel. Extravasation of the radionuclide into the tissue is the only potential complication of the procedure.

Nuclear Magnetic Resonance Imaging

Magnetic resonance imaging (MRI) is a noninvasive study that enables visualization of tumors, shunts, and soft tissues (including the heart). The child is positioned within the scanner, which creates a strong magnetic field around the patient. This causes rotation of cell nuclei at a predictable speed, which enables visualization of soft tissues better than any other noninvasive device.

The MRI scanner must be located well away from patient care areas; thus transportation of the patient to the scanner is the most problematic part of the study. Although no preparation of the patient is required, the nurse must prepare for the study by ensuring that all electrical equipment can be removed during the study (some mechanical ventilators are designed to be used during MRI studies, but many cannot be used). The child must be closely monitored throughout the study, although visibility of the child may be limited. There are no known complications of this study.

Endomyocardial Biopsy

Endomyocardial biopsy is performed during cardiac catheterization and uses a small forceps incorporated into the catheter to obtain a small specimen of the ventricular endocardium and myocardium. Histologic evaluation of the sample is then possible to contribute to the diagnosis and treatment of cardiomyopathy, myocarditis, and posttransplant rejection.

This procedure is invasive and may produce ventricular arrhythmias, ventricular perforation, pneumothorax, and hemopericardium. Preparation is the same as that required for cardiac catheterization.

Cardiac Catheterization and Angiocardiography

Cardiac catheterization involves insertion of a radiopaque catheter through an artery and/or vein into the heart. This procedure is performed under fluoroscopy so that the location and movement of the catheter can be visualized. Throughout catheterization, pressure measurements are made and oxygen saturation is recorded to provide information about blood flow patterns (including shunts) within the heart. Structures such as cardiac chambers, valves, or great vessels can be visualized through injection of a radiopaque contrast agent. Rapid sequential radiographs, called angiograms, are made to record the flow of contrast through the heart.

Therapeutic cardiac catheterization uses balloon catheters to dilate stenotic valves or vessels. Electrophysiologic studies may be used to identify intracardiac conduction pathways (particularly abnormal or accessory pathways) and sources of arrhythmias.

Box 5-26

Nursing Care of the Child Following Cardiac Catheterization

1. **Potential child/family anxiety and potential knowledge deficit:** Provide information and support, as needed
2. **Potential inadequate cardiac output and systemic perfusion:** This may be caused by progression of underlying cardiac disease, hemorrhage, cardiac perforation, tamponade, arrhythmias, or reaction to the sedation or contrast medium. Monitor systemic perfusion closely, and notify physician of signs of inadequate cardiac output, including inappropriate heart rate, diminished peripheral pulses, cool extremities, delayed capillary refill, mottled or pale or gray color, oliguria, and acidosis. Monitor catheterization site for evidence of excessive bleeding—notify physician if detected. Be prepared to support systemic perfusion as needed.
3. **Potential compromise in extremity perfusion** related to arterial or venous catheterization during procedure or hemorrhage or edema after procedure: Notify physician immediately of any compromise in *arterial perfusion* of extremity, including a pallor, mottling, diminished strength of extremity pulse, cool temperature, or delayed capillary refill. *Venous obstruction* will result in edema and possible duskiness of extremity, but capillary refill should remain brisk unless venous congestion begins to interfere with arterial circulation. Treatment for arterial compromise may require immediate pharmacologic intervention (heparin drip may be prescribed if thrombus is suspected; vasodilator therapy may be prescribed if arterial spasm is suspected) or surgical intervention. Heat may be applied to contralateral extremity (*not* to catheterized extremity) to promote reflex vasodilation. Venous obstruction may be relieved if extremity is elevated.
4. **Potential infection:** Monitor for signs of infection and sepsis. Infection may develop at catheterization site, at site of IV access, or within bloodstream. Report fever or signs of infection or sepsis to physician. Obtain cultures and administer antibiotics as ordered.
5. **Potential compromise in respiratory function** resulting from sedation, immobility, or reaction to contrast medium: Monitor pulse oximetry, respiratory rate and effort, and breath sounds and chest expansion bilaterally. Monitoring of end-tidal carbon dioxide may also be appropriate. Notify physician of any problems. Be prepared to support respiratory function as necessary.
6. **Potential alteration in renal function:** Compromise in renal function may result from low cardiac output (prerenal failure) or dehydration, or from a reaction to the contrast medium. Monitor urine output and notify physician if oliguria develops despite adequate fluid intake. Test urine for hematuria and notify physician if observed. Evaluate and maintain fluid balance.
7. **Potential pain:** Assess for signs of pain and evaluate location and severity of pain. Provide analgesia as needed and monitor effectiveness.

Potential complications of catheterization include arrhythmias, bleeding, cardiac perforation, tamponade, cerebrovascular accident, contrast agent reactions, hypercyanotic spells (if the child has cyanotic heart disease), and local vascular complications. These complications are summarized in Box 5-26.

Suggested Readings

Berman W Jr: *Handbook of pediatric ECG interpretation,* St Louis, 1991, Mosby.

Bove EL, Lloyd TR: Staged reconstruction for hypoplastic left heart syndrome: contemporary results, *Ann Surg* 224:387-395, 1996.

Castaneda AR et al, editors: *Cardiac surgery of the neonate and infant,* Philadelphia, 1994, WB Saunders.

Chameides L, Hazinski MF, editors: *Textbook of pediatric advanced life support,* Dallas, 1997, American Heart Association.

Chang AC et al: Milrinone: systemic and pulmonary hemodynamic effects in neonates after cardiac surgery, *Crit Care Med* 23:1907-1914, 1995.

Chernow B, editor: *The pharmacologic approach to the critically ill patient,* ed 3, Baltimore, 1994, Williams & Wilkins.

Cummins RO et al: Recommended guidelines for reviewing, reporting, and conducting research on in-hospital resuscitation: the in-hospital "Utstein Style," *Ann Emerg Med* 29:650-679, 1997 (also printed in *Circulation* 95:2213-2239, 1997, and *Resuscitation*).

Dajani AS et al, editors: Prevention of bacterial endocarditis: recommendations of the American Heart Association, *JAMA* 277:1794-1801, 1997.

Fink BW: *Congenital heart disease: a deductive approach to its diagnosis,* ed 3, St Louis, 1991, Mosby.

Garson A et al, editors: The science and practice of pediatric cardiology, ed 2, Baltimore, 1998, Williams & Wilkins.

Goldman AP et al: Pharmacological control of pulmonary blood flow with inhaled nitric oxide after the fenestrated Fontan operation, *Circulation* 94 (suppl II):II44-II48, 1996.

Goldstein B, Zimmerman JJ, editors: Critical care of pediatric shock, *New Horizons* 6:119-234 (entire edition).

Hazinski MF: Is pediatric resuscitation unique? Relative merits of early CPR and ventilation versus early defibrillation for young victims of cardiac arrest, *Ann Emerg Med* 25:540-543, 1995.

Hazinski MF: Pediatric evaluation and monitoring considerations. In Darovic GO, editor: *Hemodynamic monitoring: invasive and noninvasive clinical application,* ed 2, Philadelphia, 1995, WB Saunders.

Hazinski MF: Shock, multiple organ dysfunction syndrome, and burns. In McCance KL, Heuther SE, editors: *Pathophysiology: the biological basis for disease in adults and children,* ed 3, St Louis, 1998, Mosby.

Hazinski MF, Cummins RO, editors: *1998 handbook of emergency cardiac care,* Dallas, 1998, American Heart Association.

Hazinski MF et al: Outcome of cardiovascular collapse in pediatric victims of blunt trauma, *Ann Emerg Med* 23:1229-1235, 1994.

Hinshaw LB: Sepsis/septic shock: participation of the microcirculation: an abbreviated review, *Crit Care Med* 24:1072-1078, 1996.

Johns Hopkins Hospital Department of Pediatrics: *The Harriet Lane handbook,* ed 14, edited by Barone M, St Louis, 1996, Mosby.

Levin DL, Morriss FC, editors: *Essentials of pediatric intensive care,* ed 2, St Louis, 1997, Quality Medical.

Mosca RS et al: Hemodynamic characteristics of neonates following first stage palliation for hypoplastic left heart syndrome, *Circulation 92* (suppl II): II267-II271, 1995.

Nichols DG et al: *Critical heart disease in infants and children,* St Louis, 1995, Mosby.

Nichols DG et al: *Golden hour: the handbook of advanced pediatric life support,* ed 2, St Louis, 1996, Mosby.

Park MK: *The pediatric cardiology handbook,* ed 2, St Louis, 1997, Mosby.

Pollack MM, Patel KM, Ruttimann EU: Prism III: An updated pediatric risk of mortality score, *Crit Care Med* 24:743-752, 1996.

Singh-Naz N et al: Risk factors for nosocomial infections in critically ill children: a prospective cohort study, *Crit Care Med* 24:875-878, 1996.

Slonin AD et al: Cardiopulmonary resuscitation in pediatric intensive care units, *Crit Care Med* 25:1951-1955, 1997.

Vincent JL: Search for effective immunomodulating strategies against sepsis (editorial), *Lancet* 351:922-923, 1998.

Zaritsky A et al: Recommended guidelines for uniform reporting of pediatric advanced life support: the Pediatric Utstein Style. A statement for health care professionals from a task force at the American Academy of Pediatrics, the American Heart Association, and the European Resuscitation Council, *Pediatrics* 96:965-979, 1995 (also simultaneously published in *Ann Emerg Med, Circulation,* and *Resuscitation*).

Zeni F, Freeman B and Natanson C: Anti-inflammatory therapies to treat sepsis and septic shock; a reassessment (editorial), *Crit Care Med* 25:1095-1100, 1997.

6 **Pulmonary Disorders**

Essential Anatomy and Physiology

The primary functions of the respiratory system are *oxygenation* (addition of oxygen to blood) and *ventilation* (removal of carbon dioxide from blood). Respiratory function is adequate if the arterial oxygen tension (Pao_2) and carbon dioxide tension ($Paco_2$) are maintained in the normal range. Respiratory function is inadequate if these blood gas tensions are abnormal, or if normal blood gas tensions are achievable only with excessively high respiratory effort.

Oxygen (O_2) and carbon dioxide (CO_2) move between air and blood by simple diffusion across the alveolar surface. If fresh gas is not delivered to the alveoli, if blood is not delivered to alveolar capillaries, or if the alveolar surface is damaged, oxygenation or carbon dioxide elimination may be impaired.

Embryology of the Lung

A rudimentary respiratory system appears by the fourth week of gestation. Although many body systems are virtually complete by approximately 25 weeks of gestational age, the respiratory system continues to develop throughout gestation. After birth, airway dimensions and alveolar number both increase until approximately 8 years of age.

Components of the Respiratory System

There are five components of the respiratory system. Each component in the infant or child is incompletely developed or may contribute to deterioration if respiratory disease or distress develops:

- *Central nervous system control of ventilation:* Controls respiratory rate and tidal volume and responds to changes in arterial blood gases
- *Airways:* Conduct gas to and from the alveoli
- *Chest wall:* Encloses the respiratory system
- *Respiratory muscles:* Stabilize the chest and produce airflow and maintain airway patency; include the diaphragm and intercostal muscles and the muscles of the upper and lower airways
- *Lung tissue:* Alveolar surface across which oxygen uptake and carbon dioxide elimination occur

Central Nervous System Control of Ventilation

At birth, all peripheral and central chemoreceptors are present and functional. However, the newborn or young infant may respond to hypoxia with hyperpnea and then apnea. Any condition or drugs resulting in central nervous system (CNS) depression (head injury, diabetic ketoacidosis, infection, sedatives) may depress ventilation. *If the child demonstrates no response to painful stimulation, support of oxygenation and ventilation may be required.*

Airways

All conducting airways are present at birth, and the major airway branching pattern is complete.

Airways increase in size and length after birth, and alveoli continue to develop during childhood.

The upper airway of the infant and young child is compliant and may narrow during inspiration. In addition, it differs in configuration from the upper airway of the older child or adult; thus intubation of the young child requires expertise.

Glottis and Epiglottis   The glottis is more anterior and higher in the young child, and the epiglottis is longer. Therefore insertion of an endotracheal tube into the trachea requires anterior angulation of the tube or the application of cricoid pressure during intubation.

Narrowest Portion of Pharynx   The narrowest portion of the upper airway is at the level of the cricoid cartilage in the young child and at the vocal cords in the older child or adult. An endotracheal tube may pass easily through the vocal cords of the infant or young child but still be too large at the level of the cricoid cartilage.

Use of Cuffed Endotracheal Tubes   Cuffed endotracheal tubes are usually unnecessary in young children because the cricoid cartilage forms a natural seal around the tube. In addition, the airway may be injured by cuff inflation.

Airway Resistance   Resistance to airflow in any airway will increase exponentially if the airway radius decreases; thus any narrowing of the already-small pediatric airways will be significant. This resistance increases to the *fourth* power of the radius as the radius decreases during quiet breathing and to the *fifth* power of the radius as the radius decreases during times of turbulent airflow (e.g., crying). Relatively small amounts of mucus accumulation, edema or airway constriction can significantly reduce the airway radius and increase resistance to airflow and the work of breathing (Figure 6-1), particularly if airflow is turbulent.

Chest and Respiratory Muscles

The shape and compliance of the infant's chest can further impair ventilation during periods of respiratory distress. The infant's chest is round, and the ribs articulate horizontally from the back to the sternum. The intercostal muscles serve largely to

Newborn

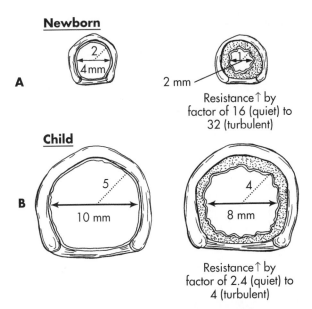

A

2 mm

Resistance↑ by
factor of 16 (quiet) to
32 (turbulent)

Child

B

Resistance↑ by
factor of 2.4 (quiet) to
4 (turbulent)

Figure 6-1 Effects of 1 mm of circumferential edema in the neonate and young adult. **A,** The neonate possesses a larynx approximately 4 mm in diameter and 2 mm in radius. If 1 mm of circumferential edema develops, it will halve the airway radius and increase resistance to airflow by a factor of 16 during quiet breathing and by a factor of approximately 32 during turbulent air flow (e.g., crying). **B,** The young adult possess a larynx approximately 10 mm in diameter and 5 mm in radius. The 1 mm of circumferential edema will reduce the radius by 20% (from 5 mm to 4 mm) and increase resistance to airflow by a factor of 2.4 during quiet breathing and by a factor of approximately 4 during turbulent air flow (e.g., crying). (From Hazinski MF: *Nursing care of the critically ill child,* ed 2, St Louis, 1992, Mosby.)

stabilize the chest wall and are not capable of lifting the ribs until approximately 8 years of age. The anterior-posterior diameter of the infant's chest cannot be increased during periods of respiratory distress. In comparison, the chest of the older child and adult is wider than it is deep, and the ribs are angled downward from back to front. During inspiration in the older child or adult, the intercostal muscles lift the ribs to increase the anterior-posterior diameter of the chest. The intercostal muscles, along with muscles of the neck, can also contribute to chest expansion during periods of res-

piratory distress. The infant's chest wall is very compliant because the ribs are cartilaginous; in contrast, the chest of the older child and adult is relatively stiff.

The diaphragm is the chief muscle of inspiration. It is innervated on each side by the phrenic nerve, which is formed by portions of the third, fourth, and fifth cervical spinal nerves. During *inspiration* the diaphragm contracts, intrathoracic pressure falls, and air is drawn into the lungs (in older children and adults the intercostal muscles lift the chest wall). During *expiration,* or exhalation, the diaphragm relaxes, intrathoracic volume decreases, and the elastic lungs recoil to preinspiratory volume (air leaves the lungs).

When the diaphragm contracts in the healthy infant or in the older child or adult, the intrathoracic pressure falls in proportion to the downward movement of the diaphragm. The fall in intrathoracic pressure results in movement of air into the lungs. In addition, in the older child or adult, the intercostal muscles contract, lifting the rib cage and preventing it from being pulled inward by the diaphragm.

When respiratory disease develops and pulmonary compliance is reduced in the infant or young child, diaphragm contraction will produce intercostal and sternal *retractions,* rather than inflation of the lungs (Figure 6-2). These retractions reduce ventilation efficiency; the diaphragm must then shorten and move much more than normal to generate a tidal volume.

The compliant chest wall of the infant or young child should expand easily outward when positive pressure ventilation is provided. Therefore, *if the chest wall does not expand bilaterally during positive pressure ventilation, positive pressure ventilation is inadequate or the airway is obstructed.* Caution should be used during hand ventilation, since the chest will expand to accommodate excessive inspiratory force and barotrauma may result.

Lung Tissue

Lung compliance (i.e., lung distensibility) is affected by surfactant and by the elasticity of lung tissue. Lung compliance is normally low in the infant and increases during childhood; lung disease or injury can further reduce lung compliance. Surfactant may be inactivated or its production de-

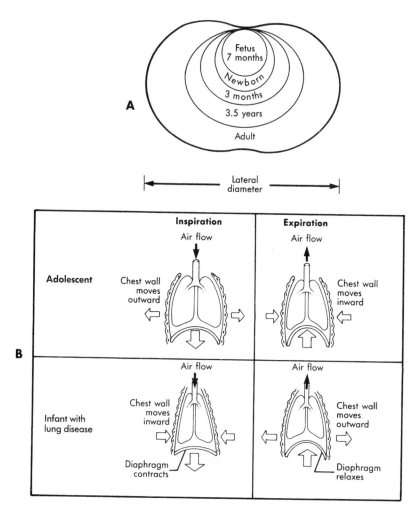

Figure 6-2   Changes in chest wall and mechanics with age. **A,** Changes in chest wall shape with age. **B,** Differences in lung mechanics caused by differences in chest wall compliance (and chest wall rigidity) in infants with lung disease and in older children and adolescents. NOTE: Arrows indicate direction of airflow, chest wall movement, and diaphragm movement. (Modified from McCance KL, Huether SE: *Pathophysiology: the biological basis for disease in adults and children,* ed 2, St. Louis, 1994, Mosby.)

creased by lung injury or disease (e.g., near-drowning, acute respiratory distress syndrome).

Pulmonary edema, infection, or inflammation also reduces gas exchange. Young infants and children with respiratory disease or injury are at risk for the development of pulmonary edema, particularly if fluid administration is excessive or if oliguria is present.

Lung Volumes

Some measurements of lung volumes may be obtained in cooperative children (usually older than 5 years) using spirometry:

- *Tidal volume (VT):* Volume of each breath. Normal VT is 6 to 10 ml/kg (VT <4 to 5 ml/kg may indicate the need for respiratory support).

- *Vital capacity (VC):* Volume of air expired after a maximal inspiratory effort. VC may be reduced by any process that reduces lung compliance (makes the lung stiffer) or by airway obstruction. Normal VC is 65 to 75 ml/kg (VC <15 to 20 ml/kg indicates the need for respiratory support).

Other lung volumes cannot be measured with spirometry but may be evaluated with specialized gas dilution techniques:

- *Functional residual capacity (FRC):* Volume of gas in the lung after a normal expiration. May increase with obstructive airway diseases such as asthma or cystic fibrosis; may decrease in patients with pulmonary fibrosis.
- *Residual volume (RV):* Volume of gas remaining in the lung after maximal expiration.

Ventilation-Perfusion Relationships

Ideally, pulmonary blood flow ($\dot{Q}$) matches alveolar ventilation ($\dot{V}_A$). However, a minor mismatch of ventilation and perfusion is normally present in the lung. The $\dot{V}_A/\dot{Q}$ mismatch may be increased when lung disease or injury is present, resulting in increased dead space ventilation or a shunt.

Minute Ventilation   Minute ventilation ($\dot{V}_E$) is the process of gas movement in and out of the lungs. Minute ventilation is a product of breathing frequency (f) and tidal volume (V_T). Ventilation is evaluated by monitoring the $Paco_2$.

Alveolar Ventilation   Alveolar ventilation ($\dot{V}_A$) is the portion of total ventilation that reaches the alveoli; this normally constitutes approximately 70% of tidal volume. The rate of carbon dioxide removal from the alveoli and the rate of oxygen delivery to the alveoli are directly dependent on alveolar ventilation.

Dead Space Ventilation   Dead space ($\dot{V}_D$) is the portion of tidal volume that does not contribute to gas exchange. This dead space includes anatomic and physiologic dead space. *Anatomic dead space*

is the volume required to fill conducting airways; this volume normally constitutes 30% of tidal volume. Since airways contain no alveoli, they do not participate in gas exchange. *Physiologic dead space* is the volume of ventilated lung that does not receive blood flow (i.e., "wasted" ventilation (Figure 6-3, *A* and *B*). Ventilation of nonperfused segments of the lung is also referred to as high $\dot{V}_A/\dot{Q}$. *Hypercarbia* may result. However, the predominant effect is wasted ventilation—ventilation that contributes little to oxygenation and carbon dioxide removal.

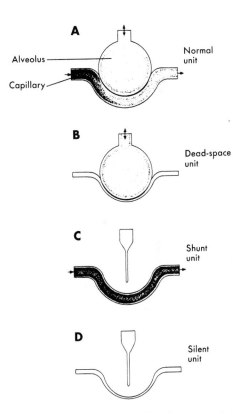

Figure 6-3   Theoretic respiratory unit with graphic representation of the relationship between ventilation and perfusion in different clinical conditions. **A,** Normal ventilation and perfusion. **B,** Normal ventilation with no perfusion. **C,** No ventilation but normal perfusion. **D,** No ventilation and no perfusion. (From Shapiro BA, Harrison RA, Walton JR: *Clinical application of blood gases,* ed 3, St Louis, 1982, Mosby.)

Hypoventilation Hypoventilation is present when there is inadequate replenishment of alveolar gas with fresh gas; the $PaCO_2$ rises, and the PaO_2 falls equivalently (see Case Study 3 on acid-base disorders later in chapter). It may be caused by respiratory depression, respiratory muscle fatigue, or airway obstruction. The PaO_2 may be increased by supplemental oxygen administration, but the hypercarbia will only be corrected if ventilation is supported (e.g., mechanical ventilation) or respiratory drive is stimulated (e.g., by naloxone administration).

When tidal volume decreases, ventilation becomes less effective. Since anatomic dead space is fixed, it will constitute a greater portion of the tidal volume, and alveolar ventilation will decrease.

Shunt A shunt (very low $\dot{V}_A/\dot{Q}>$) is present when blood enters the left atrium without passing through ventilated areas of the lung. This may result from an absolute fall in pulmonary blood flow (e.g., hypovolemic shock), an increase in pulmonary vascular resistance (i.e., pulmonary hypertension), or the development of an anatomic or physiologic shunt (Figure 6-3, C). *Shunts result in hypoxemia that cannot be corrected simply by administration of supplemental oxygen.* Continuous positive airway pressure (CPAP) or, if the patient is mechanically ventilated, positive end-expiratory pressure (PEEP) may reduce the shunt by increasing the functional residual capacity. Hypercarbia is usually *not* present because carbon dioxide is extremely soluble and diffuses readily and will be eliminated by alveoli with a more normal $\dot{V}_A/\dot{Q}$.

An *anatomic shunt* occurs when blood flow is directed away from the lungs (e.g., cyanotic congenital heart disease with right-to-left shunt). This results in hypoxemia that will not improve with oxygen administration or mechanical ventilation with PEEP; pulmonary blood flow must increase if the PaO_2 is to increase.

A *physiologic shunt* is present when blood passes through nonventilated or poorly ventilated areas of the lung (e.g., atelectatic areas). Oxygen administration alone may partially correct the hypoxemia.

In the newborn, cardiovascular and intrapulmonary shunting of blood is normal immediately after birth and is associated with shunting of blood from the pulmonary artery through the ductus arteriosus to the aorta as a result of atelectasis and edema within the lung. Perfusion of poorly ventilated areas produces hypoxemia. These shunts should disappear within a few hours or days.

Oxygen Transport

Definitions of Terms

Oxygen is carried in the blood in two ways. The majority of oxygen (97.5%) is carried in combination with hemoglobin inside red blood cells, in the form of oxyhemoglobin. A small portion of oxygen (2.5%) is carried in the dissolved state in plasma, but this is the amount measured as the PO_2 in arterial blood gases.

Arterial Oxygen Content The arterial oxygen content (CaO_2) is the volume of oxygen carried in arterial blood (milliliters of oxygen per deciliter of blood). It can be calculated by adding the oxygen bound to hemoglobin to the dissolved oxygen (Box 6-1). Normal arterial oxygen content is 18 to 20 ml O_2/dl blood.

Arterial Oxygen Tension The arterial oxygen tension (PaO_2) is the partial pressure of oxygen in arterial blood. The normal PaO_2 is approximately 100 mm Hg.

NOTE: The difference between arterial oxygen content and arterial oxygen tension is illustrated in Figure 6-4.

Oxygen Delivery Oxygen delivery ($\dot{D}O_2$) is the amount of blood delivered to the tissues per minute; it is a product of arterial oxygen content and cardiac output. It may be indexed to the body surface area (BSA):

$$\dot{D}O_2 = \text{Arterial oxygen content} \times \text{Cardiac output or index}$$

The normal $\dot{D}O_2$ (indexed) in children is 475 to 750 ml/min/m^2 BSA.

Oxygen Consumption Oxygen consumption ($\dot{V}O_2$) is the amount of oxygen consumed by tissue

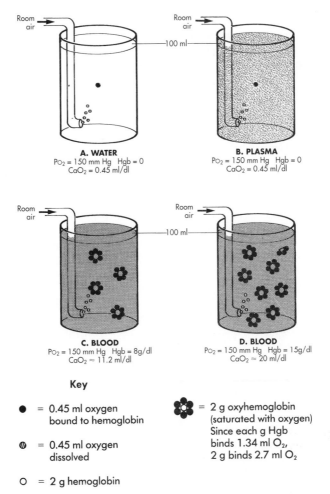

A. WATER
PO_2 = 150 mm Hg Hgb = 0
CaO_2 = 0.45 ml/dl

B. PLASMA
PO_2 = 150 mm Hg Hgb = 0
CaO_2 = 0.45 ml/dl

C. BLOOD
PO_2 = 150 mm Hg Hgb = 8g/dl
CaO_2 ≈ 11.2 ml/dl

D. BLOOD
PO_2 = 150 mm Hg Hgb = 15g/dl
CaO_2 ≈ 20 ml/dl

Key

● = 0.45 ml oxygen bound to hemoglobin

◍ = 0.45 ml oxygen dissolved

○ = 2 g hemoglobin

✿ = 2 g oxyhemoglobin (saturated with oxygen) Since each g Hgb binds 1.34 ml O_2, 2 g binds 2.7 ml O_2

Figure 6-4   Partial pressure of oxygen (Pao_2) vs. oxygen content (Cao_2) as hemoglobin concentration varies. Four beakers of fluid are in equilibrium with room air at sea level. Therefore the barometric pressure is 760 mm Hg, and the partial pressure of oxygen (Pao_2) in room air is 21% of 760 mm Hg, or approximately 150 mm Hg. **A,** Beaker A contains water. If the water is in equilibrium with room air, the Pao_2 in the water is 150 mm Hg. However, the oxygen content is only approximately 0.45 ml/dl, since this is the amount of oxygen dissolved in the water at a Pao_2 of 150 mm Hg (150 × 0.003 ml). **B,** Beaker B contains plasma. If the plasma is in equilibrium with room air, the Pao_2 of the plasma is 150 mm Hg. However, the oxygen content of the plasma is only approximately 0.45 ml/dl because this represents the amount of oxygen dissolved in the plasma at a Pao_2 of 150 mm Hg (150 × 0.003 ml). **C,** Beaker C contains whole blood with a hemoglobin of 8 g/dl. If this blood equilibrates with room air, the Pao_2 also will equal 150 mm Hg. The oxygen content of the blood is determined by the amount of oxygen dissolved in the blood (0.45ml/dl) *plus* the amount of oxygen bound to hemoglobin. Assuming the hemoglobin is fully saturated, an additional 10.7 ml of oxygen is bound to the hemoglobin; thus the total oxygen content in this fluid is 11.17 ml O_2/dl. **D,** Beaker D contains whole blood with a hemoglobin of 15 g/dl. If this blood is in equilibrium with room air approximately 0.45 ml/dl of oxygen will be dissolved in the blood, and approximately 19.5 ml/dl will be bound to hemoglobin (assuming the hemoglobin is 97% saturated), yielding a total oxygen content of 19.95 ml O_2/dl. (From Hazinski MF: *Nursing care of the critically ill child,* ed 2, St Louis, 1992, Mosby.)

Box 6-1

Calculation of Arterial Oxygen Content

Total oxygen content = O_2 bound to Hgb
                      + Dissolved O_2

The oxygen bound to hemoglobin is calculated by determining the *theoretic oxygen-carrying capacity of the blood,* or the amount of oxygen carried by the hemoglobin if the hemoglobin is fully saturated:

Oxygen capacity = Hgb concentration (mg/dl)
              $\times$ 1.34 ml O_2/g Hgb (1)

Once the patient's arterial oxygen saturation is known, the amount of oxygen bound to the hemoglobin is multiplied by the theoretic oxygen-carrying capacity:

O_2 bound to Hgb = (O_2 capacity)
              $\times$ Arterial O_2 saturation (2)

To calculate the amount of dissolved oxygen present in the blood, the child's PaO$_2$ is multiplied by 0.003 ml O_2/dl:

Dissolved oxygen = 0.003 ml O_2/dl $\times$ PaO$_2$ (3)

Finally, the total arterial oxygen content is equal to the sum of the oxygen carried by the hemoglobin and the dissolved oxygen:

Oxygen content = (Equation 2) + (Equation 3)

From Hazinski MF: *Nursing care of the critically ill child,* ed 2, St Louis, 1992, Mosby.

aerobic metabolism. It may be measured directly or calculated from arterial and venous blood samples. Normal $\dot{V}O_2$ is approximately one fourth of oxygen delivery in adults but constitutes a greater portion of oxygen delivery in children, averaging 120 to 230 ml/min/m^2 BSA (5 to 8 ml/kg/min) in the infant or child. This means that infants and children have a very small oxygen reserve. Sepsis, fever, pain, burns, and trauma increase $\dot{V}O_2$ and may result in decompensation.

Oxyhemoglobin Dissociation Curve

The relationship between PaO$_2$ and hemoglobin saturation is not a linear one; it is depicted by an S-shaped curve—the oxyhemoglobin dissociation curve (Figure 6-5). The curve contains a relatively flat portion and a relatively vertical portion.

The oxyhemoglobin dissociation curve flattens once the PaO$_2$ exceeds 80 to 100 mm Hg. At this point, the hemoglobin is almost completely saturated, and further increases in PaO$_2$ will not contribute substantially to the hemoglobin saturation or the oxygen content of blood because further increases will only contribute a small amount of oxygen dissolved in plasma (the hemoglobin is fully saturated). For example, increasing the PaO$_2$ from 100 to 300 mm Hg increases the CaO$_2$ from 18.33 ml/dl to 18.9 ml/dl—an increase of only 3% (assuming a hemoglobin concentration of 13.5 g/dl). Therefore an increase in PaO$_2$ >80 to 100 mm Hg will not significantly increase arterial oxygen content.

The oxyhemoglobin dissociation curve becomes relatively vertical when the PaO$_2$ is less than 60 mm Hg. At this point, even small decreases in the PaO$_2$ are associated with significant drops in hemoglobin saturation and arterial oxygen content.

It may be helpful to recall two important points regarding the oxyhemoglobin dissociation curve:

1. *At a normal pH, a hemoglobin saturation of 97% correlates with a PaO$_2$ of 95 mm Hg.*
2. *At a normal pH, a hemoglobin saturation of 90% correlates with a PaO$_2$ of 60 mm Hg.*

Condition 1 should correspond with an adequate oxygen content if the hemoglobin content is adequate. Condition 2 indicates the presence of hypoxemia and can only be associated with an adequate oxygen content if hemoglobin concentration is unusually high (e.g., the child with cyanotic heart disease and polycythemia).

The oxyhemoglobin dissociation curve will shift to the left or right in response to changes in body temperature, PaCO$_2$, arterial pH, or 2,3-diphosphoglycerate (2,3-DPG) in the blood. These factors can change the relationship between the PaO$_2$ and the hemoglobin saturation.

Shift to Left   The hemoglobin is better saturated at a lower PaO$_2$, but oxygen is more tightly bound

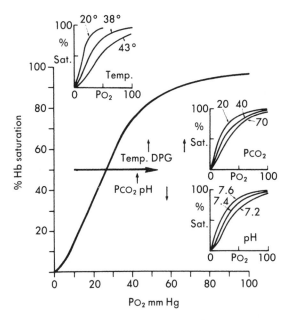

Figure 6-5 Oxyhemoglobin dissociation curve. The inset curves demonstrate shifts in the dissociation curve that result from the changes in temperature, $Paco_2$, and pH. In addition, a decrease in 2,3-diphosphoglycerate (DPG) (which is present in the neonate with large amounts of fetal hemoglobin) shifts the dissociation curve to the left, whereas an increase in 2,3,-DPG (such as occurs in children with cyanotic heart disease and polycythemia) shifts the curve to the right. (From West JB: Gas transport to the periphery. In West JB: *Respiratory physiology: the essentials,* ed 2, Baltimore, 1980, Williams & Wilkins.)

to the hemoglobin; thus oxygen release to the tissues may be impaired. Potential causes include alkalosis (rise in pH), hyperventilation (fall in $Paco_2$), or fetal hemoglobin (decreased 2,3-DPG). In an alkalotic patient a hemoglobin saturation of 90% to 93% may be associated with an adequate arterial oxygen content but significant hypoxemia (Pao_2 <60 mm Hg).

Shift to Right   The hemoglobin is less well saturated at a given Pao_2 but is also readily released to the tissues. Potential causes include acidosis (fall in pH), hypercarbia (rise in $Paco_2$, or cyanotic heart disease (increased 2,3-DPG). In a severely acidotic

patient a higher Pao_2 will be required to produce an adequate hemoglobin saturation.

Ventilation and Acid-Base Balance

Carbon dioxide is carried in the blood bound to hemoglobin or in the dissolved form. In addition, carbon dioxide may react with water to form carbonic anhydrase, or it may combine with other proteins to form carbamino compounds. Unlike the curvilinear relationship between Po_2 and the arterial oxygen content, the relationship between the $Paco_2$ and the arterial carbon dioxide content is linear.

The $Paco_2$ is directly proportional to the carbon dioxide production in the body and inversely proportional to alveolar ventilation. This has important potential consequences when interpreting the $Paco_2$, particularly in intubated patients. For example, if the patient's alveolar ventilation doubles and carbon dioxide production is constant, the $Paco_2$ will be halved. If the patient's $Paco_2$ doubles when carbon dioxide production is constant, alveolar ventilation has decreased by 50%. If carbon dioxide production increases by 50% and ventilation is fixed, the $Paco_2$ will increase by 50%.

Respiratory Acidosis   Respiratory acidosis is a fall in pH caused by hypercarbia. As the arterial Pco_2 ($Paco_2$) increases, carbon dioxide combines with water to form H_2CO_3 (carbonic acid), which then dissociates into bicarbonate ion and hydrogen ion. As more hydrogen ion is produced, acidosis results. If this condition persists for several hours or days, the kidneys will partially compensate by retaining bicarbonate to restore the pH to near-normal levels.

Metabolic alkalosis can be caused by excessive diuretic therapy in critically ill patients without adequate electrolyte intake. Metabolic alkalosis will stimulate a decrease in alveolar ventilation; thus the $Paco_2$ rises; this will begin to correct the pH to near-normal levels but represents a problem that requires treatment.

Respiratory Alkalosis   Respiratory alkalosis is a rise in pH resulting from hyperventilation and hypocarbia. As ventilation increases, hydrogen ion is eliminated. This increase in ventilation may partially compensate for the development of metabolic acidosis.

Common Clinical Conditions

Airway Obstruction

Etiology/Pathophysiology

Upper airway obstruction may result from congenital airway malformations, obstruction of the pharynx by the tongue (in the unconscious patient), aspiration of a foreign body, vocal cord weakness, enlarged tonsils, edema, or inflammation. Upper airway obstruction following extubation may produce symptoms that begin within hours after extubation and peak within 6 to 24 hours after extubation. Lower airway obstruction may be caused by airway edema, inflammation, or airway constriction.

Airway narrowing reduces the airway radius and increases resistance to airflow. If airflow (ventilation) is to be maintained, work of breathing must increase. Resistance to airflow is greater when airflow is turbulent (e.g., during crying or labored breathing) than when airflow is laminar (e.g., during quiet breathing).

Clinical Presentation

The child may compensate for a mild airway obstruction by increasing the work of breathing, so that minute ventilation remains unchanged. If, however, airway obstruction is severe, or if the child's level of consciousness is depressed, effective ventilation can be compromised, producing hypoventilation and respiratory failure. Most patients with airway obstruction demonstrate increased respiratory effort. Hypercarbia may be present, but *hypoxemia does not develop until alveolar ventilation falls.* The site and severity of airway obstruction can often be identified from the patient's clinical signs and symptoms.

Upper Airway Obstruction   Clinical signs may include inspiratory stridor, prolonged inspiratory time, and possible hoarseness and drooling. The child is often more comfortable sitting forward, and respiratory distress and agitation increase when the child is supine. The pitch of the infant's cry or voice may be altered.

Lower Airway Obstruction   Clinical signs include expiratory wheezing and prolonged expiratory time.

Mild to Moderate Airway Obstruction   Clinical signs include tachypnea, tachycardia, restlessness, and use of accessory muscles of respiration (respiratory distress). Stridor or wheezing may also be present.

Profound Airway Obstruction With Respiratory Failure   Clinical signs may include altered level of consciousness, slowing of the respiratory rate, decreased air movement, apnea or gasping, compromise in systemic perfusion, and bradycardia. Wheezing or stridor may be severe or may disappear as air movement decreases.

Management

Positioning   If the child is awake, allow the child to assume the most comfortable position. If the child is unconscious, position the child with neck extended. If the tongue obstructs the pharynx, an oral airway (for use in unconscious patients only) or a nasopharyngeal airway may be used. *Do not insert an airway if epiglottitis is suspected.*

Oxygen Administration   Administer warmed, humidified oxygen by face mask, hood, tent, or "blow-by" tubing if respiratory distress is present. Monitor the heart rate and pulse oximetry continuously, and keep the child warm and comfortable. Minimize stimulation. Note that the pulse oximeter may *not* provide an early indication of deterioration, since hypoxemia may be only a *late* sign of deterioration.

Inhalation Therapy   Racemic epinephrine (which reduces airway wall edema) may reduce upper airway obstruction related to edema or inflammation. Inhaled bronchodilators (e.g., albuterol and terbutaline) relax airway smooth muscle and are used to treat lower airway constriction (see Status Asthmaticus under Specific Diseases).

If the child with upper airway obstruction does not require high levels of supplemental oxygen, heliox may be administered to reduce the work of breathing, lessen fatigue, and possibly prevent the need for intubation. Heliox is a mixture of helium and oxygen, generally in a 70% helium/30% oxygen mixture. Since helium has a lower viscosity than oxygen or room air, it will flow readily through narrowed airways.

Response to Therapy If the child's airway obstruction is relieved by inhalation treatments, there will be a decrease in respiratory effort; improvement in color, systemic perfusion, oxyhemoglobin saturation, and responsiveness; reduction in agitation; and reduction in stridor or wheezing. *Deterioration* is present if the child's level of consciousness deteriorates or if air exchange decreases. If the respiratory rate and work of breathing decrease *despite* the continued presence of severe obstruction, the child may be tiring, and respiratory arrest may be imminent.

Indications for Intubation Elective intubation is always preferable to urgent intubation of the gasping child. The decision to intubate should be made if *clinical* signs of severe respiratory distress (poor color, altered level of consciousness, compromise in systemic perfusion) or signs of significant increase in the work of breathing or fatigue are observed. Occasionally attempts are made to support the child during a period of temporary airway obstruction, such as following extubation, if the child is closely monitored and emergency equipment is at the bedside. However, all members of the health care team should appreciate the child's critical status and identify clinical criteria for intubation.

Upper airway obstruction due to *epiglottitis* is a medical emergency. Keep the child comfortable, minimize stimulation, and plan for immediate intubation by an experienced practitioner, preferably in the operating room (see Epiglottitis under Specific Diseases).

If signs of acute deterioration are observed (slowing of the respiratory rate, bradycardia, or poor air exchange), perform hand ventilation with bag-valve-mask until intubation can be performed.

Suctioning Pulmonary secretions may produce airway obstruction and must be eliminated. This may be accomplished in several ways.

Stimulation of Cough A cough clears secretions more effectively than suctioning and should be encouraged. It may be stimulated by insertion of a catheter into the back of the pharynx of the nonintubated child. Suction may be applied to remove secretions if an effective cough results. This maneuver may produce further irritation to the larynx and *should not be performed if croup or epiglottitis is present*. It may also stimulate a gag reflex and vomiting.

Suctioning the Nonintubated Child Two people will be required to suction the unstable or resistant child. A sterile glove and catheter (see Table 6-1 for selection of catheter size), and sterile technique are required. Administer oxygen by "blow-by" tubing before, during, and immediately after the suction attempt. Apply water-soluble lubricant to the catheter before insertion. Be prepared to interrupt the suctioning and administer oxygen if the child develops bradycardia, deterioration in color or pulse oximetry, or gagging.

Hold the child's head securely, and gently introduce the catheter into the nose, toward the inferior, posterior, medial aspect of the nostril. It is helpful to gently rotate the catheter to facilitate entrance into the posterior pharynx. If the catheter does not pass freely into the nasopharynx, remove it and attempt suctioning of the other nostril.

Advance the catheter into the nasopharynx until a cough is stimulated. Apply suction to the catheter (see Table 6-1 for suction strength) as you gently rotate and withdraw the catheter. If repeated suctioning is required, allow the child to rest and

---

Table 6-1
Suction Catheter Sizes and Negative Pressure Limits for Suctioning the Nonintubated Child

Age	Size of Catheter (French)	Maximum Negative Pressure (cm H_2O)
Newborn	5-6½	−60 to −90
6 mo	8	−60 to −90
1 yr	8-10	−60 to −90
2 yr	10	−90 to −110
5 yr	12	−90 to −110
≥10 yr	12-14	−110 to −150

Modified from Hazinski MF: *Nursing care of the critically ill child*, ed 2, St Louis, 1992, Mosby.

administer oxygen before each attempt. If frequent nasal suctioning is required, consider insertion of a nasal airway; these soft rubber tubes will decrease trauma to the nasopharyngeal mucosa during suctioning.

Acid-Base Disorders

Etiology/Pathophysiology

Acid-base disorders may result from respiratory or metabolic problems and may affect many organs. These disorders are identified through arterial blood gas analysis. The practitioner must be able to interpret primary and compensatory arterial blood gas changes and be prepared to initiate appropriate treatment.

Primary acid-base disorders must be separated from *secondary* or *compensatory* acid-base disorders. Respiratory compensation for metabolic abnormalities can begin immediately if the patient is breathing spontaneously and has effective CNS function. Renal compensation for respiratory acidosis or alkalosis begins if the abnormality persists beyond 6 to 24 hours. *Compensatory mechanisms will attempt to restore the pH to near-normal levels but will **never** "overcorrect" the pH.*

Definitions of Terms

- *pH:* A reflection of blood hydrogen ion concentration. Normal: 7.4 (range: 7.35 to 7.45).
- *Acidosis:* An arterial pH <7.35.
- *Alkalosis:* An arterial pH >7.45.
- *Hypoxemia:* Pao_2 <80 mm Hg when patient is breathing room air at sea level.
- *Hypercapnia/hypercarbia:* $Paco_2$ >45 mm Hg.
- *HCO_3^-:* Body bicarbonate, regulated by the lungs (through carbon dioxide removal) and by the kidneys (through hydrogen ion and bicarbonate excretion or absorption). Normal HCO_3^- is 22 to 28 mEq/L. The bicarbonate concentration is increased with metabolic alkalosis (or metabolic compensation for respiratory acidosis) and decreased with metabolic acidosis (or metabolic compensation for respiratory alkalosis).
- *Base deficit:* A calculated number that represents the theoretic deficit of base (or excess of acid) present. A significant base deficit (more negative

than −2) indicates the presence of metabolic acidosis.
- *Base excess:* A calculated number that expresses the theoretic excess of base present (reflects metabolic alkalosis). A significant base excess (>+2) indicates metabolic alkalosis.

Clinical Presentation: Arterial Blood Gas Analysis

The clinical signs and symptoms of acid-base imbalance relate more to the underlying pathology than to the actual acid-base abnormality. Arterial blood gas analysis is performed if an imbalance is suspected. Systematic arterial blood gas analysis and prediction of the pH from the $Paco_2$ is described in Box 6-2.

Respiratory Acidosis   A primary decrease in alveolar ventilation raises the $Paco_2$ and lowers the arterial pH. Common causes include airway obstruction, central depression of respiratory drive, or respiratory muscle weakness. Renal compensation will begin within 6 to 8 hours, resulting in bicarbonate retention and a return of the pH toward normal within approximately 24 to 48 hours.

Case Study 1

A 9-month-old boy with bronchopulmonary dysplasia is admitted with a right upper lobe infiltrate and fever. Respiratory rate is 60/min. Arterial blood gas analysis in room air:

> pH: 7.33
> $Paco_2$: 72 mm Hg
> Pao_2: 52 mm Hg
> Hco_3^-: 39 mEq/L
> Base excess: +15

Interpretation: Chronic respiratory acidosis related to bronchopulmonary dysplasia. The pH is predicted from the $Paco_2$:

$$72 \text{ mm Hg} - 40 \text{ mm Hg} = 32$$
$$32 \times 0.008 = 0.256$$
$$7.4 - 0.256 = 7.14$$

Since the acidosis is not as severe as that predicted from the $Paco_2$, renal compensation has produced a metabolic alkalosis that has corrected the pH to near normal. Oxygen

Box 6-2

Systematic Arterial Blood Gas Analysis

1. Determine if the pH is acidotic, alkalotic, or normal. For simplicity, a normal pH of 7.4 is used (acidosis = pH < 7.4; alkalosis = pH > 7.4).
2. Determine if hypocarbia or hypercarbia is present. For simplicity, a normal $Paco_2$ of 40 mm Hg is used (hypercarbia = $Paco_2$ >40 mm Hg; hypocarbia = $Paco_2$ <40 mm Hg).
3. *If hypercarbia is present,* evaluate the contribution of the $Paco_2$ to the change in pH:
   a. Subtract 40 from patient's $Paco_2$.
   b. Multiply the number obtained in *a* by 0.008.
   c. Subtract the number obtained in *b* from 7.4; the resulting number is the pH predicted from the $Paco_2$.
      (1) If the patient's pH is *lower* than the predicted pH, metabolic acidosis is complicating the hypercarbia.
      (2) If the patient's pH is *higher* than the predicted pH, metabolic alkalosis (or renal compensation for respiratory acidosis) must be present.
4. *If hypocarbia is present,* evaluate the contribution of the $PaCO_2$ to the pH:
   a. Subtract the patient's $Paco_2$ from 40.
   b. Multiply the number obtained in *a* by 0.008.
   c. Add the product obtained in *b* to 7.4; the resulting number is the pH predicted from the $Paco_2$.
      (1) If the patient's pH is *higher* than the predicted pH, metabolic alkalosis must be associated with the hypocarbia.
      (2) If the patient's pH is *lower* than the predicted pH, metabolic acidosis must be associated with the hypocarbia.
5. Calculate base deficit
   a. If the patient's pH is lower than the pH predicted from the $Paco_2$, a metabolic acidosis must be present:
      (1) Subtract the predicted pH from the patient's pH (a negative number will result).
      (2) Multiply the product of *(1)* by 66. This negative number (more negative than is −2) indicates a metabolic acidosis.
   b. If the patient's pH is *higher* than the predicted pH from the $Paco_2$, a metabolic alkalosis must be present.
      (1) Subtract the predicted pH from the patient's pH (a positive number will result).
      (2) Multiply the product of *(1)* by 66. This positive number (more positive than +2) indicates a metabolic alkalosis.

---

therapy is indicated to correct the hypoxemia, but the child's ventilation is probably his baseline; therefore mechanical ventilation is probably not necessary unless his condition deteriorates.

Case Study 2

A 7-year-old child is hospitalized for an emergency appendectomy. One hour postoperatively, she is deeply asleep and difficult to arouse, with a respiratory rate of 12/min. Arterial blood gases in room air:

pH: 7.21
$Paco_2$: 64 mm Hg

Pao_2: 73 mm Hg
HCO_3^-: 25 mEq/L
Base excess: +1

Interpretation: Acute respiratory acidosis caused by hypoventilation. Note that the rise in $Paco_2$ is comparable in magnitude to the fall in the Pao_2. The pH is predicted from the $Paco_2$:

$$64 \text{ mm Hg} - 40 \text{ mm Hg} = 24$$
$$24 \times 0.008 = 0.192$$
$$7.4 - 0.192 = 7.21$$

The pH is exactly as predicted from the $Paco_2$, confirming the clinical impression of pure respiratory acidosis, resulting from hypoventilation caused by anesthesia. Alveolar ventilation must be increased. If the child cannot be awakened, administration of naloxone may be necessary. If spontaneous ventilation cannot be increased, mechanical ventilation may be required.

Respiratory Alkalosis Primary respiratory alkalosis results from an increase in alveolar ventilation, which lowers the $Paco_2$ and raises the pH. This uncommon problem may result from a response to hypoxia or from CNS disease or injury, salicylate intoxication, or overly aggressive mechanical ventilatory support. Renal compensation will begin within 6 to 8 hours, resulting in hydrogen ion retention and a return of the pH toward normal within approximately 24 to 48 hours.

Case Study 3

A 16-year-old with leukemia in remission is admitted with tachypnea (respiratory rate: 60/min) and fever. Chest radiographs reveal bilateral interstitial infiltrates. Arterial blood gases on room air:

> pH: 7.49
> $Paco_2$: 30 mm Hg
> Pao_2: 50 mm Hg
> HCO_3^-: 25 mEq/L
> Base excess: +1

Interpretation: Acute respiratory alkalosis and hyperventilation resulting from severe hypoxemia. The pH is predicted from the $Paco_2$:

> 40 mm Hg − 29 mm Hg = 11
> 11 × 0.008 = 0.088
> 7.4 + 0.088 = 7.488 = 7.49

The alkalosis (rise in pH above normal) results entirely from the fall in $Paco_2$. Oxygen therapy is indicated; if the hypoxemia is corrected, the respiratory rate, $Paco_2$, and pH may return to normal.

Metabolic Acidosis This condition results from a primary gain in acid (e.g., diabetic ketoacidosis or lactic acidosis), a fall in cardiac output, or a loss of bicarbonate ions (e.g., diarrhea) and results in a fall

in pH. If the patient is breathing spontaneously and has good CNS control of ventilation, the respiratory rate and alveolar ventilation will increase, resulting in a fall in the $Paco_2$ and a return of the pH toward normal. If the patient is sedated or ventilation is controlled or compromised, or if acidosis is severe, effective respiratory compensation cannot occur.

Case Study 4

A 6-month-old infant is admitted with 10% dehydration. He is extremely ill, lethargic, and pale, with a respiratory rate of 48/min. Arterial blood gases in room air:

> pH: 7.2
> $Paco_2$: 22 mm Hg
> Pao_2: 98 mm Hg
> HCO_3^-: 8 mEq/L
> Base deficit: −22

Interpretation: Metabolic acidosis resulting from dehydration. Respiratory compensation has partially corrected the pH, since a higher pH is predicted from the $Paco_2$:

> 40 mm Hg − 22 mm Hg = 18
> 18 × 0.008 = 0.144
> 7.4 + 0.144 = 7.54

The predicted pH from the $Paco_2$ is 7.54. The pH of 7.2 indicates metabolic acidosis, confirmed by the base deficit of −22 and the low serum bicarbonate. Treatment requires rehydration and support of ventilation if deterioration occurs.

Metabolic Alkalosis This condition results from a loss of acid (e.g., persistent vomiting) or a gain in base (e.g., hypochloremia causing renal bicarbonate retention). If the patient is breathing spontaneously, the respiratory rate and alveolar ventilation decrease; thus the $Paco_2$ increases and the pH returns toward normal. If the patient is sedated or ventilation is controlled, such compensation cannot occur.

Case Study 5

An 8-month-old infant with bronchopulmonary dysplasia is admitted to the ICU with a fever and lethargy. The infant is irritable, with dry skin and mucous membranes, and a respiratory rate of 30/min. The infant has been receiving furosemide 15 mg bid, and the mother states that she "ran out" of potassium chloride supplements last week. Arterial blood gases in room air:

pH: 7.55
$Paco_2$: 80 mm Hg
Pao_2: 80 mm Hg
HCO_3^-: 41 mEq/L
Base excess: +31

Interpretation: Chronic respiratory failure by history. The pH predicted from the $Paco_2$:

$$80 \text{ mm Hg} - 40 \text{ mm Hg} = 40$$
$$40 \times 0.008 = 0.32$$
$$7.4 - 0.32 = 7.08$$

A pH of 7.08 is predicted from the $Paco_2$. Although renal compensation may restore the pH to near normal, it will not "overcorrect" the pH to 7.55, so an additional cause of metabolic alkalosis must be present. The child's serum chloride was 88 mEq/L, and potassium was 3 mEq/L. This represents a hypochloremic and hypokalemic metabolic alkalosis; in retaining the chloride and potassium, the kidneys also retain bicarbonate and excrete hydrogen ion. The child's respiratory rate has actually decreased in an attempt to retain carbon dioxide and restore the pH to near normal. Treatment requires potassium chloride administration.

Management

Treatment of acid-base imbalance requires treatment of the underlying condition, correction of any electrolyte imbalance present, and support of oxygenation and ventilation, as needed. The child must be closely monitored to detect any deterioration and to evaluate response to therapy.

Respiratory Failure

Etiology/Pathophysiology

Respiratory failure is clinically characterized by inadequate oxygenation or ventilation. Historically, the diagnosis of respiratory failure has been con-

firmed using arterial blood gas analysis. However, *potential* respiratory failure should be identified in the child with increasing respiratory distress, and therapy may be required *before* the results of blood gas analysis are available. The diagnosis of respiratory failure can be confirmed if the child fails to respond to therapy, the child's condition deteriorates, or blood gas analysis reveals hypoxemia despite oxygen therapy, hypercarbia with acidosis, or a significant intrapulmonary shunt.

Virtually any critically ill or injured child is at risk for the development of respiratory failure. Potential causes of respiratory failure are provided in Box 6-3.

Most forms of respiratory failure are associated with a mismatching of ventilation and perfusion in the lung alveoli. Typical causes are obstruction of alveoli or airways, or a compromise of oxygen diffusion caused by pulmonary edema. These changes result in a reduction in the patient's functional

---

Box 6-3

Major Components of the Respiratory System and Potential Contribution to the Development of Respiratory Failure

Central nervous system control of ventilation: Immature in neonates; may be depressed by drugs (narcotics, barbiturates, anesthetics); may be impaired in presence of central nervous system disease, insult, or injury.

Airways: May be compromised by mucus accumulation, edema, airway constriction or closure, or airway compression. Artificial airways may become occluded or displaced.

Chest wall: May retract during episodes of respiratory distress, causing fatigue; should expand during application of positive pressure ventilation, but this may result in creation of excessive inspiratory force.

Respiratory muscles: May lack tone, power, and coordination. Any compromise in diaphragm movement or function is likely to cause hypoventilation.

Lung tissue: Pulmonary edema is likely to develop if respiratory disease or inflammation is present.

residual capacity and lung compliance; increased work of breathing; and hypoxemia, hypercarbia or both.

Clinical Presentation

Clinical Signs As noted above, a diagnosis of *potential* respiratory failure is made when signs of *respiratory distress* are observed, including tachycardia, tachypnea, increased work of breathing (retractions, nasal flaring, grunting), cyanosis or deterioration in color, altered level of consciousness, or poor systemic perfusion. These signs may indicate the need for immediate intervention.

If the respiratory or heart rate is abnormally *slow* for the patient's clinical condition, or if air entry is inadequate, deterioration is occurring. It may be necessary to institute emergency support of oxygenation and ventilation.

Physiologic Criteria Physiologic criteria used to confirm or quantify the severity of respiratory failure include hypoxemia despite oxygen therapy, hypercarbia with acidosis, and evidence of a significant pulmonary shunt (Box 6-4). These classic criteria of respiratory failure must be individually modified, however, based on the patient's baseline condition (Box 6-5). Typically these criteria are used to evaluate *trends* in status or response to therapy over time.

The *intrapulmonary shunt* can be quantified in a number of ways. It may be estimated using a shunt diagram (Figure 6-6), or by calculation of the oxygenation index ([mean airway pressure $\times$ $Fio_2 \times 100$]/Pao_2) or calculation of the Pao_2/Fio_2 ratio (should be <175 to 280 mm Hg). Occasionally the intrapulmonary shunt fraction may be calculated (Box 6-6). A significant difference between inspired oxygen and the child's arterial oxygen tension is present when perfusion of nonventilated alveoli occurs.

Pulse Oximetry Pulse oximetry allows continuous noninvasive evaluation of hemoglobin *saturation*. To determine the child's Pao_2 from pulse oximetry, the oxyhemoglobin dissociation curve must be considered (see Figure 6-5). An important relationship to remember is that *an oxyhemoglobin saturation of 90% will be associated with a* Pao_2 *of only 60 mm Hg.*

The pulse oximeter includes a photodetector with two (red and infrared) light-emitting diodes; the photodetector is aligned across a pulsatile tissue bed from the diodes. A microprocessor determines relative absorption of the red and infrared forms of light. Based on different lightabsorptive characteristics of oxygenated (saturated) and unoxygenated (desaturated) hemoglobin, the percent of oxygenated hemoglobin in the tissue bed is determined. The pulse oximeter module also provides a visual indicator of pulse strength and a digital display of the pulse rate. Audible high and low hemoglobin saturation and heart rate alarms must be set.

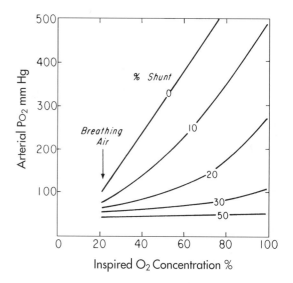

Figure 6-6 Relationship between inspired oxygen concentration and arterial oxygen tension with changing severity of intrapulmonary shunt. By comparing the patient's Fio_2 to the Pao_2, the percentage of nonfunctioning but perfused alveoli (i.e., the shunt) can be determined. Note that once the intrapulmonary shunt nears 50%, increasing the inspired oxygen concentration will produce little improvement in Pao_2; at this point, treatment must improve alveolar ventilation and/or the ventilation-perfusion ratio through the use of positive end-expiratory pressure (PEEP). Changes in cardiac output, oxygen uptake, etc., can influence the position of the shunt curves. (From West JB: *Pulmonary pathophysiology: the essentials,* ed 2, Baltimore, 1980, Williams & Wilkins.)

Box 6-4

Clinical and Physiologic Criteria of Acute Respiratory Failure

Clinical Criteria

Severe increase in respiratory effort, including severe retractions or grunting, decreased chest movement
Depressed level of consciousness
Cyanosis despite supplemental oxygen therapy
Absent or significantly decreased breath sounds
Cardiovascular signs of distress (including extreme tachypnea, peripheral vasoconstriction, mottled color)
Late signs: apnea or gasping, agonal respirations, bradycardia, or hypotension

Physiologic Criteria

Hypoxemia despite supplemental oxygen therapy (e.g., Pao_2 <75 mm Hg despite Fio_2 of 1.0)
Hypercarbia (arterial $Paco_2$ >50-75 mm Hg)
Rising oxygenation index (OI):

$$OI = \frac{(\text{Mean airway pressure in cm } H_2O) \times Fio_2 \times 100}{Pao_2}$$

OI >10 is significant, and OI > 25-35 for several hours indicates severe respiratory failure.
Falling Pao_2/Fio_2:
  Divide the arterial Po_2 by the child's fractional inspired oxygen (Fio_2). Remember that the Fio_2 is a decimal. If the number is <175-280 mm Hg, a significant shunt is present.
  Example: Pao_2 is 80 mm Hg when patient is receiving Fio_2 of 0.8 (80% oxygen).

$$Pao_2/Fio_2 = 80 \text{ mm Hg}/0.8 = 100 \text{ mm Hg}$$

  A significant shunt is present
Rising alveolar-arterial oxygen difference or gradient (A-a Do_2):

$$
\begin{aligned}
\text{A-a } Do_2 &= \text{Alveolar oxygen tension} - \text{Arterial oxygen tension} \\
&= PAo_2 \qquad\qquad\qquad - Pao_2 \\
&= [Fio_2 \text{ (Barometric pressure} - 47 \text{ mm Hg)} - Paco_2] - Pao_2
\end{aligned}
$$

Normal is <25-20 mm Hg.
Example: Pao_2 is 80 mm Hg and $Paco_2$ is 40 mm Hg when patient is receiving Fio_2 of 0.6 at sea level (barometric pressure is 760 mm Hg).

$$
\begin{aligned}
\text{A-a } Do_2 &= [0.6 \ (760 \text{ mm Hg} - 47 \text{ mm Hg)} - 40 \text{ mm Hg}] - 80 \text{ mm Hg} \\
&= [(0.6 \times 713 \text{ mm Hg)} - 40 \text{ mm Hg}] \qquad\quad - 80 \text{ mm Hg} \\
&= 388 \text{ mm Hg} \qquad\qquad\qquad\qquad\qquad\quad - 80 \text{ mm Hg} \\
&= 308 \text{ mm Hg}
\end{aligned}
$$

Rising arterial-venous oxygen difference (a-v Do_2):

$$\text{a-v } Do_2 = \text{Arterial oxygen content } (Cao_2) - \text{Mixed venous oxygen content } (C\bar{v}o_2)$$

Typically performed after patient has received Fio_2 of 1 for 15+ min. Normal is approximately 5 ml/100 dl.

Modified from Hazinski MF: *Nursing care of the critically ill child,* ed 2, St Louis, 1992, Mosby.

Box 6-5

Clinical and Physiologic Criteria for Diagnosis of Respiratory Failure in Children with Cardiopulmonary or Neuromuscular Disease

Respiratory Failure in the Child With Chronic Lung Disease

Development of acidosis

Significant increase in work of breathing

Hypoxemia or hypercarbia exceeding the child's "normal" range

Compromise in systemic perfusion (cool extremities, mottled color)

Depressed level of consciousness

Late signs: apnea or gasping, bradycardia

Respiratory Failure in the Child With Cyanotic Congenital Heart Disease

Development of metabolic acidosis

Hypoxemia exceeding the patient's "normal" range

Severe retractions or grunting

Development of hypercarbia

Late signs: apnea or gasping, compromise in systemic perfusion, bradycardia

Respiratory Failure in the Child With Neuromuscular Disease

Severe increase in respiratory effort

Weak cough, incompetent swallow or gag

Use of accessory muscles of respiration

Tidal volume <4-5 ml/kg (normal is 6-7 ml/kg)

Negative inspiratory force < -20 cm H_2O (normal is -75 to -100 cm H_2O, and forceful cough is thought to require at least -25 cm H_2O)

Vital capacity <15-20 cc/kg (normal is 65-75 cc/kg)

Respiratory Failure in the Child With Acute Exacerbation of Asthma

Peak expiratory flow rate <50% of predicted or personal best

Respiratory rate >50% above mean

Decreased alertness/responsiveness

Severe dyspnea (short phrases or single words spoken, weak cry)

Severe retractions, nasal flaring, pulsus paradoxus >20 mm Hg

Decreased breath sounds

Cyanosis, oxyhemoglobin saturation <90%

Potential hypercarbia

Modified from Hazinski MF: *Nursing care of the critically ill child,* ed 2, St Louis, 1992, Mosby.

For pulse oximetry to be useful, the signal must be strong and movement artifact must be minimized. *For the oximeter to be accurate, the heart rate detected by oximetry should be identical to the patient's heart rate.* Bedside calibration of the oximeter is not required.

Pulse oximeters are accurate over a wide range of hemoglobin saturations. However, the response time of these units to acute changes in hemoglobin saturation may vary widely. The oximeters do not recognize carboxyhemoglobin or methemoglobin and will ignore these types of hemoglobin, if present, and calculate the hemoglobin saturation as a percentage of remaining normal hemoglobin. As a result, pulse oximetry will provide an inaccurately high hemoglobin saturation for children with carbon monoxide poisoning and methemoglobinemia.

If cardiac output is normal and hemoglobin concentration is adequate, a hemoglobin saturation above 93% to 95% will be associated with adequate oxygen delivery (and a PaO_2 greater than 70 mm Hg). However, if the child's pH is maintained in the *alkalotic* range, a hemoglobin saturation below 93% to 95% will usually be associated with significant hypoxemia (PaO_2 less than 60 mm Hg), such as may develop with obstruction or displacement of the endotracheal tube. Remember, a saturation of 90% indicates mild hypoxemia (PaO_2 of 60 mm Hg) if the pH is normal. Also note that oxygen delivery can be inadequate despite a hemoglobin saturation >95% if anemia or low cardiac output is present.

Management

When *potential* respiratory failure is present, frequently evaluate the child's airway, oxygenation,

Box 6-6

Calculations to Determine Severity of Shunt

To "guesstimate" the Pa_{O_2} that should result from a given inspired oxygen, multiply the Fi_{O_2} by 500.

Example: Fi_{O_2} of 0.4 (40% oxygen) should produce a Pa_{O_2} of 200 mm Hg:

$$(0.4) \times 500 = 200 \text{ mm Hg}$$

If the Pa_{O_2} is <200 mm Hg, a significant shunt is likely to be present.

Intrapulmonary shunt fraction (Qs = flow across right-to-left shunt, Qt = cardiac output):

$$\frac{Qs}{Qt} = \frac{\text{(A-a gradient)} \times 0.003}{\text{(a-v } D_{O_2}) + \text{(A-a gradient} \times 0.003)}$$

Table 6-2
Oxygen Delivery Systems

Mode	O_2 Flow Supplied (L/min)	% Fi_{O_2} Delivered
Low-Flow Oxygen Systems		
Nasal cannula	⅛-2 (infants) 1-6 (children)	24-44
Vented O_2 mask	5-8*	24-44
Mask with reservoir	6-10*	60-99
High-Flow Oxygen Systems		
Venturi mask	As per flow valve	24-50
Nebulizer	8-10 L	30-100
Oxygen tent	15 L	24-100†
Oxygen hood	10-14 L	24-40

Modified from Johns Hopkins Hospital Department of Pediatrics: *The Harriet Lane handbook*, ed 13, edited by Johnson KB, St Louis, 1993, Mosby; data from Rogers M: Textbook of pediatric intensive care, ed 2, Baltimore, 1992, Williams & Wilkins.
*Airflows >5 L/min are required to wash out expired air from mask space.
†O_2 concentration may vary by as much as 20% from the top to the bottom of the hood.

ventilation, perfusion, and work, rate, and pattern of breathing. Administer oxygen and monitor the heart rate and pulse oximetry continuously. Position the child for maximal comfort and to provide the best oxygenation.

The goal of therapy for respiratory failure is to *maximize oxygen delivery and eliminate sufficient carbon dioxide;* this is accomplished by increasing arterial oxygen content while supporting cardiac output and ventilation. In addition, the child's *oxygen demand should be controlled:* treat fever and pain, and prevent shivering and cold stress. Minimize intrusive examinations and treatments, and encourage the parents to remain at the bedside as much as is feasible, to comfort the child.

Oxygen Administration Hypoxemia is treated with administration of warmed, humidified oxygen. Mechanical ventilation may not be required, provided that the child's respiratory effort and ventilation (reflected by the child's Pa_{CO_2}) are acceptable. Monitor and record the concentration of inspired oxygen carefully, and determine the child's response.

Methods of Oxygen Delivery If the child is unstable and cardiorespiratory deterioration has occurred, administer oxygen in the highest concentration possible. It may be necessary to support ventilation with a bag-valve-mask device (see Bag-Valve-Mask

Ventilation). If the child's respiratory effort is acceptable, supplemental oxygen may be delivered through a head hood, mask, partial or nonrebreathing mask, nasal cannula, or tent. The method of delivery is determined by the inspired oxygen required and the child's tolerance of the equipment (Table 6-2).

Oxygen Therapy With Continuous Positive Airway Pressure CPAP may be used to improve oxygenation if the patient's respiratory effort and ventilation (carbon dioxide elimination) are acceptable. CPAP will open collapsed alveoli and will move edema fluid to harmless areas of the lung. This therapy should reduce the ventilation-perfusion mismatch, reducing the alveolar-arterial oxygen gradient and improving the Pa_{O_2}.

Noninvasive Positive-Pressure Ventilation, Bilevel Positive Airway Pressure (BiPAP) BiPAP provides positive-pressure ventilatory support and continuous positive airway pressure through a nasal mask, nasal pillows, or a face mask. This form of ventilatory support does not require intubation and can be particularly useful for the treatment of chronic ventilatory failure or following weaning from mechanical ventilation. It is also used for the support of children with sleep apnea. BiPAP may be delivered by a volume- or pressure-controlled ventilator, a BiPAP circuit, or a CPAP circuit. The nasal mask, nasal pillows, or a face mask used as the patient—circuit interface should be fit securely to prevent air leaks at this interface. The ventilator provides continuous high gas flow at a pre-scribed inspired oxygen concentration and maintains positive airway pressure that cycles between high and lower positive airway pressure (hence the name "bilevel PAP"). When patient inspiratory effort is de-tected, the higher pressure is delivered until inspira-tory effort tapers; then the lower pressure is provided. The result is a set pressure for each breath. Careful system adjustment will be required to titrate inspired oxygen concentration and appropriate triggering of pressure changes by patient inspiratory effort. Patient tolerance must be closely monitored. Potential con-traindications to BPAP therapy include impaired mental status (including depressed respiratory effort or impaired airway clearance), risk of aspiration, severe hypoxemia, hemodynamic instability, or in-tolerance of nasal or face mask.

Oral or Nasal Airways   An oropharyngeal or na-sopharyngeal airway may be inserted to prevent upper airway obstruction or to facilitate removal of secre-tions. These airways are only appropriate for short-term use in children with adequate ventilation. They should be replaced by an endotracheal tube if the child's ability to maintain airway patency is in doubt.

An oropharyngeal airway may prevent occlu-sion of the pharynx by the tongue of an unconscious patient. These airways may be used to prevent biting of an orotracheal tube. An oropharyngeal airway should *not* ordinarily be inserted in a *conscious* child, since it may stimulate gagging or vomiting.

Sizing and Inserting the Oropharyngeal Airway   Place the airway on the outside of the child's cheek with the bite block segment at the lips. The end of the airway should reach the angle of the jaw (Figure 6-7). The oral airway is inserted while the tongue is depressed with a tongue blade. It may also be inserted while inverted, and then rotated in the back of the pharynx. Do not force the airway into the patient, since it may press the tongue back into the pharynx.

Nasopharyngeal airways are soft rubber or plastic tubes that provide a conduit from the nares

to the posterior pharyngeal wall. An endotracheal tube (cut so that it reaches only to the pharynx) may also be used as a nasopharyngeal airway. These airways may be used in conscious or uncon-scious children to maintain airway patency and to provide a channel for suctioning of the pharynx.

Sizing and Inserting the Nasopharyngeal Airway   The length should be equal to the distance from the nares to the outer tragus of the ear. The airway is lubricated with a water-soluble lubricant before insertion, and it should not be forced into place if resistance is encountered. These airways may easily become compressed or obstructed; fre-quent suctioning may be required.

Bag-Valve-Mask Ventilation   A manual ventilator device (bag) attached to an oxygen source and a mask of appropriate size should be present at *every* bedside in the intensive care unit (ICU)and at the bedside of any patient with cardiorespiratory dis-tress. Virtually any patient is at risk for the devel-opment of respiratory failure, and the nurse should be prepared to offer support of oxygenation and ventilation when necessary.

Hand ventilation via mask or endotracheal tube is an essential skill in the critical care unit. If venti-lation is provided with a mask, the mask size must be appropriate, and a good seal must be created between the child's face and the mask. In addition, the jaw is lifted to open the airway during the bag-mask ventilation. If the child's lung compliance is poor or airway resistance is high, it may be neces-sary to inactivate (tape or cover) the pressure "pop-off" valve on the bag to ensure delivery of adequate tidal volume. Excessive inspiratory pressures will not be conducted to the lungs during bag-valve-mask ventilation, since most of the pressure pro-vided through the bag is applied to the face.

To provide effective ventilation, the mask must fit properly over the child's nose and mouth (Figure 6-8), and the child's neck should be slightly ex-tended (unless cervical spinal injury is suspected in the trauma victim). The jaw is lifted to hold the airway open and to create a seal between the face and mask.

Hand ventilation should be synchronized with any spontaneous respiratory effort the patient demonstrates. Ventilation must be provided without generation of high peak inspiratory pres-

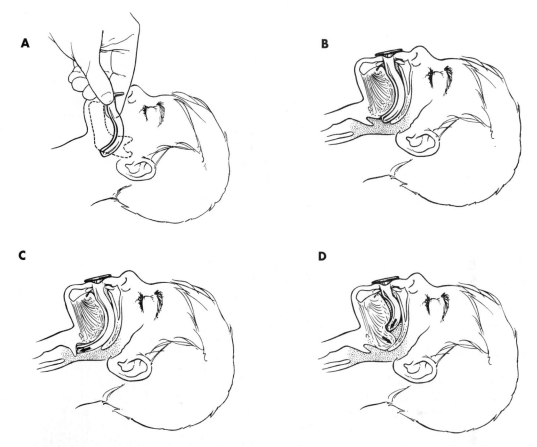

Figure 6-7 Proper oropharyngeal airway selection. **A** and **B,** An airway of the proper size should relieve obstruction caused by the tongue without damaging laryngeal structures. The appropriate size can be estimated by holding the airway next to the child's face. The tip of the airway should end just cephalad to the angle of the mandible *(broken line),* resulting in proper alignment with the glottic opening. **C,** If the oral airway inserted is too large, the tip will align posterior to the angle of the mandible and obstruct the glottic opening by pushing the epiglottis down *(arrow).* **D,** If the oral airway inserted is too small, the tip will align well above the angle of the mandible and exacerbate airway obstruction by pushing the tongue into the oropharynx *(arrows).* (From Chameides L and Hazinski MF, editors: *Textbook for pediatric advanced life support,* Dallas, 1997, American Heart Association.)

sure. This can generally be accomplished by delivering the breaths over 1 to 1.5 seconds. Short, high-pressure breaths should be avoided, because they will contribute to gastric insufflation.

Bag-valve-mask ventilation is effective if the chest expands equally and adequately bilaterally and breath sounds can be readily auscultated during each breath. Ineffective ventilation produces inadequate breath sounds bilaterally, and the chest fails to rise during ventilation.

Bag-valve-mask ventilation may produce gastric distension, which may result in vomiting and the risk of aspiration. If the child is unconscious, application of cricoid pressure will compress the esophagus, reducing or preventing further air entry into the esophagus. Insertion of a

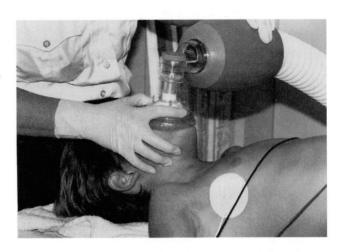

Figure 6-8 Bag-valve-mask ventilation. One hand is used to secure the mask to the face and to hold the head in a neutral position. To provide ventilation for this school-age child, the fingertips of the third, fourth, and fifth fingers are placed on the ridge of the mandible to hold the jaw forward so the airway is patent. If bag-valve-mask ventilation is provided for a smaller child (e.g., the infant or toddler), the jaw may be adequately supported with the tip of the third finger.

nasogastric tube will enable decompression of the stomach.

If ventilatory support is required, an endotracheal tube will be inserted. This will facilitate positive pressure ventilation without gastric inflation and suctioning, and will permit application of PEEP to improve oxygenation.

Manual Ventilator Bags The manual ventilator bag must have sufficient volume to ensure effective support of a patient's minute ventilation (tidal volume and respiratory rate). In general, a 230-ml bag is used for premature neonates, and a 500-ml bag is used for full-term neonates and children weighing up to 15 kg. If the child weighs more than 15 kg, a 1-L bag should generally be used. This enables delivery of effective estimated tidal volume with compression of no more than 50% of the bag volume. As a result, the bag will be able to reinflate quickly to enable ventilation at a rapid rate, if needed.

Two types of manual ventilator bags can be used to provide hand ventilation. A *self-inflating bag* is used most commonly for bag-valve-mask ventilation. These bags may also be used for hand ventilation following intubation. They do not require a source of gas, although supplementary oxygen can be provided with this bag. Without a reservoir, an oxygen concentration of 30% to 60% may be provided; if a reservoir is added to the system, 100% inspired oxygen concentration may be provided. The reservoir is available with or

without a pop-off valve. A pressure manometer may be joined to the bag to monitor airway pressure delivered (this option should be used once the child is intubated).

A *flow-inflating bag ("anesthesia bag")* may be used to provide ventilation via an endotracheal tube. It requires a continuous source of gas to inflate and greater operator skill than a self-inflating bag, but it can reliably deliver 100% oxygen. Flow through the bag and delivered airway pressure are determined by gas flow and expiratory resistance. Expiratory resistance, in turn, is controlled through adjustment of an exhalation or positive end-expiratory pressure valve. This oxygen-bag system may be joined to a pressure manometer to display the airway pressure created. The high compliance of the bag enables assessment of patient lung compliance during ventilation.

Intubation The decision to intubate is primarily a *clinical* one, often (but not always) supported by arterial blood gas measurements. Indications for intubation in the critically ill child are listed in Box 6-7 and include inability to maintain a patent airway, inadequate ventilation or oxygenation (for clinical condition), or increased work of breathing and fatigue.

Whenever possible, intubation should be accomplished on an *elective* basis, in anticipation of further deterioration in respiratory function. Respiratory arrests should *rarely* occur in the ICU, since respiratory deterioration should be promptly de-

Box 6-7

Indications for Intubation

Respiratory arrest, gasping or agonal respirations

Upper airway obstruction (stridor, significant increase in work of breathing), or potential for development of obstruction (e.g., facial trauma, inhalation injuries)

Actual or potential decrease in airway protective reflexes (e.g., compromised neurologic function)

Anticipated need for mechanical ventilatory support (e.g., acute respiratory failure, chest trauma, increased work of breathing, shock, increased intracranial pressure)

Hypoxemia despite supplemental oxygen

Inadequate ventilation

Unstable chest wall, inadequate respiratory muscle function, or severe chest trauma

From Hazinski MF: *Nursing care of the critically ill child,* ed 2, St Louis, 1992, Mosby.

tected and appropriate support provided *before* arrest occurs. An endotracheal tube of appropriate size for the patient and intubation equipment should be available near the bedside whenever cardiopulmonary deterioration is observed.

Rapid Sequence Intubation Rapid sequence intubation (RSI) is intubation with the use of paralyzing agents and sedatives, administered in rapid sequence. It is used primarily to reduce the risk of gagging and vomiting when intubation must be accomplished emergently in the child who may have a full stomach (e.g., following trauma) or increased intracranial pressure. Intubation of the conscious agitated child requires sedation and may require neuromuscular blocking agents, hypnotics, or opioids. For a comprehensive review of RSI, see the article by the Pediatric Emergency Medicine Committee of the American College of Emergency Physicians (1996). For a summary of drug choices and options for pharmacologic paralysis during intubation, see Figures 6-9 and 6-10. Vagolytic agents are often administered during intubation to prevent bradycardia.

Tube Size Tube size can be estimated from age in children beyond 1 year of age:

Endotracheal (ET) tube size (mm)

$$= \frac{\text{Age (years)}}{4} + 4$$

However, proper endotracheal tube size is most accurately estimated from the child's *length.* Length-based resuscitation tapes such as the Broselow Resuscitation Tape (Armstrong, Inc.) simplify determination of resuscitation drug dosages, as well as proper endotracheal tube and resuscitation equipment sizes. A reference table can also be used to estimate proper tube size (see inside back cover).

Equipment Before the intubation, assemble all necessary equipment at the bedside (Box 6-8). Monitor the child's heart rate continuously, using an ECG monitor with audible heart rate (QRS) tone, and pulse oximetry.

Procedure The child should be well oxygenated before and between any intubation attempts. If a short-acting muscle relaxant such as succinylcholine is administered to facilitate intubation, it may be necessary to administer atropine or glycopyrrolate (Robinul) to prevent bradycardia. Routine atropine administration without paralyzing agents is discouraged, since it may mask the development of hypoxia-induced bradycardia, resulting in undetected hypoxia.

Intubation of the critically ill child should only be attempted by individuals skilled in the technique. The nurse assisting in intubation at the head of the bed should hold the endotracheal tube (prepared with a stylet, if needed) and will provide bag-mask ventilation with 100% oxygen before and after any intubation attempt. This nurse will also suction the mouth and endotracheal tube (once inserted) if needed. The intubating physician or nurse may also require assistance in suctioning the pharynx and vocal cords just before insertion of the tube. The nurse at the head of the bed is also responsible for monitoring the patient's color, heart rate, and pulse oximetry during the intubation attempt and must advise the intubating clinician of deterioration in heart rate, oxygenation, or perfusion so that the attempt can be interrupted and hand ventilation and oxygenation can be provided.

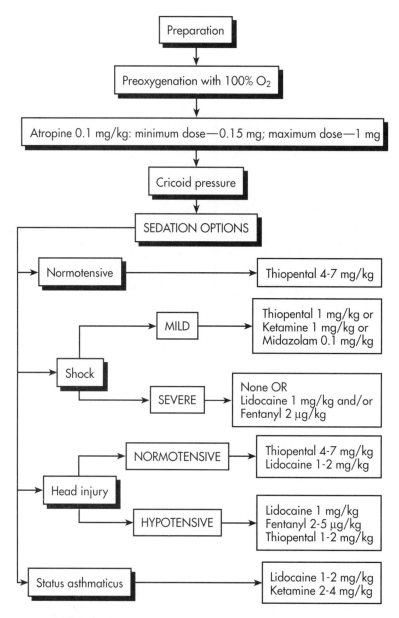

Figure 6-9 Intubation sedation algorithm. (Redrawn from Nichols DG et al, editors: *Golden hour: the handbook of advanced pediatric life support,* ed 2, St Louis, 1996, Mosby.)

If a stylet is used, it should be inserted only up to the final 1 cm of the tube; it should not extend beyond the tip of the tube. When the stylet is in proper position, the proximal end of the stylet is bent over the blue universal adapter of the endotra-cheal tube so that it will be impossible to inadvertently advance the stylet beyond the tip of the tube during intubation. If the stylet is a wire, it should be free of kinks so that it can be easily removed after successful intubation. If the endotracheal tube is

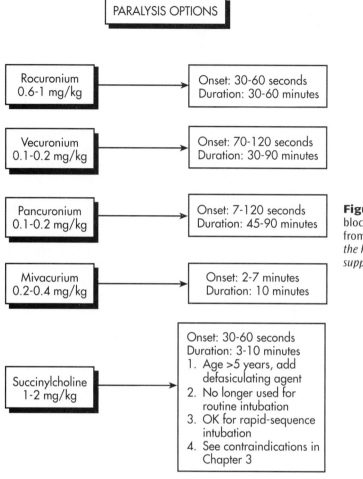

PARALYSIS OPTIONS

Rocuronium
0.6-1 mg/kg
→ Onset: 30-60 seconds
Duration: 30-60 minutes

Vecuronium
0.1-0.2 mg/kg
→ Onset: 70-120 seconds
Duration: 30-90 minutes

Pancuronium
0.1-0.2 mg/kg
→ Onset: 7-120 seconds
Duration: 45-90 minutes

Mivacurium
0.2-0.4 mg/kg
→ Onset: 2-7 minutes
Duration: 10 minutes

Succinylcholine
1-2 mg/kg
→ Onset: 30-60 seconds
Duration: 3-10 minutes
1. Age >5 years, add defasiculating agent
2. No longer used for routine intubation
3. OK for rapid-sequence intubation
4. See contraindications in Chapter 3

Figure 6-10 Selection of neuromuscular blocking agents for intubation. (Redrawn from Nichols DG et al, editors: *Golden hour: the handbook of advanced pediatric life support,* ed 2, St Louis, 1996, Mosby.)

frozen (while still in its sterile container) until just before use, a stylet may not be needed. The nurse should be prepared to apply pressure to the cricoid cartilage to facilitate entrance of the tube into the trachea.

Suction equipment must be within the reach of the nurse at the head of the bed during intubation. A large-bore suction catheter (12 or 14 French) or tonsillar suction is needed to suction the pharynx before intubation, and a suction catheter appropriate for suctioning the endotracheal tube is necessary after intubation is accomplished. Assemble tincture of benzoin (and cotton-tipped applicators, if needed) and tape torn into strips appropriate for taping of the tube at the head of the bed.

The orotracheal route is the most frequent method of endotracheal intubation performed in the ICU, because it can be accomplished rapidly and is associated with few complications. Nasotracheal intubation may be performed if it is anticipated that intubation will be required for a long period of time or if it is difficult to secure the oral airway.

If orotracheal intubation is performed, the laryngoscope blade is inserted into the trachea to control the tongue and exert pressure upward until the vocal chords are visualized. If nasotracheal intubation is performed, the tube is lubricated, gently inserted nasally, and advanced until the tip of the tube is visualized in the pharynx. The laryngoscope

Box 6-8

Equipment Needed for Intubation

Cardiac monitor with audible QRS tone

Bag, mask, and oxygen source

Endotracheal tube (estimated size for body length and age, and tubes 0.5 mm larger and smaller)

Laryngoscope blade and handle (and extra bulbs)

    Infant: 0-1 straight blade

    Small child: 1 straight blade

    Child (12-22 kg): 2 straight or curved blade

    Large child (24-30 kg): 2-3 straight or curved blade

    Adolescent (32-34 kg): 3 straight or curved blade

Stylet

    Children 3-17 kg: 6 French

    Children >17 kg: 14 French

Suction equipment

    Wall or portable suction

    Appropriate catheter to pass easily through endotracheal tube (usually the next French size above twice the endotracheal tube size in millimeters should pass readily into any endotracheal tube >3.0 mm)

    Tonsillar suction or 12-14 French suction catheter

Nasogastric tube

Tape, benzoin, water-soluble lubricant

Gloves and goggles

Paralyzing agents, sedatives, lidocaine

Magill forceps for nasotracheal intubation

From Hazinski MF: *Nursing care of the critically ill child,* ed 2, St Louis, 1992, Mosby.

blade is then used to visualize the chords, and a McGill forceps is used to advance the tube from the pharynx through the vocal cords.

The proper depth of insertion (centimeter marking on the endotracheal tube at the lip) for orotracheal intubation can be estimated from the following formula:

$$\text{Depth of insertion (cm)} = 3 \times \text{mm ET tube size}$$

Evaluation   After tube insertion, assess the position of the tube by evaluating chest expansion and breath sounds bilaterally (especially in the axillae) during hand ventilation. Listen over the child's stomach to ensure that breath sounds (indicative of possible esophageal intubation) are not heard. Proper tube position should be confirmed by a chest radiograph when the patient is stabilized.

Visual evaluation of bilateral chest expansion is best accomplished from the head or the foot of the bed. If the tube is in proper location, both sides of the chest should expand equally and adequately bilaterally. Right mainstem bronchus intubation, for example, will result in expansion of the right side of the chest with inadequate expansion of the left side of the chest.

After the tube is in place, reevaluate the tube size. Remember that the narrowest portion of the infant's larynx is below the vocal cords, at the level of the cricoid cartilage. Once the tube is placed, a hand ventilator with a pressure manometer should be used to create inspiratory pressure of 25 to 35 cm H_2O. If the *tube is of appropriate size,* a small air leak will be detectable at an inspiratory pressure of 25 to 30 cm H_2O. If the *tube is too small,* a significant air leak will be detectable at an inspiratory pressure <25 to 30 cm H_2O; although it may be possible to compensate for this air leak by increasing the tidal volume during mechanical ventilation, a large leak may necessitate tube replacement. If the *tube is too large,* a leak will not be detectable until an inspiratory pressure >30 cm H_2O is provided. An excessively large tube may contribute to the development of laryngeal edema or stenosis and may require replacement.

If the tube is in the proper position, an indelible mark is made on the tube at the lips or nares, and the tube is taped in position. If a number is visible on the tube at the lips or nares, this should be recorded on the nursing care plan. Once the endotracheal tube is taped securely in place, a chest x-ray film is obtained to confirm proper tube position, and the endotracheal tube position is adjusted accordingly. The tip of the endotracheal tube should be no lower than 1 to 2 cm above the carina and no higher than the first rib (see Figure 7-3 for examples of the radiographic evaluation of endotracheal tube location).

Securing the Tube   The endotracheal tube may be secured in a variety of ways. Regardless of the method used, tube displacement must be prevented. Factors most commonly associated with inadvertent extubation in the critically ill infant or child include the following: loose tape (slippage of the tape observed), patient agitation, and increased secretions.

Taping or retaping of the endotracheal tube must always be performed by two people. One person is responsible for holding the tube in place and immobilizing the child's head. The second person is responsible for the actual taping. This procedure should *not* be attempted by one nurse, since movement of the child can result in extubation.

The most common method of securing the endotracheal tube involves wrapping it with two pieces of tape that are anchored at two points to the child's cheeks or upper lip (not the chin). These pieces of tape are approximately 1 inch wide and 6 inches long; the pieces are cut or torn in half lengthwise for approximately 4 inches (leaving an untorn 2-inch length that remains the full width). Following application of benzoin, the untorn base of the adhesive tape is applied to the child's cheek, and one length of the torn portion is drawn across the lip and applied to the upper lip. The second length of the torn portion is drawn across the lip and wrapped around the tube at least two or three times (the end is folded over to create a removal tab). A second strip is prepared in a similar fashion and is applied from another portion of the same cheek or from the opposite direction. Auscultate breath sounds before and after tube taping or retaping, to ensure that proper tube position has been maintained.

Unintentional/spontaneous extubation may occur during movement of the patient, particularly if tension is placed on the tube by the weight of ventilator tubing. The tubing should be supported near the child's head and may be taped to a turban.

Communication With the Intubated Child The conscious child will require frequent reminders that the tube will prevent conversation and phonation. A sign board may be used if the child is able to point to letters or phrases. A simple "yes" and "no" code may be used (blink once for yes, twice for no) to enable the child to respond to questions from nurses or parents.

The awake intubated child requires some tactile stimulation and gentle touch. If the parents are unable to hold the child, they should be encouraged to sit as close to the bed as possible so that the child can see them.

The unresponsive child still requires explanations and gentle touch. The child may be able to hear but unable to signal or indicate awareness.

Causes of Deterioration in the Intubated Child The nurse must ensure that the endotracheal tube remains patent and in proper position and that the child's oxygenation and ventilation are adequate. Causes of acute deterioration in the intubated child can be recalled with the mnemonic *DOPE:*

- *D:* Displacement of the tube
- *O:* Obstruction of the tube
- *P:* Pneumothorax (or other air leaks)
- *E:* Equipment failure

Whenever the child deteriorates acutely, suspect these causes. Attempt hand ventilation and evaluate chest expansion and breath sounds. Tube displacement into the pharynx or esophagus will produce decreased breath sounds (and possibly breath sounds over the stomach). Tube displacement into a mainstem bronchus will produce a unilateral increase in breath sounds and chest expansion, with a decrease in breath sounds and chest expansion on the contralateral side. Tube obstruction will result in resistance to hand ventilation, with little or no air movement or chest expansion. Suction the tube quickly in an effort to relieve the obstruction; if the obstruction cannot be quickly eliminated, remove the tube and provide ventilation by bag and mask until reintubation can be accomplished.

Unilateral pneumothorax will produce decreased breath sounds and chest expansion on the involved side. If a tension pneumothorax is present, the mediastinum will shift away from the side of the air leak, and cardiac output may be compromised. Treatment requires immediate decompression of the pneumothorax. The diagnosis of a tension pneumothorax is often based on clinical judgment; it is often necessary to evacuate the pneumothorax before a confirmatory x-ray film can be taken, developed, and read.

Indications for Mechanical Ventilation The child with upper airway obstruction may benefit from intubation and administration of warmed, humidified inspired air or oxygen. Mechanical ventilation will be required if the hypoxemia continues despite oxygen administration, if ventilation is insufficient (hypercarbia develops), or whenever work of breathing is considered to be excessive. Mechanical hyperventilation may also be instituted to control carbon dioxide tension and to produce alkalosis in the patient with pulmonary hypertension.

Nursing Care of the Child Requiring Mechanical Ventilation

Types of Mechanical Ventilatory Support

Ventilatory support may be intermittent or continuous, short or long term, and it can use positive or negative pressure, with or without patient effort or cooperation. The type of support provided will be determined by the patient's condition and the equipment available. All clinicians must be skilled in the provision and troubleshooting of the ventilators used.

Spontaneous Ventilatory Cycle

Normal tidal volume is generated when the action of the respiratory muscles causes intraalveolar pressure to fall below atmospheric pressure. This pressure gradient is created during inspiration by contraction of the diaphragm, which enlarges intrathoracic volume and decreases intrapleural pressure. Air flows into the lungs until alveolar pressure equals atmospheric pressure; then the passive elastic recoil of the lung and thorax result in exhalation and return of the lung volume to resting state.

Negative-Pressure Ventilators

Negative-pressure ventilators are occasionally used for patients with neuromuscular disease requiring long-term ventilation. This form of ventilation creates airflow in a manner that mimics the child's spontaneous breaths. A tank or shell surrounds the child's chest, with seals around the arm and the waist. A vacuum is created within the shell to generate inspiration, and exhalation occurs passively. For this form of ventilation to be effective, the child must have a patent airway (a tracheostomy may be present) and the mechanical properties of the child's lung must be normal.

Positive-Pressure Ventilation

Positive-pressure ventilators create a pressure at the airway opening that is greater than the intraalveolar pressure, forcing pressurized gas from the ventilator unit into the lungs. This pressurized gas will flow preferentially into the areas of the lung that offer the least resistance to airflow. These areas will be the superior/anterior regions of the lung if the patient is positioned supine or semi-upright, or the areas of the lung uninvolved by disease, inflammation, or mucus obstruction.

Positive-pressure ventilators are traditionally classified according to the way in which inspiration is terminated. Most ventilators are considered to be time, pressure, volume, or flow cycled. In reality, most ventilators operate by a combination of two or three cycling modalities, and the newest generation of ventilators use microprocessors and offer a variety of cycling modalities. With all positive-pressure ventilators, exhalation is passive and is dependent on the elastic recoil of the lungs, on relatively low airway resistance, and on endotracheal tube patency (and an effective diameter). If airway resistance is high or the endotracheal tube is too small or obstructed, air trapping and hypercarbia may develop.

If a ventilator is time cycled, inspiration ends when a preset inspiratory time is reached. As a result, tidal volume is determined by the flow rate of the ventilator.

If a ventilator is pressure cycled, inspiration ceases when the preset inspiratory pressure is reached. The tidal volume delivered will be dependent on the compliance of the patient's lungs, the patient's airway resistance, and the presence or absence of a leak around the endotracheal tube.

Ventilatory Modes

Controlled Ventilation If ventilation is *controlled,* the patient cannot influence any aspect (e.g., rate, tidal volume) of ventilation or contribute to any portion of the rate or tidal volume. If ventilation is controlled, ventilatory support must be adequate to prevent any patient stimulus to breathe, or the patient must be unconscious or sedated.

Pressure Control Ventilation Pressure control ventilation is a form of controlled pressure-cycled ventilation. The variables set on the ventilator include the respiratory rate, the PEEP, and the peak inspiratory pressure. The difference between the peak inspiratory pressure and the PEEP is the ΔP, which determines tidal volume. With this form of ventilation, the mechanical ventilator provides every breath, and the patient is unable to alter the respiratory rate or tidal volume. Ventilatory support must be adequate to prevent any patient stimulus to breathe, or the patient must be neurologically depressed or pharmacologically paralyzed. Since the gas delivery by the ventilator ceases when the ΔP is reached, adjustments in the ventilator must be made as the patient's lung compliance changes, to ensure delivery of adequate tidal volume. Monitor and record the change in pressure hourly ($\Delta P =$ peak inspiratory pressure $-$ PEEP).

Advantages This form of ventilation is ideal for patients with low lung compliance (e.g., acute respiratory distress syndrome), since it may allow ventilation at lower peak inspiratory pressures than other forms of ventilation. Since gas distribution is often better than with other forms of ventilation, atelectatic areas of the lung may reexpand, resulting in improved oxygenation.

Disadvantages If variables are not appropriately adjusted when the patient's lung compliance decreases, hypoventilation may result. If the patient is conscious, sedation and possible pharmacologic paralysis are often required.

Assist/Control Ventilation If at all possible, the patient's spontaneous respiratory effort should be preserved, and the patient should be allowed to contribute to the ventilation rate or tidal volume. The classic assist/control mode of ventilation allows the patient to determine the ventilatory rate but not the tidal volume. The tidal volume and minimal respiratory rate are set; the tidal volume of all breaths will be the set tidal volume. If the patient demonstrates no spontaneous respiratory effort, the minimal respiratory rate will be delivered at the set tidal volume. Whenever the patient does begin to inspire, pressure within the system will fall; when the drop in pressure is sufficient to "trigger" a ventilation, the ventilator will cycle and deliver a positive pressure breath to the set tidal volume. The ease of patient "triggering" is determined by the sensitivity setting on the ventilator.

Advantages The patient can regulate the respiratory rate, and spontaneous respiratory effort is preserved even if the patient lacks sufficient strength to generate the full tidal volume.

Disadvantages The child is unable to regulate the tidal volume. If the trigger is too sensitive, hy-

perventilation may result; if the trigger is not sensitive enough, the patient may have to work too hard to trigger the ventilator.

Intermittent Mandatory Ventilation During *intermittent mandatory ventilation* (IMV), the patient receives a preset number of ventilator-generated breaths at a preset tidal volume and at mandatory intervals. Between mandatory breaths continuous gas flow is present in the system; thus the patient may breathe spontaneously between each mandatory positive pressure breath.

Synchronized intermittent mandatory ventilation (SIMV) also provides a preset number of breaths at a preset tidal volume, but these breaths are patient initiated (i.e., they are synchronized with the patient's spontaneous inspiration).

With either IMV or SIMV, the patient receives a minimal number of breaths at a preset tidal volume every minute. Additional breaths taken by the patient will be at a tidal volume determined by the patient's effort. Successful IMV or SIMV requires that the breaths provided by the ventilator complement the patient's spontaneous ventilation. A higher number of mandatory breaths must be provided if the patient's spontaneous ventilatory effort is minimal, and the number of mandatory breaths can be reduced as the patient's spontaneous ventilatory effort increases.

With IMV or SIMV, a continuous fresh gas flow should be present in the system from which the patient draws during spontaneous breaths. Many mechanical ventilators actually do not provide continuous gas flow through the circuit during IMV/SIMV; an inspiratory valve must be opened to enable gas flow. This valve is opened when the patient generates sufficient negative inspiratory pressure or a minimal flow within the central airway. The opening of the inspiratory valve may require excessive work for small infants and children with small tidal volumes. To eliminate this problem, a pressurized reservoir bag may be added to the inspiratory portion of the ventilator system. The child can then draw from gas in the bag during spontaneous ventilation.

Advantages Spontaneous respiratory effort is preserved; the patient controls the rate and tidal volume of some breaths. This type of ventilation may be useful for weaning.

Disadvantages   If spontaneous inspiration requires excessive effort to open the inspiratory flow valve, fatigue may develop. Spontaneous respirations may be shallow and ineffective to support ventilation.

Pressure-Support Ventilation   Pressure-support ventilation (PSV) is also known as inspiratory assist ventilation. This mode of ventilation requires patient ventilatory effort and may be used during weaning. During PSV, the respiratory rate, tidal volume, and inspiratory time are all determined by the patient. The patient initiates a breath by generating a small amount of negative pressure within the system; pressurized gas (i.e., positive pressure support) is then provided to achieve a preset airway pressure. As the patient's inspiration ceases (i.e., inspiratory flow rate declines by a certain percentage), pressure support is terminated.

Advantages   PSV can reduce patient inspiratory effort and may be useful for weaning. However, recent data suggest that significant patient work may be required to trigger the inspiratory inflation, and high patient effort may be required throughout the ventilatory cycle.

Disadvantages   Inspiratory support must be properly adjusted for the resistance offered by the endotracheal tube and ventilator circuit; excessively high triggering pressures or low inspiratory flows will increase the work of breathing. A large air leak around the tube precludes successful PSV. Finally, it may be difficult to adjust the ventilator for a tachypneic infant.

Alternative Modes of Ventilatory Support

High-Frequency Ventilation   High-frequency ventilation (HFV) uses rapid respiratory rates (300 to 3000/min) at tidal volumes smaller than dead space to achieve adequate oxygenation and ventilation. The theoretic advantage of HFV is that it avoids large increases in airway pressure that are required with conventional mechanical ventilation to produce large tidal volumes.

HFV has been effective in individual patients in the treatment of bronchopleural fistulas and in the support of patients with severe, dilated cardiomyopathies or diaphragm hernia., Although HFV has not been associated with a reduced incidence of barotrauma or a reduced incidence of chronic lung disease compared with conventional mechanical ventilation, it may be useful in patients with severe respiratory failure.

Jet Ventilation   An injection catheter within the lumen of the central airway pulses gas under high pressure at a cycling rate. Tidal volume varies with jet driving pressure, frequency, and dwell time. Exhalation is passive.

High-Frequency Oscillatory Ventilation   High-frequency oscillatory (HFO) ventilation uses a piston to move a very small volume of gas to and from the alveoli at extremely high frequencies (500 to 3000 cycles/min). The effective tidal volume delivered is determined by airway resistances. Carbon dioxide elimination is, in turn, influenced by the effective tidal volume delivered and by vibration frequency.

Extracorporeal Membrane Oxygenation   Extracorporeal membrane oxygenation (ECMO) therapy provides support of cardiac or pulmonary function (or both) using external cardiopulmonary bypass with a membrane oxygenator. This system may be used to provide temporary support for the infant or child with *acute* cardiac or respiratory failure.

Suggested indications for use of ECMO support include reversible acute respiratory failure unresponsive to conventional mechanical ventilatory support. Several methods of ECMO support may be provided. All forms require removal of venous blood from the body, oxygenation and carbon dioxide removal, warming of the blood in the oxygenator, and return of the blood to the body. Cannulas must be inserted to conduct the patient's blood to the oxygenator and to return blood to the patient.

Venovenous ECMO diverts patient venous blood to the oxygenator and returns the oxygenated blood to the patient's right atrium or to a large vein. This form of ECMO support may be used in the treatment of respiratory failure, but it requires good cardiac function, since the patient's heart is still responsible for ejection of normal cardiac output.

Venoarterial ECMO diverts venous blood to the oxygenator and returns the blood to the patient's arterial circulation (the carotid artery in infants or another large artery in the child). This form of ECMO therapy can provide total cardiac and pulmonary support.

During ECMO therapy, at least one nurse and one perfusionist must remain at the bedside at all times to monitor the patient and the ECMO equipment. Adequate analgesia and sedation must also be provided. Mechanical ventilation is required at minimal settings to prevent the development of atelectasis. Cannula dislodgment or tubing separation can result in immediate hemorrhage; thus the cannula must be secured, and all tubing must be visible at all times.

The patient must be anticoagulated during ECMO therapy, with an activated coagulation time (ACT) of approximately 180 to 200 seconds (normal is approximately 80 to 130 seconds). If lower flows are used during ECMO, the ACT is maintained at a higher level (e.g., ACT is maintained at ≥240 seconds when the flow rate is <100 ml/min) to reduce the risk of thrombus formation. Although anticoagulant-impregnated ECMO circuits have become commercially available, they are still not widely used.

When venoarterial ECMO therapy is provided, the blood is returned to the patient at a mean pressure, rather than a pulsatile one. Therefore, unless the patient's heart contributes a significant portion of cardiac output, peripheral pulses will not be palpable. However, the mean arterial pressure should still be maintained at a satisfactory level.

Complications of ECMO therapy include bleeding, mechanical or technical problems, and infection. Neurologic sequelae in neonates (including intracranial hemorrhage) have been reported.

Although ECMO therapy has been lifesaving for some patients with severe respiratory failure, its overall value has remained controversial, since there have been no randomized, controlled clinical trials demonstrating its efficacy. For further information regarding ECMO therapy, see Chapters 5 and 14 of *Nursing Care of the Critically Ill Child* (Hazinski, 1992). Survival following ECMO support for pediatric respiratory failure is significantly lower than survival following ECMO support of persistent pulmonary hypertension of the newborn or following diaphragm hernia repair (Green, 1996).

Positive End-Expiratory Pressure

Positive End-Expiratory Pressure (PEEP) is required in the treatment of hypoxemic patients unresponsive to mechanical ventilation with supplementary oxygen. PEEP is used in the care of intubated patients, whereas continuous positive airway pressure (CPAP) is used for patients who are breathing spontaneously. The physiologic effects of PEEP and CPAP are identical, although the following text refers only to PEEP.

Therapeutic Effects of Positive End-Expiratory Pressure PEEP increases or maintains lung air space volume; it increases functional residual capacity and opens (recruits) atelectatic areas of the lung, reducing intrapulmonary shunting. As a result, the patient's arterial oxygen content and arterial oxygen tension should rise.

PEEP redistributes lung water. It moves pulmonary edema fluid into harmless areas of the lung so that it will no longer interfere with gas exchange.

PEEP therapy may also maintain inspiratory muscles in a position of relative mechanical advantage; thus the work of inspiration may be reduced if the patient breathes spontaneously.

Detrimental Effects of Positive End-Expiratory Pressure PEEP increases intrathoracic pressure and may impede systemic venous return and distort left ventricular geometry. These changes may all reduce cardiac output, especially if hypovolemia is present. PEEP may increase pulmonary vascular resistance, increasing right-to-left shunts in children with congenital heart disease. High levels of PEEP may produce alveolar hyperinflation and increase the risk of air leaks. Finally, high levels of PEEP (exceeding 8 to 12 cm H_2O) may impede cerebral venous return and contribute to increased intracranial pressure.

Determination of Optimal Positive End-Expiratory Pressure The ideal PEEP is the *lowest PEEP consistent with maximal oxygen delivery* and often is associated with maximal pulmonary compliance (Box 6-9). Although high levels of PEEP may increase arterial oxygen *content,* they may result in a fall in oxygen *delivery* if cardiac output is compromised (oxygen delivery = arterial oxygen content × cardiac output or index). The optimal PEEP will reduce the intrapulmonary shunt so that arterial oxygenation increases without sig-

Box 6-9

Characteristics Associated With "Optimal" Positive End-Expiratory Pressure

"Optimal positive end-expiratory pressure (PEEP)" is *lowest* PEEP consistent with *maximal oxygen delivery* at lowest inspired oxygen concentration.

Maintains Pao_2 >60 mm Hg and hemoglobin saturation >90% with Fio_2 <0.5.

Does not significantly depress cardiac output or compromise systemic perfusion (consider fluid, inotropes).

Maintains highest mixed venous oxygen tension or saturation.

Reduces intrapulmonary shunt.

Increases lung compliance.

"Optimal" PEEP *does not* correlate with highest Pao_2 or hemoglobin saturation.

From Hazinski MF: *Nursing care of the critically ill child*, ed 2, St Louis, 1992, Mosby.

nificant depression in cardiac output or systemic perfusion.

PEEP therapy is often adjusted during PEEP studies to determine the best level of PEEP. Oxygen delivery is assessed as the PEEP is increased in a stair-step fashion by 2 to 4 cm H_2O each time. If a thermodilution cardiac output pulmonary artery catheter is in place, an arterial blood gas is drawn simultaneously with determination of thermodilution cardiac output calculation approximately 20 minutes after the PEEP is changed. The oxygen delivery can then be calculated as follows:

$$\dot{D}o_2 = \text{Arterial oxygen content} \times \text{Cardiac output}$$

If a pulmonary artery catheter is not in place, PEEP is adjusted by calculation of arterial oxygen content and careful evaluation of the child's systemic perfusion. If excessive levels of PEEP are compromising cardiac output, the child's color, perfusion of extremities, and urine output will deteriorate. If systemic perfusion is only mildly compromised, volume or inotrope administration may

*Use cardiac index for $\dot{D}o_2$ (I).

restore perfusion. In general, adjustment of PEEP to levels as high as 10 to 12 cm H_2O may be accomplished using noninvasive assessment of cardiac output. If higher levels of PEEP are required, invasive monitoring of cardiac output (e.g., pulmonary artery catheter) should be considered.

Optimal PEEP therapy may also be identified through evaluation of static lung compliance. To evaluate compliance, the ventilator circuit tubing is occluded briefly at the end of inspiration to create a plateau pressure:

$$\text{Compliance} = \frac{\text{Volume change (ml)}}{\text{Pressure change (cm } H_2O)}$$
$$= \frac{\text{Tidal volume}}{\text{Plateau pressure} - \text{PEEP}}$$

Case Study 6:

The following variables were obtained during a PEEP study performed for a 2-year-old child with acute respiratory distress syndrome following an episode of sepsis. During the trial, the child received 90% inspired oxygen, and the hemoglobin concentration was 15 g/dl.

10:00 AM: PEEP 4 cm H_2O, Pao_2 54 mm Hg
Hemoglobin (Hgb) saturation 85%
Cardiac index 3.74 L/min/m^2 BSA
10:30 AM: PEEP 8 cm H_2O, Pao_2 60 mm Hg
Hgb saturation 90%
Cardiac index 3.73 L/min/m^2 BSA
11:00 AM: PEEP 12 cm H_2O, Pao_2 62 mm Hg
Hgb saturation 93%
Cardiac index 3.19 L/min/m^2 BSA

Which PEEP is associated with the best oxygen delivery?

PEEP of 4 cm H_2O:

(O_2 content: 17.2 ml O_2/dl)
  $\times$ (Cardiac output: 3.74 L/min/m^2)
= Oxygen delivery of 643 ml O_2/min/m^2 BSA

PEEP of 8 cm H_2O:

(O_2 content: 18.3 ml O_2/dl)
  $\times$ (Cardiac output: 3.73 L/min/m^2)
= Oxygen delivery of 678 ml O_2/min/m^2 BSA

PEEP of 12 cm H_2O:

(O_2 content: 18.9 ml O_2/dl)
 $\times$ (Cardiac output: 3.19 L/min/ m²)
= Oxygen delivery of 603 ml O_2/min/m² BSA

Discussion: PEEP of 8 cm H_2O provides maximal oxygen delivery. Although the PEEP of 12 cm H_2O increased oxygen content substantially, it also resulted in a fall in cardiac index, which produced an overall fall in oxygen delivery.

PEEP therapy is often increased to correct hypoxemia so that high levels of inspired oxygen can be reduced. However, both high airway pressures *and* high levels of inspired oxygen may be detrimental. Therefore it is important to attempt to support the patient's oxygen delivery and to use no higher inspired oxygen concentration *and* PEEP than is absolutely necessary to maintain tissue oxygenation.

Maintaining Positive End-Expiratory Pressure During Suctioning   Whenever the child demonstrates significant hypoxemia and requires PEEP therapy, that level of PEEP should be maintained even during suctioning. The PEEP (and its therapeutic effects) can be lost if the ventilator circuit is opened to atmospheric pressure, and 20 to 30 minutes or longer may be required to regain the therapeutic effects provided by PEEP therapy. PEEP can be maintained through use of a closed suction system (such as that manufactured by Ballard Systems) or by attachment of a Boude valve (creating a seal around the suction catheter to prevent loss of PEEP).

Inadvertent Positive End-Expiratory Pressure   Inadvertent or intrinsic PEEP (also called "auto-PEEP") can develop during mechanical ventilation when the ventilator inspiratory cycle begins before the previous exhalation has been completed. Potential causes include airflow obstruction resulting in air trapping, inadequate exhalation time, or malfunction of the exhalation or PEEP valve on the ventilator.

Inadvertent PEEP should be suspected if the patient's chest does not appear to fall during exhalation and if the carbon dioxide tension begins to rise. The patient may also demonstrate increased work of breathing when spontaneous ventilation is allowed. Inadvertent PEEP may be corrected by increasing the exhalation time or by correcting the faulty ventilator valve.

Tapering of Positive End-Expiratory Pressure   When PEEP therapy is weaned, the PEEP should be gradually reduced in increments of 1 to 2 cm H_2O as tolerated. If the child's oxygen delivery remains acceptable for several hours, the PEEP is reduced again. A PEEP of +2 to +4 cm H_2O should probably be maintained while the endotracheal tube is in place, since this mimics physiologic PEEP (that produced by talking, coughing, etc.).

Choosing Values for Ventilator Parameters

Although there are many kinds of ventilators and many modes of ventilation, the goals of mechanical ventilation are always the same: to maintain normal gas exchange, to avoid air leaks and oxygen injury, and to maintain oxygen delivery until the lung injury resolves. Initial values or settings of ventilator parameters are listed in Table 6-3. During positive pressure ventilation, the child's chest must rise; *inadequate chest expansion or inadequate breath sounds indicate inadequate ventilation, and the cause must be identified.*

Initial values for ventilator parameters are just that—initial. Evaluate the patient's oxygenation and ventilation, and make changes as needed. Whenever vital signs are recorded, check the following ventilator parameters:

- Respiratory rate (RR)—include patient-generated and ventilator-generated values
- Tidal volume (and chest expansion)
- Minute ventilation ($\dot{V}_T \times$ RR)
- Pressure limit control
- Peak inspiratory pressure or ΔP (change in pressure)
- Inspired oxygen concentration
- PEEP

Fluid Therapy and Nutritional Support During Mechanical Ventilation

The child with respiratory failure is at risk for the development of pulmonary edema resulting from increased capillary permeability. In addition, posi-

Table 6-3
Suggested Values of Ventilator Parameters* for Initiation of Conventional Mechanical Ventilation

| Age | Respiratory Rate | Tidal Volume† | Peak Inspiratory Pressure† | | Inspiration-Expiration (I:E) Ratio |
			Normal Lungs	Diseased Lungs	
Newborn	30-40	10-20 cc/kg	15-20 cm H_2O	20-30+ cm H_2O	1:2 (1.5:1 or 1:1 may be needed if interstitial lung disease is present)
Infant	20-30	10-20 cc/kg	15-30 cm H_2O	30-40+ cm H_2O	
Child	18-25	10-20 cc/kg	20-30 cm H_2O	30-40+ cm H_2O	
Older child	12-22	10-15 cc/kg	25-35 cm H_2O	30-40+ cm H_2O	

Modified from Hazinski MF: *Nursing care of the critically ill child*, ed 2, St Louis, 1992, Mosby.
*The parameters should always be modified according to the patient's clinical condition. Once mechanical ventilation is begun, the nurse should continuously monitor the child's response to the ventilatory support.
†These parameters should be adjusted after consideration of the resistance (or compliance) within the ventilator circuit (including tubing).

tive pressure ventilation is associated with increased levels of circulating antidiuretic hormone (ADH); thus the kidneys will retain free water. For these reasons, the child with respiratory failure should receive approximately 66% to 75% of calculated maintenance fluid requirements once intravascular volume and systemic perfusion are adequate. Generous fluid administration may contribute to the development of pulmonary edema and worsening of respiratory failure.

The child's maintenance caloric requirements should be calculated, with appropriate modifications made for the presence of fever, hypermetabolic state, and decreased activity. Since the respiratory quotient of carbohydrates exceeds that of fat, it may be advisable to provide a high proportion of the child's calories in the form of fat. Sudden administration of a large quantity of carbohydrates may increase carbon dioxide production and result in hypercarbia and worsening of respiratory failure in a previously stable ventilated patient (this is seldom a problem in pediatric patients except during long-term therapy with IMV). Intravenous (IV) lipid emulsions are typically avoided when severe respiratory failure is present, since they elevate serum triglyceride levels and may contribute to a compromise in gas exchange and increased hypoxemia.

Feeding will increase carbon dioxide production; thus appropriate adjustments may be required in ventilatory support if tube feedings are begun following a period of inadequate nutrition. For further information regarding nutritional support, see Chapter 10.

Nutrition may be provided with nasogastric feedings unless gastroesophageal reflux is present. If reflux is present, transpyloric feedings should be considered. Tube feedings can be provided even in the presence of pharmacologic paralysis, provided that bowel sounds are present. If tube feeding is not tolerated, parenteral nutrition should be provided.

Nonventilatory Methods of Improving Oxygen Supply-Demand Ratio

Systemic oxygenation may be improved with sedation/paralysis to reduce patient respiratory effort (with appropriate support provided), position, hemoglobin concentration, and environment. Any of these therapies may improve oxygen delivery or minimize oxygen demand:

- *Sedation and neuromuscular blockade:* Reduction or elimination of the work of breathing may be helpful (see Chapter 3). Paralysis is occasionally necessary if it is impossible to synchronize the child's spontaneous ventilation with mechanical ventilatory support. If high peak inspiratory pressures are created during mechanical ventilation, paralysis prevents the child from generating even higher pressures while coughing or struggling "against" the ventilator; such paralysis may reduce the risk of spontaneous pneumothorax in these patients (see Chapter 3). Paralyzing agents should only be provided in conjunction with sedatives and analgesics, however.

- *Analgesia and pain control:* Pain control may minimize oxygen requirements (see Chapter 3).
- *Patient position:* The best perfused segments of the lung will be dependent; the best oxygenated segments will be superior. If unilateral lung disease is present, best oxygenation will occur with the "good" lung "down." Infants with severe lung disease may improve oxygenation and ventilation when placed in the prone or side-lying position. There are no firm rules regarding positioning; therefore the nurse should be aware of the potential effects of body position on gas exchange and note these effects when they are observed.
- *Hemoglobin concentration:* No ideal hemoglobin concentration has been determined; an increased hemoglobin concentration increases oxygen-carrying capacity and oxygen delivery but also increases blood viscosity. As a general rule, avoid anemia and maintain the hemoglobin at approximately 12 to 15 mg/dl, with the hematocrit approximately 35% to 40%.
- *Neutral thermal environment:* Maintaining a neutral thermal environment will minimize the neonate's oxygen consumption.

Assessment of the Child During Mechanical Ventilation

The use of a mechanical ventilator does not ensure that the child is being ventilated. The effectiveness of ventilation must constantly be evaluated through physical examination and interpretation of arterial blood gases. The objective impression that the child "looks good" or "looks bad" is as important (if not more so) than any other assessment. The vital signs should be appropriate for the clinical condition.

Clinical Assessment

Evaluate the child's clinical condition and effectiveness of oxygenation and ventilation continuously. The following questions may be helpful:

- Is the child fighting the ventilator? If so, provide hand ventilation, evaluate tube position and patency, and rule out pneumothorax and equipment failure.
- Is the heart rate too fast or too slow for the clinical condition? Extreme tachycardia or bradycardia may indicate hypoxemia, air leak, or low cardiac output.
- Is the blood pressure appropriate? Hypertension or hypotension may indicate hypoxia or pain.
- Are the child's color and perfusion acceptable? Deterioration in color or perfusion may indicate hypoxia and respiratory insufficiency.
- Is the chest rising symmetrically with each ventilation? Chest expansion should be equal and adequate bilaterally.
- Are breath sounds equal and adequate bilaterally? Unilateral pathology such as pneumothorax or effusion may change the pitch rather than the intensity of breath sounds.
- Is the child's level of consciousness appropriate for the clinical condition? Extreme irritability or lethargy should be investigated.
- Are the child's hemoglobin saturation (per pulse oximetry) and arterial blood gases appropriate? Monitor for evidence of hypoxemia.
- Is the child's end-tidal CO_2 ($P_{ET}CO_2$) stable and appropriate? A fall in $P_{ET}CO_2$ may indicate extubation; a rise may indicate inadequate ventilation.

If the child's condition deteriorates suddenly, provide hand ventilation and evaluate tube position and patency, as well as bilateral breath sounds. The most common causes of sudden deterioration in the intubated child are *D*isplaced tube, *O*bstructed tube, *P*neumothorax, and *E*quipment failure ("DOPE").

Laboratory Assessment

Use laboratory values to reinforce the clinical impression. The following data may be useful:

1. *Arterial blood gases:* For information regarding interpretation, see Common Clinical Conditions.
2. *Pulse oximetry:* Provides a continuous display of the child's hemoglobin saturation. Values may not immediately reflect rapid or severe decreases in hemoglobin saturation.

3. $P_{ET}CO_2$: Provides a continuous display of partial pressure of carbon dioxide in expired air. This should approximate the $Paco_2$ unless there is a ventilation-perfusion mismatch, dead space ventilation, or shunt.
   a. *Sudden decrease in $P_{ET}CO_2$ to near zero values:* Rule out extubation, leak (tube too small), complete endotracheal tube obstruction.
   b. *Decrease in $P_{ET}CO_2$:* Decrease in cardiac output or pulmonary blood flow.
   c. *Gradual rise in $P_{ET}CO_2$:* Inadequate ventilation.
4. *Chest radiographs:* Often performed daily to assess progression of the disease state. Check endotracheal tube placement (see Figure 7-3, p. 362).

Airway Humidification and Suctioning

Humidification

Intubation bypasses the patient's natural gas humidifier, the upper airway. As a result, the inspired gas must be humidified before it is delivered to the patient. Airway humidification is particularly important during HFV. Inadequate humidification of inspired air may result in increased volume and viscosity of secretions, and it increases the risk of airway obstruction, including endotracheal tube obstruction. If an increase in the quantity or viscosity of secretions is observed, evaluate the effectiveness of the humidification system.

Gas delivered through an endotracheal tube should be 100% humidified and warmed to near body temperature, depending on the infant's size:

- Neonates: 32° to 34° C
- Infants and young children: 30° to 32° C
- Adolescents: 28° to 30° C

Monitor the temperature in the inspiratory ventilator tubing near the patient. Inadequate heat in the circuit may result in condensation of water within the tubing and inadequate delivery of humidified gas to the patient. Excessive heat in the circuit can result in water condensation within the tubing, bronchospasm, and elevation in the patient's body temperature (Williams, 1996).

Suctioning

Secretions must be removed by suction when the patient is intubated. However, suctioning is a much less effective method of secretion removal than the patient's intrinsic cough.

The goal of suctioning is maintenance of endotracheal tube patency. Therefore suctioning should be performed whenever there is evidence of accumulation of secretions or whenever there is a question of tube obstruction. This means that the need for suctioning must be determined individually; "routine" suctioning should not be performed. Patients with bacterial tracheitis or bronchiolitis may require suctioning every few minutes, whereas the comatose patient with normal lungs may require suctioning only once in several hours. Unnecessary or careless suctioning should not be performed and may cause mucosal damage and stimulate additional mucus production.

Equipment required for the procedure includes a suction catheter (estimate appropriate size by doubling the endotracheal tube size and use the next French size). If the child is unstable, two persons are required to perform the suctioning: one person provides hand ventilation (or adjusts the mechanical ventilator to increase ventilation) and monitors the patient during the suctioning; the second person performs gentle suctioning using sterile technique.

Auscultate breath sounds before and after suctioning to verify tube patency, tube position, adequate secretion removal, and absence of pneumothorax.

Provide preoxygenation and hyperventilation immediately before the introduction of the suction catheter into the endotracheal tube. This preoxygenation can be accomplished through use of manual ventilation or by increasing the respiratory rate and inspired oxygen concentration (baseline Fio_2 + 10%, or use of 100% oxygen, per unit policy) provided by mechanical ventilation. If the child requires a PEEP ≥8 cm H_2O, that PEEP should be maintained during suctioning through use of a closed suction system or a Boude valve.

The peak inspiratory pressure generated during the presuctioning hyperventilation should approximately equal the proximal airway pressure generated during mechanical ventilation. Excessive inspiratory pressures should be avoided because they may result in pneumothorax or barotrauma.

Routine instillation of normal saline into the endotracheal tube before suctioning may not be necessary if the inspired air is adequately humidified, because secretions will usually be thin. If secretions are thick or tenacious, instillation of 0.5 to 2 ml of normal saline before suctioning may facilitate their removal.

The goal of endotracheal tube suctioning is maintenance or restoration of tube patency—*the suction catheter should only be inserted just beyond the tip of the endotracheal tube, and not to the carina or into a mainstem bronchus.*

Throughout the suctioning procedure, closely monitor the child's heart rate, color, and blood pressure. Discontinue suctioning and provide ventilation and oxygen if deterioration is observed. Provide manual ventilation following suctioning to prevent the development of atelectasis and reverse any hypoxia or hypercarbia that may have developed.

Weaning From Mechanical Ventilation

Weaning Options

Weaning is the gradual withdrawal of mechanical ventilatory support. It should be considered when the child's underlying disease process resolves, the blood gases improve, sedation is no longer required, and cardiopulmonary function is stable. In general, a spontaneous tidal volume of >5 ml/kg, a vital capacity >10 ml/kg, and a PEEP <4 cm H_2O are required before extubation can be considered.

The three most common methods of weaning are IMV/SIMV, the use of a T-piece, and PSV. In general, when any form of weaning is used, the time the child receives conventional ventilation is reduced and the opportunity for spontaneous ventilation with IMV/SIMV, T-piece, or PSV is lengthened. Monitor the child closely for evidence of increased work of breathing, upper airway obstruction (stridor), hypercarbia, hypoxemia, hypoventilation, or fatigue. Noninvasive monitoring, particularly pulse oximetry and $P_{ET}CO_2$, will provide valuable adjuncts to intermittent arterial blood gas analysis.

Extubation

The decision to extubate the patient is made when neither mechanical ventilation nor intubation is necessary. This decision usually requires a satisfactory $PaCO_2$, chest radiograph, and hematocrit; effective cough and respiratory effort; absence of sedation; and good cardiorespiratory, neurologic, and renal function. Predictors of extubation failure include poor respiratory effort, need for high peak inspiratory pressure and support before extubation, low dynamic compliance, and decreased inspiratory drive (Khan, Brown, and Venkataraman, 1996).

Before extubation is accomplished, equipment for reintubation must be assembled at the bedside (see Box 6-8). A source of humidified oxygen should also be available at the bedside. Gastric tube feedings are usually withheld for 1 to 2 hours before extubation so that the stomach is empty should reintubation be required. Suction the endotracheal tube immediately before extubation (with appropriate presuctioning and postsuctioning oxygenation and ventilation).

Administration of dexamethasone (0.5 mg/kg; maximum: 10 mg) IV every 6 hours for four to six doses may reduce the frequency of postextubation upper airway obstruction. Specifically, the frequency of stridor, increased work of breathing, and need for epinephrine inhalation may all be reduced by the dexamethasone administration (Anene et al., 1996).

If upper airway obstruction develops after extubation, inhaled nebulized saline, racemic epinephrine, or heliox may be used (see Airway Obstruction under Common Clinical Conditions). Pulse oximetry and arterial blood gas analysis will be useful in monitoring oxygenation and ventilation following extubation, although increased respiratory effort may determine the need for reintubation.

Monitor the child closely for 24 hours following extubation for signs of upper airway obstruction: tachycardia, tachypnea, hoarseness, stridor, prolonged inspiratory time, increased work of breathing, and decreased air movement. Postextubation laryngeal edema is usually maximal 6 to 24 hours after extubation. Be prepared to assist with reintubation if needed.

Complications of Intubation and Mechanical Ventilation

Complications of Intubation

The most common complication of intubation is post-extubation laryngeal and subglottic edema. Additional potential complications of intubation include tracheal mucosal ulceration, vocal cord injury, granuloma or polyp formation, and vocal cord paralysis. Factors contributing to the development of postextubation edema and other sequelae are:

- Traumatic intubation
- Excessively large endotracheal tube (Air leak is not observed with provision of 25 to 30 cm H_2O inspiratory pressure.)
- Tube movement in trachea during intubation period (tube or head moves frequently)
- Inadequate humidification of inspired air, inadequate suctioning
- Prolonged orotracheal intubation
- Presence of respiratory infection during intubation period

Pneumonia and Aspiration

Hospital-acquired pneumonia and infection are common among intubated patients, and the risk of infection increases with the duration of the ICU stay, as well as the duration of intubation. Nosocomial infections may develop in as many as 42% of intubated patients. Risk factors for pneumonia include poor handwashing technique among health care personnel, inadequate sterilization of equipment, and break in sterile suction technique (e.g., during suctioning). The presence of underlying diseases such as bronchopulmonary dysplasia or immune deficiency may also increase the risk of nosocomial pneumonia.

Oxygen Toxicity

Prolonged breathing of high levels of inspired oxygen can result in the development of acute lung injury called oxygen toxicity. This toxicity is thought to result from the formation of high concentrations of oxygen-derived free radicals, which have potent oxidizing powers that can damage lung cells. Free radicals can initiate or perpetuate reactions that affect cell membrane permeability and produce cellular injury.

The effects of oxygen toxicity in the lung of the patient with respiratory failure are often difficult to separate from the effects of the patient's underlying disease or injury resulting from positive pressure ventilation. The functional result of these pathologic changes is the development of pulmonary edema and, with prolonged oxygen exposure, progressive pulmonary interstitial fibrosis.

The dose and duration of exposure that will produce oxygen toxicity is unknown. If underlying lung disease is present, or if the oxygen is administered at high pressures, tolerance for high or even moderate levels of inspired oxygen may be diminished considerably.

To prevent oxygen toxicity, *the minimal inspired oxygen concentration consistent with adequate tissue oxygenation should be administered.* Frequently PEEP is increased to levels sufficient to enable reduction of the inspired oxygen concentration to less than 40%. However, PEEP may be as harmful to the lung as administration of high levels of supplementary inspired oxygen. Oxygen administration should never be avoided in the patient with profound hypoxemia because of fear of oxygen toxicity; any toxic effects of oxygen at that point will be conjectural, whereas the effects of systemic hypoxia are well known. Oxygen administration should always be adjusted according to either blood gas analysis or pulse oximetry. The inspired oxygen concentration and patient response should be recorded.

To minimize oxygen requirements, the child's oxygen consumption must be minimized. Treat fever and pain, prevent shivering, and consider pharmacologic paralysis if the child's work of breathing is high during mechanical ventilatory support. It may be possible to reduce levels of inspired oxygen if the patient's oxygen requirements are kept minimal.

Complications of Positive-Pressure Ventilation

Positive-pressure ventilation results in increased airway pressures and increased intrathoracic pressure, which may affect cardiovascular and respiratory functions. Positive pressure ventilation may decrease systemic and pulmonary venous return to the heart and compress the great vessels, with a consequent fall in cardiac output. This fall is particularly likely if hypovolemia is present. In addition,

> ## Box 6-10
>
> ## Complications of Intubation and Positive Pressure Ventilation
>
> ### Complications of Intubation
> Postintubation upper airway edema/injury
> Pneumonia and infection
>
> ### Complications of Oxygen Therapy and Positive Pressure Ventilation
> Oxygen toxicity
> Barotrauma related to positive pressure ventilation
> Compromise in systemic venous return/decreased cardiac output
> Fluid retention
>
> ### Complications of Critical Illness
> (Including stress ulcer, nutritional compromise, hazards of immobility)

positive pressure ventilation may increase ADH secretion, which will promote water retention and also affect intravascular volume and osmolality (Box 6-10).

Positive pressure ventilation may produce barotrauma, including pneumothorax, pneumopericardium, and pneumomediastinum. The risk of tension pneumothorax is high whenever positive pressure ventilation produces high peak inspiratory or mean airway pressures. Clinical signs of tension pneumothorax include sudden deterioration in color, systemic perfusion, and oxygenation; decreased breath sounds and chest expansion on the side of the pneumothorax; and a shift of heart sounds away from the pneumothorax. A tension pneumothorax must be immediately evacuated using a large over-the-needle catheter inserted into the second intercostal space, over the third rib in the midclavicular line. The catheter may be joined to a short segment of IV extension tubing, with immersion of the tip of the tubing 2 cm into a sterile water bottle (this creates a 2-cm H_2O underwater seal). Following the release of a gush of air, a chest tube is inserted. Necessary equipment for pneumothorax evacuation should be assembled at the bedside when the risk of air leak is high.

Respiratory Physical Therapy Techniques
Chest Physiotherapy

Chest physiotherapy may assist the removal of lung secretions and help maintain normal airway function. Oxygen administration or bronchodilator inhalation may be required during treatments.

Chest physiotherapy requires use of a series of four techniques: positioning of the patient, percussion, vibration, and patient cough. These techniques promote deep breathing, effective coughing, and removal of airway secretions. The patient's condition and tolerance must be carefully monitored throughout the procedure. Contraindications to chest physiotherapy include status asthmaticus, presence of retained foreign bodies, displaced or fractured ribs, severe hemoptysis, and pulmonary hemorrhage. The frequency and duration of chest physiotherapy must be tailored to each patient. It should not be performed within 1 hour of meals.

Detailed presentation of chest physiotherapy is beyond the scope of this book; for further information, see pp. 454-458 of *Nursing Care of the Critically Ill Child* (Hazinski, 1992). A summary of basic techniques is provided here:

- *Postural drainage:* Gravity is used to promote tracheobronchial drainage. Position the child with the targeted portion of the lung superior to other lung segments. The remaining techniques are applied to the targeted lung segment during postural drainage.
- *Percussion or clapping:* Performed with a cupped hand or soft face mask to move secretions to large airways where they can be evacuated.
- *Vibration:* Application of a shaking motion over the draining bronchopulmonary segment. It is also designed to move secretions toward large airways.

Incentive Spirometry

Incentive spirometry is intended to augment chest physiotherapy. It is used to prevent or treat atelectasis. A variety of aids are available to visually display the child's inspiratory effort, and target goals may be set. The child may also accomplish incentive spirometry by blowing bubbles or blowing paper cups across a bedside table.

Other Devices

Patients with chronic suppurative lung diseases such as cystic fibrosis or chronic bronchiectasis may benefit from devices that improve mucociliary clearance. An example of this is a "flutter valve," which patients can be taught to use.

Nursing Care Plan

Box 6-11 lists potential patient problems and highlights nursing care.

Specific Diseases

Status Asthmaticus

Etiology/Pathophysiology

Asthma is the most common chronic illness in childhood and is defined as reversible airway obstruction caused by airway inflammation and bronchial hyperreactivity, and obstruction of airways by thick mucus. Inflammatory cell infiltration and subsequent mediator release are responsible for the bronchial inflammation and hyperreactivity, increased mucus production, and airway edema. Expiratory airflow limitation causes air trapping and forces the patient to breathe at a high lung volume where lung compliance is diminished, thereby increasing the work of breathing.

Status asthmaticus is the exacerbation of asthma symptoms unresponsive to conventional outpatient or emergency room therapy. The work of breathing is very high, and hypoxemia develops. As lung compliance decreases, the child with asthma must generate high negative pressures on inspiration, subjecting the pulmonary circulation to increased transmural pressure. This creates the potential for pulmonary edema.

Hypoxemia, secondary to ventilation-perfusion mismatch, is common in status asthmaticus. Persistence of hypoxemia and subsequent anaerobic cellular metabolism may result in metabolic acidosis. Severe asthma is associated with the development of hypercarbia and respiratory acidosis.

Clinical Presentation

Acute exacerbations of asthma are characterized by worsening of symptoms, including dyspnea, wheezing, and a productive cough. The child may exhibit tachypnea, use of accessory muscles, and prolonged expiration. As the attack progresses, decreased air movement can produce decreased breath sounds, muffled cough, decreased wheezing, and somnolence. Hypoxia may cause agitation or combativeness. A decreased level of consciousness is usually indicative of the development of respiratory failure and impending respiratory arrest.

Clinical examination alone cannot reliably differentiate mild from severe exacerbations, and physiologic assessments may be helpful (Table 6-4). The evaluation of peak expiratory flow rate (PEFR) may be a useful part of comprehensive asthma management.

A decrease in PEFR to <80% of predicted or personal best is an early indication of deterioration. Hypoxemia is usually not present during mild exacerbation of asthma; if the hemoglobin saturation falls to <90%, the exacerbation is severe. Hypercarbia and combined metabolic and respiratory acidosis also indicate a severe exacerbation.

The use of sternocleidomastoid muscles during inspiration correlates well with a PEFR <50% of predicted and moderate to severe exacerbation. Although pulsus paradoxus >20 mm Hg is associated with moderate to severe exacerbation, it may be impossible to obtain in tachypneic infants or uncooperative children.

Management

The immediate goal of therapy is relief of airway obstruction, and restoration of oxygenation and ventilation. Humidified supplemental oxygen is administered as needed. Acute bronchospasm in the child with status asthmaticus is treated with inhaled beta-adrenergic agonist drugs (e.g., albuterol, 0.15 mg/kg) and IV administration of corticosteroids. Oral steroid administration is possible when the child is stable. IV methylxanthines (aminophylline/theophylline), past mainstays of therapy, are rarely used because they can produce significant side effects and do not offer significant therapeutic advantages.

Aerosolized bronchodilators (beta-adrenergic agonists) diluted with normal saline should be delivered with the prescribed FiO_2, ensuring that the oxygen flow is adequate to meet respiratory demand. The aerosols may be administered as

Box 6-11

Nursing Care of the Child Requiring Mechanical Ventilatory Support

General Comments: The nurse is responsible for ensuring that ventilatory support is effective. The child's compliant chest should expand during positive pressure ventilation. If the chest does not rise, positive pressure ventilation is probably ineffective. The nurse must also ensure that emergency respiratory support equipment (including hand ventilator, mask, oxygen source, additional endotracheal tubes, and intubation equipment) is readily available.

1. **Potential ineffective breathing pattern,** possibly caused by *"DOPE" (tube displacement, tube obstruction, pneumothorax and other complications of ventilation, or equipment failure).*
   a. Monitor child's color, responsiveness, and clinical appearance. If there is evidence of acute deterioration, be prepared to provide hand ventilation and assess position and patency of endotracheal tube, rule out pneumothorax (and tension pneumothorax) through clinical examination, and evaluate equipment function. See problem 2.
   b. Ensure that chest expands equally and adequately bilaterally and that breath sounds are adequate during every inspiration.
   c. Verify ventilatory variables hourly and check them (after completion of *a* and *b* above) if there is any deterioration in patient's condition. Check connections of all tubing hourly and with change in patient's condition. All tubing should be visible at all times. Ensure that all visual and audible alarms are active at all times (or only temporarily silenced during activities such as suctioning).
   d. Evaluate arterial blood gases, including noninvasive analysis (pulse oximetry and end-tidal carbon dioxide). Inspired oxygen concentration should be lowest concentration necessary to prevent hypoxemia.
   e. Positive end-expiratory pressure (PEEP) may be needed if a significant intrapulmonary shunt is present, to improve oxygenation. Monitor PEEP and peak inspiratory pressure (PIP) and exhaled tidal volume: A sudden *rise in PIP* with a volume-cycled ventilator may indicate reduced lung compliance or pneumothorax. A *rise in PEEP* may indicate inadvertent PEEP produced by obstruction to exhalation or malfunction or maladjustment of ventilator. *Loss of PEEP* may occur with spontaneous patient inspiration, leak around endotracheal tube, or leak in system.

2. **Potential ineffective airway clearance or breathing pattern** related to potential tube displacement or obstruction, or pneumothorax. If these signs develop, remove patient from ventilator, provide hand ventilation, and notify physician immediately. Treatment of tension pneumothorax should not await chest radiograph (it is a clinical, not a radiographic, diagnosis).
   a. Assess child's general appearance and clinical condition at a minimum of hourly intervals; monitor chest expansion and breath sounds bilaterally.
   b. Suction endotracheal tube as needed to maintain patency and remove tube secretions. Two people are required to suction unstable patient.
   c. Monitor for evidence of *tube displacement:* respiratory distress, agitation, deterioration in color or perfusion, or altered level of consciousness; inadequate chest expansion or breath sounds unilaterally (if mainstem bronchus migration) or bilaterally (with extubation); decrease in pulse oximetry, end-tidal carbon dioxide, or arterial blood gases; change in point of endotracheal tube that is present at lips or nares (mark tube at edge of lips or nares with indelible marker and monitor mark and record number on tube near lips or nares in nursing notes to enable detection of tube movement). Note the most common conditions preceding spontaneous extubation: vigorous coughing or movement of child, loose tape, or large volume of secretions.

Continued

Box 6-11

Nursing Care of the Child Requiring Mechanical Ventilatory Support—cont'd

d. Monitor for evidence of *tube obstruction*: respiratory distress, agitation, deterioration in color or perfusion, or altered level of consciousness; inadequate chest expansion or breath sounds; rise in arterial carbon dioxide tension or reduced end-tidal carbon dioxide; rattle, shudder, or other inspiratory sounds; increased PIP or increased resistance to hand ventilation; possible deterioration in Pao_2, pulse oximetry, or vital signs.

e. Monitor for signs of *pneumothorax*: deterioration in clinical appearance, oxygenation, or vital signs; decreased chest expansion or breath sounds with increased resistance to hand ventilation; deviation of trachea and point of maximal impulse away from side of suspected pneumothorax. Tension pneumothorax will produce a fall in cardiac output and systemic perfusion. Note that if child requires ventilation at high pressures, development of pneumothorax or tension pneumothorax is a strong possibility. Equipment needed to tap air from chest or chest tubes should be present at bedside.

4. **Potential hypoxemia,** which may be caused by inadequate ventilatory support, pulmonary edema, acute respiratory distress syndrome, endotracheal tube displacement, tube obstruction, tension pneumothorax, or failure of mechanical ventilator system.

5. **Potential restlessness,** which may be caused by hypoxemia, hypercapnia, respiratory efforts that are asynchronous with ventilator support, sleep deprivation, fear, or pain. Identify and treat cause.

6. **Potential hypoventilation,** which may be related to development of atelectasis, inadequate spontaneous respiratory effort, inappropriate mechanical ventilatory support, increased pulmonary secretions, decreased mobility, or inappropriate weaning. Clinical signs include inadequate chest expansion, breath sounds, and possible hypoxemia. Treatment requires evaluation and potential adjustment in mechanical ventilatory support, change in patient position, and potential incentive spirometry.

7. **Potential compromise in systemic perfusion,** which may be caused by impedance in systemic venous return, hypovolemia, hypoxemia, or tension pneumothorax. Identify and treat cause.

8. **Potential infection,** which may be caused by multiple invasive catheters and lines, colonization of respiratory tract, or break in aseptic/sterile technique during suctioning. Clinical signs include fever, altered secretions, and pulmonary congestion. Treatment includes prevention of infection when possible, early detection of infection, and treatment with antimicrobials.

9. **Potential difficulty weaning,** which may be caused by muscle weakness, poor nutrition, failure of resolution of pulmonary disease, excessive secretions, or neurologic impairment in cough or gag. Treatment is to identify and rectify the cause.

10. **Potential patient anxiety,** which may be caused by hypoxemia, hypercarbia, respiratory distress, underlying disease, pain, or separation from parents. Rule out hypoxemia and "DOPE" (see problem 1). Pain should be treated, and sedation may be needed, but do not assume that pain is the cause until hypoxemia and "DOPE" have been ruled out.

11. **Potential compromise in nutrition.** Provide enteral feeding as soon as possible. Provide maintenance calories (for age and condition) and appropriate fluid intake.

Table 6-4
Estimation of Severity of Acute Exacerbation in the Child With Asthma

Sign/Symptom	Mild	Moderate	Severe
Peak expiratory flow rate	70%-90% predicted or baseline	50%-70% predicted or baseline	<50% predicted or baseline
Respiratory rate	Normal to 30% above mean	30%-50% increase above mean	>50% increase above mean
Alertness	Normal	Normal	May be decreased
Dyspnea	Absent or mild, speaks in complete sentences	Moderate, speaks in phrases or partial sentences	Severe, speaks only in single words or short phrases
Accessory muscle use	No retractions to mild intercostal retractions	Moderate intercostal retractions with tracheosternal retractions, use of sternocleidomastoid muscles, chest hyperinflation	Moderate intercostal retractions, tracheosternal retractions with nasal flaring during inspiration, chest hyperinflation
Color	Good	Pale	Possibly cyanotic
Auscultation	End-expiratory wheeze only	Inspiratory and expiratory wheezing	Breath sounds inaudible
Oxygen saturation	>95%	90%-95%	<90%
Pao_2	↓	↓↓	↓↓↓
pH	High (alkalotic)	Normal	Low (acidotic)
Acid-base status	Respiratory alkalosis	Normal	Metabolic and respiratory acidosis
$Paco_2$	<35 (↓)	<40 (normal)	>40 (↑)

Modified from Bergman DA, Chairperson, Provisional Committee on Quality Improvement, American Academy of Pediatrics: Practice parameter: the office management of acute exacerbations of asthma in children, *Pediatrics* 93:119-126, 1994.
*Oxygen saturation values will have to be adjusted for altitude. These values assume that the patient is at sea level.

often as every 20 minutes, although continuous administration usually provides better relief of bronchospasm (Table 6-5). Monitor the child's appearance and heart rate during inhalation therapy.

Hydrocortisone is administered as an IV bolus loading dose of 10 mg/kg (maximum dose: 300 mg), then 10 mg/kg daily divided every 6 hours. Methylprednisolone may also be administered (2 to 4 mg/kg as a bolus, then 1 to 2 mg/kg every 4 to 6 hours).

Continuous *IV* administration of a beta-adrenergic agonist may be considered if continuous inhalation therapy cannot be provided (e.g., the child removes the mask) or is ineffective. For the rare occasion when aminophylline infusion is used, the infusion dose is determined by the child's age and then adjusted for the presence of cardiovascular or hepatic dysfunction. The aminophylline (theophylline) level should be checked during infusion

(therapeutic levels: 10 to 20 mg/L). The infusion should be maintained but not increased until steady state has been reached (approximately 12 hours). If the serum levels are inadequate, administration of 1mg/kg bolus of aminophylline will increase the serum theophylline level by 2 mg/L, but serum levels should be checked whenever the dose is increased.

If oxygen, corticosteroids, and inhaled beta-adrenergic agonists do not improve the child's condition, IV terbutaline or isoproterenol may be administered continuously at 0.1 to 0.25 μg/kg/min. Monitor closely for the development of tachycardia and arrhythmias. IV magnesium sulfate and inhaled ipratropium bromide are other agents that are occasionally used to treat bronchospasm, but the efficacy of these agents is under investigation; thus the drugs are not yet widely accepted.

IV fluids are usually administered at approximately 66% to 75% of calculated maintenance re-

Table 6-5
Bronchodilator Agents for Nebulization (in 2.5 ml Normal Saline)*

Name (Brand Name)	Concentration	Dose
Terbutaline (Brethine, Bricanyl)	1 mg/ml†	0.2 mg/kg (maximum: 10 mg) q30min × 3
Metaproterenol (Alupent, Metaprel)	50 mg/ml	0.5 mg/kg (maximum: 15 mg) q30min × 3
Albuterol (Ventolin, Proventil)	5 mg/ml	1st dose: 0.15 mg/kg (maximum: 2 mg), then 0.05 mg/kg (maximum: 2 mg) q20min or continuously
Ipratropium (Atrovent)	—	1-2 puffs q6h

Modified from Nichols DG et al, editors: *Golden hour: the handbook of advanced pediatric life support,* ed 2, St Louis, 1996, Mosby.
*Nebulizers driven with 5-10 L/min O_2
†Approved by FDA for parenteral use, but also effective as aerosol. Do not dilute further.

quirements unless dehydration or hypovolemia is present. Excessive amounts of IV fluids should not be administered, since the patient is already at risk for the development of pulmonary edema. Monitor fluid intake and output carefully.

Chest physiotherapy is contraindicated during acute asthma, since it may aggravate the child. However, percussion and postural drainage can be instituted when the child's airway obstruction begins to resolve, as indicated by the onset of a loose, moist cough.

Children with asthma require close medical follow-up to control baseline disease and to reduce the frequency and severity of status asthmaticus. Patient and family education and the prophylactic use of inhaled antiinflammatory agents can prevent or treat mild exacerbations of asthma and may prevent the development of severe exacerbations. Teaching information can be obtained from local chapters of the American Lung Association.

Acute Respiratory Distress Syndrome
Etiology/Pathophysiology

Acute respiratory distress syndrome (ARDS) is a complication of acute lung insult (e.g., trauma or sepsis) that produces respiratory failure associated with diffuse alveolar injury and increased permeability pulmonary edema. ARDS injury evolves in three stages: a latent period (6 to 48 hours after injury), a period of acute respiratory failure, and a chronic/recuperative period.

1. *Latent phase:* Acute lung injury occurs. The patient may appear clinically normal, but damage to the alveolar-capillary membrane has occurred, and pulmonary edema is developing.
2. *Acute respiratory failure phase:* Many mediators (e.g., arachidonic acid metabolites) have been secreted or formed that exacerbate the pulmonary damage. Progressive pulmonary edema causes intrapulmonary shunting and hypoxemia, as well as decreased lung compliance and increased work of breathing. Surfactant inactivation results in increased surface tension in alveoli and increased tendency toward collapse (atelectasis).
3. *Chronic phase:* This phase is characterized by type II pneumocyte proliferation, fibrin infiltration, and diffuse alveolar fibrosis. The lung begins to heal but may also become fibrotic. During this phase, complications of acute therapy, such as oxygen toxicity or pulmonary fibrosis, may develop.

Clinical Presentation

Initial signs may be only those of the initial insult (e.g., pneumonia, drug overdose, aspiration episode, sepsis, kerosene ingestion, etc.). Hyperventilation, hypocapnia, and respiratory alkalosis may be observed as pulmonary edema stimulates lung receptors to increase the respiratory rate. A chest radiograph may reveal pulmonary interstitial edema with fine reticular infiltrates.

Acute respiratory failure is associated with hypoxemia, tachypnea, and increased respiratory effort. Intrapulmonary shunting may produce hypoxemia unresponsive to oxygen administration. Intubation and mechanical ventilatory support are often required. Hypercapnia is not a common feature of ARDS, although it may develop when ARDS is severe. Pulmonary hypertension and bronchoconstriction may also be present.

Management

Management of ARDS requires support of oxygenation and ventilatory function so that oxygen delivery is optimized. If mechanical ventilation is required, an arterial catheter should be placed to enable continuous evaluation of mean arterial pressure and provide ready access for arterial blood gas sampling.

Oxygen, Ventilation, and Positive End-Expiratory Pressure Supplemental oxygen administration should improve arterial oxygen saturation unless intrapulmonary shunting is severe. Persistent hypoxemia despite supplemental oxygen or a significant increase in respiratory effort is an indication that intubation and mechanical ventilatory support may be required. Anemia should be treated to maintain hemoglobin concentration and oxygen-carrying capacity.

PEEP therapy and mechanical ventilatory support should be adjusted to maximize oxygen delivery (oxygen delivery = arterial oxygen content × cardiac output; oxygen delivery indexed = arterial oxygen content × cardiac index). PEEP should increase arterial oxygen content without significantly depressing cardiac output (see Box 6-9, p. 320).

If PEEP significantly compromises cardiac output and systemic perfusion, oxygen delivery will fall. Signs of decreased systemic perfusion include a deterioration in the child's color, cooling of the child's extremities, delayed capillary refill, and reduction in urine volume. If high levels of PEEP are required to maintain arterial oxygenation, a thermodilution cardiac output pulmonary artery catheter may be inserted to enable calculation of cardiac output so that trends in oxygen delivery can be evaluated as therapy is modified. (see Positive End-Expiratory Pressure under Nursing Care of the Child Requiring Mechanical Ventilation, p. 319).

Mechanical ventilation is generally adjusted to allow a mild to moderate hypercarbia if cardiovascular function is good and severe acidosis is not produced. This is termed *permissive hypercapnia.* Permissive hypercapnia may enable reduction in minute ventilation (particularly the tidal volume and peak inspiratory pressure) and may prevent or reduce barotrauma. Although initially the hypercarbia will produce a respiratory acidosis, within 6 to 24 hours renal bicarbonate retention will begin to restore the pH to near normal.

Sedation and Muscle Relaxants Sedation may facilitate control of ventilation and reduction of peak inspiratory pressures. Pharmacologic muscle paralysis should be considered if the patient is "fighting" the ventilator, if high peak inspiratory pressures are present, or if hypoxemia is severe. Pharmacologic paralysis not only eliminates the work of breathing, it will also permit the mechanical ventilator to function more effectively. Patients should not be paralyzed without analgesia or sedation (see Figure 6-10 and Chapter 3).

Suctioning When the patient is unstable, suctioning must be performed by two health care providers. If the child is receiving high levels of PEEP, these levels of PEEP must be maintained during suctioning through use of a closed suction system or a Boude valve.

Preparation for Treatment of Pneumothorax Whenever high peak inspiratory pressures are required to maintain oxygenation and ventilation, the development of a pneumothorax should be anticipated. In fact, under these conditions, the sudden development of hypoxemia (sudden cyanosis, bradycardia, or a fall in hemoglobin saturation per pulse oximetry) or deterioration in systemic perfusion should be presumed to be caused by a tension pneumothorax until this complication has been ruled out. An 18- to 20-gauge over-the-needle catheter and chest tube equipment should be assembled at the bedside.

Signs of *tension pneumothorax* include a unilateral decrease in chest expansion and breath sounds, hypoxemia, compromise in systemic perfusion, and mediastinal shift away from the side of the pneumothorax. Tension pneumothoraces may cause acute and abrupt deterioration, requiring urgent intervention, or they may be subacute with time to confirm by chest radiograph (see Figure 12-3 for an illustration of chest tube insertion).

Minimization of Oxygen Demands Treat fever and pain, since both will increase oxygen consumption. Cold stress will increase the neonate's oxygen consumption and may contribute to deterioration; therefore maintain the young infant in a neutral thermal environment. As noted earlier, pharmacologic paralysis (with analgesia) may reduce the oxygen consumption by respiratory muscles and will enable better ventilatory control of the child with severe respiratory failure.

The hypoxemic child is likely to be irritable and frightened. Explanations should be provided before any procedure is performed, and the child should always be sedated when pharmacologic paralysis is necessary.

Supportive Care If cardiac output and systemic perfusion are acceptable (i.e., the child is euvolemic), fluid intake is generally limited to approximately 50 to 60 ml/kg/day. Remember that drug administration, blood transfusion, and catheter flushes all contribute to fluid intake, and excessive fluid administration may contribute to worsening pulmonary edema. Diuretic therapy may be helpful in the treatment of pulmonary edema.

Monitor the child's systemic perfusion closely. The urine volume and skin perfusion are helpful indicators of the effectiveness of end-organ perfusion. If systemic perfusion is compromised by positive pressure ventilation or high levels of PEEP, volume administration or inotropic support (dopamine at 4 to 8 μg/kg/min) may be required to restore perfusion to satisfactory levels.

Children with ARDS are at high risk for developing secondary infection. Good handwashing technique must be practiced by every member of the health care team, and appropriate clean or aseptic technique must be used for all procedures. Monitor the child closely for evidence of infection and sepsis, including fever, tachycardia, elevation or depression in the white blood cell count, thrombocytopenia, or altered level of consciousness. Infants may demonstrate temperature instability, rather than fever. Blood cultures should be drawn if infection is suspected, and parenteral antibiotic therapy may be initiated or changed.

Provide nutritional support as soon as possible. Ensure delivery of sufficient calories to meet resting needs, with appropriate adjustments for fever, increased catabolic state, wound healing, and reduced activity. Calories in the form of fats should be administered to prevent the need for high levels of carbohydrate administration, since the respiratory quotient (carbon dioxide produced during metabolism) of carbohydrates is almost twice that of fats.

Tube feedings provide an ideal method of delivering adequate nutrition, but IV alimentation should be considered if tube feedings are not tolerated. IV lipid emulsions should probably not be administered during the acute phase of ARDS, since they may elevate serum triglyceride levels, which will contribute to a compromise in gas exchange and increased hypoxemia.

Recent Developments in Therapy Alternative methods of oxygenation and ventilation continue to be explored. Liquid ventilation with perfluorocarbon (Perflubron) uses a liquid polymer that binds and releases large amounts of oxygen and can deliver oxygen to the alveoli at much lower surface tensions than gas. However, this technique requires continued investigation before commercial use.

Aerosolized surfactant has dramatically reduced the acute mortality from newborn hyaline membrane disease (see Respiratory Distress Syndrome). It has been less effective in the treatment of pediatric hypoxemic respiratory failure associated with surfactant washout or inactivation, including ARDS and near-drowning.

Nitric oxide is useful in the treatment of persistent pulmonary hypertension of the newborn (PPHN) and has reduced the need for ECMO of these infants. Clinical trials of nitric oxide therapy for treatment of pulmonary hypertension or respiratory failure with intrapulmonary shunting have documented beneficial effects of this therapy (see Pulmonary Hypertension and Chapter 5, p. 211).

Respiratory Distress Syndrome

Etiology/Pathophysiology

Respiratory distress syndrome (RDS), also called hyaline membrane disease, is a neonatal lung disease caused by deficiency, absence, or inactivation of lung surfactant. Although premature infants with birth weights <1500 g are most frequently affected, even term infants can develop RDS.

Surfactant is a complex substance consisting of lipids and proteins, formed by alveolar type II cells (type II pneumocytes). Since surfactant decreases surface tension at the air-fluid interface, insufficient surfactant results in atelectasis and decreased lung compliance. The net result of RDS in the neonate is progressive atelectasis, hypoxemia, increased work of breathing, and respiratory insufficiency. Pulmonary hypertension can result from prolonged alveolar hypoxia and acidosis.

Clinical Presentation

The infant with RDS usually exhibits moderate to severe respiratory distress shortly after birth. Clinical signs include tachypnea, nasal flaring, retractions, and cyanosis in room air. An expiratory grunt may also be present. Hypoxia is associated with respiratory acidosis; as the infant's condition deteriorates, systemic perfusion is compromised and metabolic acidosis develops. The chest radiograph may reveal the characteristic ground-glass appearance of the lung fields with air bronchograms indicative of atelectasis.

Management

Prevention of RDS by prevention of premature births is the most effective form of therapy. If the premature birth cannot be prevented, administration of dexamethasone to the mother 24 hours before premature delivery will increase surfactant synthesis in the neonate and will reduce the incidence and severity of RDS.

Oxygen therapy is mandatory. If respiratory effort is adequate, CPAP may be provided by nasal cannula to reduce the intrapulmonary shunt and eliminate hypoxemia. Intubation and ventilation with PEEP will often be required for very immature infants and for large infants who develop severe respiratory distress.

Since the lung compliance of the neonate with RDS is poor and the lung is immature in other ways, positive pressure ventilation of any kind may produce barotrauma, including tension pneumothorax and pneumomediastinum. Pneumothorax in the neonate with RDS will produce sudden onset of severe hypoxemia and bradycardia. Signs of pneu-

momediastinum include mediastinal displacement on chest radiographs, hypoxemia, and hypercapnia; a crunch may be heard over the mediastinum or palpated over the sternum.

Intratracheal administration of either human or artificial surfactant has substantially reduced acute mortality from RDS in very premature infants and may reduce the severity of respiratory failure. However, exogenous surfactant has not been effective in reducing the incidence of chronic lung disease; thus it has not reduced the number of infants with bronchopulmonary dysplasia.

Bronchopulmonary Dysplasia

Etiology/Pathophysiology

Bronchopulmonary dysplasia (BPD) is a chronic lung disease occurring in infants born prematurely who have survived neonatal respiratory failure and its therapy (including high inspired oxygen concentration and positive pressure ventilation). By definition, BPD is present if the infant is oxygen dependent and demonstrates physical and radiologic evidence of lung disease at 1 month of age (or 36 weeks postconceptual age).

BPD is associated with reduced lung compliance, increased airway resistance, and severe expiratory flow limitation due to edema, fibrosis, and small airway inflammation. Both hyperinflation and atelectasis are present; ventilation-perfusion mismatch results in alveolar hypoventilation, hypercapnia, and hypoxemia.

Sequelae of chronic alveolar hypoxia may include increased pulmonary vascular resistance, pulmonary hypertension, and cor pulmonale (see Pulmonary Hypertension and Chapter 5, p. 211). Supplemental oxygen is an essential component of therapy when hypoxemia is present, to prevent alveolar hypoxia.

Clinical Presentation

The infant with BPD often demonstrates a barrel chest, tachypnea, retractions, and failure to thrive. In the most severely affected infants, digital clubbing is present and signals a very poor prognosis. The chest radiograph often shows scattered linear infiltrates and patchy areas of hyperinflation.

Arterial blood gases will reveal a compensated respiratory acidosis. Renal retention of bicarbonate restores the arterial pH to near normal despite the presence of hypercarbia; note that renal compensation will never *overcompensate* to produce an alkalotic pH. If respiratory failure worsens from the baseline (e.g., caused by pneumonia), a significant acidosis will develop, indicating that the respiratory failure has acutely outstripped renal compensation. Hypoxemia should not be present if appropriate oxygen therapy is provided.

An *alkalotic* arterial pH represents a complication of diuretic therapy, rather than renal "overcompensation." This alkalosis is not always associated with hypokalemia or hypochloremia but should be considered in any infant who receives chronic furosemide therapy without concomitant potassium chloride supplementation.

Infants with BPD are often hospitalized for increased respiratory distress associated with respiratory infections. Therefore symptoms of *potential* respiratory failure are likely to be present, including increased respiratory effort. Hypercapnia or hypoxemia beyond the child's baseline values, associated with an acidotic pH, indicate probable acute respiratory deterioration (failure). Be alert for signs of congestive heart failure, including tachycardia, tachypnea, hepatomegaly, periorbital or sacral edema, decreased urine output, and decreased peripheral perfusion.

Management

The goal of therapy is maintenance of adequate ventilation and oxygenation. This is achieved through administration of oxygen, diuretics, bronchodilators, steroids, and nutritional support. Postnatal administration of dexamethasone to the neonate with RDS may improve pulmonary status and may minimize lung injury, but its long-term value remains unproved.

Supplemental oxygen will promote adequate tissue oxygenation and avoid pulmonary vascular and cardiac complications. Oxygen requirements may vary during wakefulness, sleep, crying, and feeding; thus oxygen administration should be adjusted carefully, based on monitoring of oxygen saturations by pulse oximetry. Supplemental oxygen should not be "weaned" if doing so creates even intermittent hypoxemia, because this will be associated with alveolar hypoxia and may stimulate the development of pulmonary hypertension.

Hospitalization is often required for decompensation associated with respiratory infections, particularly during the fall and winter months, when respiratory viruses (e.g., respiratory syncytial virus [RSV]) are prevalent. Mechanical ventilatory support will be required if worsening hypoxemia or hypercarbia is associated with significant acidosis or apnea, or if increased work of breathing with signs of fatigue develop. Ventilatory support for chronically hypercarbic infants should be provided to restore the pH to baseline levels, rather than reducing the carbon dioxide levels or raising the pH to "normal." Adequate exhalation time is required during mechanical ventilation to prevent air trapping (Figure 6-11).

Diuretic therapy may improve lung function, but serum electrolytes and pH must be closely monitored to prevent the development of hypochloremic or hypokalemic metabolic alkalosis. Formation of renal calculi has also been associated with furosemide administration; therefore examine the urine at intervals for hematuria and hypercalciuria.

Beta-agonists, particularly the inhaled bronchodilators (e.g., albuterol) may be prescribed for infants with BPD and recurrent wheezing. Steroids may be indicated for the treatment of exacerbations of reactive airway disease, which are seen in older infants with chronic BPD.

Optimal nutritional support is essential for recovery of the infant with BPD, but this support may be difficult to attain. High caloric intake must be provided in limited fluid volume. In addition, many infants with BPD demonstrate gastro-esophageal reflux or swallowing dysfunction. Whenever possible, these infants should be fed in a quiet environment. Gastric or nasojejunal tube feedings may be necessary to supplement oral feedings.

The family will require extensive support, since BPD is a chronic illness characterized by periodic acute exacerbations. Approximately half of all children with BPD will require rehospitalization during the first 2 years after discharge from the newborn unit, but most infants will demonstrate clinical improvement during the first year of life. The parents must be taught the need for long-term follow-up care and regular respiratory evaluation. The parents should also be cautioned about the hazards of tobacco smoke exposure, wood stoves, and other inhaled irritants.

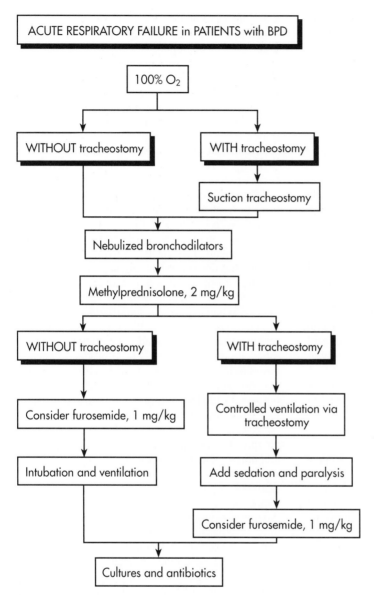

Figure 6-11 Management of patients with bronchopulmonary dysplasia (BPD) and acute respiratory failure. (Redrawn from Nichols DG et al, editors: *Golden hour: the handbook of advanced pediatric life support,* ed 2, St Louis, 1996, Mosby.)

Congenital Diaphragm Hernia

Etiology/Pathophysiology

Diaphragm hernia is a congenital defect in the diaphragm that results in a communication between the thoracic and abdominal cavities during fetal life. In the majority of patients (>85%), the left side of the diaphragm is affected. Abdominal organs enter the chest in utero and interfere with growth and development of both lungs, resulting in varying degrees of pulmonary hypoplasia. Most neonates with congenital diaphragm hernia (CDH) develop severe respiratory insufficiency and require surgery during the first days of life.

In infants with CDH, alveolar hypoxia and acidosis produce increased pulmonary vascular resistance. This typically results in right to left shunting through the ductus arteriosus. This condition is referred to as persistent fetal circulation (PFC) or persistent pulmonary hypertension of the newborn (PPHN). It produces worsening hypoxemia and acidosis and may result in right ventricular failure (see Pulmonary Hypertension and discussion of shock in Chapter 5).

Clinical Presentation

The neonate with CDH has a barrel chest with a flat or sunken abdomen. Tachypnea and respiratory distress, including nasal flaring, severe retractions, cyanosis, and respiratory acidosis, are present. Decreased lung compliance is apparent following intubation, since high inspiratory pressures will be required during hand ventilation and mechanical ventilation. The differential diagnosis includes pneumothorax, lung cysts, or large pleural effusion.

Arterial blood gas analysis is consistent with respiratory failure, including hypoxemia and respiratory acidosis. The chest radiograph is usually diagnostic; loops of bowel are visible in the left side of the chest, and the mediastinum is shifted into the right side. Echocardiography may be used to evaluate the severity of pulmonary hypertension.

Management

Support of oxygenation and ventilation is required. The neonate is intubated, mechanically ventilated, and sedated (pharmacologic paralysis is often provided—see Chapter 3) and placed in semi-Fowler's position. A nasogastric tube is inserted to decompress the stomach. Surgical intervention is required.

Before and after surgery, mechanical support of oxygenation and ventilation may include conventional mechanical ventilation, high-frequency ventilation, or extracorporeal membrane oxygenation (ECMO). ECMO may be used to stabilize the infant before surgical intervention and may also be used intraoperatively and postoperatively.

The goal of therapy is improvement in oxygenation and arterial pH. If alveolar hypoxia and acidosis persist, pulmonary hypertension will remain severe and will promote right-to-left shunting and progressive hypoxemia and acidosis.

The pulmonary vascular bed will be very reactive preoperatively and postoperatively. Factors that cause pulmonary vasoconstriction should be avoided, and factors that cause pulmonary vasodilation should be supported. The care of the child with pulmonary hypertension is summarized under Pulmonary Hypertension and Chapter 5, p. 211.

A mild alkalosis (pH 7.5) is maintained through mild hyperventilation, administration of sodium bicarbonate, or both. Alveolar oxygenation is supported through mechanical ventilation, and the effectiveness of oxygenation is evaluated with pulse oximetry. Two people are required for suctioning, to prevent the development of hypoxia.

Recently, inhaled nitric oxide (NO) has been used to treat neonatal pulmonary hypertension in patients with CDH, as well as in other infants with persistent pulmonary hypertension caused by sepsis, pneumonia, or RDS. Nitric oxide is an endothelial-derived relaxing factor, a naturally occurring vasodilator that is produced in lung capillary cells and that acts to dilate vascular smooth muscle. When it is administered in inhaled form and produces pulmonary vasodilation, it is metabolized within seconds or is bound to hemoglobin; thus in moderate doses it is unlikely to produce systemic vasodilation. Use of nitric oxide has improved oxygenation and reduced the need for ECMO in newborns with PPHN and has been particularly useful following surgical correction of CDH (see p. 211).

Because neonates with CDH have small, noncompliant lungs (particularly on the side with the diaphragm defect), they are at risk for the development of pneumothorax preoperatively and postoperatively. Signs of tension pneumothorax include hypertension, tachycardia, sudden decrease in hemoglobin saturation and oxygenation, asymmetry of chest expansion during positive pressure ventilation, decreased or absent unilateral breath sounds, and tracheal deviation. A chest radiograph can confirm the diagnosis. Decompression of the pneumothorax with a needle or chest tube insertion is often necessary.

Pulmonary Hypertension

Etiology/Pathophysiology

Pulmonary hypertension is caused by an increase in pulmonary artery resistance, which may be a primary condition of unknown etiology or secondary to infection, RDS, chronic alveolar hypoxia from any cause, asphyxia, congenital heart disease, or congenital lung malformations. Secondary pulmonary hypertension can be caused by an increase in the volume of pulmonary blood flow, by an increase in the pressure of pulmonary blood flow, or from obstruction to pulmonary venous return or left atrial blood flow (e.g., mitral stenosis). If the pulmonary hypertension persists, structural changes in the pulmonary arteries develop and can become permanent and progressive. These changes are called pulmonary vascular disease.

Eisenmenger's Syndrome   If severe pulmonary hypertension is caused by a congenital heart or vascular malformation causing a left-to-right or aorta–to–pulmonary artery shunt, the direction of the shunt may reverse to become a right-to-left shunt (or a pulmonary artery–to–aorta shunt). This reversal of shunt direction is called Eisenmenger's syndrome and indicates the presence of severe and probably irreversible pulmonary hypertension.

Cor Pulmonale   Cor pulmonale is heart failure resulting from pulmonary hypertension. This complication can develop in children with chronic lung disease. It may be prevented if oxygen administration is adjusted to prevent hypoxemia and alveolar hypoxia.

Clinical Presentation

The patient with pulmonary hypertension may be asymptomatic or may demonstrate symptoms of the primary condition. For example, the child with a congenital heart defect may develop congestive heart failure from the defect. When pulmonary hypertension is severe, hypoxemia, dyspnea, and decreased exercise tolerance develop. Pulmonary hypertension can be diagnosed by echocardiography or by direct measurement of pulmonary artery pressure with a pulmonary artery catheter or during cardiac catheterization. Evaluation of structural changes in the pulmonary arteries requires a biopsy, which may be accomplished through a thoracotomy or thoracoscopy.

The development of Eisenmenger's syndrome is associated with the development of cyanosis indicating a right-to-left shunt in the child with congenital heart disease that formerly produced a left-to-right shunt. Right heart failure and cor pulmonale in the child with pulmonary hypertension is characterized by tachycardia, reduced ejection fraction, systemic venous engorgement, and signs of adrenergic compensation, including peripheral vasoconstriction, decreased urine output, and diaphoresis. Cor pulmonale may be reversible, or it may be chronic or severe and progressive.

Management

Treatment of pulmonary hypertension requires elimination of factors that promote pulmonary vasoconstriction and administration of oxygen or other agents that promote pulmonary vasodilation:

- *Pulmonary vasoconstrictors:* Alveolar hypoxia, acidosis, hypothermia, hyperinflation, and agitation
- *Pulmonary vasodilators:* Oxygen, alkalosis, normothermia, sedation, prevention of hyperinflation, and experimental therapies, including inhaled nitric oxide, and calcium channel blockers

Treatment of primary pulmonary hypertension is supportive. The only curative therapy is a lung or heart-lung transplant. Treatment of secondary pulmonary hypertension requires identification and treatment of the cause. For example, cardiovascular surgery may be required to eliminate a source of hypertensive pulmonary blood flow. Postoperative pulmonary hypertension may lead to postoperative instability, requiring careful support of oxygenation with mechanical ventilation, sedation (narcotics and possibly anesthetic agents may be required), maintenance of a mild metabolic or respiratory alkalosis (pH 7.5), reduction in stimulation, and possible administration of pulmonary vasodilators.

Nitric oxide is an endothelium-derived relaxing factor. It is produced in lung capillary cells, and it acts in vascular smooth muscle cells to promote pulmonary vasodilation. It may be administered by inhalation to promote selective pulmonary vasodilation. Since this vasodilator is delivered by inhalation, it dilates pulmonary arteries near the best ventilated alveoli, improving the match of ventilation and perfusion. It is metabolized within seconds or is bound by hemoglobin; thus it usually will not produce systemic vasodilation in moderate doses. Nitric oxide has improved the clinical course of newborns with persistent pulmonary hypertension and now may be used to treat pediatric pulmonary hypertension following cardiovascular surgery (with research protocol).

Nitric oxide is delivered via a mechanical ventilator. A dose of 10 to 80 parts per million (ppm) is provided, although a response is usually obtained with lower doses. A positive response includes pulmonary vasodilation, a decrease in pulmonary artery pressure, and an improvement in oxygenation. Methemoglobin may be formed during nitric oxide therapy; thus levels of methemoglobin are monitored during therapy. Therapy should be halted or reduced if the methemoglobin level exceeds 20% of total hemoglobin. Since the pulse oximeter does not recognize methemoglobin, pulse oximetry will not be accurate in the presence of >5% methemoglobinemia.

During mechanical ventilation, suctioning may cause abrupt and severe deterioration. Two health care professionals should be used to suction the patient, since alveolar hypoxia and deterioration may occur during suctioning. One professional provides hand ventilation and monitors the patient's color, heart rate, and pulse oximetry while the second professional only suctions efficiently. If deterioration occurs during suctioning, the suctioning attempt should be interrupted to provide oxygenation.

For further information regarding manipulation of pulmonary vascular resistance, see Chapter 5, p. 211.

Croup (Laryngotracheobronchitis)

Etiology/Pathophysiology

Croup refers to the clinical syndrome of stridor, cough, and hoarseness that results from laryngeal inflammation and edema causing upper airway narrowing. Infectious laryngotracheobronchitis (LTB) is usually viral in origin. Viral LTB is most common and occurs predominantly in children 3 months to 3 years of age. It may be caused by parainfluenza (60%), RSV, adenovirus, or influenza. Bacterial LTB is rare but can be caused by *Staphylococcus aureus* or *Corynebacterium diphtheriae*. Noninfectious croup may result from laryngotracheomalacia, asthma, angioneurotic edema, hemangioma, foreign body aspiration, vocal cord weakness, an extrinsic mass, or subglottic stenosis following endotracheal intubation.

The subglottic region is the narrowest segment of the child's upper airway. It consists of a richly vascularized area surrounded by the rigid ring of the cricoid cartilage. When infection or irritation produces edema, the cartilage limits external expansion of the tissue, and the airway lumen is narrowed. In addition, the subglottic edema may limit vocal cord abduction during inspiration, further increasing airway resistance. Inflammatory secretions may also contribute to the airway obstruction.

Clinical Presentation

A history of rhinitis, mild fever, malaise, and anorexia for 2 to 3 days usually precedes the development of respiratory signs. The onset of croup is heralded by the development of a barking cough and hoarseness. The child appears restless and anxious and may demonstrate inspiratory stridor. Since the airway obstruction increases resistance to airflow, sternal retractions, a sign of increased respiratory effort, will be present. Diminished breath sounds and adventitious sounds may be noted on auscultation.

Ventilation-perfusion mismatch results from inflammation of the small airways (bronchiolitis). Hypercapnia, hypoxemia, tachycardia, and respiratory acidosis may develop if airway obstruction is severe.

The differential diagnosis of acute LTB includes epiglottitis, foreign body aspiration, retropharyngeal or peritonsillar abscess, bacterial tracheitis, diphtheria, trauma, allergic reaction, angioneurotic edema, or tumor (Table 6-6). The most important diagnostic study performed for the child with croup is a lateral radiograph of the neck, which is performed to *rule out* epiglottitis, retropharyngeal abscess, and foreign body airway obstruction, rather than to diagnose croup. It will reveal a normal epiglottis and edema of the subglottic tracheal soft tissues. Direct examination of the oropharynx should be performed only by a physician skilled in airway management (see Epiglottitis).

Management

Treatment of LTB is largely supportive and includes oxygen therapy plus measures that comfort the child and facilitate airflow until the inflammation resolves. Maintenance of a patent airway is essential.

Table 6-6
Diagnostic Features of Infectious Causes of Stridor

	Viral Croup	Epiglottitis	Bacterial Tracheitis	Retropharyngeal Abscess
History				
Age	2 months-4 years	3-6 years (up to adult)	2-4 years	Children-adults
Prodrome	None or upper respiratory tract infection	None	Upper respiratory tract infection	Pharyngitis, trauma
Onset	Gradual	Fulminant	Variable	Slow
Dysphagia	±	+++	±	+++
Signs:				
Fever	Low grade	High, toxic	High, toxic	Variable
Stridor	+++	++	+++	+
Drooling	−	+++	±	+++
Posture	Lying	Sitting	Variable	Variable
Tests:				
WBC	<10,000	>10,000	>10,000	>10,000
X-ray	Subglottic narrowing	Swollen supraglottis	Subglottic irregularity	Widened retropharynx
Cultures	Parainfluenza, respiratory syncytial virus	*Haemophilus influenzae,* streptococcus	*Staphylococcus aureus*	Staphylococcus, streptococcus, anaerobes

Modified from Nichols DG et al, editors: *Golden hour: the handbook of advanced pediatric life support,* ed 2, St Louis, 1996, Mosby.

Keep the child as quiet and comfortable as possible, and prevent crying and agitation, which create turbulent airflow and increase resistance to airflow and respiratory effort. Encourage the parents to remain at the bedside to decrease the child's agitation. Do not perform painful procedures until the diagnosis is confirmed (i.e., epiglottitis is ruled out) and airway patency can be monitored.

Equipment for intubation and possible tracheostomy should be readily available at the bedside. Consider intubation if the child demonstrates increased work of breathing (particularly if associated with signs of fatigue), heart rate consistently greater than 160 beats/min, circumoral pallor, increased agitation, apprehension, or decreased level of consciousness.

Respiratory distress may be minimized by the administration of humidified oxygen. Pulse oximetry will enable detection of hypoxemia and can guide the titration of oxygen therapy.

Monitor the child's heart rate and rhythm, as well as respiratory rate, depth, and pattern, including severity of retractions and nasal flaring. Extreme tachycardia or bradycardia may indicate the development of hypoxemia. A decrease in hoarseness, periodic breathing, or slowing of the respiratory rate may indicate respiratory muscle fatigue. Arterial blood samples for blood gas analysis may be obtained if the child's condition warrants it, but frequent arterial punctures should be avoided if possible because they cause further agitation.

Monitor the child's body temperature and administer antipyretics as ordered for fever >38.5° C. Administer IV fluids if respiratory distress or deterioration preclude adequate oral intake or if dehydration is present. Avoid fluid overload, however, because it can cause or worsen pulmonary edema. The urine specific gravity and daily evaluation of body weight provide good indicators of the child's level of hydration.

Racemic epinephrine may be administered by inhalation to reduce airway edema and airway resistance and to improve clinical symptoms of respiratory distress. Hourly treatments may occasionally be necessary. Side effects include tachycardia and irritability.

Heliox, a mixture of 30% oxygen and 70% helium, may be administered. Since the density of helium is lower than the density of air or oxygen, the helium will flow rapidly through the narrowed upper airway. Heliox inhalation may decrease the work of breathing, lessen fatigue, and possibly prevent intubation. However, it cannot be used if the child requires >30% to 40% supplemental oxygen.

Parenteral corticosteroids are probably indicated for severely affected patients. Steroid administration (dexamethasone, 0.6 mg/kg) will produce symptomatic improvement (improvement in color, air entry, stridor, and retractions) and may improve oxygenation and decrease the length of hospital stay.

Epiglottitis

Etiology/Pathophysiology

Epiglottitis is a medical emergency characterized by severe airway obstruction caused by inflammation and swelling of the epiglottis, false cords, and aryepiglottic folds. Complete occlusion of the airway may be precipitated by stimulation of the gag reflex, traumatic examination of the upper airway, or suctioning.

Epiglottitis is most common in children 3 to 6 years of age, and until recently, *Haemophilus influenzae* was the most common causative organism. With the introduction of the *H. influenzae* B vaccine, epiglottitis is now rare in immunized individuals. Uncommon causes of epiglottitis include group A beta streptococcus, pneumococcus, *Staphylococcus aureus,* and nontypable *H. influenzae* strains.

Clinical Presentation

The clinical course of epiglottis is typically rapid. The child often demonstrates a muffled voice and weak cough, in contrast to the barking cough and hoarseness that are observed in patients with LTB.

Other signs and symptoms (see Table 6-6) include high fever (above 39° C), sore throat, drooling, and dysphagia. Swelling of the epiglottis produces signs of progressive airway obstruction, including inspiratory stridor, sternal retractions, tachycardia, and decreased breath sounds. The child is often anxious, preferring to sit and lean forward. Late signs of hypoxia include listlessness, cyanosis, and cardiac arrhythmias, including bradycardia and premature ventricular contractions.

A lateral radiograph of the neck shows the epiglottis as a large, rounded soft tissue mass at the base of the tongue. Definitive diagnosis is established through direct examination of the upper airway, but this should only occur in the operating room just before intubation. The epiglottis is cherry red and swollen.

Management

The child with suspected epiglottitis must be kept quiet and undisturbed until intubation can be accomplished by skilled personnel in the operating room or other controlled area. Personnel qualified to perform emergency intubation or tracheostomy must be present. The child's primary caretakers should remain with the child, if possible, to reduce the child's anxiety. Minimize stimulation or agitation of the child to prevent episodes of crying. The child will probably be most comfortable held in the arms of a person known to him or her.

Oxygen can be administered by simple "blow-by" technique or through a loosely fitting mask, but it should not be forced on the child. Older children with severe epiglottitis may prefer to sit upright, with the hands out in front of the trunk and the neck thrust forward. The child should *not* be forced into the supine position, since this may compromise diaphragm excursion and air movement and may precipitate crying and laryngospasm.

Monitor the child's oxygenation and respiratory status closely. Assess the rate and depth of respiration and the presence of retractions; observe for nasal flaring and stridor; and evaluate the child's color and air movement. If a significant increase in work of breathing or deterioration in air movement is observed, notify a physician immediately; it may be necessary to accelerate plans for intubation.

Intubation and tracheostomy equipment (including laryngoscope blades with working bulbs, tube, lidocaine jelly, and tracheostomy tray) of the proper size should be placed at the bedside. *Inspection of the upper airway should generally not be performed at the bedside. If it is necessary to examine the airway, someone skilled in intubation must be present at the bedside with all equipment for an urgent intubation readily available.* Stimulus of a gag reflex (e.g., during insertion of a tongue blade or suction catheter) should be avoided as it may induce laryngospasm or increase edema, resulting in acute airway obstruction. Occasionally intubation cannot be accomplished once laryngospasm has occurred, and creation of a tracheostomy may be required.

If the lateral neck radiograph suggests epiglottitis, immediate endotracheal intubation is performed by skilled personnel, usually in the operating room. The red, swollen epiglottis is visualized as the tube is inserted—this confirms the diagnosis. It may be necessary to insert an endotracheal tube that is one size smaller than normal for the child's age and body length, since the radius of the child's airway is compromised by swelling.

If cardiorespiratory arrest should occur before an artificial airway has been secured, bag-mask ventilation with 100% oxygen (an FiO_2 of 1.00) should be attempted. Ventilation may not be effective if inflammation is severe or if the child struggles. If the child loses consciousness, it may be possible to provide effective bag-valve-mask ventilation. If airway obstruction prevents this ventilation, a cricothyrotomy may occasionally be performed. A large-bore needle (13 to 15 gauge) is inserted into the cricothyroid area and is joined to a standard 15-mm blue endotracheal tube adapter. This cricothyrotomy will enable delivery of *oxygen* but will not effectively remove *carbon dioxide;* thus hypercarbia will likely result.

Once intubation is accomplished, low-pressure mechanical ventilation is provided with 25% to 40% inspired oxygen (FiO_2 of 0.25 to 0.40). The endotracheal tube must be taped securely in place, since spontaneous extubation can be a life-threatening event (reintubation can be extremely difficult). Sedation may be necessary if oxygen administration and establishment of a patient airway do not eliminate the patient's agitation. Extubation can usually be accomplished within 48 to 72 hours after antibiotic therapy is started.

Provide adequate fluid and caloric intake. Withhold oral fluids before intubation to reduce the possibility of vomiting and aspiration during intubation. IV fluids will ensure adequate hydration. Immediately after extubation, the child should receive nothing by mouth for 4 or more hours, until the health team is certain that reintubation will not be required. Once the child has demonstrated tolerance of extubation, oral fluids may again be provided.

Bronchiolitis

Etiology/Pathophysiology

Bronchiolitis is a lower respiratory tract viral illness, predominantly caused by RSV but also associated with adenovirus, influenza, and parainfluenza. The peak incidence of illness occurs from midwinter to early spring and typically affects infants less than 18 months of age. Bronchiolitis may be severe in infants with chronic lung or cardiovascular disease.

Bronchiolitis is characterized by inflammation of the bronchioles, increased mucus production, airway edema, small airway obstruction, and air trapping. Air trapping, in turn, creates an increase in functional residual capacity, causing the infant to breathe at a higher lung volume, which reduces lung compliance and increases the work of breathing. Multiple areas of atelectasis produce ventilation-perfusion mismatch with resultant hypoxia and hypercarbia.

Clinical Presentation

Diagnosis is based primarily on clinical observations and knowledge of community outbreaks. A typical history includes 2 to 5 days of upper respiratory tract infection and fever, followed by development of tachypnea, wheezing, crackles, and retractions. Episodes of apnea and/or cyanosis may also be observed. Lung hyperinflation may produce a palpable liver. The diagnosis of RSV bronchiolitis can be made by culture of infected secretions or by techniques that detect RSV antigen (including ELISA).

The chest radiograph demonstrates hyperinflation, a flattened diaphragm, and atelectasis. Hypoxemia may be detected using pulse oximetry, and both hypoxemia and hypercarbia may be detected by arterial blood gas sampling.

Management

There is no specific therapy for acute bronchiolitis regardless of etiology. Treatment is largely supportive, ensuring adequate oxygenation with ventilatory support as needed. Monitor the infant's respiratory status closely and be alert for signs of respiratory fatigue, respiratory failure, or apnea. Signs of *potential* respiratory failure include an increase in respiratory effort, cyanosis, and mottled color. The child with potential respiratory failure requires administration of humidified oxygen and reduction of oxygen demand. Keep the infant warm and comfortable, and minimize stimulation.

Aerosolized beta-adrenergic agonists, such as albuterol or terbutaline, may result in symptomatic improvement. Treatment with corticosteroids is controversial but may be useful if the infant has a past history of wheezing or asthma.

Adequate hydration is maintained by the IV route; the tachypneic, distressed infant should receive nothing by mouth. Bronchiolitis is highly contagious, and hospital personnel, adults, and children can be easily infected. Contact and/or respiratory isolation is recommended for children with bronchiolitis.

Ribavirin is an antiviral agent that may be administered to infants with confirmed RSV infection; administration of this agent should be provided according to established hospital protocol. The efficacy of ribavirin is controversial, however, and it is no longer used in some centers. It is administered by a small-particle aerosol generator (SPAG) while the infant is breathing spontaneously, or it may be administered through the ventilator circuit during mechanical ventilation (use of special filters is required). If ribavirin is administered during mechanical ventilation, monitor for evidence of airway or ventilator circuit obstruction and be prepared to provide hand ventilation if circuit obstruction develops. Adverse reactions to ribavirin therapy include anemia, conjunctivitis, and rash. Since the teratogenic effects of ribavirin are unknown, pregnant nurses should not care for the infant receiving this therapy.

Pneumonia
Pathophysiology

Pneumonia is an infection or inflammation of the lung, The causative agent is most commonly infectious, including viruses, bacteria, or, rarely, fungi. Pneumonia can also be caused by aspiration and resultant inflammation.

Causative agents of pneumonia vary with the age and clinical condition of the child:

1. Neonatal pneumonia
   a. Congenital: cytomegalovirus, herpes simplex, rubella, or toxoplasma
   b. Acquired: *Chlamydia trachomatis,* group B streptococcus, or gram-negative enterobacillus such as *Escherichia coli* or *Klebsiella* organisms
2. All age groups: viral pneumonia (influenza, RSV, parainfluenza virus, or adenovirus) most common
3. Children older than age 5: possibly *Mycoplasma pneumoniae*
4. Bacterial pneumonia in otherwise healthy children: pneumococcus *(Streptococcus pneumoniae),* streptococcus, or staphylococcus
5. Pneumonia in the immunocompromised child: *Pneumocystis carinii, Candida* species, or *Aspergillus* organisms

Pneumonia can be classified as lobar, bronchopneumonia, or interstitial pneumonia on the basis of clinical and radiographic evidence. In lobar pneumonia one or more lobes are involved. Interstitial pneumonia is associated with bilateral alveolar inflammation.

Clinical Presentation

Clinically, it may be difficult to distinguish bacterial from viral pneumonia:

- *Viral pneumonia:* Often preceded by symptoms of upper respiratory tract infection. Diffuse interstitial infiltrate is present on the chest radiograph.
- *Bacterial pneumonia:* Often characterized by high fever and sudden onset or may follow a viral illness. Lobar consolidation or pleural

effusion is often present on the chest radiograph.

Generally, infants and younger children tend to develop more severe symptoms of respiratory infection than older children. In addition, the natural history of the illness may differ in infants because of the anatomic differences of the infant lung.

Possible signs and symptoms of respiratory infection include:

- Fever or (in young infants) hypothermia
- Respiratory symptoms: cough, tachypnea, chest pain, retractions, nasal flaring, cyanosis, crackles, dullness to percussion, change in pitch or intensity of breath sounds over an area of consolidation
- Change in behavior: irritability, restlessness, lethargy
- Gastrointestinal symptoms: anorexia, vomiting, diarrhea, abdominal pain

A specific pathogen is identified by blood culture, pleural fluid culture, or culture of lower respiratory tract secretions by bronchoscopy. Sputum cultures are generally unreliable. Open-lung biopsy is occasionally necessary to establish a diagnosis in immunocompromised patients or when the patient has not responded clinically to broad-spectrum antibiotic therapy.

Management

Treatment of pneumonia requires respiratory assessment and general supportive care, including oxygen. Antimicrobial agents are provided if a bacterial etiology is suspected. If the child is immunosuppressed, broad-spectrum antimicrobial therapy is instituted before a pathogen is isolated, and antibiotic therapy is reassessed after culture results are obtained.

Evaluate the child's respiratory rate and effort, color, gas exchange, and breath sounds. Auscultate lung fields frequently and be alert to the development or worsening of adventitious sounds, or alteration in the pitch or intensity of breath sounds. Once any area of consolidation or congestion is identified, monitor for evidence of clearing or exacerbation. Significant changes should be reported

to the physician. If deterioration in respiratory function occurs, intubation and mechanical ventilatory support may be required.

Suctioning may be necessary to assist in the removal of secretions if the child's cough is ineffective. Chest physiotherapy may aid in mobilization of secretions if there is lobar consolidation and hypoxemia is present, or if neuromuscular disease or other conditions prevent an effective cough.

If unilateral pneumonia is present, position the child with the involved lobe on top to provide postural drainage; this position may also improve systemic oxygenation because the uninvolved lung is better perfused (but less well ventilated) in the dependent position. However, the child's individual response should be assessed.

Monitor the child's body temperature and treat fever with antipyretics. Monitor the child's fluid status through evaluation of systemic perfusion, and urine volume and specific gravity. If the child's circulating blood volume is adequate (i.e., significant dehydration is not present), the child's fluid intake is generally limited to approximately two thirds of calculated maintenance fluids. Fever will increase insensible water losses; thus a slight increase in fluid intake (75% maintenance fluids) may be necessary. Viral pneumonia requires contact isolation, which includes the use of masks for those close to the patient, use of gowns if soiling of clothing by secretions is likely, and use of gloves if infected material is likely to be touched. Handwashing must be performed before and after *every* contact with the patient, patient equipment, or bedclothes. Infective or contaminated material must be disposed of in properly marked bags.

Complications of pneumonia (especially staphylococcal pneumonia) include the development of empyema, lung abscess, and pleural effusion. Rarely, pyopneumothorax and tension pneumothorax can develop. If pleural fluid accumulation in the chest is detected by auscultation, chest radiograph, or ultrasound, a thoracentesis is performed and the fluid obtained is cultured. Continuous chest drainage may be necessary when purulent fluid is aspirated.

Once the child's respiratory status is stable, oral feedings can be resumed, and the IV fluid administration rate should be reduced accordingly. As the child continues to improve, a diet appropriate for age can be provided.

Prophylaxis may prevent some episodes of pneumonia. Children and adolescents with human immunodeficiency virus (HIV) infection and low CD4+ cell counts may receive lifetime prophylaxis against *Pneumocystis carinii* using trimethoprim-sulfamethoxazole or aerosolized pentamidine.

Aspiration Pneumonia

Etiology/Pathophysiology

Aspiration pneumonia occurs when food, pharyngeal or gastrointestinal secretions, or volatile compounds enter the lung and cause inflammation or a chemical pneumonitis. The risk of aspiration pneumonia is increased in patients with an impaired level of consciousness or impaired neuromuscular control. Complications resulting from aspiration of particulate matter is discussed under Foreign Body Aspiration (immediately following).

Aspiration pneumonia may be classified according to the type of substance aspirated. The severity of the lung injury is dependent on the acidity, the volatility, and the viscosity of the aspirated material, as well as the presence of bacteria. Aspiration can result in a bacterial pneumonia or a chemical pneumonitis, particularly following aspiration of gastric acid or hydrocarbons (kerosene, furniture polish, etc.). Inert fluids, including saline, saliva, water, barium, and many nasogastric feeding solutions, may not produce a chemical pneumonitis or infection but may decrease lung compliance and cause hypoxemia.

Pulmonary hemorrhage, necrosis, surfactant inactivation, and pulmonary edema may occur following aspiration, resulting in abnormal compliance and V/Q mismatching. In its most severe form, aspiration syndromes can lead to respiratory failure and ARDS. The classification and clinical signs of the most common forms of hydrocarbon aspiration are listed in Table 6-7.

Clinical Presentation

Aspiration of gastric contents may produce immediate pulmonary symptoms that worsen over the first 24 hours. Cough, vomiting, tachypnea, dyspnea, rales (crackles), wheezing, and cyanosis may be noted, as well as pulmonary edema and hemoptysis. Fever usually results from a chemical pneumonitis and does not necessarily indicate the presence of a bacterial infection.

Clinical signs of aspiration of oral secretions may not be distinguishable from other forms of acute bacterial pneumonia. If vegetable matter has been aspirated (nuts, carrots, or popcorn), symptoms may not appear for several weeks following the episode. There may be an increased cough, fever, and foul-smelling sputum.

The chest radiograph may not reveal signs of the aspiration for several hours, but then changes may appear and worsen over the first 72 hours. Clearing may then be observed, although some abnormalities may persist for 4 to 6 weeks. Initial perihilar densities are present, which progress to consolidation. Air trapping and formation of pneumatoceles and cysts may rarely develop. Infiltrates may be present in any lobe but are most likely to be observed in the right upper lobe of the supine, intubated patient.

Management

In the event of hydrocarbon ingestion/aspiration, it is essential to identify the material and estimate the amount ingested. In general, vomiting should *not* be induced following the aspiration of most hydrocarbons, since further aspiration may occur. However, a poison control center should be consulted immediately, and their recommendations followed. Assess pulmonary, cardiac, neurologic, gastrointestinal, and renal status closely for evidence of toxicity.

Treatment is primarily supportive, including monitoring of blood gases and oxyhemoglobin saturation, management of bronchospasm and arrhythmias, mechanical ventilation, and support of oxygenation. Risk of air leaks is high; therefore be alert for the development of signs of pneumothorax, pneumomediastinum, and pneumopericardium. Treatment is similar to that described for ARDS (see Acute Respiratory Distress Syndrome, p. 332 and Nursing Care of the Child Requiring Mechanical Ventilation, p. 316).

The risk of aspiration is increased when obtunded or tachypneic patients are fed or when critically ill infants are overfed. In these patients prevention of aspiration pneumonia is essential.

Table 6-7
Clinical Features and Toxic Manifestations Following Aspiration of Common Hydrocarbons

Classification	Examples	Toxic Manifestations
Aliphatics (low-viscosity hydro-carbons)	Petroleum ether Gasoline Naphtha (lighter fluid, cleaning fluid, paint thinner) Kerosene (fuel, lighter fluid, painter thinner) Mineral seal oil (furniture polish)	Most commonly ingested, most likely to cause pulmonary toxicity Chemical pneumonitis CNS depression (due to hypoxemia) Coma, respiratory arrest GI irritant Myocardial dysfunction
Aromatic	Benzene, toluene, xylene, naphthalene, aniline Nail polish removers Degreasing cleaners Lacquers	Chemical pneumonitis Cardiac arrhythmias Excitement, delirium, seizures, hypertonicity, hyperreflexia secondary to systemic absorption via lung, skin, or gut
Halogenated	Carbon tetrachloride Tetrachloroethane Trichloromethane PCBs (polychlorinated biphenyls) This group most commonly used as solvents, antiseptics, propellants, refrigerants, and fumigants	Pulmonary and CNS toxicity less likely Hepatic and renal damage
Hydrocarbons combined with toxic additives		Toxicity dependent on additives
Hydrocarbons (high viscosity)	Lubricating oil Mineral oil Petroleum jelly Grease, tar	Much less likely to cause chemical pneumonitis, minimal absorption secondary to very high viscosity

From Hazinski MF: *Nursing care of the critically ill child,* ed 2, St Louis, 1992, Mosby.

Positioning of the infant or child with the right side down following feedings may reduce the possibility of aspiration and promote the movement of gastric contents into the duodenum. Elevate the head of the child's bed during and after every feeding if gastroesophageal reflux is suspected.

When nasogastric feedings are administered by continuous infusion, monitor the child closely, since an infusion pump will continue to infuse the feeding material even when the child is vomiting. Use of Y-tubing (with one arm of the Y serving as a vent) during infusion of feedings will allow reflux if the child vomits. Feedings should be advanced very gradually in both volume and concentration.

Before each intermittent nasogastric feeding, some centers recommend the aspiration of gastric contents and measurement of total residual undi-gested feedings. If the child continues to retain significant amounts of residual formula between each feeding, the volume or the concentration of the formula should be reduced, or the time between feedings should be increased.

Foreign Body Aspiration

Etiology/Pathophysiology

Aspiration of a foreign body presents a serious and potentially fatal problem. The severity of the foreign body aspiration (FBA) is determined by the type of object aspirated, and the location and extent of airway obstruction produced. Prompt recognition of the problem and effective removal of the object are essential.

The greatest risk of FBA occurs in the older infant and toddler. Items aspirated include inorganic objects such as plastic toys and earrings, as well as vegetable matter, such as hot dogs, nuts, peanuts, seeds, and uncooked vegetables.

Clinical Presentation

The possibility of FBA should be considered in any child who has an *acute* onset of respiratory distress. Laryngotracheal foreign bodies result in the acute onset of dyspnea, cough, and stridor; bronchial foreign bodies produce cough, decreased air entry, wheezing, and dyspnea. Cyanosis may also develop. Other, less common findings are hoarseness, chest pain, and recurrent respiratory tract infections. Foreign bodies lodged in the esophagus can cause significant respiratory distress and dysphagia.

Initial diagnostic testing includes an anteroposterior and lateral chest radiograph. A normal chest radiograph does not exclude the possibility of a foreign body aspiration. Although metallic objects will be visible on chest radiographs, nonmetallic objects are usually not visible. When a single foreign body is lodged in a single bronchus, unilateral obstructive emphysema will be seen on chest radiographs, particularly when inspiratory films are compared with expiratory films. Chest fluoroscopy may reveal a shift of the mediastinum on inspiration.

Management

The most effective intervention for acute aspiration of a foreign body in the airway is immediate removal of the object via rigid bronchoscopy. Before removal, the child should be kept calm and should be monitored to ensure that the airway remains patent. The child's vital signs and degree of respiratory distress are monitored, and oxygen is administered if necessary. Signs of deterioration include changes in heart rate and respiratory rate, increased severity and distribution of sternal retractions, pallor or cyanosis, loss of ability to speak, and drooling. Keep emergency equipment for intubation at the bedside.

Following removal of the object, monitor the heart rate and respiratory rate and effort. Signs of upper airway obstruction may result from edema at the site of the foreign body removal. If upper airway obstruction develops, an increase in respiratory distress will be seen, and intubation and mechanical ventilatory support may be required.

Following removal of the foreign body, chest physiotherapy may be helpful for several days, particularly if the object was lodged beyond the mainstem bronchus or if signs of infection are present. Aspirated vegetable material may break apart during removal and lodge distally; repeat bronchoscopy may be necessary if symptoms persist.

Near-Drowning

Etiology/Pathophysiology

Drowning is defined as submersion resulting in asphyxia and death within 24 hours, whereas near-drowning is defined as submersion resulting in the need for hospitalization, but not resulting in death within 24 hours. For practical purposes, most children who arrive in the ICU following submersion are classified as near-drowning victims, whether or not they survive 24 hours.

Near-drowning is one of the leading causes of death in children 1 to 4 years of age in the United States. It is also responsible for permanent and devastating neurologic sequelae in many survivors.

The majority of drownings and near-drownings are preventable. Most children drown in the home bathtub or home swimming pool. The single most important factor in preventing submersion is continuous adult observation during baths and swimming. A circumferential fence with a self-closing, self-latching gate will discourage entrance into the pool area but does not eliminate the need for adult supervision. The home should not form one of the barriers to the pool, since it is easy for a small child to open a house door to gain entrance to the pool area. Nonrigid pool covers and pool alarms are ineffective in preventing near-drowning.

All parents should know cardiopulmonary resuscitation (CPR), and this is especially true for parents in homes with swimming pools. Children should be taught not to swim alone and to watch out for each other.

Drowning and near-drowning may occur in fresh or salt water; the type of fluid aspirated is not usually significant clinically, because only a brief duration of submersion and a small quantity of fluid aspiration is necessary to produce asphyxia.

Anoxia rather than aspiration is responsible for most of the severe cardiopulmonary and neurologic complications.

Anoxia, laryngospasm, and any aspiration of fluid can cause inflammation, airway obstruction, collapse of the small airways, and an ARDS-type picture. Pulmonary capillary membrane permeability increases, producing pulmonary edema. Hypercapnia and hypoxemia with combined metabolic and respiratory acidosis develop. Surfactant washout and inactivation contribute to the development of atelectasis and intrapulmonary shunting.

The severity of neurologic sequelae following near-drowning is related to the duration of submersion, the temperature of the water, and the time that elapses before effective CPR (including basic life support) and advanced life support (including intubation) are provided. The time of submersion as reported by bystanders is notoriously unreliable, however, so it is often impossible to determine the duration of cardiopulmonary arrest.

Very small children may survive prolonged submersion in *icy* (<5° C) water because the child becomes rapidly hypothermic, reducing oxygen consumption. However, submersion beyond 5 minutes is usually associated with severe neurologic damage.

Clinical Presentation

Poor prognostic indicators for children submerged in *non*-icy waters include:

- Absence of perfusing cardiac rhythm on arrival in the emergency department (ED)—includes asystole
- Submersion duration >5 minutes or CPR duration >25 minutes
- Glasgow Coma Scale score <4 with unresponsive pupils within the first 12 to 24 hours in the ICU

The child's clinical condition and indications of severity of anoxic insult must be evaluated on arrival in the ED. On the basis of this information and discussions with the parents, the need for further aggressive resuscitation should be carefully considered.

If the child is breathing spontaneously, signs of pulmonary edema and respiratory distress (tachycardia, tachypnea, stridor, retractions) may develop, particularly within the first 8 to 12 hours after submersion.

If ventilatory support is provided, decreased lung compliance will be apparent. Auscultation may reveal pulmonary congestion and decreased lung aeration bilaterally. Rales may be heard.

Moderate hypoxemia may initially be accompanied by hypocapnia if spontaneous ventilation is restored. If ventilation-perfusion abnormalities are severe, severe hypoxemia with metabolic acidosis and hypercapnia will develop.

Management

If the child has a perfusing cardiac rhythm on arrival in the ICU, the goal of therapy is to maintain oxygen delivery through support of cardiovascular and pulmonary function. Elective intubation is performed if significant respiratory distress, diminished level of consciousness, or increased volume of secretions is present, since these factors may contribute to the development of airway obstruction following submersion.

The child with near-drowning is likely to develop ARDS; thus the need for intubation and mechanical ventilation with PEEP should be anticipated (see Acute Respiratory Distress Syndrome).

For further information regarding the neurologic sequelae of near-drowning, see Chapters 8 and 12 in this book and Chapters 6, 8, and 12 in *Nursing Care of the Critically Ill Child* (Hazinski, 1992).

If the child arrives in the ICU in full cardiopulmonary arrest, resuscitation is initially continued while the child's primary physician confirms the presence of asystole despite intubation and good resuscitation technique and informs the parents of the child's poor prognosis. At that time, the primary physician will determine if aggressive resuscitation is to continue. If resuscitation is discontinued, the child's body should be prepared so that the parents can visit the child for the last time (see Chapter 4). If the child's parents have agreed to potential organ donation, resuscitation and aggressive support is continued in an attempt to restore sufficient organ perfusion to enable pronouncement of brain death and organ donation (see Chapter 8). Occasionally, aggressive support of oxygenation and perfusion may restore sufficient perfusion to the brain stem to prevent brain death pronouncement. If brain death pronouncement is not possible but devastating neurologic damage is apparent, withdrawal of ventilatory support may be recommended to the parents.

Chest Trauma

Etiology/Pathophysiology

Trauma may involve damage to the chest wall, lungs, airways, esophagus, diaphragm, or heart. Blunt trauma is most common in children, although penetrating injuries caused by gunshot wounds or knives are increasing in frequency.

Rib fractures are relatively uncommon following blunt trauma in children because the rib cage of the child is more compliant and more resilient than the rib cage of the adult. Therefore significant parenchymal or other internal thoracic injury may be present *without* external manifestations of injury. If rib fractures *are* present, they indicate severe injury, and pneumothorax, hemothorax, or pulmonary contusion is likely to be present. A flail chest is a relatively uncommon but serious complication of multiple rib fractures and results in paradoxical movement of an unstable portion of the chest wall.

Other forms of chest trauma include pericardial tamponade, fracture of the sternum, rupture of the larynx, and lacerations of the trachea, bronchi, heart, or intrathoracic vessels. These injuries are likely to produce secondary complications, including airway obstruction, tension pneumothorax, hemothorax, and shock.

Clinical Presentation and Management

The most common complications of chest trauma are airway obstruction, tension pneumothorax, hemothorax, cardiac tamponade, pulmonary contusion, and shock. Because these problems must be anticipated and promptly treated, information regarding assessment is presented with management.

Every trauma victim requires simultaneous cervical spine immobilization and control of the airway, support of ventilation, and shock resuscitation. Urgent surgical exploration may also be indicated. In general, patients with penetrating torso wounds below the intermammary line and anterior to the midaxillary line undergo emergent exploratory thoracotomy. In addition, surgical exploration is indicated for persistent shock or hemorrhage despite transfusion and application of external pressure (see Chapter 12).

Airway obstruction is treated with intubation and mechanical ventilatory support. Simultaneous protection of the cervical spine is mandatory. If the airway obstruction is beyond the depth of the endotracheal tube, bronchoscopy may be required.

A tension pneumothorax constitutes a medical emergency and requires immediate decompression. It produces diminished chest expansion and breath sounds on the side of the pneumothorax, deviation of the mediastinum away from the pneumothorax, and a decrease in cardiac output and systemic perfusion. Decompression can be rapidly accomplished through insertion of an 18- to 20-gauge needle into the second intercostal space, over the top of the third rib, in the midclavicular line of the affected side, or into the fourth or fifth intercostal space in the anterior axillary line. Successful decompression will result in a gush of air from the chest. Chest tube insertion is then performed (see Figure 12-3, p. 594).

A hemothorax is treated with chest tube insertion and replacement of blood loss, as needed. Surgical exploration is indicated if significant or continuous hemorrhage occurs or if damage to mediastinal structures or blood vessels is suspected.

Shock is treated with bolus administration of both crystalloids (20 ml/kg of lactated Ringer's solution or normal saline, administered over approximately 15 to 20 minutes) and blood (packed red blood cells, 10 ml/kg, administered over approximately 15 to 20 minutes). These fluids are administered in a 3:1 crystalloid-colloid ratio and repeated as needed (see Figure 12-6). Hypotension will not be present until the child has lost approximately 25% of circulating blood volume acutely; thus the presence of hypotension indicates significant blood loss and patient decompensation (see Chapter 12, p. 585, for information regarding resuscitation). Hemodynamic instability despite repeated boluses of crystalloid plus two boluses of blood, and significant ongoing blood loss are potential indications for urgent surgical exploration.

Cardiac tamponade produces signs of inadequate systemic perfusion, including tachycardia, tachypnea, diminished peripheral pulses, and delayed capillary refill despite volume resuscitation. Hepatomegaly may also be present, eliminating hypovolemia from the differential diagnosis of shock. Theoretically, pulsus paradoxus (a fall in systolic arterial pressure by >8 to 10 mm Hg during spontaneous inspiration) and muffled heart tones may be observed, but these are difficult to appreciate during resuscitation of the child in shock. Cardiac tamponade may be confirmed through use of echocardiography and must be treated with immediate decompression (see Figure 12-4, Pericardiocentesis, p. 600).

Cardiac contusion should be suspected in any child with a history of blunt chest trauma. A 12-lead ECG and quantification of cardiac isoenzymes will enable identification of cardiac contusion. Treatment is supportive (volume therapy and vasoactive drug therapy).

Open chest wounds result in entry of air into the thorax (development of progressive pneumothorax) during spontaneous respiration. These wounds must be sealed immediately with aseptic technique and will require later surgical exploration.

Pulmonary contusions are treated supportively. ARDS may develop, requiring mechanical ventilation with supplemental oxygen and PEEP.

Common Diagnostic Tests

There are many pulmonary function tests that are clinically useful but impractical in the critical care setting. This section focuses on those tests of pulmonary function that are performed in the critical care unit.

Physical Examination

The most important diagnostic tool for the assessment of respiratory function is the physical examination. The child's respiratory rate, pattern, degree of effort, chest expansion, and breath sounds will usually reveal the presence of injury, disease, or potential respiratory failure.

Chest Radiograph

The chest radiograph is used frequently to evaluate the critically ill or injured child. See Chapter 7 for further information.

Bronchoscopy

Flexible and rigid bronchoscopy allows direct visualization of the larynx and larger airways and facilitates sampling of secretions or tissue for culture, special stains, and cytology. Transbronchial biopsy is often used to diagnose rejection following lung transplantation. Although rigid bronchoscopes have been available for years, the development of small flexible fiberoptic bronchoscopes has resulted in increased use of this diagnostic tool at the bedside. Rarely, the flexible bronchoscope can be used to facilitate intubation of the patient with craniofacial trauma or craniofacial malformation.

In preparation for bronchoscopy, the child receives nothing by mouth or via nasogastric tube for 4 to 6 hours before the procedure. If a nasogastric tube is in place, the stomach is emptied. Analgesia, anesthesia, or sedation will be prescribed (see Chapter 3). Flexible bronchoscopy can be performed at the bedside, whereas rigid bronchoscopy is generally performed using general anesthesia in the operating room.

The bronchoscope is introduced either nasally or orally. During mechanical ventilation, flexible bronchoscopy is performed using a special T-adaptor to enable continuous ventilation. Cardiovascular and pulmonary status are closely monitored during the procedure.

Complications of bronchoscopy are rare and include laryngospasm, hemoptysis, and vocal cord injury. In addition, transient upper airway edema may develop.

A transbronchial biopsy is performed during bronchoscopy using general anesthesia; it can be performed at the bedside in the critical care unit. A biopsy forceps is then inserted through the bronchoscope, and the desired tissue sample is obtained. Complications of this procedure are much less common than those experienced following open lung biopsy and include pneumothorax, transient pyrexia, and dyspnea.

Thoracoscopy

Video-assisted thoracic surgery (VATS) may be used for thoracoscopic biopsy (thoracoscopy) of the pleura or lung without the need for a thoracotomy; lung resection can also be accomplished with this technique. General anesthesia is usually

---

Box 6-12

Evaluation of Ulnar Collateral Flow: Allen Test and Doppler Flow

Modified Allen Test

1. Compress/clench the child's hand several times.
2. Elevate the hand above the heart and compress/clench the hand tightly.
3. Occlude both the ulnar and radial arteries and lower the hand to the level of the heart.
4. Open the hand but *do not* hyperextend the fingers. Release pressure over the ulnar artery. If color returns to the hand within 6 seconds while the radial artery remains occluded, the Allen test is *negative,* and circulation through the ulnar artery and palmar arch is thought to be adequate. If the hand fails to reperfuse within 6 seconds, the Allen test is *positive,* and flow through the ulnar artery and palmar arch may be inadequate if the radial artery becomes obstructed.

Doppler Flow Evaluation

1. Place a Doppler probe between the heads of the third and fourth metacarpals on the palm of the hand, perpendicular to the palm.
2. Advance the probe proximally until the pulsatile signal is maximal.
3. Occlude the radial artery while monitoring the Doppler signal. If the pulsatile signal is unchanged or increases in intensity, ulnar and palmar arch circulation are probably adequate. If the pulsatile sound diminishes in intensity, flow through the ulnar artery and palmar arch or collateral circulation may be inadequate if the radial artery becomes obstructed.

Location of Radial Artery

A Doppler flow probe may be used to locate the radial artery and confirm catheter placement. A fiberoptic light source may be placed under the wrist (or foot) of small infants to locate arterial flow.

From Chamerdes L, Hazinski MF: *Textbook of pediatric advanced life support,* Dallas, 1997, The American Heart Association.

---

provided, although the procedure may be performed with analgesia and sedation. During VATS thoracoscopy, the biopsied lung is collapsed, and ventilation of the other lung must be sufficient to maintain gas exchange during the procedure. Three 1-inch skin incisions are made, and three instruments are inserted into the chest: one instrument inflates the chest cavity with carbon dioxide (creating a pneumothorax and collapsing the lung), the second instrument is a video thoracoscope to guide the procedure, and the third instrument is the biopsy forceps. At the end of the procedure, the biopsied lung is reinflated, and the instruments are removed.

Assessment of Arterial Blood Gases

Blood Sampling and Blood Gas Analysis

The effectiveness of gas exchange is best evaluated by measuring the pH, Po_2, and Pco_2 of arterial blood. It is also possible to assess "arterialized" capillary samples, but analysis of the Pao_2 by this method may be unreliable.

Arterial Sampling   The vessels used most frequently for arterial sampling are the umbilical artery in neonates and the brachial, radial, and femoral arteries in infants and children. Although occasional puncture may be performed to obtain blood samples, an arterial catheter should be placed to facilitate blood sampling if severe cardiorespiratory disease is present, if continuous observation of blood pressure is required, or if frequent arterial sampling will be necessary.

The blood sample is collected into a syringe that contains liquid or solid heparin. As little as 0.2 ml of blood can be used for blood gas analysis if the "micro" method of analysis is performed.

Before puncture of the radial artery in the wrist, an Allen test may be performed to evaluate effectiveness of ulnar collateral flow in the hand (Box 6-12). A local anesthetic (1% to 2% lidocaine or topical anesthetic cream) is applied at the skin puncture site. The skin is scrubbed with a povidone-iodine solution, and, of course, gloves are worn during the procedure.

The arterial puncture is made at a 45-degree angle, and the artery is entered with the bevel of the needle pointing downward. When the artery is entered, blood will appear in the syringe. Following collection of the sample, the arterial puncture site is covered with dry gauze and pressure is applied for at least 5 minutes to ensure that bleeding has ceased. If a femoral puncture is performed, pressure is applied for 5 to 15 minutes.

All bubbles must be eliminated from the arterial sample before it is analyzed. The syringe is rotated to mix the sample with heparin. The blood gas syringe is closed with an airtight stopper, and the sample is placed on ice. Analysis should be performed immediately.

Complications of arterial puncture include arterial spasm or hematoma formation. These can lead to subsequent occlusion of the artery and compromise of perfusion to the distal extremity.

Capillary Sampling for Blood Gas Analysis Although an accurate P_{CO_2} and pH can be obtained with a capillary sample, the P_{O_2} will be lower than the child's arterial P_{O_2} (P_{aO_2}). If shock or other causes of poor systemic perfusion are present, the capillary P_{O_2} will be much lower than the P_{aO_2}; thus this form of blood sampling should not be relied on in the management of the child with cardiorespiratory instability.

The best area for the capillary stick is one that is highly vascularized. The infant's heel, earlobe, finger, or toe is usually used. Heel stick specimens may be obtained from the medial portion of the heel, but only before the infant has begun to walk; once the infant begins to walk, calluses form on the heel, making this site unsuitable for sampling.

The sample area must be warmed for approximately 10 minutes to increase blood flow to the area; this "arterializes" the capillary blood. A puncture wound is made with a lance or scalpel blade so that blood flows freely from the sample site. The blood is collected in a heparinized 0.2-ml capillary tube. The tube is sealed and placed on ice. Analysis should be performed immediately.

Complications of repeated capillary sticks are rare but include infection. Osteomyelitis has been reported in neonates following heel stick sampling.

Venous Samples Venous blood may be used for blood gas analysis, but interpretation of the P_{O_2} and P_{CO_2} is difficult. The venous pH may be monitored, but it will be lower than the arterial pH in the critically ill child.

Pulmonary Artery Samples Pulmonary artery blood obtained through a pulmonary artery catheter provides a true mixed venous blood sample. If arterial blood and pulmonary artery blood are obtained and analyzed simultaneously, the arterial-venous oxygen content difference (a-v D_{O_2}) can be calculated using the Fick equation (see Chapter 5).

Continuous monitoring of mixed venous oxygen saturation is now possible using a pulmonary artery catheter containing a fiberoptic for spectrophotometry. This technique uses characteristics of light *reflection* from the hemoglobin in the pulmonary artery in a manner similar to the analysis of light *absorption* using pulse oximetry. Continuous monitoring of this mixed venous oxygen saturation (S_{vO_2}) enables detection of any change in the balance of oxygen supply and demand.

Noninvasive Monitoring of Blood Gases

Pulse Oximetry The saturation of hemoglobin in arterial blood can be continuously monitored using a pulse oximeter. These devices are extremely useful when properly applied and accurately interpreted.

The pulse oximeter measures the patient's hemoglobin *saturation,* which can range between 10% and 100%. The relationship between the patient's hemoglobin saturation and arterial oxygen tension is illustrated by the oxyhemoglobin dissociation curve (see Figure 6-5). Effects of the pH on this curve must also be considered. For example, at a normal blood pH, a hemoglobin saturation above 93% to 95% indicates a P_{aO_2} of greater than 70 mm Hg. However, if the patient is alkalotic (e.g., for the treatment of pulmonary hypertension), a hemoglobin saturation of 93% to 95% may be associated with a P_{aO_2} of 60 mm Hg or less.

Pulse oximeters require pulsatile flow to operate properly, and they are highly sensitive to movement artifact. The instrument probe is placed on the finger, toe, foot, hand, or earlobe and may be housed in a clip or on an adhesive strip. The probe consists of two light-emitting diodes, which are placed on one side of the pulsatile tissue bed; these diodes transmit light through the tissue to a photodetector placed directly across the tissue bed from them. A microprocessor in the base unit determines the absorption of red and infrared light by the tissue, to determine the percent of oxygenated hemoglobin present in the tissue bed. The pulse rate is also displayed by the monitor. The oximeter is only accurate when it traces the pulse rate accurately.

Excess ambient light or excessive patient movement can result in artifact and an audible alarm. Nail polish should be removed before the pulse oximeter is placed over a fingertip. Tissue burns may result if a probe from one manufacturer is used with a base unit from a different manufacturer, if a probe with a cracked casing is used, or if tissue perfusion is extremely poor. When poor tissue perfusion is present, the probe site should be changed every 4 to 6 hours.

Pulse oximeters will not recognize carboxyhemoglobin or methemoglobin; thus they may demonstrate a falsely high hemoglobin saturation in the presence of carbon monoxide poisoning or methemoglobinemia. In the presence of these diseases, the hemoglobin saturation should be measured by co-oximeter in the blood gas laboratory.

End-Tidal Carbon Dioxide Monitoring The amount of carbon dioxide in exhaled air can be monitored continuously with a variety of devices; most commonly, exhaled air is analyzed continuously using an infrared carbon dioxide sensor or a mass spectrometer. If the patient is breathing spontaneously, the sampling catheter can be placed inside the nostril (e.g., through a nasal cannula) or tracheostomy stoma.

The P_{CO_2} of expired air at end-expiration is approximately equal to the alveolar P_{CO_2}; in patients with normal lungs the alveolar P_{CO_2} is the same as the Pa_{CO_2}. As a result, the end-tidal carbon dioxide ($P_{ET}CO_2$) may replace or substitute for repeated arterial blood gas analysis during weaning of patients from mechanical ventilation and during care of children with chronic lung disease.

Although it is relatively simple to measure P_{CO_2} in a gas sample, it is extremely difficult to obtain a true alveolar gas sample uncontaminated by dead space gas or ambient air. If the $P_{ET}CO_2$ is to be used, the Pa_{CO_2} and the $P_{ET}CO_2$ are evaluated simultaneously to determine their relationship. In general, changes in the $P_{ET}CO_2$ will accurately reflect trends in the Pa_{CO_2} even if significant lung

disease is present. The $P_{ET}CO_2$ will correlate poorly with the Pa_{CO_2} in the presence of interstitial lung disease, however.

Potential explanations for changes in the $P_{ET}CO_2$ in the *intubated* patient include:

- *Sudden decrease in $P_{ET}CO_2$:* Tube obstruction or extubation
- *Gradual fall in the $P_{ET}CO_2$ to nonzero levels:* Leak around the endotracheal tube, partial airway obstruction, or a fall in cardiac output or lung perfusion
- *Rise in the $P_{ET}CO_2$:* Hypoventilation or partial airway obstruction

Assessment of Lung Volumes and Flows

Simple measurements of various lung volumes and capacities can be performed at the bedside to provide an objective estimate of the child's respiratory status:

- *Vital capacity (VC):* VC is the maximum amount of air that can be exhaled after a maximum inspiratory effort. A handheld spirometer is joined to a mouthpiece, endotracheal tube, or ventilator tubing. The child is instructed to take the deepest breath possible and then, with the spirometer attached, exhale the air as quickly, forcefully, and completely as possible. Normal VC is 65 to 75 ml/kg; assisted ventilation is often required if VC is <15 ml/kg. Poor patient effort or an inadequate seal around the airway may result in falsely low measurements.
- *Tidal volume (VT):* The tidal volume is the volume of air moved in each breath. A handheld spirometer is joined to a mouthpiece, endotracheal tube, or ventilator tubing. The total volume inspired over a minute is divided by the respiratory rate to obtain an average tidal volume. Predicted VT is 6 to 7 ml/kg. VT <4 to 5 ml/kg may indicate significant airway obstruction or inadequate respiratory effort to sustain spontaneous ventilation. A normal tidal volume does not exclude the presence of severe lung, chest wall, or respiratory muscle disease.
- *Inspiratory occlusion pressure (inspiratory force):* Measurement of inspiratory force

may be helpful in the assessment of patients with neuromuscular disease. Measurement can be made through mechanical ventilation tubing or via tubing attached to a face mask. The inspiratory tubing or port is occluded, and the child's maximal inspiratory force is measured using a standard pressure transducer. Normal inspiratory force is -75 to -100 cm H_2O. A negative inspiratory force of < -20 cm H_2O suggests that a significant mechanical limitation to spontaneous breathing may be present.

- *Lung compliance:* Lung compliance is defined as the change in lung volume per unit change in transpulmonary pressure (ml/cm H_2O) when the lungs are motionless. In the clinical setting, the compliance of the lung and chest wall are often measured together during mechanical ventilation.
- *Static lung compliance:* An inspiratory hold is applied (the exhalation tubing is occluded) after a known volume is delivered by the ventilator. To compute compliance, the pressure at that volume is recorded and the tidal volume is divided by the measured pressure.
- *Dynamic lung compliance:* Dynamic lung compliance equals tidal volume divided by peak inspiratory pressure (this is the ratio of change in volume to change in pressure between points of zero flow at the end of inspiration and expiration). In healthy children static and dynamic lung compliance are similar. If reduced lung compliance is present, a higher pressure will be required to deliver the desired tidal volume.

Conclusions

While these diagnostic tests may be clinically useful, *physical examination and arterial blood gas analysis provide the most rapid, complete, and objective estimate of pulmonary function.* Nothing can replace the careful observations of a skilled clinician.

Suggested Readings

Abman SH et al: Acute effects of inhaled nitric oxide in children with severe hypoxemic respiratory failure, *J Pediatr* 124:881-888, 1994.

Anene O et al: Dexamethasone for the prevention of postextubation airway obstruction: a prospective, randomized, double-blind placebo-controlled trial, *Crit Care Med* 24:1666-1669, 1996.

Barnett PLJ et al: Intravenous versus oral corticosteroids in the management of acute asthma in children, *Ann Emerg Med* 29:212-217, 1997.

Bergman DA, Chairperson, Provisional Committee on Quality Improvement, American Academy of Pediatrics: Practice parameter: the office management of acute exacerbations of asthma in children, *Pediatrics* 93:119-126, 1994.

Chatburn RI, El-Kharib M, Blumer JI: Benchmark data for the outcome of mechanical ventilation in a pediatric intensive care unit, *Resp Care* 42:221-225, 1997.

Demirakça et al: Inhaled Nitric oxide in neonatal and pediatric acute respiratory distress syndrome: dose response, prolonged inhalation, and weaning, *Crit Care Med* 24:1913-1919, 1996.

Green TP et al: The impact of extracorporeal membrane oxygenation on survival in pediatric patients with acute respiratory failure, *Crit Care Med* 24:323-329, 1996.

Harrison AM et al: Comparison of simultaneously obtained arterial and capillary blood gases in pediatric intensive care unit patients, *Crit Care Med* 25:1904-1908, 1997.

Hazinski MF: *Nursing care of the critically ill child,* ed 2, St Louis, 1992, Mosby.

Hillberg RE, Johnson DC: Noninvasive ventilation, *N Engl J Med* 337:1746-1752, 1997.

Khan N, Brown A, Venkataraman ST: Predictors of extubation success and failure in mechanically ventilated infants and children, *Crit Care Med* 24:1568-1579, 1996.

Kirby TJ: Thoracoscopy: rebirth of an old technique, *Clin Pulm Med* 1:165-173, 1994.

Makela MJ, Martsola J, Ruuskanen O: Respiratory syncytial virus infection in children, *Curr Opin Pediatr* 6:17-22, 1994.

Meert KL et al: Aerosolized ribavirin in mechanically ventilated children with respiratory syncytial virus lower respiratory tract disease: a prospective, double-blind randomized trial, *Crit Care Med* 22:566-572, 1994.

Moler FW et al: Extracorporeal life support for severe pediatric respiratory failure: an updated experience, 1991-1993, *J Pediatr* 124:875-880, 1994.

Murphy S, Kelly HW: Asthma, inflammation, and airway hyperresponsiveness in children, *Curr Opin Pediatr* 5:255-265, 1993.

Navas L et al: Network on infections in Canada: improved outcome of respiratory syncytial virus infection in a high-risk hospitalized population of Canadian children, *J Pediatr* 121:348-354, 1992.

Padman R, Lawless ST, Kettrick RG: Noninvasive ventilation via bilevel positive airway support in pediatric practice, *Crit Care Med* 26:169-173, 1998.

Pediatric Emergency Medicine Committee of the American College of Emergency Physicians: Rapid-sequence intubation of the pediatric patient, *Ann Emerg Med* 28:55-74, 1996.

Qareshi F, Zaritsky A, Lakkis H: Efficacy of nebulized ipratropium in severely asthmatic children, *Crit Care Med* 29:205-211, 1997.

Randolph AG, Wang EE: Ribavirin for respiratory syncytial virus lower respiratory tract infection: a systematic overview, *Arch Pediatr Adolesc Med* 150:942-947, 1996.

Sarnaik AP et al: Predicting the outcome in children with severe acute respiratory failure treated with high-frequency ventilation, *Crit Care Med* 24:1396-1402, 1996.

Stark JM: Lung infections in children, *Curr Opin Pediatr* 5:273-280, 1993.

Tobias JD, Garrett JS: Therapeutic options for severe refractory status asthmaticus: inhalational anesthetic agents, extracorporeal membrane oxygenation and helium/oxygen ventilation, *Paediatric Anaesth* 7:47-57, 1997.

US Department of Health and Human Services, Public Health Service National Institutes of Health, National Heart, Lung, and Blood Institute: Practical guide for the diagnosis and management of asthma: managing asthma exacerbations at home, in the emergency department, and in the hospital, NIH Publication No. 97-403, Bethesda, 1997, US Department of Health and Human Services.

Whitehead B et al: Technique and use of transbronchial biopsy in children and adolescents, *Pediatr Pulmonol* 12:240-246, 1992.

Williams R et al: Relationship between the humidity and temperature of inspired gas and the function of the airway mucosa, *Crit Care Med* 24:1920-1929, 1996.

Willson DF et al: Calf's lung surfactant extract in acute hypoxemic respiratory failure in children, *Crit Care Med* 24:1316-1322, 1996.

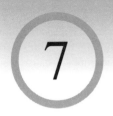

Chest X-Ray Interpretation

Pearls

◆ Use the chest radiograph in conjunction with careful clinical examination.

◆ Develop a systematic method of reviewing chest radiographs and use that format every time you view a film.

◆ Loss of the cardiac silhouette indicates lung opacification (pneumonia, atelectasis).

◆ Free air shifts to superior portions of the chest, whereas free fluid tends to shift to dependent (inferior) portions of the chest.

◆ Atelectasis represents volume *loss;* therefore structures often shift toward it.

◆ Pneumothorax represents volume *gain;* therefore structures often shift away from it.

Additional Helpful Chapters
Chapter 5: Cardiovascular Disorders
Chapter 6: Pulmonary Disorders

Introduction

A basic understanding of the chest radiograph can aid in the assessment and care of critically ill patients. The nurse may be the first person to see a chest film after it has been processed and should thus be able to recognize changes in the radiograph to ensure early detection of pulmonary disorders and complications of, and response to, therapy. Of course, the *chest films should be used only in conjunction with careful physical assessment.* The purpose of this chapter is to present the basic concepts used in the interpretation of chest radiographs and the application of these concepts to the care of the critically ill child.

Because radiographs are a common diagnostic study in critical care units, health care providers often become lax in shielding themselves and their patients from scattered radiation. The nurse should always wear a lead shield if it is necessary to remain at the bedside during x-ray examinations and should always be certain that the child has a gonadal shield in place. Pregnant nurses should check hospital policy regarding protection during patient x-ray examinations. If it is necessary to hold the child during x-ray examinations, lead gloves should be worn.

Definition of Terms

X-rays are a form of short-wavelength energy; images are produced when an x-ray beam is directed through an object to a film cassette. The image produced is determined by the composition, or *density,* of the object through which the beam passes. *Radiopaque/radiodense objects* (e.g., metal or bone) block or absorb a significant part of the x-ray beam; thus a *white shadow is produced* on the x-ray film. *Radiolucent objects* (e.g., gas or air density) do not block very much of the x-ray beam; thus *a black image appears* on the x-ray film. The four major categories of densities are listed in Table 7-1.

Bones contain a large amount of calcium; thus they are nearly as dense as metal, producing a

white image on radiographs. Body tissues and cavities containing water (including the heart) will produce a light image on radiographs because their density is consistent with water. Because fat (including muscle) does not block much of the x-ray beam, it appears dark gray on radiographs. Since gas or air absorbs very little of the x-ray beam, it appears black on radiographs.

Table 7-1
Radiographic Appearance of Materials

Material	Density	Radiologic Appearance
Metal	Most radiopaque/radiodense	White image
Water	Moderately radiopaque/radiodense	Light image
Fat	Mildly radiopaque/fairly radiolucent	Dark gray image
Gas/air	Least radiopaque/most radiolucent	Black image

Box 7-1

Most Common Views Used for Chest Radiographs

Upright Posteroanterior (PA) Film

Obtained in the radiology department.

X-ray beam is directed from the back of the patient, through the patient, to a film in front of the patient.

Anteroposterior (AP) Film

Most common film obtained in the pediatric intensive care unit (PICU).

Film cassette is placed behind the patient, and beam is directed from the front of the patient, through the patient, to the cassette.

Should be obtained with the patient sitting upright in bed but may be obtained with the patient supine (should be indicated). Heart size tends to appear larger on AP than on PA films.

NOTE: When a PA or AP film is obtained, evaluation of lateral relationships is possible, but evaluation of anterior-posterior relationships (depth) of structures cannot be determined, because this dimension is compressed. If anterior-posterior relation-

ships must be evaluated, a lateral film is obtained.

Lateral Film

Patient is upright, and film is directed from one side of the patient, through the patient, to a cassette placed on the other side of the patient. Image is labeled according to the side nearest the x-ray tube.

NOTE: Lateral views enable evaluation of depth or anterior-posterior relationships of structures, but not of lateral relationships, since this dimension is compressed.

Lateral Decubitus Film

Patient is positioned on the side.

Film cassette is placed at the patient's back, and x-ray is aimed horizontally (parallel to the floor), through the patient.

Provides best image of air-fluid levels in the lung. Image is labeled according to the side on which the patient is lying.

All parts of the body contain one or more of the four densities. The juxtaposition of body parts or chambers of differing densities creates contrasts on the radiograph, and the position, size, and shape of structures can be evaluated.

When objects of varying densities are in contact, the differences in their images creates a *silhouette*. The absence of an expected silhouette suggests the presence of abnormal tissue densities, often indicating pathology.

An *x-ray film creates a two-dimensional image of three-dimensional objects as it compresses the image onto one plane.* As a result, it is impossible to evaluate the depth of structures through which the beam passes. The most common views used for chest radiographs are listed in Box 7-1; the views are usually labeled according to the part of the body *nearest* the x-ray tube.

Interpretation of Film Technique

The evaluation of the chest radiograph requires knowledge of the exposure conditions of the film, the angle of the x-ray beam, and the alignment and position of the patient (Figure 7-1). If the patient and the x-ray beam are properly positioned, the x-ray beam will be perpendicular to the x-ray cassette and to the horizontal or vertical axis of the patient. If either the patient or the beam is slanted, an oblique view will be

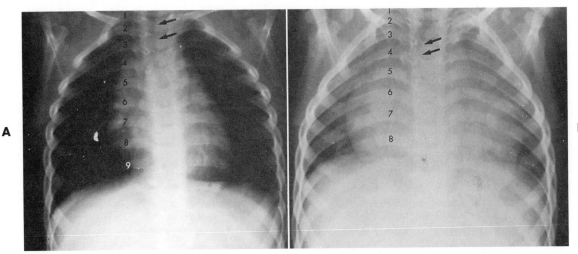

A **B**

Figure 7-1 Nomal chest films obtained from the same child during inspiration and expiration. **A,** Inspiratory phase. Nine ribs can be counted above the diaphragm, indicating good inspiration. Alignment is good (note similarity of clavicles). Penetration of film is good (all vertebral bodies are visible; some pulmonary vascular markings can be seen). Intercostal spaces are equal; both sides of the diaphragm are visible. Mediastinum and trachea are straight *(arrows)*. Heart borders are sharply defined, and heart size is normal. Pulmonary vascular markings are visible in proximal two thirds of lung fields (normal). **B,** Expiratory phase. Only eight ribs are visible above the diaphragm (see numbers on ribs), indicating inadequate lung expansion. Alignment is good. Penetration of film is good. Intercostal spaces are narrow because expiration is occurring. Both sides of the diaphragm are hazy, and left hemidiaphragm is not readily identifiable. Mediastinum appears widened, and trachea seems to buckle to the right *(arrows)*. Heart appears much larger than in **A,** and heart borders are obliterated, but this is caused by expiration and reduction in apparent lung volume. Silhouette sign appears to be present, cardiothoracic size calculated from this view would be large, and pulmonary vascular markings appear prominent, but these are all artifacts caused by expiration. (Courtesy Dr. H. Rex Gardner, Rush Presbyterian Saint Luke's Hospital, Chicago. From Hazinski MF: *Nursing care of the critically ill child,* ed 2, St Louis, 1992, Mosby.)

obtained, and structures farthest from the beam will be shortened while those closest to the beam will be enlarged.

1. *X-ray position:* If the x-ray beam is properly positioned, the apexes of both lungs should be visible above both clavicles.
2. *Patient position:* If the patient is properly positioned, the clavicles should be straight and of equal size; if the patient is rotated, one side of the chest image (and one clavicle) will appear larger than the other. Any *free air* present in the chest will accumulate at the *superior* portions of the lung, and *free fluid* will accumulate in *dependent* portions of the lung; thus it is essential to determine if the patient was supine or upright when the film was taken:
   a. If the patient is *supine* when the film is taken, any free fluid will pool along the back of the lungs, and free air will accumulate along the front of the chest and diaphragm.
   b. If the patient is *upright* when the film is taken, free fluid will accumulate along the diaphragm, and free air will rise to the apexes of the lungs.
3. *Film exposure:* If the film is properly exposed, the vertebral bodies will be clearly visible. If the film is underpenetrated (underexposed), all of the images on the film will appear lighter; if the film is overpenetrated (overexposed), all of the images will be darkened.
4. *Degree of inspiration:* Unless otherwise indicated, all chest films should be obtained during inspiration. With good inspiration and chest expansion, 9 to 10 ribs will be visible above the diaphragm. If maximal inspiration is not present, the lungs may appear more congested (since they are not maximally filled with air) and the trachea may buckle to the right (see Figure 7-1).

Interpretation of Chest Films

It is good practice to develop a routine when viewing chest films (Box 7-2). The most important aspect of film review is that *all* aspects of the film must be evaluated. In addition, the film will be most valuable when it is compared with the patient's previous films so that changes can be appreciated.

Radiographic Evaluation of Equipment Location

Endotracheal Tube Location

If the child is intubated, the position of the endotracheal (ET) tube should be checked first (Figure 7-2). The radiopaque tip should be positioned approximately 1 to 2 cm above the carina or approximately at the level of the child's third rib.

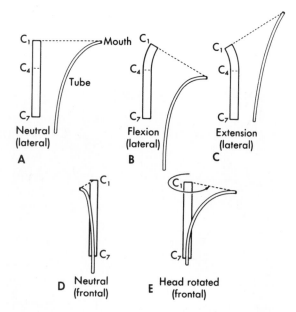

Figure 7-2   Proposed mechanism of orotracheal tube movement with changes in head position in the infant and young child. This movement must be considered when evaluating endotracheal (ET) tube position on the chest radiograph. The upper cervical vertebrae *(C1 to C4)* primarily provide neck flexion and extension, and head rotation. The lower cervical spine *(C4 to C7)* is fairly fixed. A functional lever arm is created between the anterior maxilla and the upper cervical spine; this lever arm moves the ET tube when the head moves. **A,** Neutral position, lateral view. **B,** Flexion of neck, lateral view (pushes ET tube further into trachea). **C,** Extension of neck, lateral view (pulls ET tube upward by a lever arm effect). **D,** Neutral position, frontal view. **E,** Lateral rotation, frontal view (displaces ET tube upward and further out of trachea). (From Donn SM, Kuhns LR: Mechanisms of endotracheal tube movement with change of head position in the neonate, *Pediatr Radiol* 9:39, 1980.)

Box 7-2

An Organized Approach to Chest X-Ray Interpretation

1. Technique

Check alignment, position (check clavicles).

Check degree of inspiration (full = 9-10 ribs).

Check penetration (vertebral bodies visualized).

2. Soft Tissues of Chest and Neck

Check for subcutaneous emphysema.

Examine extrathoracic structures.

3. Bony Thorax and Intercostal Spaces

Examine clavicles, scapula, ribs, humeri, and cervical and thoracic vertebrae.

Check for bony fractures.

Evaluate width of intercostal spaces (should be equal).

4. Diaphragm and Area Below Diaphragm

Note clarity and position of diaphragm (check for elevation).

Check for location of gastric bubble (normal: patient's left).

5. Pleura and Costophrenic Angles

Check for fluid or air between pleural layers (between bony thorax and lung).

Costophrenic angle should be sharp.

6. Mediastinum

Borders should be sharp.

Check for lateral shift.

7. Trachea

Should be straight (buckling to the left in expiratory film may be observed if left aortic arch is present).

Check for narrowing.

8. Heart and Great Vessels

Borders of heart and aorta should be distinct.

Obliteration of heart borders is *silhouette* sign (see Table 7-1).

Measure *cardiothoracic ratio* (normal: approximately 0.5).

9. Lung Fields

Compare right with left.

Note presence and location of any opacification.

Look for air-fluid levels.

10. Hili and Pulmonary Vascularity

Vascularity is most prominent at hili.

Peripheral pulmonary vascular markings normally are visible in proximal two thirds of lung fields (note if markings are increased or decreased).

Prominent but hazy pulmonary vascular markings may result from pulmonary edema or pulmonary venous congestion.

11. Check Location and Continuity of All Tubes, Wires, and Catheters

Evaluate endotracheal tube position in light of head position.

Tip of endotracheal tube should be at level of third rib (1-2 cm above carina).

12. Compare With Previous Films

Data from Hazinski MF: *Nursing care of the critically ill child,* ed 2, St Louis, 1992, Mosby.

Since the position of an orotracheal tube will change relative to the position of the child's head (see Figure 7-2), the child's head should be in neutral position when the x-ray film is obtained. If the head is not in neutral position:

- Neck *flexion* will move the tip of the *ET tube further into the trachea.*
- Neck *extension or rotation* will move the tip of the *ET tube out of the trachea.*

If the tip of the ET tube is located too close to the carina, it can easily slip into a mainstem bronchus. Right mainstem bronchus intubation can result in right upper lobe (RUL) or left lung atelectasis. RUL atelectasis develops because the ET tube blocks the entrance of the RUL bronchus into the right mainstem bronchus (Figure 7-3, *A*). Left lung atelectasis can develop because the right lung is preferentially ventilated (Figure 7-3, *B*). Note that *ET tube displacement is not a radiographic diagnosis, but one*

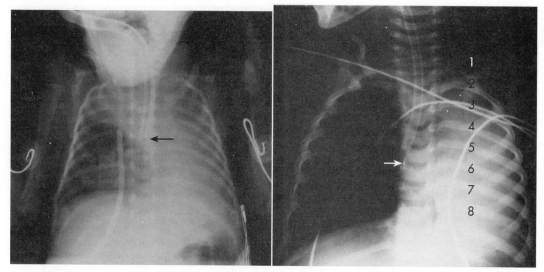

Figure 7-3 Consequences of ET tube migration. **A,** Right mainstem bronchus intubation resulting in right upper lobe (RUL) atelectasis. The ET tube is clearly inserted beyond the carina and beyond the level of the third rib and has moved into the right mainstem bronchus *(arrow)*. This has resulted in obstruction in the branch of the bronchus supplying the RUL, causing RUL atelectasis to develop. The tube should be withdrawn to proper position 1 to 2 cm above the carina. Note that the infant's neck is flexed, with the chin resting on the chest; this head position would tend to move the tip of the ET tube further into the trachea/bronchus. **B,** Right mainstem bronchus intubation resulting in left lung atelectasis. Note that the tip of the ET tube is well beyond the level of the carina, into the right bronchus *(arrow),* and the entire left lung is opacified (atelectasis). The bedside nurse noted decreased breath sounds and chest expansion on the left and loud breath sounds on the right. The ET tube was withdrawn 4 cm. (**B** From Hazinski MF: *Nursing care of the critically ill child,* ed 2, St Louis, 1992, Mosby.)

that should be recognized by clinical examination; loud breath sounds and hyperdynamic chest expansion are typically noted on the side where mainstem bronchus intubation has occurred, and decreased breath sounds and inadequate chest expansion are present on the opposite side.

Location of Vascular Catheters, Tubes, and Wires

Assess the location of any central venous, pulmonary artery, or intracardiac catheters. Trace the lines along their entire length, since they may migrate distally or advance into inappropriate areas. For example, an internal jugular catheter may migrate into the head during insertion instead of toward the heart; a pulmonary artery catheter may move into the main pulmonary artery; or a right atrial catheter may fall into the right ventricle. Often such catheter migration will be detected by a change in monitored pressure or waveform.

REMEMBER: Anteroposterior (AP) or posteroanterior (PA) films will enable evaluation of lateral relationships of catheters and tubes to other structures but will not allow determination of anterior-posterior relationships, since this dimension is compressed (Figure 7-4). If the AP location of a catheter or tube in the chest must be evaluated, a lateral film may be obtained.

Central Venous Catheter

The central venous catheter tip should lie within the superior or inferior vena cava (SVC or IVC) or

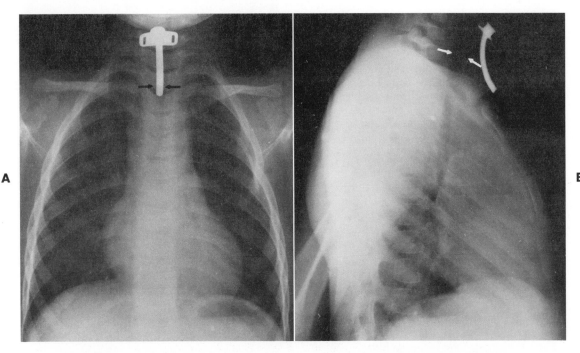

Figure 7-4 Appearance of tracheostomy tube on AP and lateral chest radiographs. These films were obtained when the nurse noted difficulty in inserting the tracheostomy tube and noted inadequate breath sounds when hand ventilation was provided via the tube. Breath sounds were adequate during spontaneous ventilation. **A,** AP view. Lung expansion appears adequate, and the tracheostomy tube appears to be in the midline of the trachea *(arrows)*. **B,** Lateral view. The air density of the trachea is visible *(arrows)*, and it is apparent that the tracheostomy tube has been inserted subcutaneously (it is not in the trachea at all). (Courtesy Dr. Andrew K. Poznanski, Children's Memorial Hospital, Chicago. From Hazinski MF: *Nursing care of the critically ill child,* ed 2, St Louis, 1992, Mosby.)

at the SVC–right atrial junction (Figure 7-5). Occasionally the catheter passes from the SVC through the right atrium into the IVC or from the SVC into the right atrium and then into the right ventricle. The catheter may also migrate deep into the right atrium. If such migration occurs, the catheter should be repositioned.

Pulmonary Artery Catheter

The pulmonary artery catheter tip should be positioned in a distal portion of the pulmonary artery that is posterior and inferior to the heart, and specifically inferior to the left atrium. If the patient is supine, it will not be possible to determine whether the catheter tip is in front of or behind the heart on an AP or PA film. However, it will be pos-

sible to evaluate whether the tip is in a distal pulmonary artery (Figure 7-6). A lateral view will enable evaluation of the location of the catheter tip in relation to the left atrium. Waveform analysis will aid in determination of the catheter tip location.

Umbilical Venous and Arterial Catheters

An umbilical *venous* catheter will track from the umbilicus upward (in the front of the abdomen) and then into the IVC, which is located along the right of the patient's vertebral column (Figure 7-7, **A** and **B**). The catheter is typically inserted just until a good blood return is obtained (approximately 1 to 4 cm). Advancement of the tip into the portal vein or hepatic circulation is avoided, because it creates

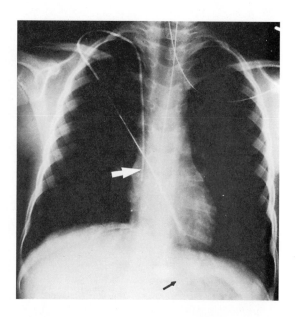

Figure 7-5   Evaluation of central venous catheter and nasogastric tube placement. This postoperative chest x-ray film is normal: chest expansion is good, lungs are clear, heart size is normal, and pulmonary vascular markings are normal. A central venous catheter is in place with the tip resting in the right atrium *(arrow)*. A nasogastric tube is in place *(small arrow)*. (From Hazinski MF: *Nursing care of the critically ill child,* ed 2, St Louis, 1992, Mosby.)

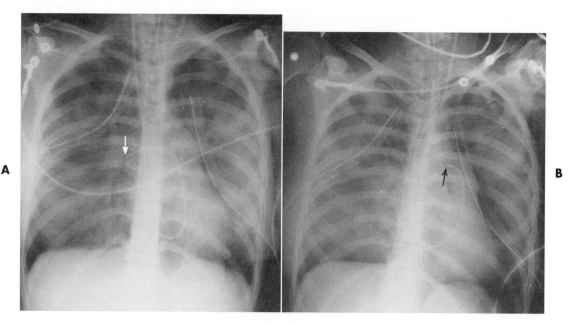

Figure 7-6   Evaluation of pulmonary artery catheter placement. **A,** This child has acute respiratory distress syndrome following trauma. Note bilateral pulmonary infiltrates/edema and bilateral chest tubes. The tip of the ET tube is slightly high, located at the level of the second rib. The tip of the pulmonary artery catheter is located beyond the main pulmonary artery, in a branch of the right pulmonary artery *(arrow)*. The pulmonary wedge waveform varies minimally between inspiration and expiration and is consistent with a wedge in a good location (zone III). **B,** The pulmonary artery wedge waveform changed in appearance (from **A**) and began to vary widely between inspiration and expiration. The tip of the pulmonary artery catheter has fallen back into the main pulmonary artery *(arrow)*. It was necessary to reposition the catheter tip.

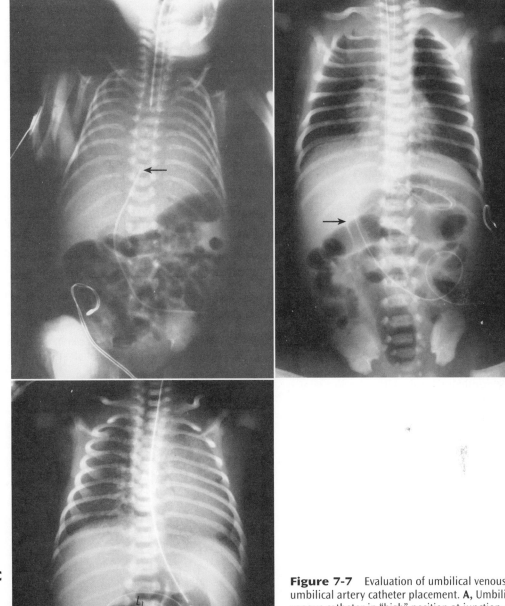

Figure 7-7 Evaluation of umbilical venous and umbilical artery catheter placement. **A,** Umbilical venous catheter in "high" position at junction of inferior vena cava and right atrium *(arrow)*. This is very high placement, which is acceptable, but not optimal; if the catheter is advanced further, there is a risk of right atrial perforation. If the catheter is withdrawn 1 to 2 cm, it will reside within the hepatic circulation. **B,** Umbilical venous catheter in hepatic circulation *(arrow)*. This catheter should be withdrawn, since infusion of a high osmolality solution may injure the liver. **C,** Umbilical artery catheter in proper position. The tip of this catheter *(arrow)* is at approximately the level of the third or fourth lumbar vertebra (proper position).

the possibility that hypertonic or alkaline solutions infused via the catheter will infuse directly into the portal vein (Figure 7-7, *A* and *B*).

An umbilical *artery* catheter will track from the umbilicus downward and then into the aorta, which is located on the patient's left of the vertebral column. The catheter tip is advanced until it enters the descending aorta, to prevent obstruction of the femoral or iliac arteries (Figure 7-7, *C*).

Nasogastric and Nasojejunal Tubes

The nasogastric tube should be traced down the esophagus into the stomach. The tip of the tube should reside within the stomach, and all ports (breaks in the radiopaque catheter line) should be located within the stomach (note normal location of nasogastric tubes in Figure 7-5). If a nasojejunal tube is placed, the tip should be located to the patient's right of midline, indicating passage beyond the pyloric sphincter of the stomach.

Pacing Wires

The location and integrity of any pacing wires should be verified. Occasionally a pacing wire is dislodged or fractured.

Common Radiographic Abnormalities in Pediatric Critical Care

Air Space Disease

The term *air space disease* indicates abnormal (nonair) densities *in* the lung, in contrast to abnormal densities in the chest (e.g., pneumothorax, hemothorax). Air space disease densities generally indicate the development of lung disease, atelectasis, tumor, edema, or hemorrhage in the lung. Opacification produced by intrapulmonary (air space) disease must be differentiated from that produced by pleural space fluid accumulation, since the therapies for each will differ. Note that the position of the patient can be helpful in distinguishing the two. If the patient with a pleural effusion is supine, the effusion may "layer out" behind the lung and may be difficult to differentiate from air

space disease (see Pleural Fluid under Pleural Fluid or Air). If the patient is upright, free fluid may accumulate along the diaphragm and be difficult to differentiate from diaphragm elevation caused by atelectasis.

Pneumonia

Pneumonia can initially produce a patchy infiltration with fluffy margins, although it may later produce more segmental or lobar disease, with more homogeneous opacification of the involved area of the lung. Identification of an air bronchogram within the area of the pneumonia confirms that the opacification is intrapulmonary (Figure 7-8).

Normally the fluid-filled heart creates a silhouette against the air-filled lungs. Obliteration of this silhouette can only be caused by opacification of the portion of the lung adjacent to the heart. If pneumonia causes obliteration of a cardiac border, the pneumonia must be in contact with the heart, and opacified portions of the lung can be identified by the portion of the cardiac silhouette that is obliterated (Table 7-2).

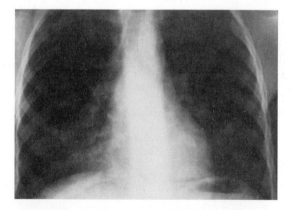

Figure 7-8 Right middle lobe pneumonia. Note the hazy opacification along the right heart border. This opacification is caused by the fluid density of the pneumonia obliterating the silhouette of the heart against the lung. This silhouette sign enables localization of the pneumonia to the right middle lobe. (Courtesy Dr. H. Rex Gardner, Rush Presbyterian Saint Luke's Medical Center, Chicago. From Hazinski MF: *Nursing care of the critically ill child*, ed 2, St Louis, 1992, Mosby.)

Table 7-2
Significance of the Silhouette Sign: Obliteration of Cardiac Silhouette by Lung Opacification

Obliterated Heart Border or Structure	Opacified Lung Segment
Upper portion of right heart border and ascending aorta	Right upper lobe (RUL)
Most of right heart border	Right middle lobe (RML)
Right diaphragm	Right lower lobe (RLL)
Aortic knob (and upper left heart border)	Left upper lobe (LUL)
Most of left heart border	Lingula
Left diaphragm	Left lower lobe (LLL)

From Hazinski MF: *Nursing care of the critically ill child*, ed 2, St Louis, 1992, Mosby.

Box 7-3

Radiographic Appearance of Common Pneumonias

Streptococcus pneumoniae: Lobar consolidation common. Empyema or pneumatocele may develop.
Haemophilus pneumoniae: Frequently associated with pleural effusion; may be associated with empyema or pneumatocele.
Staphylococcus pneumoniae: Most common in infants younger than 1 year of age. Pneumonia typically involves the right lung and may cause development of pneumatoceles or abscesses.
Pneumocystic carinii: Must be suspected in immunologically compromised patient presenting with fever and respiratory distress. Pneumonia produces perihilar congestion and then peripheral intrapulmonary involvement; soon assumes an alveolar and interstitial distribution. In patients with acquired immunodeficiency syndrome (AIDS), appearance may be atypical.
Aspiration pneumonia: Typically develops in the portion of the lung that was dependent at the time of aspiration; results in patchy opacification in the lung bases and perihilar infiltrations.

Some pneumonias have characteristic radiographic appearances (Box 7-3). This appearance can aid in the clinical diagnosis.

Atelectasis

Atelectasis is collapse of a portion of the lung and is usually caused by airway obstruction. The obstruction can result from a foreign body, a mucus plug, exudate, or compression of the airway by another thoracic structure (see Figure 7-3, A—the ET tube obstructs the RUL bronchus, resulting in RUL atelectasis). The absence of air results in opacification of that portion of the lung. If atelectasis is present adjacent to the heart, it may produce obliteration of a portion of the cardiac silhouette; by determining the portion of the cardiac silhouette that is lost, the location of the atelectasis can be identified (see Table 7-2).

Atelectasis represents a *volume loss* in the chest; thus the trachea, mediastinum, and intrathoracic structures in that hemithorax shift *toward* the area of atelectasis. In addition, the hemidiaphragm on the involved side is elevated, and the intercostal spaces on the involved side narrow. By comparison, the uninvolved lung may become hyperinflated, and a widening of intercostal spaces may be observed on the uninvolved side (Figure 7-9).

Lung Abscesses and Pneumatoceles

Lung abscesses and pneumatoceles can complicate pneumonia. Both produce circumscribed collections of air within the lungs.

Emphysema

Emphysema is distension of the lung, with air trapping. This problem represents increased volume in that lung; thus the diaphragm on the involved side is often flattened, and the trachea and mediastinum shift away from that side.

Pleural Fluid or Air

Pleural Fluid

Pleural fluid accumulation can result from pleural effusion; a chylothorax, hemothorax, or hydrothorax; or a pleural reaction. Free pleural fluid characteristically assumes a *dependent* position in the

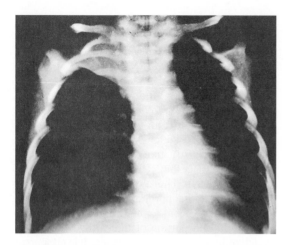

Figure 7-9   Atelectasis. Note opacification of the right upper lobe. Because atelectasis represents collapse of a portion of the lung (volume loss), other structures have shifted toward the involved area. The right hemidiaphragm is elevated, and the hilum of the right lung is shifted upward. (Courtesy Dr. H. Rex Gardner, Rush Presbyterian Saint Luke's Medical Center, Chicago. From Hazinski MF: *Nursing care of the critically ill child,* ed 2, St Louis, 1992, Mosby.)

chest: if the patient is upright, the fluid will accumulate along the diaphragm. Small-volume fluid accumulation may merely produce a blunting of the costophrenic angle, whereas significant fluid accumulation will make the diaphragm appear to be elevated (Figure 7-10, *A*). If the patient is supine, the fluid may "layer out" along the back of the lung and may be difficult to distinguish from intrapulmonary disease.

Significant fluid accumulation creates an increase in volume and thus may cause mediastinal structures to shift away from the involved side. A lateral decubitus film will help identify and quantify the free fluid in the thorax (Figure 7-10, *B*)

Pneumothorax

Pneumothorax is the accumulation of free air between the lung and the chest wall. Since this air contains no tissue or blood vessels, it appears hyperlucent compared with normal lung tissue. Often a margin is apparent around the pneumothorax.

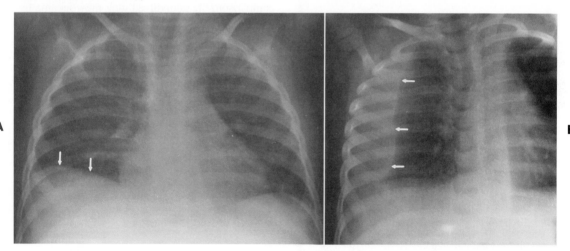

A   B

Figure 7-10   Pleural effusion. This 3-year-old developed tachypnea and increased respiratory effort, with decreased breath sounds and chest expansion on the right side. **A,** Upright AP film. This is apparently a good inspiratory film (9 to 10 ribs visible on left side, 8 to 9 on right side). The right lung field is smaller than the left. This may be caused by fluid accumulation along the diaphragm (arrows) or atelectasis with elevation of the diaphragm toward the area of volume loss. **B,** Right lateral decubitus film. Once patient lies on the right side, the free pleural fluid accumulates toward that dependent side *(arrows)*. (Courtesy Dr. Andrew K. Poznanski, Children's Memorial Hospital, Chicago. From Hazinski MF: *Nursing care of the critically ill child,* ed 2, St Louis, 1992, Mosby.)

Free air (pneumothorax) will tend to accumulate in superior portions of the chest. Therefore, if the child is upright when the film is taken, the free air will accumulate along the apexes of the lung (Figure 7-11, *A*). If the child is supine, the free air will accumulate along the diaphragm and the anterior chest—a small pneumothorax may be difficult to identify from a supine radiograph.

A pneumothorax represents a volume *gain*. It may collapse a portion of the underlying lung (which occasionally can be identified), but the air occupies volume; thus the diaphragm on the involved side is often flattened, and the trachea and mediastinum shift away from the pneumothorax.

A *tension pneumothorax* is a cardiopulmonary emergency, caused by the significant accumulation of air in the chest and resulting in compromise of venous return to the heart and a decrease in cardiac output (Figure 7-11, *B*). The trachea and mediastinum will shift away from the side of the pneumothorax. The *diagnosis of tension pneumothorax is a clinical diagnosis, not a radiographic one—* the pneumothorax should usually be decompressed before the time is taken to obtain, develop, and read a chest x-ray film.

Pneumopericardium

A pneumopericardium is a collection of air within the pericardial sac surrounding the heart. It will appear as a radiolucent border between the radiopaque pericardial sac and the radiopaque heart. If the pneumopericardium is significant, it can produce effects similar to cardiac tamponade; if cardiac output is compromised, the pneumopericardium must be evacuated on an urgent basis.

Special Techniques: Fluoroscopy

Fluoroscopy provides a dynamic image of the structures examined. It is used for evaluation of structures or organ movement (e.g., the diaphragm), or for localization of pathology.

Fluoroscopy is generally performed in the radiology department, although it may be performed at the bedside of the critically ill child. Videotapes are

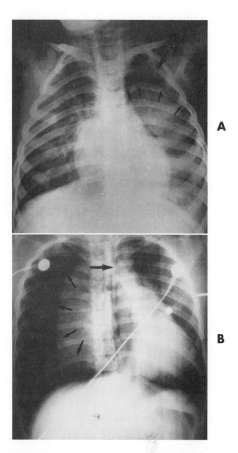

Figure 7-11   Pneumothorax. A pneumothorax can often be detected as a radiolucent (black) area between the chest wall and the combined air-fluid density of the lungs. **A,** Left pneumothorax and third rib fracture in upright AP film. The third rib was fractured *(large arrow)* when the child was involved in a bicycle crash. Note the border between the lung and the pneumothorax *(small arrows)*. The pneumothorax accumulates near the apex or top of the lung when the child is upright. **B,** Tension pneumothorax caused by blunt chest trauma. Although no ribs are fractured, a significant chest injury has occurred. The pneumothorax occupies volume; thus structures such as the heart and trachea *(large arrow)* are shifted away from the pneumothorax. The right lung is largely collapsed (see small arrows demarcating border between lung and pneumothorax). *A tension pneumothorax is a clinical diagnosis, not a radiographic one.* This film was obtained while preparations were underway to decompress the pneumothorax on an urgent basis. (**A** courtesy Dr. Andrew K. Poznanski, Children's Memorial Hospital, Chicago.)

usually made to enable later viewing and analysis. Gonadal shielding is required for the child and the attendant nurse.

Conclusions

Chest radiographs are a valuable adjunct to assessment of the critically ill child when they are used in conjunction with careful clinical examination. If a systematic method of reviewing radiographs is developed and used, the nurse will be able to confirm clinical impressions, evaluate catheter and tube position, evaluate the patient's response to therapy, and identify pathology.

Suggested Readings

Felson B, Weinstein AS, Spitz HB: *Principles of chest roentgenology: a programmed text,* ed 2, Philadelphia, 1970, WB Saunders.

Heller RM et al: *Exercises in diagnostic radiology,* ed 2, Philadelphia, 1987, WB Saunders.

Kuhns LR, Poznanski AK: Endotracheal tube position in the infant, *J Pediatr* 78:991, 1981.

Poznanski AK: The chest. In Poznanski AK, editor: *Practical approaches to pediatric radiology,* ed 2, St Louis, 1976, Mosby.

Silverman FN, Kuhn JP: *Essentials of Caffey's pediatric x-ray diagnosis,* St Louis, 1989, Mosby.

8 Neurologic Disorders

Mary Fran Hazinski, Cathy Headrick, Derek Bruce

Pearls

- Early signs of increased intracranial pressure (ICP) may be subtle in the infant and child; "classic" signs of increased ICP (hypertension, bradycardia, and apnea) may only develop when herniation is imminent.
- Young children with closed head injury present with diffuse signs of injury more often than adults and may demonstrate more complete recovery from such injury than adults; as a result, the approach to the care of the child with closed head injury tends to be very aggressive.
- Head trauma produces a primary insult. Patient outcome will likely be further compromised if secondary insults, such as hypoxemia or hypotension, develop.
- When the child is unconscious, the most important section of the Glasgow Coma Scale (GCS) is the motor score; yet this section is often incompletely or incorrectly performed. The GCS should be evaluated in the same way by all members of the health care team so that trends in the patient's condition will be recognized.
- Increased ICP is often associated with maldistribution of cerebral blood flow. Inadequate blood *flow* may be present in areas of the brain despite an adequate calculated cerebral perfusion *pressure.*
- Seizures may be difficult to detect if neuromuscular blockers are administered.
- Spinal cord injury may be present in children without radiographic abnormalities.
- The potential for organ donation should be considered whenever devastating neurologic injury occurs, and parents should be offered the option of vascular organ donation whenever brain death pronouncement is made. The option of nonvascular organs (corneas, bones, heart valves) should be offered when pronouncement of death is anticipated (brain death pronouncement not required).

Additional Helpful Chapters

Introduction

This chapter provides an overview of relevant neurologic anatomy, physiology, and pathophysiology. In addition, it describes assessment and interventions appropriate for the critically ill child with neurologic disease or injury. A major focus of this chapter is the recognition and management of increased intracranial pressure.

Essential Anatomy and Physiology

Axial Skeleton

The *axial skeleton* consists of the bones of the skull and vertebral column; it protects the central nervous system (CNS), including the brain and spinal cord. The frontal, temporal, parietal, and occipital bones form the *cranial vault*. The floor of this vault is composed of three bony compartments: the anterior, middle, and posterior *fossae*. These fossae and the parts of the brain they contain are used to designate areas of injury or disease (Table 8-1):

- *Anterior fossa:* Contains frontal lobes of brain
- *Middle fossa:* Contains hypothalamus, pituitary gland, upper brain stem, and temporal lobes
- *Posterior fossa:* Contains brain stem, pons, medulla, and cerebellum

Blood vessels and cranial nerves enter and leave the skull through small openings in the skull; each opening is called a *foramen.* The posterior fossa contains the *foramen magnum,* through which the brain stem and spinal cord join. Lesions in this area, such as those produced by cervical neck trauma, can interrupt vital brain functions and nerve pathways to and from the brain. Cerebrospinal fluid (CSF) and the vertebral arteries also pass through the foramen magnum.

At birth, the skull plates are not fused; they are separated by nonossified spaces, called sutures, and *fontanelles.* Normally, the posterior fontanelle closes at approximately 2 months of age, and the anterior fontanelle closes at approximately 16 to 18 months of age. *Microcephaly,* failure of brain growth, may result in early fusion of the skull bones. Conversely, *craniosynostosis,* or premature fusion of the bones, can produce microcephaly, since brain growth is inhibited.

A space-occupying lesion in the skull, such as a tumor or hydrocephalus, may cause the fontanelles to bulge. If intracranial volume or pressure is chronically increased, the bones of the skull may separate, even after fusion. This produces an increase in head circumference.

Meninges

Three membranes, *the meninges,* surround the brain and spinal column. These membranes and the spaces between them serve important roles in normal physiology and pathophysiology:

- *Dura mater:* Outermost membrane, consisting of tough connective tissue lining the endocranial vault. Folds in the dura mater

Table 8-1
Contents of Cranial Fossae

Fossa	Brain	Cranial Nerves	Arteries
Anterior fossa	Frontal lobes	Olfactory	Anterior cerebral
Middle fossa	Temporal lobes	Optic	Carotids
	Hypothalamus		Middle cerebral
	Pituitary gland		
Posterior fossa	Brain stem	III-XII	Basilar
	Pons		Vertebrals
	Medulla		
	Cerebellum		

create divisions in the intracranial contents. The largest fold is the *tentorium cerebelli;* intracranial lesions are divided into those that occur above this fold (supratentorial lesions) and those that occur below it (infratentorial lesions).

- *Subdural space:* Contains bridging veins from the cortex to the venous sinuses. Serious head trauma can rupture these vessels, causing a subdural hematoma.
- *Arachnoid:* Middle membrane, consisting of spiderlike tissue that covers the surface of the brain and spinal cord to the exit of the spinal cord roots.
- *Subarachnoid space:* Just under the arachnoid membrane; contains CSF. Head injury may result in the accumulation of blood in this space, called a subarachnoid hemorrhage (SAH), which may obstruct CSF flow or prevent its reabsorption.
- *Pia mater:* Third and innermost membrane that follows the contour of the brain and spinal cord.

Brain

The brain is divided into three major areas: the *cerebrum,* the *brain stem,* and the *cerebellum.* The divisions of the brain and their major functions are presented briefly here.

Cerebrum

The cerebrum consists of the cerebral cortex and cerebral hemispheres, the thalamus, the hypothalamus, the basal ganglia, and the olfactory and optic nerves. The cerebral cortex consists of the convoluted gray matter that forms the outermost layer of the brain. It consists largely of specialized neurons that process and respond to specific stimuli; this area performs the higher functions of the human brain. As a result, it continues to develop beyond infancy and childhood.

The *cerebral hemispheres* are two mirror-image portions of the brain that consist largely of the cerebral cortex and fiber tracts. In general, the cerebral hemispheres govern the function of and receive sensations from the contralateral side of the body. The cerebral hemispheres are connected by a wide band of nerve fibers called the *corpus callosum.* These nerve fibers allow the brain to function

as a single unit despite the fact that it is divided into two hemispheres.

The *thalamus* borders and surrounds the third ventricle and is composed of gray matter. The gray matter serves as a major integrating center for afferent impulses from the body to the cerebral cortex. The thalamus is the center for the primitive appreciation of pain, temperature, and tactile sensations.

The *hypothalamus* lies beneath the thalamus and near the optic chiasm. This is the chief region for subcortical integration of sympathetic and parasympathetic activities. The hypothalamus secretes hormones that are important in the control of visceral activities, maintenance of water balance and metabolism, regulation of body temperature, and endocrine gland secretion. Two hormones, *vasopressin* (antidiuretic hormone [ADH], also known as arginine vasopressin [AVP]) and *oxytocin,* are synthesized by the hypothalamus and transmitted in nerve tracts to the posterior pituitary gland, which releases them.

The anterior pituitary gland, called the *adenohypophysis,* secretes hormones that control endocrine glands throughout the body. These hormones include growth hormone (somatotrophin), adrenocorticotropic hormone (ACTH), thyroid-stimulating hormone (TSH), melanocyte-stimulating hormone, and others. Injury to or disease of the hypothalamus or the pituitary can produce a wide variety of neuroendocrine problems and can result in fluid and electrolyte imbalance and growth disturbances.

The *basal ganglia* are paired masses of gray matter deep within the cerebral hemispheres. They contain the nuclei of neurons and networks of tracts that control aspects of motor function. This system selects motor messages from lower pathways for interpretation and transmission to the cerebral cortex. Interference with neurotransmission to this area, such as that associated with cerebral palsy or Parkinson's disease, results in disturbances in intentional movement and involuntary movements.

Brain Stem

The brain stem is located at the base of the skull and is the major nerve pathway between the cerebral cortex and the spinal cord. The three major divisions of the brain stem are the *midbrain,* the *pons,* and the *medulla;* together they control many involuntary but essential functions of the body:

- *Midbrain:* Consists of fibers that join the upper and lower brain stem. It is the center for reticular activity and assimilates some sensory input from the lower neurons before it is relayed to the cortex.
- *Pons:* Contains fiber tracts connecting the medulla oblongata and cerebellum with upper portions of the brain. It is the origin of the abducens, facial, trigeminal, and acoustic cranial nerves.
- *Medulla oblongata:* Contains critical regulatory centers for cardiovascular and respiratory functions; thus disease or injury here may be life threatening. It is also the site of decussation (crossing) of many corticospinal motor neurons. It transmits messages to and from the spinal pathways for interpretation by and reaction of the cortex. The glossopharyngeal, vagus, spinal accessory, and hypoglossal cranial nerves originate here.

Cerebellum

The cerebellum is located in the posterior fossa, directly below the occipital lobe. It consists of two hemispheres that contain gray matter. This area of the brain integrates voluntary movement.

Cranial Nerves

The cranial nerves are 12 pairs of peripheral nerves that arise from the brain; each has a specific motor or sensory function, and four cranial nerves have parasympathetic functions. Cranial nerve function can be lost as a result of lesions near the origin of the cranial nerve or following direct injury to the cranial nerve itself. Evaluation of cranial nerve function may enable location of and determination of the severity of a specific CNS disease or injury (Table 8-2). Evaluation of cranial nerve function becomes extremely important when evaluation of higher brain functions is impaired because the patient is comatose or unresponsive.

Spinal Cord

The spinal cord is a cylindric structure composed of neurons and nerve fibers that join the medulla at the foramen magnum and extend to the level of the second lumbar vertebra. The spinal cord (like the brain) is surrounded by the pia mater, the CSF, the arachnoid, and the dura mater.

The spinal cord contains gray and white material. The gray matter consists of cell bodies and cell nuclei, and the white matter consists of nerve fibers, which are grouped into tracts. The gray matter in the spinal cord is shaped like a butterfly with anterior and posterior projections called the anterior horn and the posterior horn.

Peripheral sensory nerves carry impulses to the posterior horn through the dorsal root of the spinal column, where they synapse or communicate with other neurons that will carry information up the spinal column or to other neurons at the same level of the spinal column. *Lower motor neurons* are located in the anterior horn of the spinal column. The lower motor neurons affect motor activity and receive input from the brain, as well as from other neurons within the spinal cord. Injury to the brain or higher levels of the spinal cord may result in loss of inhibition to the lower motor neurons, causing spastic paralysis. Motor neural axons exit as the ventral root.

Spinal cord reflexes consist of responses to stimuli that can be generated within the spinal cord; these reflexes *do not* require input from the brain. For example, when the patellar tendon is tapped with a reflex hammer, reflexive contraction of the rectus femoris results. When the bottom of the foot is stroked, the foot may withdraw from the stimulus. Since these reflexes can all occur at the spinal cord level, they may continue despite spinal cord transection, brain injury, or brain death.

Central Nervous System Circulation and Perfusion

Cerebral Circulation

The brain requires a constant supply of oxygen and substrates for energy. In addition, adequate circulation is required to remove carbon dioxide and other metabolites from the brain. The brain requires approximately 18% of the total body oxygen content, and it receives approximately 25% of the child's cardiac output. If the brain is deprived of oxygen for even a few minutes, brain ischemia can

Table 8-2
Cranial Nerves: Function, Potential Mechanism of Injury, and Assessment

Cranial Nerve	Function	Mechanism of Injury	Assessment
I. Olfactory	Smell	Fracture of cribiform plate or ethmoid area (rare) Brain death	Apply simple odors (difficult to test reliably in young children).
II. Optic*	Vision	Direct trauma to orbit or globe; fracture involving optic foramen (relatively common); increased incracranial pressure (ICP) Brain death	Ask child to describe objects near and far and also ask for identification of colors. Test each eye separately, and assess ability of child to see object moving into visual field from periphery.
III. Oculomotor*	Pupil constriction, movement of eye and eyelid	Pressure of herniating uncus on nerve or fracture involving cavernous sinus Brain death	Both pupils should constrict in response to light as light is applied to each. Consensual constriction (constriction in response to light directed to contralateral eye) should also be observed. Eyes should be able to move to follow moving object throughout visual field, and eyelids should raise equally when eyes are open. Damage to sympathetic nervous system fibers (Horner's syndrome) results in parasympathetic dominance and pupil constriction associated with ipsilateral ptosis (drooping eyelid). Ptosis and lateral downward deviation of eye with pupil dilation and decreased response to light are typical signs of oculomotor injury. Always record pupil size in millimeters.
IV. Trochlear*	Movement of eye (superior oblique muscle)	Injury near course of nerve in area of brain stem or fracture of orbit (uncommon) Brain death	Assess ability of eyes to track object throughout visual field. Damage to this nerve prevents eyes from moving downward and medially. Diplopia may also be present.
V. Trigeminal	Sensation to most of face and movement of jaw (mastication)	Direct injury to terminal branches, particularly to fibers of second division in roof of maxillary sinus Brain death	Apply soft and sharp objects to skin of face (as patient's eyes are covered) and assess sensation (test above eye, upper lip, and lower lip and chin to test all three branches). Motor functions are intact if child can clench and move jaw and chew food.
VI. Abducens*	Lateral movement of eye	Injury near brain stem and course of nerve (uncommon) Brain death	Assess eye movement within socket, tracking an object throughout visual field. Assess conjugate eye movement by moving object close to patient—both eyes should track object and move together as object is tracked throughout visual field. Patient may instinctively turn head toward weakened muscle to prevent diplopia.

From Hazinski MF: *Nursing care of the critically ill child,* ed 2, St Louis, 1992, Mosby; data from McCance K, Huether SE, editors: *Pathophysiology: the biological basis for disease in adults and children,* St Louis, 1990, Mosby; Rudy EB: *Advanced neurological and neurosurgical nursing,* St Louis, 1984, Mosby; Seidel HM et al, editors: *Mosby's guide to physical examination,* St Louis, 1987, Mosby; Thompson JM et al, editors: *Mosby's manual of clinical nursing,* ed 2, St Louis, 1989, Mosby; and Slota MC: Pediatric neurological assessment, *Crit Care Nurse* 3(6):106, 1983.
*Innervation to eye muscles is generally tested simultaneously, and cranial nerves controlling lateral gaze (III and VI) *must* be intact to obtain a *normal* or *positive* "Doll's eyes" response (oculocephalic reflex) and "cold water calorics" response (oculovestibular reflex).

Continued

Table 8-2

Cranial Nerves: Function, Potential Mechanism of Injury, and Assessment—cont'd

Cranial Nerve	Function	Mechanism of Injury	Assessment
VII. Facial	Motor innervation of face (forehead, eyes, and mouth) and sensation to anterior two thirds of tongue (sweet/bitter discrimination) Tearing	Fracture of temporal bone, laceration in area of parotid gland Brain death	Ask child to "make faces" (demonstrate) and assess symmetry of face. Utilize sugar, salt, vinegar to test taste on front of tongue. Tearing with cry should be present.
VIII. Vestibulo-cochlear (acoustic)	Hearing and equilibrium	Fracture of petrous portion of temporal bone (often injured with cranial nerve VII) Brain death	Check gross hearing by clapping hands (startle reflex should be observed in infants, blink reflex should occur with sudden sound). Test fine hearing through use of ticking watch or tuning fork. Vestibular division of this nerve is tested for response to *"cold water calorics"* and *"doll's eyes"* response. Both of these reflexes require that cranial nerve innervation controlling lateral gaze (cranial nerves III and VI) be intact for normal response. *Cold water calorics* (oculovestibular reflex)— instillation of cold water in ear should stimulate cranial nerves VIII, III, and VI, producing lateral nystagmus (*do not perform this test if patient is conscious*—this is typically performed to document absence of any cranial nerve function). *"Doll's eyes"* maneuver (oculo-cephalic reflex) also tests the vestibular portion of cranial nerve VIII, as well as cranial nerves III and VI (lateral gaze)—as the patient's head is turned, eyes should shift in sockets in direction *opposite* head rotation.
IX. Glossopha-ryngeal	Motor fibers to throat and voluntary muscles of swallowing, speech Taste to posterior one third of tongue	Brain stem injury or deep laceration of neck Brain death	Evaluate swallow, cough, and gag (tests cranial nerves IX and X simultaneously). Child's clarity of speech should also be evaluated.

From Hazinski MF: *Nursing care of the critically ill child,* ed 2, St Louis, 1992, Mosby; data from McCance K, Huether SE, editors: *Pathophysiology: the biological basis for disease in adults and chilren,* St Louis, 1990, Mosby; Rudy EB: *Advanced neurological and neurosurgical nursing,* St Louis, 1984, Mosby; Seidel HM et al, editors: *Mosby's guide to physical examination,* St Louis, 1987, Mosby; Thompson JM et al, editors: *Mosby's manual of clinical nursing,* ed 2, St Louis, 1989, Mosby; and Slota MC: Pediatric neurological assessment, *Crit Care Nurse* 3(6):106, 1983.

Table 8-2
Cranial Nerves: Function, Potential Mechanism of Injury, and Assessment—cont'd

Cranial Nerve	Function	Mechanism of Injury	Assessment
X. Vagus	Sensory and motor impulses for pharynx, as well as parasympathetic fibers to abdomen	Brain stem injury, deep laceration of neck (rare) Brain death	Test as above, particularly cough and gag reflex.
XI. Spinal accessory	Motor innervation of sternocleidomastoid, upper trapezius	Laceration of neck (rare) Brain death	Ask child to turn head as you palpate sternocleidomastoid, and to shrug shoulders as you feel trapezius muscles contract.
XII. Hypoglossal	Innervation of tongue	Neck laceration associated with injury of major vessels Brain death	Ask child to stick out tongue. Pinch nose of infant, and mouth should open and tip of tongue should rise in midline.

Table 8-3
Cerebral Circulation: Vascular Supply

Artery	Area of Supply
Right and left carotid arteries	Cerebral hemispheres and basal ganglia
Circle of Willis	Anterior communicating artery and posterior communicating arteries join basilar artery to carotid artery, completing an anastomotic circle
Right and left vertebral arteries	Spinal cord (anterior spinal artery), medulla, and inferior cerebellum
Basilar artery	Pons, midbrain, and upper cerebellum
Spinal radicular arteries	Spinal cord

develop. Because cells of the CNS do not regenerate, significant ischemic insult may result in permanent neurologic dysfunction or brain death.

The cerebral arterial circulation arises from the two vertebral arteries and from the right and left internal carotid arteries (Table 8-3). Venous drainage from the brain flows primarily into large vascular channels within the dura, known as dural sinuses, that ultimately drain into the internal jugular veins.

The arterial supply of the spinal cord begins from paired spinal arteries that arise from the vertebral arteries at the level of the foramen magnum. In addition, the spinal cord is perfused from branches of the intercostal arteries that arise from the thoracic aorta.

A cerebrovascular accident, or stroke, is a sudden compromise in perfusion to an area of the brain (Box 8-1). Strokes are uncommon in children but may result from congenital arteriovenous malformations or from complications of sickle cell anemia or leukemia with hyperleukocytosis. *Arteriovenous malformations* are abnormal connections between cerebral arteries and veins, most commonly involving branches of the middle cerebral artery. The high volume of venous return may produce congestive heart failure. More commonly, the high-volume, high-pressure flow of blood from the artery into the vein results in dilation of the vein; rupture of the vein produces an intracranial hemorrhage, which is often fatal.

Box 8-1

Causes of Stroke in Children

Neonatal Strokes

Hypoxic-ischemic insult
Polycythemia
Disseminated intravascular coagulation
Carotid artery injury (birth trauma)

Strokes During Childhood

Hypoxic-ischemic insult (including status epilepticus
  or cardiopulmonary arrest)
Hemoglobin or coagulation disorders
  Sickle cell thrombotic vasoocclusive crisis
  Protein S
  Protein C
  Antithrombin III deficiency
Congenital heart disease:
  Cyanotic heart disease; increased risk associated
    with the following:
    Hematocrit >60% (polycythemia and dehydra-
      tion increase risk)
    Microcytic anemia
    Sepsis
    Endocarditis, particularly of valves in any blood
      flow pathway that mixes with systemic arte-
      rial blood flow
  Acyanotic heart disease; increased risk associated
    with the following:
    Thrombus or vegetation, particularly of aortic
      and mitral valves or any valves in any blood
      flow pathway that mixes with systemic arte-
      rial blood flow
    Atrial fibrillation
Disorders of brain circulation
  Posterior circulation neurovascular syndrome

Arteriovenous malformation
Cerebral aneurysms
Vasculopathies
  Systemic lupus erythematosus
  Arteritis
  Periarteritis
  Postmeningitis vasculitis or thrombophlebitis
Malignancies
  Cerebral metastasis
  Hyperleukocytosis
  Disseminated intravascular coagulation
  Homocystinuria
  Chemotherapy complications
Neurocutaneous syndromes
  Neurofibromatosis
  Sturge-Weber syndrome
  Tuberous sclerosis
Trauma
  Intracerebral hemorrhage
  Injury to carotid artery (blunt or penetrating
    trauma)
  Venous occlusion
Infectious disease
  Cat-scratch disease
  Mycoplasma pneumoniae
  Sinovenous occlusion: infections of the ears, mas-
    toids, or sinuses

Data from Dean JM, Rogers MC: Cerebrovascular disease
and hypertensive encephalopathy. In Rogers MC, editor:
Textbook of pediatric intensive care, ed 3, Baltimore, 1996,
Williams & Wilkins; and Fuchs SM: Paralysis and
hemiplegia. In Barkin RM, editor: *Pediatric emergency
medicine,* ed 2, St Louis, 1997, Mosby.

Blood-Brain Barrier

The *blood-brain barrier* is the name given to the cerebral capillary walls and the glial astrocyte cells that protect neural tissues from circulating toxins or potentially harmful alterations in the extracellular milieu. The capillary membranes and the glial investment around the capillaries are relatively impermeable; thus they can protect the cerebral tissue from exposure to wide fluctuations in acid-base balance or ionic composition and can prevent the entry of antigenic or toxic material into the brain. Many drugs, including some contrast agents and

antibiotics, do not cross the blood-brain barrier. However, because the blood-brain barrier is freely permeable to water, rapid changes in the intravascular osmolality can affect cerebral hydration and function. The immature brain does not have adequate development of glial cells; thus the blood-brain barrier is incomplete in young infants.

Factors Affecting Cerebral Perfusion

Cerebral blood flow (CBF) is the blood that is in transit through the brain; this term is commonly used to describe the cerebral arterial flow perfusing the brain. *Cerebral blood volume (CBV)* is the total amount of blood in the intracranial vault at any one time, including both arterial and venous blood.

Normal CBF in adults is approximately 50 to 60 ml/100 g brain tissue/min. The normal quantity of CBF in children is unknown but is estimated:

- Healthy neonate: 40 ml/10 g brain tissue/min
- Child 1 to 9 years: 75 to 110 ml/110 g brain tissue/min
- Adolescent: 50 ml/100 g brain tissue/min

The absolute quantity of CBF is not as important as the relationship between CBF (including oxygen and substrate delivery) and cerebral metabolic requirements; CBF must increase as cerebral metabolism and need for oxygen increase and can decrease toward normal when metabolism and oxygen requirements are reduced toward normal. Inadequate or excessive CBF may produce complications.

Head injury and some encephalopathies may result in CBF that is not matched to metabolic requirements. This uncoupling between cerebral oxygen demand and cerebral oxygen delivery can contribute to regional cerebral ischemia or to areas of excessive CBV and increased intracranial pressure (ICP).

Seizures (particularly status epilepticus) increase the cerebral oxygen demand. This increase in oxygen demand can stimulate an increase in CBF and can produce an increase in ICP in patients who already have increased intracranial volume (e.g., patients with head injury). If CBF cannot increase commensurate with demand, ischemia can result.

If CBF is severely reduced, ischemia results, and cerebral cellular metabolic functions will be compromised and may cease. If ischemia continues, cerebral cellular membranes will become more permeable, and cerebral cellular uptake of water will occur. Profound ischemia may result in permanent neurologic dysfunction or brain death.

Cerebral Venous Return

Cerebral venous return must equal cerebral arterial flow, or CBV will increase and ICP may rise. If intracranial volume increases (e.g., from increased brain or CSF volume or tumor), cerebral venous

---

Box 8-2

Factors Controlling Cerebral Blood Flow

Pressure autoregulation: Constant blood flow is maintained despite a change in arterial blood pressure.

Metabolic autoregulation: Local blood flow is increased to match increased local metabolic needs (e.g., in response to seizures).

Arterial carbon dioxide: Cerebral blood flow increases when the $Paco_2$ increases.

Arterial oxygen tension: Cerebral blood flow increases when the Pao_2 falls below 50-55 mm Hg.

Biochemical alterations: Cerebral blood flow will increase in response to an increase in potassium, calcium, hydrogen ions, cytokines, adenosine, and nitric oxide.

---

blood can be displaced out of the intracranial vault to enable compensation for that volume, preventing a rise in ICP.

Cerebral venous return may be obstructed by compression or thrombosis of the internal jugular vein (e.g., by extremely high ICP or turning of the head) or by obstruction of superior vena caval flow (e.g., tension pneumothorax). Increased ICP may compress cerebral veins, impeding cerebral venous return.

Autoregulation

CBF is normally maintained at a constant level by a process of *cerebral autoregulation;* the tone and resistance in the cerebral arteries is constantly adjusted in response to local tissue biochemical changes and arterial pressure (Box 8-2). Autoregulation is essential to maintenance of cerebral perfusion and function over a wide variety of clinical conditions (e.g., arterial hypertension or hypotension). Severe alterations in systemic arterial blood pressure will exceed the limits of autoregulatory compensation, however, and further changes in arterial pressure will be associated with changes in the arterial pressure and flow.

Autoregulation may be compromised or destroyed following severe traumatic or anoxic head injury. If cerebral autoregulation is lost, CBF becomes passively related to the mean arterial pressure (MAP), and a fall in MAP will result in a decrease in cerebral perfusion.

Effects of Arterial Blood Gases   CBF is affected by changes in arterial carbon dioxide tension and by profound hypoxemia.

Carbon Dioxide Response   CBF is normally directly related to the arterial carbon dioxide tension; as the $Paco_2$ rises, cerebral arteries dilate and CBF increases. Hypocarbia, on the other hand, constricts cerebral arteries and reduces CBF. *Mild hyperventilation may be used in the treatment of patients with head injury to reduce the CBF, to decrease CBV and ICP.*

Extreme hypocarbia should be avoided, if possible, for a variety of reasons. Severe hypocarbia can reduce CBF and create cerebral ischemia. In addition, hypocarbia and alkalosis will shift the oxyhemoglobin dissociation curve to the left; although the hemoglobin will be better saturated at lower arterial oxygen tensions, hemoglobin release of oxygen to the tissues is made more difficult. Finally, "rebound" cerebral arterial dilation has been documented in laboratory animals if carbon dioxide levels are normalized abruptly following prolonged hyperventilation; thus normalization of carbon dioxide levels should be accomplished slowly during therapy.

The vasoconstrictive response to hypocarbia may be minimal or absent in some patients. Loss of carbon dioxide reactivity has been linked with poor outcome following closed head injury and may be observed following an ischemic insult.

Oxygen Response   CBF is unchanged over the normal range of arterial oxygen tension (Pao_2). However, severe hypoxemia (Pao_2 <50 to 55 mm Hg) will produce cerebral arterial dilation and an increase in CBF. Tissue hypoxia and acidosis will also result in cerebral arterial dilation. If the child with head injury is hyperventilated (this practice has recently become less common), the shift in the oxyhemoglobin dissociation curve means that the hemoglobin saturation may be acceptable (90% to 93%) despite the development of hypoxemia (Pao_2 <60 mm Hg). Therefore, when monitoring pulse oximetry in a hypocarbic or alkalotic patient, remember that a mild reduction in hemoglobin saturation may indicate significant hypoxemia.

Hemoglobin saturation should be maintained at >95% in alkalotic patients if hypoxemia is to be avoided.

Cerebral Perfusion Pressure

Cerebral perfusion pressure (CPP) is the difference between the cerebral arterial pressure and the ICP. It is calculated and estimated clinically by the following formula:

$$CPP = MAP - ICP$$

The CPP will fall if there is an uncompensated fall in mean systemic arterial pressure or an uncompensated rise in mean ICP or if both occur simultaneously. The calculated CPP can be maintained despite a rise in ICP if the mean arterial pressure (MAP) rises commensurate with a rise in ICP. Such compensation may or may not be associated with effective CBF and cerebral *perfusion.* The normal range of CPP in adults is approximately 80 to 100 mm Hg but is unknown in children.

A minimum CPP of 40 to 60 mm Hg is probably required for effective cerebral perfusion; however, this number is not absolute, since perfusion is determined by blood *flow,* not blood *pressure. A "normal" CPP does not guarantee effective cerebral perfusion.* A clinical correlate of CPP in the patient with increased ICP might be the MAP in the patient with shock. The patient with a "normal" CPP may still have inadequate cerebral perfusion, just as the patient with impaired cardiovascular function and a "normal" blood pressure may still have inadequate systemic perfusion. Shock may be present with a "normal" blood pressure, and cerebral ischemia may be present with a "normal" CPP. A low CPP is definitely worrisome, but "normal" CPP is not reassuring in the presence of intracranial hypertension and clinical deterioration.

Case Study

A 5-year-old boy is hospitalized with a closed head injury after being struck by an automobile. An ICP monitor is placed, and the initial ICP measurement is 10 mm Hg with a MAP of 65 mm Hg. The child demonstrates purposeful response to painful stimulation and brisk pupil response to light bilaterally but does not open his eyes or follow commands.

Late that night, the child becomes tachycardic and hypertensive, the right pupil dilates, and the child becomes unresponsive to painful stimulation. At that time, the ICP is 40 mm Hg and the MAP is 95 mm Hg.

Calculate the CPP for each set of measurements provided. Which measurements are associated with the highest CPP? (Answer: identical, 55 mm Hg.) *Which measurements are associated with evidence of better cerebral perfusion and function?* (Answer: first set.)

Evaluation of Cerebral Blood Flow

Qualitative radioisotope scans have been performed for a number of years to determine *presence* or *absence* of CBF. *Quantitative* CBF measurements can be performed using cold xenon markers, but such measurements may not be easily performed at the bedside of the critically ill patient. A variety of invasive techniques may be used at the bedside to monitor *trends* in CBF.

Jugular venous bulb cannulation can enable calculation of the arteriovenous content difference as an indicator of CBF. An arteriovenous oxygen tension difference of approximately 22 to 23 mm Hg is thought to be associated with acceptable cerebral perfusion. Inhaled nitrous oxide or injected radioactive isotopes may also be used as indicators if simultaneous arterial and venous sampling can be accomplished. If inhaled radioactive xenon is used as an indicator, the arterial concentration can be assumed to equal the inhaled concentration; thus an arterial sample is not required for the calculations. However, the exhaled radioactive xenon must be captured.

Jugular venous bulb cannulation may also be performed to sample jugular venous oxygen tension and saturation. A small (e.g., 4 French) fiberoptic catheter can be inserted in the jugular venous bulb to monitor continuous jugular venous oxygen saturations; normal jugular venous oxygen saturation is approximately 65% to 70%. A jugular venous oxygen saturation of <50% is thought to indicate extreme compromise in cerebral perfusion and poor outcome. An increase in jugular venous oxygen saturation (e.g., >75%) probably indicates an increase in CBF.

Cerebrospinal Fluid Circulation

The CSF is a clear, colorless liquid that is produced in the ventricles and in specialized capillaries within the CNS. CSF circulates in the subarachnoid space and through the ventricles and the central canal of the spinal cord. It provides buoyancy to reduce the effective weight of the brain, and it cushions the CNS from injury. It also acts as a lymphatic system for the brain.

CSF is formed primarily by the choroid plexuses and circulates through the ventricles and through the subarachnoid space surrounding the brain and spinal cord. It is reabsorbed by the subarachnoid villi in the subarachnoid space (Figure 8-1).

CSF is not a mere filtrate of plasma. It contains water, oxygen, carbon dioxide, sodium, potassium, chloride, glucose, a small amount of protein, and an occasional lymphocyte (Table 8-4). Red blood cells are only present in a CSF sample if a traumatic tap was performed or if cerebral hemorrhage has occurred. Generally, CSF is hypertonic to blood, but its changes in osmolality will parallel those of blood.

Intracranial Pressure and Volume Relationships

Monroe-Kellie Hypothesis

For all practical purposes, the skull is a rigid structure, which limits the total potential intracranial volume. The ICP is determined by the intracranial volume and intracranial compliance (the change in pressure resulting from a change in volume). Although the infant's skull can expand to accommodate *gradual* and minor increases in intracranial volume (e.g., a slow-growing brain tumor), the skull *cannot* expand rapidly to accommodate acute or significant increases in intracranial volume (e.g., a significant intracranial hemorrhage).

The intracranial contents include the *brain,* the *blood,* and *cerebrospinal fluid.* The intracranial volume, therefore, is equal to the sum of the volumes of these substances:

$$\text{Intracranial volume} = \text{Brain}_{vol} + \text{Blood}_{vol} + \text{CSF}_{vol} + \text{Mass (if any)}$$

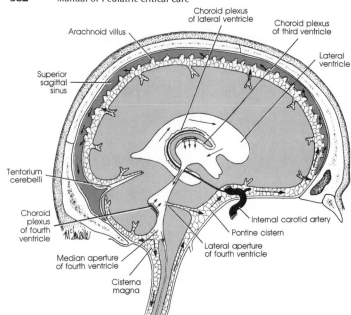

Formation:
80% choroid plexus capillaries
20% cerebral tissue

Circulation:
Lateral ventricles to third ventricle through foramen of Munro;
Through the aqueduct from third to fourth ventricle;
Through the lateral foraminae of Luschka and central foramen of Magendie from the fourth ventricle to the subarachnoid space;
Down the spinal canal then over the cerebral hemispheres

Absorption:
Into the venous sinuses through the arachnoid villi
From the spinal nerve roots

Figure 8-1   Cerebrospinal fluid (CSF) circulation. CSF is secreted from the floor of the lateral ventricles. After circulation through the ventricles and cisterns around the spinal cord, the fluid is reabsorbed by the arachnoid villi in the subarachnoid space. (From Nolte J: *The human brain,* St Louis, 1991, Mosby.)

Table 8-4
Normal Cerebrospinal Fluid Contents in Children

	Neonates		
	Preterm	**Term**	**Patients >6 Mo of Age**
WBC/mm^3			
Mean	9	8	2.6 $\pm$ 2.45
$\pm$2 SD	0-25	0-22	0-4 $\pm$ 2
PMNs* (%)	57	61	71 $\pm$ 1.36
Protein (mg/100 ml)			
Mean	115	90	<40
Range	65-150	20-170	
Glucose (mg/100 ml)			
Mean	50	52	>40
Range	24-63	34-119	
CSF/blood glucose (%)			
Mean	74	81	50
Range	55-150	44-248	40-60

From Hazinski MF: *Nursing care of the critically ill child,* ed 2, St Louis, 1992, Mosby; modified from Hieber JP: Encephalitis/meningitis. In Levin DL, Morriss FC, Moore GC editor: *A practical guide to pediatric intensive care,* ed 2, St Louis, 1984, Mosby; and Protnoy JM, Olson LC: Normal cerebrospinal fluid values in children: another look, *Pediatrics* 75:484, 1985.
*Polymorphonuclear leukocytes.

If the volume of any of the intracranial contents increases without a commensurate and compensatory decrease in the volume of other substances in the intracranial vault, ICP will rise.

Brain

The brain occupies most (80%) of the intracranial space; it is noncompressible, but it is somewhat movable within the cranium. If significant pressure gradients develop within the cranium or between the intracranial space and the spinal column, *cerebral herniation* can occur. Brain stem herniation through the foramen magnum produces brain death.

Brain volume may increase as a result of *cerebral edema* (an increase in brain water content). This edema may result from a hypoxic/ischemic insult and increased cell membrane permeability, or it may be caused by an extravascular fluid shift associated with a sudden drop in serum osmolality (e.g., a decrease in the serum sodium level). Brain volume can also increase as a result of an increase in CBF, such as may occur in some areas of the brain following head trauma. This increase in brain blood flow is often referred to as brain "swelling" or *hyperemic cerebral edema.*

Cerebral Blood Volume and Blood Flow

CBV constitutes approximately 7% to 10% of the total intracranial volume. CBF normally matches cerebral metabolic requirements and is also influenced by the biochemical environment in brain tissue. As noted earlier, CBF may increase in some areas of the brain following head injury and may exceed metabolic demand. In other areas of the brain, blood flow may be inadequate, producing ischemia.

Some of the CBV is contained in venous capacitance vessels and is shifted out of the intracranial vault during periods of increased intracranial volume. Hyperventilation may produce cerebral venous constriction and displacement of this venous capacitance blood.

If the volume of other intracranial contents increases significantly and ICP rises, CBF can be compromised. Cessation of CBF results in brain death.

Cerebrospinal Fluid

CSF normally constitutes 7% to 10% of the total intracranial volume and remains constant provided that production is matched by absorption. CSF accumulation can result from obstruction to CSF flow (e.g., obstructive hydrocephalus, such as following meningitis) or reduction in CSF reabsorption (e.g., communicating hydrocephalus, such as following subarachnoid hemorrhage).

CSF is the material most easily displaced from the intracranial vault as compensation for an increase in intracranial volume. CSF may also be removed from the intracranial vault by a shunt or placement of a ventricular drain.

Normal Intracranial Pressure

The ICP is the pressure exerted by the intracranial contents. Normal ICP is approximately 4 to 15 mm Hg and is not static. It can be transiently increased by anything that acutely increases cerebral venous pressure (such as vigorous coughing or a Valsalva maneuver), or movement from an upright to a reclining position.

When the volume of the brain, cerebral blood, or CSF increases, intracranial volume may increase. Initially, ICP may remain low if another intracranial substance (e.g., cerebral venous blood or CSF) can be displaced from the skull. This compensation is limited; if intracranial volume continues to increase, ICP will ultimately rise. Once the limits of compensation have been reached, progressively smaller incremental increases in volume will be associated with progressively more significant increases in ICP.

Intracranial Pressure Monitoring

ICP monitoring enables determination of the ICP and calculation of the CPP. It is useful in assessment of the child at risk for the development of increased ICP, particularly when the child is unconscious. In these children the clinical examination is not helpful in detecting early signs of increased ICP. ICP monitoring also enables evaluation of the child's response to therapy.

Indications   ICP monitoring should be initiated for:

- *Deep coma:* Glasgow Coma Scale (GCS) score of 3, 4, or 5 (acute)
- *Coma plus cardiovascular instability:* GCS 7 with shock

- *Unstable patient or required diagnostic studies:* GCS of 6, 7, or 8 plus unstable clinical course or prolonged diagnostic studies required (e.g., computed tomography [CT] scan with contrast).
- *CSF drainage required:* acute posttraumatic hydrocephalus or other indication for CSF drainage. Requires insertion of intraventricular catheter.

ICP monitoring is useful as an adjunct to the clinical assessment of the patient. It is also extremely helpful in the evaluation of trends in the patient's condition, particularly in response to therapy. For trends in the ICP to be useful, ICP monitoring must be performed in exactly the same way by each nurse, so that errors in ICP monitoring are eliminated or standardized. ICP measurements should never be evaluated in isolation; they should always be interpreted in conjunction with the patient's clinical appearance.

Methods   The ICP can be monitored in a variety of ways; the system used will be determined by the size of the patient's ventricles and whether or not CSF drainage is required (Table 8-5).

Fluid-Filled System/Ventriculostomy   The original method of ICP monitoring (the "gold standard") is the intraventricular monitor. In the past, this method of ICP monitoring was thought to be most accurate. A standard fluid-filled system and transducer is used, which must be zeroed, leveled,

and calibrated at regular intervals. Although use of a ventricular catheter is required if drainage of CSF is needed, it carries the highest risk of infection (ventriculitis). Ventriculitis develops in 7% to 15% of patients who undergo ventricular ICP monitoring and is most likely to develop if the catheter remains in place >72 hours. Ventricular bleeding may also develop during catheterization. Aspiration should *not* be performed through a ventricular catheter, since it may produce tearing of choroid plexus vessels and uncontrollable intracranial hemorrhage.

In recent years, the accuracy of the fiberoptic and microsensor systems has approached that of the traditional intraventricular monitoring systems, with a lower risk of complications. These newer systems can be placed in the parenchyma of the brain; thus the risk of ventriculitis is lower.

Fiberoptic Systems   These systems use a fiberoptic catheter. A beam of light is sent down the catheter, and the ICP is determined by the distortion of the light beam produced by the pressure on the tip of the catheter. These catheters may be placed in the ventricle (they may include a CSF drainage port) or in the parenchyma of the brain. The catheters are stiff and fragile and must be "zeroed" to atmospheric pressure before insertion.

Microsensor Devices   These systems are placed in the parenchyma of the brain or in the subdural space. Each catheter contains a microminiature silicon strain gauge sensor in the tip and electrical connectors at the other end. The strain gauge transducer converts the ICP to an electrical signal right at the tip of the catheter; thus there is no concern regarding leveling of the transducer. This catheter must be "zeroed" to atmospheric pressure before insertion but requires no additional "zeroing" following insertion. The bedside ICP monitor is calibrated to the bedside cardiac monitor and screen frequently during use. The microsensor ICP catheters are softer and less fragile than the fiberoptic catheters.

Zeroing and Calibration   Every ICP monitoring system must be "zeroed" and calibrated according to the manufacturer's specifications (Box 8-3).

Fluid-Filled Systems   The transducer must be "zeroed" before insertion and during every shift (more often if the transducer level or the patient's

Table 8-5
Intracranial Pressure Monitoring: Choice of Devices

Size of Ventricles, Requirements	Device
Enlarged Ventricles Cerebrospinal fluid drainage required	Ventricular catheter with drainage system
Slit Ventricles Monitoring only	Fiberoptic or microsensor device or ventricular catheter without drainage system

Box 8-3

Calibration of Intracranial Pressure Monitoring Devices

Microprocessor Device

NOTE: *The catheter is zeroed before insertion and following separation and reattachment of catheter with monitor only;* the interface box and bedside monitor are calibrated at the time of catheter insertion and daily.

1. To zero the catheter (this is accomplished before patient insertion):
   a. Connect the intracranial pressure (ICP) interface box to the gray patient cable and the gray patient cable to the sterile microprocessor cable (obtained from the sterile package and handed to you by the neurosurgeon). Some interface boxes must be turned to "transducer" at this point, whereas others are to remain off until the next step (1-b) is completed.
   b. Without contaminating the sterile insertion field, pour sterile normal saline into the bottom of the sterile plastic microsensor package. The physician (using sterile gloves and technique) will lay the tip of the microsensor in the saline.
   c. Some interface monitors are to be turned on at this point. All interface boxes should be zeroed at this point. A black knob may be turned until the ICP value on the monitor reads zero (it usually begins close to 500); this black knob should then be locked using the switch under the knob.
   d. After zeroing, the Codman interface box displays a three-digit "zero-reference value." This value should be recorded on the patient's chart and nursing Kardex, since it will be used if replacement of the system's cables and monitor is required.
   e. Once the interface box is "zeroed," it may be necessary to press "menu/enter."
   f. The physician places the catheter.
2. The bedside monitor should be joined to the ICP catheter and to the ICP interface box:
   a. Put the interface box on "standby;" press "zero" on the bedside monitor. The ICP display should read zero. When the monitor displays zero, press "menu/enter" on the interface box. You will then be prompted to calibrate the monitors.
   b. To calibrate the interface box and monitor: press the "100" button on the interface box. The interface monitor and bedside monitor should both display "100 mm Hg." Once this calibration is performed, press "menu/enter."
   c. The system is ready for monitoring. The interface box should be calibrated with the bedside monitor once daily. The catheter is "zeroed" only before insertion.

Fiberoptic Monitoring System

1. Join the ICP monitoring computer to the connector tubing and to the bedside monitor.
2. During catheter insertion, join the distal end of the catheter to the connector port of the fiberoptic monitoring system.
   a. Calibration of the fiberoptic catheter: Use the small screwdriver supplied with the catheter to zero the system before *insertion of the catheter into the patient.*
   b. Calibrate the ICP computer to the bedside monitor, using the calibration button on the ICP monitor (as the button is depressed, an ICP of 20, 40, 100, and 200 mm Hg will be displayed on the ICP monitor—these numbers should coincide with the display on the bedside monitor). Calibrate the bedside monitor accordingly. This calibration can be performed at any time.

Fluid-Filled Monitoring System

1. Flush tubing and stopcocks with irrigant fluid.
2. Determine the zero reference point and place the transducer at that level. Open the stopcock to air and zero the transducer. Maintain the transducer at that level for pressure measurements.
3. Join a 2-foot segment of noncompliant tubing to the zeroing stopcock—this segment is used as calibration tubing. Flush this tubing segment with irrigant fluid and open the distal end to air. Turn the stopcock open between this tubing segment and the transducer.

Continued

Box 8-3

Calibration of Intracranial Pressure Monitoring Devices—cont'd

a. Lower the distal tip to the zero reference point—the monitor should indicate 0 mm Hg pressure.
b. Elevate the tip of the tubing segment exactly 27.2 cm above the zero reference point—the monitor should indicate pressure of 20 mm Hg (the column of water

27.2 cm above the zero reference point creates a 27.2 cm H_2O pressure, which equals 20 mm Hg).
4. Turn the stopcock off to the calibration tubing and open to the ICP catheter.
5. The system is ready for monitoring.

---

position is changed). If there is any question of accuracy, mechanical calibration of the transducer can be accomplished using a water-filled tubing (1.36 cm H_2O = 1 mm Hg) or mercury manometer. If the transducer is joined by tubing to a patient, use of a water-filled manometer is the preferred calibration method. The transducer is typically placed at the level of the outer canthus of the eye (the level of the lateral ventricles).

The CPP is routinely calculated during ICP monitoring as the difference between the MAP and the ICP. If a fluid-filled ICP monitoring system is used, the zero reference point for both monitoring systems should be identical. If the ICP transducer zero reference point is located above the arterial pressure transducer zero reference point (as happens if the ICP transducer is leveled at the head and the arterial transducer is leveled at the heart, and the head of the bed is elevated), the calculated CPP will be falsely high (if the ICP transducer is 13.6 cm above the arterial transducer, this will result in a CPP that is 10 mm Hg too high).

In order for the ICP and arterial transducers to be at the same height, the arterial transducer should ideally be "zeroed" and placed at the level of the cerebral ventricles. Since this practice represents a departure from normal nursing technique and requires leveling of the arterial transducer differently for the child with head injury than is required for the child with heart disease or respiratory failure, unit policy must address this issue. In many intensive care units (ICUs), the arterial transducer is leveled at the right atrium in the conventional fashion, and allowances are made for the inaccuracy of the CPP calculation. Since the ICP measurement and CPP

calculation are used for trending, this practice is acceptable provided that it is consistent throughout the pediatric intensive care unit.

Fiberoptic Systems The fiberoptic catheters can only be zeroed before insertion. The ICP monitor digital display must be calibrated with a bedside monitor before insertion and at least every shift (or anytime the patient is disconnected from the bedside monitor). Fiberoptic monitoring systems contain no fluid and do not use transducers; thus leveling of a transducer is not required. This eliminates any concern regarding the relationship between the ICP monitoring system and the arterial transducer during calculation of the CPP.

Microsensor Devices The catheter tip transducer is only "zeroed" before insertion and following any separation and rejoining of the catheter with the monitor. The catheter is joined to the transducer and "zeroed" with the terminal 3 inches of the catheter tip lying submerged in a well (provided with the sterile package), covered in 0.5 to 1 inch of sterile water or normal saline. A connector housing joins the catheter to the monitor cable, and the zero reference value displayed when the catheter is zeroed is recorded there; thus if the patient is separated from the monitor, the system can be rezeroed while the catheter remains in place. The ICP monitor must be calibrated to 20 and 100 mm Hg and to the bedside monitor before use and once a day.

Nursing Responsibilities Safety and reliability of the ICP monitoring system must be ensured. The trend in the ICP is usually more important than any single measurement; thus it is essential that all nurses in the unit practice the same techniques for zeroing, leveling (if appropriate), and calibration of the ICP monitoring system.

Safety and Consistency Aseptic technique is required during catheter insertion and manipulation of the system. Minimize the frequency of breaks in the system (e.g., during changing of ventricular drainage collection bags), which will compromise sterility. Dress the catheter entrance site with an occlusive dressing.

Ensure that the transducer is appropriately "zeroed" and leveled (if a fluid-filled system is used), and mechanically calibrated (see Box 8-3). All stopcocks must be visible—check to ensure that all are turned in the proper direction. *Never* aspirate a ventricular drainage catheter—intraventricular hemorrhage may result.

Obtain specific orders regarding actions to be taken when the ICP rises (e.g., administer mannitol if ICP is >25 mm Hg). Fluid-filled ICP tubing systems should *not* be continuously irrigated.

Simultaneous Intracranial Pressure Monitoring and Ventricular Drainage Obtain orders regarding the height of the drainage system above the ventricle (typically the drainage drip chamber is placed 27.2 to 35 cm above the ventricle so that it will spontaneously drain when the ICP is >20 to 25 mm Hg). Determine if the stopcock is to remain "open" to allow continuous drainage of CSF from the ventricle and the collection system, or if intermittent drainage is to be performed when the ICP is >25 mm Hg (Figure 8-2). Note that if continuous drainage is performed with a drainage system 27.2 cm above the ventricle, drainage will prevent the ICP from exceeding 20 mm Hg (the drainage system will effectively "vent" pressure).

Recording Trends in Intracranial Pressure No single ICP measurement is consistently deleterious to all patients, but trends in the ICP can indicate

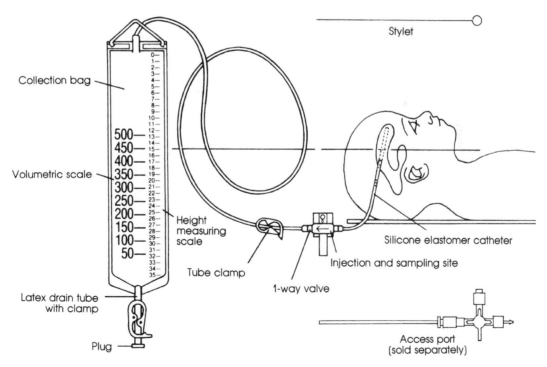

Figure 8-2 Intracranial pressure (ICP) monitor with external ventricular drainage system for controlled drainage of CSF. The Holter-Hausner system is depicted here, although several devices are currently marketed. The drainage port is depicted 15 cm above the ventricles. (Courtesy Phoenix Biomedical Corp., Bridgeport, Pa. From Hazinski MF: *Nursing care of the critically ill child,* ed 2, St Louis, 1992, Mosby.)

deterioration, particularly when they occur in conjunction with clinical deterioration. Any increase in ICP associated with clinical deterioration is very worrisome, and spontaneous spikes in ICP are generally more worrisome than those that occur only in response to stimulation (e.g., suctioning or venipuncture). When intracranial compliance is poor, the ICP spikes will be higher and will occur spontaneously. The average ICP will also increase. As the child recovers, the ICP spikes will only occur with stimulation, and the average ICP will decrease.

The charting of the ICP should indicate spikes occurring, as well as whether these spikes occur spontaneously or in response to stimulation only (Box 8-4). Elevation in ICP associated with a fall in CPP is also worrisome. Although the CPP may be misleading, and although there is no general agreement on the minimal CPP required in infants and children, attempts are generally made to maintain the CPP >50 mm Hg.

Common Clinical Conditions

Increased Intracranial Pressure

Etiology/Pathophysiology

Increased ICP is a symptom of an uncompensated rise in intracranial volume. Although the increased ICP can result from brain injury or disease, increased ICP itself can cause further intracranial injury, including brain distortion or herniation,

compromise or elimination of cerebral perfusion, or change in neurotransmitter levels.

Increased ICP is often treated as a single clinical entity when it has a variety of causes that will influence the selection and efficacy of therapy.

- *Traumatic increased ICP:* Typically results from a maldistribution of cerebral blood flow (CBF) and peaks within 24 to 48 hours after the insult.
- *Hypoxic/ischemic increased ICP:* Results from an increase in cerebral water content; the ICP may peak as late as 48 to 72 hours or more after the initial insult. An ICP >20 mm Hg in the child with an anoxic insult is thought to be a sign of a devastating insult rather than a treatable problem.

Increased ICP can result from either a *primary* or *secondary insult.* The *primary insult* may include trauma, a thromboembolic event or hemorrhage, or hypoxia/ischemia. This insult disrupts brain function and cannot be reversed, since it has already occurred by the time the child arrives in the emergency department or ICU. However, *secondary insults* can occur minutes, hours, or days after the primary insult and can cause new cerebral injury or extend existing injury. Secondary insult may be caused by cardiorespiratory compromise and resulting hypotension, hypoxemia, or hypercarbia, or by status epilepticus. These insults must be prevented or promptly detected and treated.

Normal ICP is approximately 4 to 15 mm Hg, and an ICP exceeding 20 mm Hg usually constitutes increased ICP. The ICP can be measured with a variety of devices, including fluid-filled transducer monitoring systems, fiberoptic catheters, and microprocessor devices.

Brain Volume An increase in brain volume results from cerebral swelling (increased or maldistributed blood flow) or cerebral edema (increased water content). *Brain swelling* is the term used to refer to maldistributed CBF that may include excessive flow to some areas of the brain within 24 to 48 hours after head trauma. This maldistributed flow results from formation or activation of a variety of mediators that contribute to vasodilation and increased capillary permeability in some parts of the brain and vasoconstriction and inadequate blood flow in other parts of the brain.

Increased Cerebral Blood Volume Increased CBV can result from increased CBF, obstruction to cerebral venous return, or an intracranial hemorrhage. CBF to some areas of the brain following head injury may be increased. CBV may also increase in response to hypercarbia or significant hypoxemia in association with some encephalopathies.

Increased CBV associated with obstruction to cerebral venous return can result from jugular venous obstruction (e.g., clot formation, compression of the jugular vein, or extremely high intrathoracic pressure). Arteriovenous malformations are the most common congenital, nontraumatic cause of intracranial hemorrhage and increased CBV in children.

Cerebrospinal Fluid Accumulation CSF accumulation can result from obstruction to CSF flow or a compromise in CSF reabsorption and, rarely, by increased CSF production. Potential causes are:

1. *Obstruction to CSF flow (obstructive hydrocephalus):* Can result from occlusion of the aqueduct of Sylvius by:
   a. Inflammatory cells (following meningitis)
   b. Fragments of red blood cells following intraventricular bleeding (this may cause acute or late hydrocephalus in trauma patients)
   c. Compression of the third and fourth ventricles by tumor

   Treatment requires insertion of a drain or shunt.

2. *Decreased CSF reabsorption (communicating hydrocephalus):* May be associated with head trauma and significant subarachnoid hemorrhage.
3. *Increased CSF production:* A choroid plexus tumor is a rare cause of communicating hydrocephalus.

Mass Lesions Intracranial tumors are one of the most common forms of childhood malignancy. Tumors are most frequently infratentorial and are

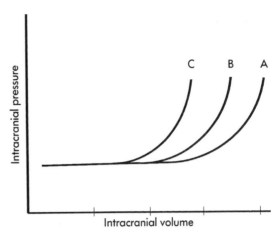

Figure 8-3 Intracranial pressure-volume curves. The change in ICP resulting from an increase in intracranial volume is not linear and will be related to intracranial compliance. Initially, when an increase in intracranial volume develops, other intracranial contents are displaced out of the intracranial vault or compressed to prevent an increase in ICP. When the limits of compensation or compliance have been reached, the same increase in volume (**A**) is better tolerated than a more rapid increase in volume (**B**). Once the ICP begins to rise, then smaller increases in volume will produce a rise in ICP in the future (**C**).

often located near or in the brain stem (see Intracranial Tumors under Specific Diseases, p. 434). Water accumulation (edema) may complicate the mass effect of the tumor, contributing to further increase in intracranial volume.

Intracranial Compliance The relationship between intracranial volume and ICP is illustrated by a pressure-volume curve (Figure 8-3). The shape of this curve reflects *intracranial compliance,* which is the change in ICP that occurs with a given increase in intracranial volume. If the curve is virtually horizontal, intracranial compliance is high, and an increase in intracranial volume will initially be tolerated without a significant change in ICP. If the curve is virtually vertical, intracranial compliance is very low, and even a small rise in intracranial volume will produce a significant rise in ICP.

When intracranial compliance is high, an increase in the volume of brain, blood, or CSF (or mass lesion) results in displacement of venous capacitance blood from the intracranial vault and displacement of CSF into the subarachnoid space along the spinal column (unless obstructive hydrocephalus is present). Initially these compensatory mechanisms enable tolerance of the increased volume of one component of the intracranial vault without an increase in ICP.

Once the limits of compensation have been reached, however, intracranial compliance is reduced. Further increase in intracranial volume will result in a rise in ICP. The increase in ICP then becomes nearly exponential; progressively smaller rises in intracranial volume will produce progressively greater rises in ICP.

Compliance is affected by time and by preceding rises in intracranial volume (see Figure 8-3). Gradual rises in intracranial volume (e.g., with a brain tumor) enable accommodation of a greater volume than if the increase in volume is acute (e.g., with intracranial hemorrhage). Frequent increases in intracranial volume will decrease intracranial compliance; thus the ICP will rise with smaller increases in intracranial volume in the future.

Biochemical Mediators A primary neurologic injury or insult can result in the formation or release of free oxygen radicals and excitatory neurotransmitters (e.g., glutamate and aspartate) and liberation of intracellular calcium. These substances can all contribute to maldistribution of CBF and secondary neurologic injury.

Free oxygen radicals are formed as a result of lipid peroxidation through a variety of pathways, including arachidonic acid metabolism (these mediators have been implicated in the pathophysiology of septic shock; see Table 5-10). These radicals can alter cell membrane permeability, resulting in cell injury or death.

Excitatory neurotransmitters and excessive intracellular calcium alter cellular calcium influx in some brain cells, rendering them hypermetabolic. Although endogenous protective mechanisms exist to eliminate these harmful substances, protective mechanisms may be overwhelmed when severe brain injury or insult is present.

Clinical Presentation

The child with increased ICP typically demonstrates an alteration in level of consciousness (LOC); pupil dilation with decreased response to light; changes in heart rate, blood pressure, and respiratory rate or pattern; and abnormal motor activity or reflexes (Box 8-5). The child may complain of headache or nausea and may vomit, particularly in the morning or after moving from a reclining to an upright position.

Evaluation of Cardiorespiratory Function The neurologic evaluation includes evaluation of cardiopulmonary function. Always evaluate vital signs in light of the patient's clinical condition—tachycardia and tachypnea are usually more appropriate in critically ill children than a "normal" heart rate and respiratory rate.

Evaluation of Airway, Oxygenation Increased ICP may be associated with a decrease in LOC and inability to protect the airway. In addition, apnea or hypoventilation may produce hypoxemia or hypercarbia, resulting in cerebral artery dilation and an increase in CBF with a further rise in ICP.

Box 8-5

Signs and Symptoms of Increased Intracranial Pressure

Change in Level of Consciousness
Irritability, then lethargy
Confusion, disorientation
Decreased responsiveness (decreased eye contact; decreased response to parents, to pain)
Reduced ability to follow commands (hold up two fingers, wiggle toes, stick out tongue)

Pupil Dilation With Decreased Response to Light

Reduced Spontaneous Movement or Deterioration in Reflexive Posturing
Purposeful movement deteriorates
Decorticate posturing, then
Decerebrate posturing, then
Flaccid response to pain

Cushing's Triad (Hypertension, Bradycardia, Apnea) May Occur Only as Late Sign

Modified from Hazinski MF: *Nursing care of the critically ill child,* ed 2, St Louis, 1992, Mosby.

Evaluation of Systemic Perfusion   If systemic perfusion is poor, cerebral perfusion is likely to be compromised. Signs of poor perfusion may include an inappropriately rapid or slow heart rate (bradycardia is most common), diminished intensity of peripheral pulses, delayed capillary refill despite a warm ambient temperature, and cool extremities. The skin may be mottled in appearance. Shock resuscitation must be provided to ensure that cerebral perfusion is optimized (see Shock, p. 140).

Hypotension is usually associated with inadequate systemic (and possibly cerebral) perfusion, but perfusion may be inadequate despite a normal blood pressure. Hypotension beyond 1 year of age is a systolic blood pressure ≤70 mm Hg plus twice the child's age in years. Hypotension following head trauma can be associated with a worsening neurologic outcome; therefore it must be prevented or promptly detected and treated. *Hypertension* may develop as a compensatory mechanism to maintain cerebral perfusion in patients with an increase in ICP but may also be a sign of pain or fear.

Evaluation of Level of Consciousness, Responsiveness   Evaluation of LOC is probably the single most important aspect of assessment of the child with increased ICP. It should be evaluated at frequent intervals, using consistent terminology. Any scoring system must be used in the same way by all members of the health care team in order that trends in the patient's condition can be immediately identified. Reevaluation should occur whenever changes are observed in the ICP, central perfusion pressure (CPP), or clinical appearance. Excessive *irritability* or *lethargy* must be investigated. Hints to evaluate LOC:

- Signs of decreased LOC in infants may include lethargy, decreased eye contact, poor visual tracking, and change in feeding behavior (including vomiting).
- *Decreased response to frightening or painful procedures is usually abnormal and often indicates cardiorespiratory or neurologic compromise.*
- Record information about the child's favorite activities, family members, and companions to evaluate accuracy of the child's responsiveness.

- *Stupor* is present if the child responds only to the most noxious stimuli (e.g., painful stimulus).
- *Coma* is present if the child cannot be aroused despite application of strong external stimuli (e.g., painful stimulus).

Glasgow Coma Scale   The GCS is probably the most consistently used system to score neurologic responsiveness (Table 8-6), through evaluation of motor activity, verbal responses, and eye opening following simple stimuli or commands. A score of 3 to 15 is achieved. The lowest possible score, a 3, is assigned to the patient who is flaccid and unresponsive to any stimulus. If the patient is unconscious, the lowest scores possible (1 point each) will be achieved for eye opening and verbal responses; thus the critical portion of the GCS will be determined by the motor response, particularly the child's response to painful stimulus. This portion of the GCS must be carefully assessed, and the child's best response recorded.

Any scale or patient condition scoring system is most useful if it enables evaluation of trends in the patient's condition over time. Therefore the scale must be applied in exactly the same way by everyone. The scale can also be incorporated into the nursing care flow sheet so that the information is readily accessible.

If the child's response to pain decreases, look for other clinical signs of neurologic deterioration, including apnea (or change in breathing pattern), hypertension, tachycardia, or bradycardia. Deterioration should be reported to a physician immediately.

Motor Response   *Purposeful* spontaneous movements, rather than *reflexive* responses, must be elicited. Increased ICP may produce decreased motor function, or abnormal posturing or reflexes. With progressive deterioration, flaccid paralysis will result.

- *Ability to follow commands:* This is assessed first. Ask the child to hold up two fingers, stick out his or her tongue, or wiggle toes—these are actions that can *not* be accomplished by reflex. Do not ask the child to squeeze your hand, since reflex curling of the fingers can occur. If the child can follow commands, a motor score of 6 applies.

Table 8-6
Modified Glasgow Coma Scale for Infants and Children

	Child	Infant	Score
Eye opening	Spontaneous	Spontaneous	4
	To verbal stimuli	To verbal stimuli	3
	To pain only	To pain only	2
	No response	No response	1
Verbal response	Oriented, appropriate	Coos and babbles	5
	Confused	Irritable cries	4
	Inappropriate words	Cries to pain	3
	Incomprehensible words or nonspecific sounds	Moans to pain	2
	No response	No response	1
Motor response	Obeys commands	Moves spontaneously and purposefully	6
	Localizes painful stimulus	Withdraws to touch	5
	Withdraws in response to pain	Withdraws in response to pain	4
	Flexion in response to pain	Decorticate posturing (abnormal flexion) in response to pain	3
	Extension in response to pain	Decerebrate posturing (abnormal extension) in response to pain	2
	No response	No response	1

From Hazinski MF: *Nursing care of the critically ill child,* ed 2, St Louis, 1992, Mosby; modified from Davis RJ et al: Head and spinal cord injury. In Rogers MC, editor: *Textbook of pediatric intensive care,* Baltimore, 1987, Williams & Wilkins; James H, Anas N, Perkin RM: *Brain insults in infants and children,* New York, 1985, Grune & Stratton; and Morray JP et al: Coma scale for use in brain-injured children, *Critical Care Med* 12:1018, 1984.

- *Localization of pain:* Apply a *central* pain stimulus to the head, neck, or trunk above the nipple line. Rub the sternum or pinch the trapezius and look for a *purposeful* movement of the child's hands (should be unrestrained) toward the stimulus. *Nonpurposeful* movements, such as arching of the shoulders or groaning, cannot be scored here. Usually, if the patient is sufficiently responsive to groan, further stimulus will elicit a purposeful response. If the best response of the child is localization of pain, a motor score of 5 applies.
- *Withdrawal from pain:* Apply *peripheral* painful stimuli to the medial aspects of each extremity to determine if the child *withdraws* from the stimulus. Purposeful withdrawal occurs when the child *abducts* each extremity after the *medial* aspect of the extremity is pinched. If abduction/withdrawal is the child's best response, a motor score of 4 applies. Note that reflex withdrawal from a very peripheral stimulus, such as pinching

the toe or finger or stroking the bottom of the foot, can be accomplished through a reflex spinal arc and should *not* be interpreted as a purposeful withdrawal.
- *Decorticate posturing in response to pain:* Arms flex, draw toward midline; legs extend. If this is the child's best response, a motor score of 3 applies.
- *Decerebrate posturing in response to pain:* Arms and legs extend. If this is the child's best response, a motor score of 2 applies.
- *Flaccid response to pain:* No movement is observed when a painful stimulus is applied. If the child demonstrates no response to painful stimulus, a motor score of 1 applies.

Abnormal motor activity may be observed that is not included in the GCS, and this should be recorded and reported to a physician:

- *Hemiparesis or hemiplegia:* May develop on the side opposite the brain injury or insult (e.g., a left temporal depressed skull fracture may result in compromise of movement and sensation on the right side).

- *Quadriplegia:* Typically results from cervical spine injury and results in loss of movement in all four extremities.
- *Spasticity:* May result from increased ICP, cerebral palsy, or loss of inhibition to lower motor neurons.
- *Seizures:* Not a primary sign of increased ICP but may contribute to a rise in ICP or complicate management. Status epilepticus increases cerebral metabolic demand and thus must be treated. Consider subclinical status epilepticus as a potential cause of unexplained deterioration in the child with increased ICP (see Status Epilepticus).

Eye Opening   The GCS evaluates eye opening, and scoring is determined by the amount of stimulus required to stimulate the eye opening (see Table 8-6).

Verbal Response   This portion of the GCS is impossible to assess in the intubated or preverbal child without some adjustment of criteria. Modifications in this portion of the score have been proposed for preverbal children (see Table 8-6). While the child is intubated, this portion of the GCS may be ignored, but the intubation should be noted on the chart.

Evaluation of Cranial Nerves   Many cranial nerves can be evaluated during routine nursing activities (see Table 8-2). *Loss* of previously demonstrated cranial nerve function requires immediate investigation, since it may indicate neurologic deterioration.

Cranial Nerve III   The pupils are normally the same size bilaterally, and pupil constriction is normally brisk with consensual constriction in response to light (e.g., shine a light into the left pupil, and both the left and right pupils constrict). Increased ICP or uncal herniation (e.g., lateral shift of the temporal lobe) may result in compression of the oculomotor nerve, with resultant pupil dilation and decreased constrictive response to light. If the intracranial lesion is *unilateral,* pupil dilation will usually occur on the same side as the lesion. The awake child may complain of blurred vision or

diplopia. Potential alterations in pupil size or response to light or eye movement include:

- *Pupil dilation:* May be caused by increased ICP, hypothermia, or administration of atropine or large doses of sympathomimetic drugs or mydriatic drops.
- *Unilateral ptosis:* May result from oculomotor nerve compression and increased ICP. Pupil dilation with decreased response to light will also be observed.
- *Blindness:* Pupil(s) will not constrict in response to light.
- *Meiosis (pupil constriction):* May result from hemorrhage in or dysfunction of the pons, from poisoning, or from large doses of morphine sulfate. May also occur as a result of Horner's syndrome.
- *Horner's syndrome:* Unilateral ptosis, meiosis, and anhydrosis resulting from ipsilateral interruption of sympathetic nervous system fibers (can occur following cardiovascular surgery). Horner's syndrome will affect the side of the interrupted sympathetic nervous system fibers (e.g., the side of surgery), but both pupils should still respond briskly to light.

Cranial Nerves II, III, IV, and VI   If the child is awake and tracks objects across and up and down in a visual field, these cranial nerves are probably intact.

Cranial Nerves VII, VIII, and XI   Wrinkling of the forehead when coughing indicates function of the facial nerve (cranial nerve VII). If the child startles to noise, the acoustic nerve is functioning (cranial nerve VIII). A gag reflex during suctioning or placement of a nasogastric tube or shrugging of the shoulders and upper arms indicates function of cranial nerve XI.

Cushing's Reflex   Cushing's reflex is an association of clinical signs that may indicate increased ICP. The development of this reflex indicates *profound compromise in perfusion of the brain stem,* and it may appear only when cerebral brain stem herniation is imminent. This reflex consists of an increase in systolic arterial blood pressure, bradycardia, and apnea.

Papilledema   Papilledema is edema of the optic nerve or disc, resulting in engorged and pulseless retinal veins. Papilledema does not develop acutely (within hours); if it is present, the ICP has been elevated for 48 hours or more.

Diagnostic Tests   ICP monitoring and careful clinical assessment provide the most useful information about the child's neurologic status. The CT scan is extremely helpful in determining the severity of head injury, in localizing mass lesions or intracranial bleeding, or in determining the presence of diffuse cerebral edema, infarction, or evidence of anoxic injury. The CT scan is used in the acute management of the patient with increased ICP to evaluate the presence and severity of cerebral edema or swelling. If the third and fourth ventricles and basilar cisterns are widely patent and visible on the CT scan, the patient's intracranial volume has probably not yet reached the limits of compensation, although the ICP may be high. If the third and fourth ventricles are collapsed and the basilar cisterns are obliterated, however, it is likely that the patient has reached the limits of compensation; further increase in intracranial volume is likely to produce a profound increase in ICP, and cerebral herniation may result. Collapse of the lateral ventricles (in the absence of an external CSF drain) may also indicate exhaustion of compensatory mechanisms.

A quantitative or qualitative radioactive cerebral perfusion scan may be performed to evaluate brain blood flow or to confirm absence of brain blood flow as part of brain death pronouncement. This study requires injecting a radioactive isotope and imaging to document the quantity or absence of circulation of the compound in the brain.

Management

The goals of management of increased ICP are:

1. Maintain effective cerebral perfusion through maintenance of excellent systemic perfusion and control of ICP
2. Preserve cerebral function
3. Prevent secondary insults to the brain

Secondary insults include hypoxia, hypotension, fluid and electrolyte imbalance, and seizures. An adequate airway, effective oxygenation and ventilation, and adequate blood pressure and perfusion *must* be maintained—too often, the condition of the child with increased ICP deteriorates as a result of inattention to the basics of critical care. Poor outcome following closed head injury has been linked with documented hypoxemia or hypotension during the first days following the injury.

Optimal therapy for increased ICP requires identification of the specific cause of the problem and selection of therapy aimed at that specific cause. If that therapy fails to control the ICP, then additional therapy is added (Table 8-7 and Figure 8-4). All causes of increased ICP are not treated identically. Although increased ICP resulting from traumatic brain injury may respond to the measures described here, there is no evidence that increased

Table 8-7
Management of Raised Intracranial Pressure of Known Etiology

Increased CSF	Increased Blood Volume	Increased Brain Volume	Significant Mass Lesion	Persistent, Increased ICP Despite Selective Therapy
Head up Drainage Steroids Acetazolamide (Diamox) Mannitol	Head up Hyperventilation* Metabolic suppression Hypothermia	Head up Steroids Mannitol Surgery	Surgical removal Hyperventilation* Mannitol Steroids	Head up Head midline Hyperventilation* Muscle paralysis Sedation Mannitol Hypothermia Arterial hypertension

Mild rather than extreme hyperventilation is now advocated (see p. 397).

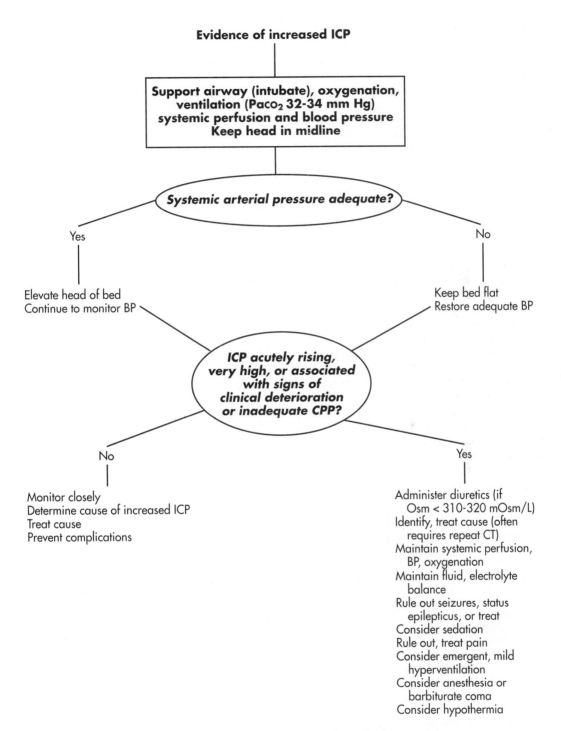

Figure 8-4   Initial management of increased ICP of unknown etiology.

ICP resulting from anoxic cerebral injury will be affected by these measures.

Assessment and Support of Airway and Ventilation Assess the child's airway. If the child is obtunded or demonstrates decreased response to painful stimulation, consider elective intubation to prevent possible airway obstruction or respiratory arrest. Intubation should also be performed if hypoventilation, hypoxemia, hypercarbia, or signs of increased ICP are observed (these indications are summarized in Box 8-6). If the child is responsive, sedation is required. If the trauma victim is thought to have a full stomach, rapid sequence intubation is used, although succinylcholine may be avoided because it may increase CBF and ICP.

Ensure effective oxygenation and ventilation throughout the care of the child with increased ICP. The PaO_2 should be maintained at 80 to 100 mm Hg with an oxyhemoglobin saturation of 97% to 99%, and hypoxia must be prevented. A normocarbia or a very *mild* hypocarbia is generally maintained ($PaCO_2$ of approximately 32 to 34 mm Hg) to control CBF. Extreme hyperventilation is avoided except under emergent conditions, since it may severely reduce CBF, creating cerebral ischemia in some parts of the brain (see Reduction in Cerebral Blood Volume). If a mild respiratory alkalosis is maintained, hemoglobin saturation should be maintained at 98% to 99%; hemoglobin saturation

<93% in alkalotic patients is associated with hypoxemia. Suctioning should be performed skillfully by two nurses to prevent the development of hypercarbia and hypoxemia.

If the child coughs frequently or struggles "against" the ventilator, peak and mean airway pressures will rise and may impede cerebral venous return and contribute to increased CBV and increased ICP. It may be necessary to administer paralyzing agents (with analgesics) to ensure effective control of ventilation.

Assessment and Support of Systemic Perfusion Evaluate the child's systemic perfusion virtually constantly. If systemic perfusion is poor, support of appropriate heart rate, intravascular volume, myocardial function, and vascular resistance is required. Intravenous (IV) fluids are administered as needed to ensure adequate intravascular volume relative to the vascular space. Fluid administered to improve systemic perfusion or blood volume should be delivered by bolus (over 15 to 20 minutes), and nonglucose, isotonic fluids (normal saline, lactated Ringer's solution, or colloids) should be used. Dextrose-containing fluids with one-half normal saline (0.45% NaCl) may be used to deliver maintenance fluids or dilute medications, since such fluids will replace insensible water losses. Dextrose-and-water solutions are avoided, since they may contribute to abrupt lowering of the serum sodium resulting in an extravascular fluid shift.

Myocardial dysfunction may result from cardiac contusion in trauma patients, or it may complicate barbiturate administration. Barbiturate administration also produces vasodilation, which may compromise blood pressure. Sympathomimetic drug infusion is indicated for either myocardial dysfunction or vasodilation that compromises blood pressure or systemic perfusion. Dopamine or epinephrine are usually preferred. Dobutamine is not the drug of choice for the vasodilated and hypotensive patient, because the beta-2 adrenergic effects of dobutamine may result in peripheral vasodilation and worsening of the hypotension. If the ICP rises whenever the systemic arterial pressure rises, cerebral autoregulation may be lost, and the patient's prognosis is very poor.

Box 8-6

Indications for Intubation in the Child With Head Injury or Increased Intracranial Pressure

Impaired airway clearance or compromise in protective reflexes (weak cough, gag)
Hypoventilation
Hypoxemia or hypercarbia
Evidence of increased intracranial pressure
Associated shock, pulmonary failure

From Hazinski MF: *Nursing care of the critically ill child*, ed 2, St Louis, 1992, Mosby.

Evaluation of Cerebral Perfusion: Jugular Venous Oxygen Saturation and Arteriovenous Oxygen Difference A major goal of therapy for increased ICP is to match CBF and cerebral oxygen delivery to cerebral oxygen utilization and requirements. Ideally, this is done through evaluation of CBF rather than simply ICP. CBF may be grossly evaluated and quantified using cold xenon scans. Intermittent or continuous evaluation of the jugular venous oxygen saturation can be used to evaluate arteriovenous oxygen content difference and to evaluate the balance between CBF and cerebral utilization of oxygen. In general, a decrease in the jugular venous oxygen saturation indicates an undesirable decrease in cerebral oxygen delivery or increase in cerebral oxygen utilization (Box 8-7). A jugular venous oxygen saturation <50% has been linked with poor outcome in adults with head injury.

Reduction in Cerebral Blood Volume When increased ICP is caused by trauma or encephalopa-

thy, CBF does not match metabolic requirements. It may be excessive in some areas of the brain but inadequate (causing ischemia) in other areas of the brain. Acute reduction in CBF and CBV can be achieved with hyperventilation, but extreme hypocarbia is generally avoided in order to prevent the development of ischemia. Under emergent conditions before intubation, acute hyperventilation may be provided with bag and mask, but intubation and mechanical ventilatory support are ultimately required.

Mild Hyperventilation When increased ICP is present, the arterial oxygen and carbon dioxide tensions should be controlled with mechanical ventilatory support. Hand ventilation should not be the primary method to control carbon dioxide tension and ICP, since extreme hypocarbia and cerebral ischemia may be created during these times. Mechanical ventilatory support is manipulated to maintain the arterial carbon dioxide tension at approximately 32 to 34 mm Hg. In addition, hypoxemia is avoided; the arterial oxygen tension is maintained at 80 to 100 mm Hg; and hemoglobin saturation is maintained at 97% to 99%.

Hyperventilation and respiratory alkalosis shift the child's oxyhemoglobin dissociation curve *to the left;* thus the hemoglobin will be well saturated at relatively low arterial oxygen tensions. This means that in the hyperventilated patient, a hemoglobin saturation of 90% may be associated with a PaO_2 of 50 to 60 mm Hg—this degree of hypoxemia will produce cerebral artery dilation and may contribute to an increased ICP. Therefore the hemoglobin saturation should be monitored continuously using pulse oximetry, and it should be maintained at 97% to 99% saturation.

Skillful pulmonary support and suction technique are required to prevent hypoxemia and any rise in $PaCO_2$. Assess breath sounds frequently and prevent or promptly treat atelectasis and hypoventilation. Pharmacologic paralysis (with analgesia) may be necessary to control ventilation. If possible, avoid high peak inspiratory and positive end-expiratory pressures, since they may contribute to obstruction of cerebral venous return. Monitor for evidence of pneumothorax, since cerebral venous

---

Box 8-7

Factors Causing a Fall in Jugular Venous Oxygen Saturation

Fall in Cerebral Oxygen Delivery

Fall in cerebral blood flow
- Increase in intracranial pressure
- Fall in cardiac output (inadequate heart rate, inadequate intravascular volume relative to vascular space, decreased myocardial function, extreme vasodilation)
- Fall in arterial blood pressure (hypovolemia, myocardial dysfunction, vasodilation)

Fall in hemoglobin saturation (hypoxemia)
- Suctioning
- Hypoventilation
- Atelectasis
- Tube obstruction

Fall in hemoglobin concentration (e.g., anemia or hemorrhage)

Increase in Cerebral Oxygen Consumption

Seizures or status epilepticus
Fever
Sepsis

return can be impeded by a significant increase in intrathoracic pressure.

Elevation of Head of Bed Enhancement of cerebral venous return will contribute to reduction in CBV. If arterial blood pressure is adequate, elevate the head of the bed (no more than 30 degrees). Keep the head in midline—turning of the head may increase the ICP.

If the child's ICP continues to increase despite oxygenation and ventilation, administration of diuretics or osmotic agents may be necessary. The nurse should also notify a physician if hand ventilation is necessary to control the ICP, since this suggests the need for additional therapy.

Maintenance and Manipulation of Serum Osmolality Maintain the osmolality at approximately 300 to 310 mOsm/L (normal osmolality is 272 to 300 mOsm/L). Prevent rapid reduction in serum sodium and osmolality (e.g., caused by administration of a large volume of hypotonic fluid or the undetected development of the syndrome of inappropriate antidiuretic hormone secretion [SIADH]). An acute fall in serum sodium or osmolality will result in an extravascular free water shift (into the interstitial spaces), contributing to cerebral edema. There is no evidence that maintenance of a constantly high intravascular osmolality will result in a continuous intravascular fluid shift. In fact, serum osmolality exceeding 320 mOsm/L may be detrimental.

Monitor the child's serum electrolytes closely during therapy. Since osmotic diuresis results in loss of free water and electrolytes, electrolyte imbalance can rapidly develop.

Fluid Administration Once shock resuscitation is accomplished and the child's intravascular volume is adequate, approximately one half to two thirds of standard "maintenance" fluid requirements (Table 8-8) are administered in the form of one-half normal saline (0.45% NaCl). This will maintain the serum sodium and osmolality even if SIADH is present. Remember that children with head trauma or increased ICP are at risk for the development of SIADH—if it develops, treatment consists of limitation of fluid intake (see Syndrome of Inappropriate Antidiuretic Hormone Secretion). Avoid hypotonic fluid (5% dextrose and water, or solutions of 0.2% NaCl), since it may abruptly de-

Table 8-8
Estimation of Maintenance Fluid Requirements in Children

Weight	Formula
Body Weight Daily Maintenance Formula	
Neonate (<72 hr)	60-100 ml/kg
0-10 kg	100 ml/kg
11-20 kg	1000 ml for first 10 kg + 50 ml/kg for kg 11-20
21-30 kg	1500 ml for first 20 kg + 25 ml/kg for kg 21-30
Body Weight Hourly Maintenance Formula	
0-10 kg	4 ml/kg/hr
11-20 kg	40 ml/hr for first 10 kg + 2 ml/kg/hr for kg 11-20
21-30 kg	60 ml/hr for first 20 kg + 1 ml/kg/hr for kg 21-30
Body Surface Area Formula	
1500 ml/m² body surface area/day	
Insensible Water Losses	
300 ml/m² body surface area/day	

From Hazinski MF: *Nursing care of the critically ill child,* ed 2, St Louis, 1992, Mosby.
note: This table enables calculation of generous maintenance fluid requirements for normal children. Children with increased intracranial pressure, particularly if it is associated with trauma or surgery, are likely to retain free water. As a result, once intravascular volume is adequate, the child will likely require no more than 50% to 67% of the calculated maintenance fluid requirements. Hypotonic fluids are avoided.

crease serum sodium and osmolality, resulting in an extravascular fluid shift.

Estimation of Serum Osmolality Monitor the patient's serum osmolality closely; it may be measured in the laboratory or estimated from the formula listed in Box 8-8. Note that the formula does not reflect changes in osmolality resulting from administered osmotic agents. Osmotic agents are usually withheld if the serum osmolality exceeds 310 mOsm/L, and a physician should be notified if the serum osmolality exceeds 315 to 320 mOsm/L.

Diuretic and Osmotic Agents Intravascular volume and osmolality may be manipulated with diuretics or osmotic agents. Furosemide is the diuretic that is most frequently used during the first

---

Box 8-8

Estimation of Serum Osmolality

$$2 \times [Na^+] = \underline{\hspace{1cm}}$$
$$+ [Glucose] \div 18 = +\underline{\hspace{1cm}}$$
$$+ [BUN] \div 2.8 = +\underline{\hspace{1cm}}$$
$$= \underline{\hspace{1cm}} \text{ mOsm/L}$$

(Normal: 272-300 mOsm/L)

NOTE: This formula does not reflect changes in serum osmolality associated with administration of osmotic agents or associated with hyperlipidemia.

Modified from Hazinski MF: *Nursing care of the critically ill child,* ed 2, St Louis, 1992, Mosby.

---

24 to 48 hours of injury; it can be administered alone or in combination with osmotic diuretics. A dose of 1 mg/kg IV of furosemide produces an acute free water diuresis within minutes; since free water is excreted in excess of sodium, serum osmolality is maintained. In addition, furosemide decreases venous tone and reduces production of CSF. This drug will produce potassium excretion; thus the serum potassium level must be closely monitored (a fall should be anticipated), and potassium chloride administration may be required.

Osmotic agents are administered to produce an acute, transient rise in intravascular osmolality, producing a shift of free water from the interstitial space to the intravascular space. This free water is then eliminated by the kidneys.

Mannitol is useful for treatment of increased ICP because it produces both osmotic diuresis and cerebral vasoconstriction; it therefore may reduce increased ICP and CBV by two mechanisms. It must be filtered before use (to prevent infusion of crystals), and it is administered over 5 to 20 minutes, in a dose of 0.15 to 0.3 g/kg/dose. Diuresis is typically observed within 10 to 20 minutes, although the ICP may fall more quickly following administration. Higher doses of mannitol (1 g/kg) are reserved for emergency control of intracranial hypertension.

Mannitol administration (particularly in higher doses) may transiently *increase* cerebral intravas-cular volume and contribute to a brief rise in ICP. Following administration and a decrease in ICP, the ICP may rise again to higher pressures, the so-called rebound effect. This elevation in ICP, associated with a relatively high CPP, is thought to develop in dehydrated patients.

Hypertonic (3% to 29.2%) saline may be used as an osmotic agent to promote osmotic diuresis. It may also be administered to treat conditions associated with an acute reduction in serum sodium and osmolality and resulting cerebral edema (e.g., SIADH resulting in seizures). Hypertonic saline is used intermittently to produce diuresis. Use of this therapy to *maintain* a consistently high serum osmolality is of no demonstrable benefit. Frequent doses may produce extremely high serum sodium concentration and osmolality and has been reported to contribute to the development of agranulocytopenia.

Glycerol is an osmotic diuretic that may be administered in doses identical to mannitol (0.15 to 0.3 g/kg). It is a smaller molecule than mannitol and contains smaller, more osmotically active particles than mannitol; thus it may result in a greater diuretic effect. Potential side effects of glycerol include intravascular hemolysis and an increase in serum triglyceride.

Urea (30%) is an osmotic diuretic; 1 g/kg every 4 to 6 hours may be administered. The use of urea is often limited because it is contraindicated in the presence of renal or liver disease. Potential side effects include hypotension, nausea, vomiting, headaches, syncope, and dizziness. Tissue sloughing may occur if the drug enters subcutaneous tissue; thus central venous administration is recommended.

Concentrated glucose solutions (D_{25} or D_{50}) may be used to create osmotic diuresis, but their use should be reserved for children with documented hypoglycemia. *Hyper*glycemia is common following head injury and has been associated with increased morbidity and mortality.

Drainage of Cerebrospinal Fluid   If CSF circulation is obstructed or CSF reabsorption is inhibited in the child with increased ICP, CSF drainage may be required. Obstructive hydrocephalus may result from head injury complicated by an intraventricular bleed or third- or fourth-ventricle compression; and communicating hydrocephalus may result from head injury complicated by subarachnoid hemorrhage.

Temporary CSF drainage is achieved by insertion of an intraventricular catheter with a drainage port. Permanent drainage of CSF from the intracranial vault is achieved through surgical insertion of a ventriculoperitoneal shunt. If a shunt is placed, monitor for signs of increased ICP indicating potential shunt malfunction and note in the nursing care plan if the shunt must be "pumped" to maintain function.

If the ICP is extremely high, the third and fourth ventricles will collapse and CSF will accumulate in the lateral ventricles, contributing to a further rise in ICP. Under these conditions CSF drainage may reduce the ICP. However, when the ICP is extremely high, the ventricles may collapse around the drainage/monitoring catheter, preventing further CSF drainage.

In the absence of posttraumatic hydrocephalus, routine drainage of CSF to reduce the ICP is controversial. If CSF pathways are patent, CSF displacement from the intracranial vault should occur spontaneously when the ICP rises. Therefore CSF drainage may be unnecessary and may introduce the risk of infection, hemorrhage, and upward herniation of the brain.

General Supportive Care and Control of Oxygen Requirements

The patient with increased ICP is intubated and mechanically ventilated.

Analgesia   Pain can contribute to a rise in ICP. If the child has multisystem trauma and is responsive, analgesia is required. If the patient is agitated or the work of breathing is high, pharmacologic paralysis (with analgesia) will eliminate the work of breathing during mechanical ventilation.

Anesthetic agents (lidocaine, fentanyl, barbiturates) may be administered to reduce the cerebral metabolic rate and improve the cerebral oxygen delivery-supply relationship. These agents will reduce the ICP, but their effect on morbidity and mortality is unknown.

Temperature Regulation   Fever increases cerebral metabolic and oxygen requirements and should thus be treated with antipyretics. A cold environmental temperature will stimulate nonshiver-

ing thermogenesis and increase oxygen consumption in the young infant. Mild hypothermia may be created to reduce oxygen demand, but shivering must be prevented (muscle relaxants may be used). See Hypothermia.

Seizure Control   Seizures will increase CBF and the metabolic rate, and they should be treated. Prophylactic anticonvulsants may be prescribed for the child with head injury, particularly if the child demonstrates *risk factors for posttraumatic seizures:*

- Severe head injury
- Diffuse cerebral edema
- Acute subdural hematoma
- Open, depressed skull fracture

Status epilepticus may create an acute and severe rise in ICP and should be suspected in any child with head injury who demonstrates sudden neurologic deterioration, pupil dilation, and fluctuation in vital signs. Subclinical seizures/status epilepticus may cause acute deterioration and may require an EEG for diagnosis. Status epilepticus must be treated promptly with anticonvulsants.

Nutritional Support   Nutritional support should be provided as soon as possible. Enteral feeding is preferable to parenteral alimentation. Nasogastric feedings may be provided if the child demonstrates an effective cough and gag reflex; nasojejunal feedings may be provided even if the child is unconscious. Parenteral alimentation should be provided until systemic and gastrointestinal perfusion is stable and enteral nutrition can be accomplished.

Barbiturate Therapy   Barbiturate therapy may be prescribed if severe intracranial hypertension is unresponsive to maximal oxygenation, ventilation, diuresis, sedation, and analgesia. Although *prophylactic* barbiturate therapy has not been shown to reduce morbidity or mortality following head injury, barbiturate therapy has been associated with successful treatment of some children with refractory intracranial hypertension. As a result, barbiturate therapy may be used to treat refractory intracranial hypertension. There is *no evidence that barbiturate coma improves survival or outcome of patients with ischemic cerebral insult;* thus barbiturate coma is not used for these patients.

The anesthetic effects of the barbiturates reduce the cerebral metabolic rate and oxygen consumption and make the patient less responsive to external stimuli; thus the ICP will fall. However, barbiturates can depress cardiovascular function and produce systemic vasodilation. These effects can reduce the mean arterial pressure (MAP) and cerebral perfusion pressure. When barbiturates are administered, cardiovascular function must be monitored and supported carefully. An arterial line and central venous pressure monitoring catheter should be in place so that intravascular volume status and arterial pressure can be evaluated. If vasodilation develops, bolus administration of intravascular fluids may be necessary. If the MAP falls and circulating blood volume is judged to be adequate, vasopressors are administered. A continuous infusion of dopamine (5 to 10 μg/kg/min; higher doses may be required to produce vasoconstriction), epinephrine, or norepinephrine (0.3 μg/kg/min or more may be required) is prepared at the bedside and administered as needed to maintain the systemic perfusion and MAP.

Thiopental, phenobarbital, or pentobarbital is administered to induce coma. Thiopental is most often used for short-term anesthesia, and pentobarbital is usually preferred for continuous infusion, since it has a shorter half-life than phenobarbital and may thus be weaned more readily. The barbiturate dose is:

- *Initial loading dose:* 2 to 5 mg/kg.
- *Continuous infusion:* 1 mg/kg/hr or hourly dose of 0.5 to 3 mg/kg. The dosage should be increased until coma is achieved (confirmed by burst suppression on the bedside electroencephalogram [EEG] or obliteration of any clinical response to painful stimuli). Cranial nerve function may also be obliterated (pupils may constrict minimally in response to light).
- *Target serum level (pentobarbital):* 20 to 40 μg/ml (or 2 to 4 mg/dl).

In general, the barbiturates are administered to produce clinical improvement (reduction in signs of increased ICP, reduction in actual ICP, or both). This may require obliteration of clinical responsiveness. The serum barbiturate level should be monitored, although therapy may be limited by the cardiovascular depression produced even before therapeutic drug levels of the barbiturate are achieved. Although hypotension may be corrected by administration of sympathomimetic drugs, maximal sympathomimetic support is often limited by tachycardia or significant vasoconstriction. Thus barbiturate therapy requires titration to produce maximal therapeutic effects with minimal side or toxic effects.

Barbiturates obliterate most neurologic function, although brain stem evoked potentials may be evaluated. As a result, the diagnosis of brain death will require withdrawal of the barbiturate or performance of confirmatory tests to evaluate CBF (e.g., cerebral perfusion scan). The barbiturate level must be subtherapeutic before an EEG can be performed to confirm brain death. It will take several days for the barbiturate level to fall from therapeutic levels.

If the ICP is effectively controlled, the barbiturate therapy may be weaned within 24 to 36 hours. During reduction in the barbiturate dose, the patient's ICP, MAP, CPP, and neurologic function must be closely monitored. As the child becomes more responsive, provision of analgesics will likely be required.

Steroids, "Lazeroids," and Modulation of Neurotransmitters Free oxygen radicals, excitatory neurotransmitters, and excess intracellular calcium contribute to secondary injury following ischemic or traumatic brain insults. However, inhibitors of free oxygen radicals (e.g., superoxide dismutase) have had only limited success in the treatment of traumatic or ischemic brain injury, perhaps in part because they have limited ability to penetrate the blood-brain barrier. Steroidlike compounds, the 21-aminosteroids ("lazeroids"), do decrease free oxygen radical formation and intracellular calcium accumulation and have shown promise in laboratory and limited clinical trials. Their efficacy in the treatment of cerebral ischemia, head trauma, and subarachnoid hemorrhage is currently under investigation. Calcium channel blockers have not been shown to improve outcome of ischemic or traumatic insult.

Hypothermia More than a decade ago, moderate hypothermia was a standard part of the management of increased ICP complicating either traumatic or ischemic insult; however, its efficacy was never clinically evaluated. Hypothermia was linked with an increased incidence of sepsis in near-drowning victims; this effect was thought to be related to a decrease in granulocyte formation and function. Hypothermia (reducing body temperature to 32° to 34° C) is again being used to reduce cerebral oxygen demand and possibly exert some protective effect on the brain when a rise in ICP is unresponsive to other therapy. Mild (34° C) or moderate (32° to 34° C) hypothermia may be used (Marion et al., 1993; Shiozaki et al., 1993). The hypothermia may be induced through surface cooling, gastric lavage, or both. Administration of muscle relaxants and possibly paralytic agents may be required to prevent shivering.

Weaning From Support   As the child's condition improves, and the ICP is controlled and the CPP is maintained, therapies may be gradually tapered. In general, pentobarbital or other anesthetics are tapered first, and ventilatory support (particularly control of the $Paco_2$ and oxygenation) is tapered last, as tolerated. Only one change in therapy should be made at a time, and the child's response must be evaluated before additional changes are made. If the ICP rises again, it may be necessary to reinstitute a therapy and stabilize the patient for 12 to 24 hours before additional changes are made.

Psychosocial Support   Throughout the child's care, the child and family require compassionate support. While the child requires intensive physical care, attention is naturally focused on supporting the child's survival. However, the family is simultaneously attempting to cope with the possibility of the child's death or long-term disability. Additional nurses, chaplains, and social workers should be enlisted to ensure that the family has the support they need. The more people involved in the child's care, the more important it is that there be consistency in communication. It is often helpful if a few physicians and nurses are consistently responsible for communication with the family.

The child can often hear despite the presence of coma or administration of pharmacologic paralyzing agents. As a result, explanations must be pro-

vided to the child throughout care. If the child is dying, the child and family must be prepared (see Chapter 4).

If the need for extended rehabilitative therapy is anticipated, this therapy should be initiated as soon as possible. Occupational and rehabilitative therapists should begin therapy in the ICU and may prevent some complications of increased ICP or coma (e.g., hazards of immobility).

Coma

Etiology/Pathophysiology

A patient's LOC is normal when he or she is aware of the environment, can be aroused from sleep, and is oriented (as age appropriate) to time, place, and person. A decreased LOC is present if the child is abnormally lethargic or confused, or if the child is not appropriately oriented to time and place. Decreased LOC can be further divided into stupor and coma:

- *Stupor:* The child can be aroused only through application of strong external stimuli.
- *Coma:* The child cannot be aroused despite application of strong external stimuli (see Table 8-6).

Coma is described as the lack of eye opening and verbal response for ≥6 hours following a cerebral insult. It can result from CNS inflammation, head injury, cerebral edema, mass lesions, hypoxia, electrolyte or acid base imbalances, or drug toxicity. Causes of coma are often divided into structural (trauma, mass lesion) or metabolic (hepatic encephalopathy). Treatment of all forms of coma requires evaluation and support of cardiorespiratory function. In addition, treatment of structural coma is aimed at preventing or limiting increased ICP, whereas treatment of metabolic coma is aimed at eliminating the toxin and its effects.

Clinical Presentation

The comatose child demonstrates no observable response to external stimuli. Abnormal posturing may be observed. Cranial nerve function may be impaired, and reflexes may disappear. Ultimately, brain stem dysfunction may develop, and cardiorespiratory compromise may be observed.

Assessment of the comatose child should include all aspects of assessment described under Increased Intracranial Pressure, p. 390. The following should be assessed at least hourly when the child is unstable and whenever the child's clinical condition changes:

- LOC
- Vital signs (including blood pressure) and systemic perfusion
- Pupil size and response to light
- GCS
- Cranial nerve function

Assessment of cranial nerve function is extremely important when the child is comatose, since higher brain function cannot be assessed. Most cranial nerves can be assessed during routine nursing care (see Table 8-2):

- *Cranial nerves III, IV, and VI:* Eye movement, pupil constriction in response to light
- *Cranial nerve VII:* Facial grimace
- *Cranial nerves IX and X:* Cough and gag reflexes during suctioning

The oculocephalic reflex and the oculovestibular reflex may be lost as a result of drug toxicity, metabolic dysfunction, or brain death. Evaluation of these reflexes is part of the clinical examination to confirm brain death and is described under Brain Death, p. 412.

Common reflexes and body movement should be evaluated:

1. *Corneal reflex:* Stroking of the eyelashes or peripheral cornea should produce brisk blink; absence of reflex usually indicates brain stem injury.
2. *Tonic neck reflex:* When the infant is supine and the head is rapidly turned to the side, the ipsilateral arm and leg extend while the contralateral arm and leg flex. This reflex is normal in infants 2 to 6 months of age but abnormal beyond 9 months of age.

3. *Deep tendon reflexes:* May be exaggerated or may be accompanied by clonus (rhythmic flexion and contraction after flexion of the wrist or ankle) if cerebral hemisphere injury or diffuse metabolic disorder is present.
4. *Movement:* Limb movements should be described as purposeful, nonpurposeful, or consistent with seizure activity.
5. *Purposeful movement:* When a *central* painful stimulus is provided, the child attempts to grab the hand applying the stimulus. This movement is considered purposeful localization of pain. When the *medial* aspect of each extremity is pinched, the child normally *abducts* or *withdraws* the extremity from the midline and from the painful stimulus. This movement is considered *purposeful withdrawal.* Note that flexion and adduction (movement toward the midline) are not necessarily purposeful and may indicate decorticate posturing. Flexion/withdrawal from a *peripheral* stimulus may result only from a spinal reflex arc and does *not* indicate purposeful withdrawal.
6. *Posturing:* Decorticate or decerebrate posturing may be observed:
   a. *Decorticate posturing:* Arms flex at elbows; legs extended with plantar flexion at ankles. All four extremities are tightly adducted, although the ankles may be externally rotated.
   b. *Decerebrate posturing:* Arms and legs extend. The wrists are flexed, and the arms are at the sides, rather than pulled toward midline
7. *Seizures:* Must be described, timed, and, if persistent, treated.

Evaluate the child's respiratory rate and pattern and the effectiveness of oxygenation and ventilation. Many of the conditions that cause coma may alter the respiratory pattern or depress respiratory function. The most common respiratory patterns include:

- *Cheyne-Stokes respirations:* Alternating bradypnea and hyperpnea

- *Central neurogenic hyperventilation:* Constant rapid respiratory rate without physiologic stimulus (no hypoxemia or hypercapnia)
- *Apneustic breathing:* Prolonged inspiration and expiration
- *Cluster breathing:* Very irregular breathing (associated with apnea)
- *Ataxic breathing:* Extremely irregular breathing

The comatose child may develop upper airway obstruction (the tongue or secretions obstruct the pharynx), hypoventilation, or apnea. Signs of upper airway obstruction include decreased air movement, stridor, and upper airway congestion. The work of breathing may increase, although respiratory depression may also be observed. Ensure that the child's oxygenation and ventilation are adequate. Pulse oximetry enables continuous noninvasive evaluation of oxygenation but *does not evaluate ventilation.* End-tidal carbon dioxide monitors may be used to evaluate ventilation. Nonspecific signs of respiratory distress include an inappropriately rapid or slow respiratory rate, decreased air movement, retractions, stridor or wheezing, tachycardia (bradycardia is even more worrisome), and poor perfusion. Indications for intubation in the comatose child include inability to maintain a patent airway (including loss of cough or gag reflexes), increased ICP, hypoventilation, apnea, hypoxemia, and hypercarbia.

Whenever the child is admitted with coma of unknown etiology, the first urine specimen obtained should be sent for drug screening and toxicology. In addition, blood samples are drawn for analysis of arterial blood gases, serum electrolyte concentration (including glucose), and blood cultures. Child abuse and trauma must also be ruled out. A CT scan may reveal evidence of trauma, intracranial hemorrhage, or local or diffuse cerebral edema. If the child is stable, magnetic resonance imaging (MRI) can provide detailed imaging of the brain and spinal cord. An EEG may be ordered to rule out the presence of subclinical seizures (see Common Diagnostic Tests, p. 441). A lumbar puncture will be performed if meningitis is suspected.

Predictors of a poor prognosis following prolonged coma (particularly nontraumatic coma) during childhood include absence of spontaneous respirations, flaccidity, fixed pupils, presence of decorticate or decerebrate posturing, and presence of deep coma for more than 2 weeks.

Management

Principles of Assessment and Care The management of the comatose child is largely supportive. The child's neurologic and cardiorespiratory function must be closely monitored, and any deterioration (particularly increased ICP, shock, or respiratory failure) must be reported to a physician immediately.

- *If increased ICP is detected:* Provide oxygenation and mild hyperventilation with bag and mask until intubation and mechanical ventilation can be initiated. Consider use of osmotic diuretics.
- *If respiratory failure develops:* Suction the upper airway as needed. Assist with intubation and mechanical ventilation as necessary (if in doubt, intubate).
- Nutritional support is mandatory, and the hazards of immobility must be prevented.

Support of Cardiorespiratory Function If the child is unable to cough effectively, suction the upper airway as needed. Position the patient so that secretions pool in the cheek rather than in the pharynx. A nasopharyngeal airway or oropharyngeal airway may be required to maintain airway patency, and intubation is occasionally required.

Ensure effectiveness of air movement and chest expansion. Position the child for maximum airway patency with the neck slightly extended; elevate the head of the bed.

Monitor the child's heart rate, systemic perfusion, oxygenation (pulse oximetry), and carbon dioxide elimination. Hypoxia or hypercarbia may not produce any overt signs of distress in the comatose child. Therefore the nurse must monitor for nonspecific signs of deterioration, including a change in systemic perfusion, color, heart rate, and, of course, noninvasive blood gas indicators. If upper airway obstruction develops or hypoventilation or apnea is observed, elective intubation and mechanical ventilation are probably required.

Coma and immobility may produce venous pooling and redistribution of circulating blood volume. Orthostatic hypotension may be observed. Treatment may require volume administration.

Monitor the child's fluid intake and output. Once systemic perfusion and circulating blood volume are adequate, avoid excessive volume administration.

Nutritional Support   Develop a plan for provision of adequate caloric intake as soon as the child arrives in the unit. If systemic perfusion is adequate, enteral nutrition may be attempted. Begin with a small volume and dilute concentration (preferably elemental formula), and advance as tolerated. If cough and gag reflex are present, nasogastric feeding may be attempted; transpyloric feeding is appropriate if cough and gag reflexes are absent, to prevent regurgitation and aspiration. Feeding may be initiated despite hypoactive bowel sounds, although the child's tolerance must be carefully assessed. Signs of feeding intolerance include gastric distension, vomiting, diarrhea, and increased gastric residuals. These signs indicate the need to reduce the volume or concentration of the feeding (see p. 523).

If enteral feeding cannot be accomplished, parenteral nutrition must be provided. If inadequate calories, proteins, and vitamins are provided, the child will develop a negative nitrogen balance and protein deficiency, and wound healing will be delayed; also, the risk of infection will be increased. Nutritional compromise may delay weaning from mechanical ventilation.

Stool softeners should be provided as needed to prevent constipation or bowel impaction, and use of glycerin suppositories may be required. Chart stool output consistently.

Prevention of the Hazards of Immobility   Referral to an occupational and physical therapist should be accomplished as soon as possible so that active and passive range-of-motion exercises can begin. High-top sneakers and wrist and ankle splints should be obtained to support these joints and prevent contractures and pressure sores.

Skin care must be meticulous to prevent the development of pressure sores. Keep the skin as dry as possible, and inspect it several times daily. The use of convoluted foam mattresses or alternating support beds should prevent skin breakdown.

The risk of infection is high if multiple invasive monitoring and drainage catheters are used. Ensure good handwashing technique by health care providers and practice scrupulous aseptic and sterile technique during insertion of catheters and dressing changes. Inspect all wounds and skin puncture sites carefully for evidence of inflammation. Signs of infection include erythema or wound drainage, fever or hypothermia, or leukocytosis (see discussion of septic shock, p. 140). If infection is suspected, obtain appropriate cultures and initiate antimicrobial therapy as indicated.

The comatose child usually demonstrates both bowel and bladder incontinence. If a urinary catheter is in place, catheter care is required to minimize the risk of urinary tract infection (UTI)— monitor for cloudy urine and consider urinalysis and urine culture if UTI is suspected.

If the child's blink reflex is not intact, lubricate the corneas with ophthalmic ointment. It may be necessary to patch the eyes to protect the corneas.

Cleanse the child's mouth several times daily to prevent the development of gingivitis or dental caries. Such cleansing may reduce bacterial colonization of the mouth and pharyngeal secretions.

Psychosocial Support   *The comatose child may hear any or all of the conversations at the bedside;* therefore be careful to avoid frightening terminology or discussions at the bedside. At all times, assume that the child can hear; explain all procedures and noises to the child, and offer comfort and encouragement.

Provide the family with consistent information. It may be helpful to reduce the number of nursing and medical staff responsible for providing new information. Regular conferences with the family allow the staff and the family to ask and answer questions. If the child's recovery is doubtful, the family should be prepared for the news. If withdrawal of support is considered on the basis of futility, the family must participate in the decision. If a pronouncement of brain death is made, however, family consent for withdrawal of support should *not* be requested, since the brain death pronouncement is final and nonnegotiable (see Brain Death and Organ Donation, p. 411).

Status Epilepticus

Etiology/Pathophysiology

Status epilepticus (SE) is characterized by a prolonged or frequently repeated seizure activity that effectively creates a fixed and lasting epileptic condition. In clinical practice it is defined as a single generalized, tonic-clonic seizure lasting ≥10 minutes without intervening return of consciousness.

The most common causes of SE in children are high fever secondary to an infection outside of the CNS, and sudden discontinuation of an anticonvulsant drug. Additional causes of SE in children include meningitis, encephalitis, metabolic disorders (e.g., hypoxia, hypoglycemia), toxic ingestion, or head injury. In approximately half of the children who develop SE, no specific cause is identified.

SE constitutes a medical emergency because sustained convulsions can increase CBF and cerebral oxygen consumption and can result in permanent brain damage. It is important to note that many of the sequelae attributed to SE actually result from progression of the patient's underlying condition. If SE is effectively treated, neurologic sequelae can often be prevented or minimized.

Sustained seizure activity increases the adenosine triphosphate (ATP) requirements of neurons because the constant electrical activity requires an extremely active sodium-potassium pump. This increase in cerebral oxygen requirement will increase CBF and may complicate the management of increased ICP. In addition, tissue oxygen requirements are increased by constant muscle contraction and relaxation; thus lactic acidosis or increased systemic oxygen consumption may result.

Clinical Presentation

When seizure activity is suspected, note the time of the onset of the seizure activity, any precipitating factors, any progression of the seizure, and the seizure duration. Seizures should be described rather than labeled, but several types of seizures may be recognized:

1. *Partial (focal) seizures*
   a. *Simple:* Can produce motor, sensory, or autonomic manifestations, but decrease in LOC does not occur.
   b. *Complex:* Psychomotor or temporal lobe seizures with impaired consciousness. May include combinations of simple manifestations, automatisms, or psychic phenomena.
   c. *Evolving:* Simple or complex seizures may evolve into generalized seizures.
2. *Generalized seizures*
   a. *Absence:* Periods of confusion or decreased LOC or stupor *not* associated with abnormal muscle activity. This form of SE most commonly develops in children with persistent *petit mal* seizures and is rarely associated with acute CNS pathology. The EEG shows bilateral, regular, generalized, symmetric spikes.
   b. *Tonic-clonic (grand mal):* May be intermittent seizures or SE. Tonic and clonic seizures may occur independently. The EEG shows focal spikes.
   c. *Myoclonic:* Bilateral extensor and/or flexor muscle contractions. This form of SE is generally related to degenerative brain disease, toxic encephalopathy, and anoxic brain damage. The EEG shows many spikes with slow background activity.
   d. *Atonic:* Loss of muscle tone with loss of consciousness.

Critically ill children with neurologic, cardiorespiratory, or multisystem disease are at risk for the development of cerebral injury, anoxia, or metabolic imbalances that may produce seizures. *Seizure activity or SE may be impossible to detect during pharmacologic paralysis unless an EEG is performed.* Paralyzing agents will suppress myoclonic or tonic-clonic muscle activity, masking seizure activity. Seizures must therefore be suspected and ruled out whenever the child demonstrates tachycardia or alternating tachycardia and bradycardia, wide fluctuations in blood pressure, poor systemic perfusion, nystagmus, or pupil dilation. An EEG must be obtained to confirm or rule out the seizures.

During the EEG, hyperventilation may be performed to unmask subclinical seizures. The hyperventilation-reduced CBF and the mild ischemia it produces may make seizures appear on the EEG.

Management

Treatment of SE requires maintenance of vital functions, abolition of the seizures, and elimination of any precipitating factors. A protocol must be followed for the treatment of SE to ensure that anticonvulsant therapy is provided in a logical sequence to control seizures while minimizing effects on cardiorespiratory function. Depression of cardiorespiratory function must be anticipated and corrected with intubation and mechanical ventilatory support, if necessary. The therapy should not produce more complications than the SE.

During the seizure activity the child is placed on a flat, soft surface with no hard or sharp objects nearby. If the patient's bed is used, it may be necessary to pad the side rails.

Support of Cardiorespiratory Function Assess and support the child's airway, breathing, and systemic perfusion. If the child is breathing spontaneously, position the child with the airway extended and the head turned to the side; elevate the head of the bed to maximize diaphragm excursion. *There is no need to insert anything in the patient's mouth during seizures* unless tongue or cheek biting results in significant bleeding. Forced insertion of a tongue blade or airway may produce broken teeth or oral lacerations.

If the child becomes apneic or demonstrates hypoventilation or respiratory distress during the SE or its therapy, provide bag-mask ventilation until intubation is accomplished. A nasogastric tube may be placed before intubation to empty the stomach and reduce the risk of vomiting and aspiration during intubation. If muscle relaxants or anesthetics are provided during intubation, these must be noted, since they will affect (or eliminate) motor activity and neurologic responses.

Assess and support systemic perfusion. Bradycardia or hypotension must be treated promptly. Venous access must be achieved as quickly as possible to provide a route of administration for fluid therapy and medication and to enable blood sampling for chemistries and toxicology. Correct documented metabolic derangements (e.g., hypoglycemia, hyponatremia) immediately.

Evaluate the child's core body temperature. A high fever should be reduced with antipyretics and a cooling blanket.

Perform a rapid neurologic examination to identify any reversible or progressive causes of the SE. If signs of increased ICP are present, oxygenation and ventilation are supported (the child should be intubated, and mechanical ventilation provided), and administration of osmotic diuretics should be considered.

Anticonvulsant Therapy The drugs used for the treatment of SE will be determined by hospital protocol and the child's history of response to the drugs. In general, milder, short-acting drugs are initially provided; if the SE is not controlled, more potent drugs with anesthetic properties are provided. If the child is breathing spontaneously, elective intubation should be planned, since respiratory depression is likely to develop.

Most anticonvulsant drugs will produce chemical burns if they extravasate into tissues; thus they should be administered through a secure IV catheter in a large vein. Intramuscular injection is not recommended because absorption is unpredictable. The dosage, peak effect, and therapeutic serum level of the most common anticonvulsants are listed in Table 8-9.

Diazepam (Valium) is widely used in initial management of seizures (dose: 0.25 to 0.3 mg/kg IV). It should be effective within 1 to 5 minutes. The short serum half-life of the drug (7 minutes) often mandates repeat dosing within 15-minute intervals, which should be anticipated to produce respiratory depression. If repeated dosing is required, consider the addition of a longer-acting anticonvulsant. Side effects include hypotension, bradycardia, laryngospasm, and respiratory depression.

Lorazepam (Ativan) has a rapid (2- to 3-minute) onset of action, with a longer duration of effects than that of diazepam; thus it may be preferable to that drug. It is administered intravenously in a dose of 0.03 to 0.10 mg/kg over 1 to 3 minutes, and it may be repeated at 10- to 15-minute intervals. This drug may produce respiratory depression, although the incidence of this complication is lower with lorazepam than with diazepam. Be prepared to institute respiratory support, if needed.

Phenytoin (Dilantin) is the primary nonsedative anticonvulsant used in children (dose: 10 to 15 mg/kg IV). Its major disadvantage is the potential for cardiovascular compromise. The onset of

Table 8-9
Anticonvulsant Therapy for Treatment of Pediatric Status Epilepticus

Drug (Trade Name)	Dosage	Peak Effect	Therapeutic Serum Level
Diazepam (Valium)	0.25-0.3 mg/kg IV (maximum: 10 mg)	1-5 min (half-life 7 min)	
Lorazepam (Ativan)	0.03-0.1 mg/kg IV (maximum: 4 mg)	60-90 min (onset within 2-3 min)	20-40 ng/ml
Phenobarbital (Luminal)	5 mg/kg/dose IV for three doses or 20 mg/kg (maximum: 390 mg)	½-1 hr (range: 24 hr)	15-40 μg/ml
Phenytoin (Dilantin)	10-15 mg/kg IV	10 min (range: 24 hr)	10-25 μg/ml
Valproic acid (Depakene)	10-20 mg/kg enema	2-4 hr	50 mg/L
Paraldehyde (rarely used)	15 ml/kg IV or 0.3 ml/kg rectally	Immediate	—
General Anesthesia*			
Thiopental sodium (Pentothal) or pentobarbital sodium (Nembutol)	2-4 mg/kg loading dose plus continuous infusion to maintain EEG burst suppression (typically 0.5-3.0 mg/kg/hr)		20-40 μg/ml or 2-4 mg/dl
Phenobarbitol also may be utilized			

From Hazinski MF: *Nursing care of the critically ill child,* ed 2, St Louis, 1992, Mosby.
*Not to be instituted without proper monitoring of hemodynamic status. Monitor closely for hypotension, compromise of cardiovascular function.

action is approximately 15 to 20 minutes, with a long half-life. This drug is incompatible with many IV drugs and should not be mixed with dextrose solutions. Side effects include myocardial depression; bradycardia, heart block, and other arrhythmias; and cardiac arrest.

Phenobarbital is widely used for treatment of seizures in children because it has a long serum half-life and wide therapeutic range (dose: 5 mg/kg/dose IV × 3). The onset of action in the brain may occur within minutes, although peak concentrations may not develop for 30 to 60 minutes. Because it acts synergistically with diazepam, these drugs are often administered together (the phenobarbital dose is lowered). Side effects include respiratory depression, bronchospasm, apnea, bradycardia, hypotension, and sedation. Sedative effects prevent meaningful neurologic evaluation for several hours after administration.

Valproic acid (Depakene) may provide effective anticonvulsant effects but can only be administered through the gastrointestinal tract, resulting in a slow onset of action (2 to 4 hours). It must be ad-

ministered orally or through a nasogastric or rectal tube. It can be well absorbed rectally, using a 1:1 dilution of valproated syrup (250 mg/5 ml) mixed with tap water. A loading dose of 10 to 20 mg/kg is administered as a retention enema. Potential complications include liver dysfunction (liver enzyme concentrations should be closely monitored) and a possible increase in the plasma concentrations of other anticonvulsants.

Paraldehyde may be used to treat SE refractory to other anticonvulsants. It can be administered intravenously, rectally, or intramuscularly, although the IV drug is no longer available. A rectal dose is generally used by mixing paraldehyde 2:1 with peanut, cottonseed, or olive oil. The dose may be repeated every 2 to 4 hours. Side effects are uncommon but include potential cardiac, respiratory, renal, and hepatic toxins. This drug is excreted through the lungs.

Barbiturate Coma If SE is unresponsive to the anticonvulsant drugs just described, the patient may be transferred to a unit or facility where careful and intensive hemodynamic and EEG monitoring can be performed. Control of SE may then be attempted by administration of barbiturates to induce coma. Before these drugs are administered, the child should be intubated and mechanically ventilated, and an arterial line and central venous catheter are inserted. High doses of barbiturates may produce myocardial depression, vasodilation, and hypotension. The child's intravascular volume should be supported, and volume expanders should be readily available. A sympathomimetic infusion (e.g., dopamine, norepinephrine, or epinephrine) should be prepared for use if hypotension or myocardial dysfunction develop.

A loading dose of the barbiturate is administered, followed by a continuous or hourly infusion of pentobarbital or thiopental sodium administered in doses sufficient to induce coma and maintain burst suppression on the EEG. Thiopental sodium is often preferred over phenobarbital because thiopental has a shorter half-life. Monitor the child's blood pressure and systemic perfusion as the barbiturate dose is increased and provide volume therapy or vasopressor support as needed to maintain systemic perfusion. Once the child's seizures are controlled, plans regarding long-term anticonvulsant prophylaxis should be made.

Surgery If there is a seizure focus identified by the EEG plus a focal lesion on an MRI scan, a positive emission tomography (PET) scan, or a single photon emission computer tomography (SPECT) scan, local surgical resection of the epileptic focus may be indicated.

Syndrome of Inappropriate Antidiuretic Hormone Secretion

Etiology/Pathophysiology

The syndrome of inappropriate antidiuretic hormone secretion (SIADH) is a syndrome of secretion of ADH in the absence of a physiologic stimulus. ADH is normally formed in the supraoptic and paraventricular nuclei in the hypothalamus and is released primarily in response to a rise in serum osmolality and also in response to significant hypotension or hypovolemia. ADH increases the permeability of the renal collecting ducts to water, so that free water is retained, urine volume is reduced, and urine concentration is increased. If ADH continues to be secreted in the absence of a physiologic stimulus, free water intoxication, with a fall in the serum sodium level and osmolality, will develop.

SIADH may develop in any patient who sustains inflammation of, injury to, or compression of the pituitary gland (e.g., meningitis, head trauma), or following ingestion of drugs or development of an ADH-secreting tumor. SIADH has been linked with respiratory failure and positive pressure ventilation and has been reported postoperatively. Sudden volume loss or fluid shift or hypotension may produce ADH secretion, but these physiologic stimuli represent appropriate rather than inappropriate ADH secretion.

Clinical Presentation

The diagnosis of SIADH requires the absence of adrenal or renal disease and otherwise normal pituitary function. The diagnosis should be suspected in the patient at risk when hyponatremia develops in the presence of a relatively low urine volume. SIADH is confirmed when a urine electrolyte analysis reveals a high urine osmolality and urine sodium concentration in the presence of a low serum osmolality and sodium concentration. If ADH secretion is *appropriate,* when the serum osmolality and sodium concentration are low, ADH secretion should decrease and free water should be excreted by the kidneys; thus the urine osmolality and sodium concentration should be lower than the serum osmolality and sodium. Signs of water intoxication and hyponatremia may be observed, including lethargy, stupor, seizures, and coma.

Management

The treatment of SIADH is fluid restriction (to 30% to 70% of calculated maintenance requirements). The diagnosis of SIADH is reconfirmed when the serum sodium rises in response to fluid restriction. Throughout therapy, the child's LOC, neurologic function, and systemic perfusion must be closely monitored.

If profound hyponatremia produces neurologic symptoms such as seizures or decreased LOC, hypertonic saline (3% sodium chloride, 3 to 5 ml/kg) may be administered. A loop diuretic (furosemide, 1 to 2 mg/kg) may also be provided to enhance free water excretion. Avoid rapid correction of hyponatremia, since this may cause compensatory fluid shifts. An increase of approximately 1 mEq/hr is generally targeted.

Administration of lithium carbonate or demeclocycline (dimethyl chlortetracycline) may be indicated if chronic SIADH develops. These drugs inhibit the effect of ADH on the renal collecting tubules.

Diabetes Insipidus

Etiology/Pathophysiology

Diabetes insipidus (DI) results from the decreased production or decreased renal response to vasopressin. There are two major types of DI:

- *Central (neurogenic) DI:* Decreased production of vasopressin, which results from brain death, head injuries, CNS infections, intraventricular hemorrhage, or neurosurgery near the pituitary gland (e.g., resection of a craniopharyngioma)
- *Nephrogenic DI:* Defect in the kidney's ability to respond to circulating ADH

The following discussion pertains only to neurogenic DI—see p. 465 for information regarding nephrogenic DI.

When ADH is not synthesized by the hypothalamus or when the pituitary stalk is damaged, circulating ADH levels are negligible. As a result, the renal collecting tubules remain impermeable to water; thus no free water is reabsorbed from the collecting tubules, and large amounts of water are lost in the urine. The intravascular volume is quickly depleted unless replacement fluids are provided. In addition, hemoconcentration develops. Fluid will shift from the interstitial space into the intravascular space in response to the osmotic gradient, and this fluid is quickly lost in the urine. Intravascular volume depletion stimulates aldosterone secretion, resulting in sodium retention and further hypernatremia.

Typically, the child is hospitalized and is dependent on the bedside nurse to ensure adequate fluid replacement. If the child is ambulatory and

old enough to obtain fluid independently, the child may compensate for the DI with ingestion of large quantities of fluid. Infants will be unable to do so.

Clinical Presentation

Pathognomonic signs of DI include:

- Polyuria with an extremely low (<1.005) urine specific gravity and osmolality
- Rising serum sodium and osmolality

In addition, hypovolemia develops if urine fluid losses are not replaced (signs include a compromise in systemic perfusion, tachycardia, and a fall in central venous pressure). Mucous membranes will be parched, and the anterior fontanelle (in infants) will be depressed. Signs of hypernatremic hypovolemic shock include diminished peripheral pulses, prolonged capillary refill (despite a warm ambient temperature), metabolic acidosis, and (late) hypotension. Urine output often remains high until renal perfusion is severely compromised.

The awake, communicative child will complain of thirst.

Management

Management of DI consists of three elements:

- Evaluation and support of intravascular volume, systemic perfusion, and fluid and electrolyte balance
- Immediate replacement of urinary fluid and electrolyte losses
- Provision of exogenous ADH

Support of Intravascular Volume, Systemic Perfusion, and Fluid and Electrolyte Balance Determine if shock is present, and monitor serum electrolyte concentration (particularly serum sodium). Insert two large-bore venous catheters; if possible, one catheter should enable central venous pressure monitoring. Treat hypovolemic shock with one or more boluses of 2.5% dextrose and 0.45% NaCl until the child's perfusion improves and central venous pressure is 3 to 5 mm Hg. Improvement in systemic perfusion is indicated by strengthening of peripheral pulses, warming of extremities, reduction in capillary refill time, and improvement in the child's LOC.

Aggressive volume therapy is required until signs of shock are corrected and urine volume tapers. If hypernatremia is present, avoid rapid reduction in the serum sodium concentration, since it can result in complications, including cerebral edema, seizures, or cerebral hemorrhage. The serum sodium can be safely lowered by approximately 10 mEq/L/day or by 1 mEq/L in any 1 hour.

Evaluate the child's serum sodium and osmolality, and urine sodium, osmolality, and specific gravity. Determine the urine specific gravity at least hourly and every 15 to 30 minutes following administration of ADH (to evaluate response to the ADH).

Replacement of Fluid and Electrolyte Losses
Establish reliable IV access (consider intraosseous access, particularly for children younger than 6 years of age), including a central venous pressure monitoring line if possible. If the child is incontinent or in shock, insertion of a urinary catheter is recommended.

Maintain accurate records of fluid intake and output. The child's urine output should be totaled every 15 to 30 minutes, and the volume of fluid lost in the urine should be replaced with 2.5% dextrose and 0.2% NaCl during the next 15 to 30 minutes. If urine volume remains high, replacement with one-eighth or one-sixteenth normal saline may be needed, but these fluids must be specially mixed by the hospital pharmacy. Fluid used to replace urine output must be administered *in addition to maintenance fluid requirements*. If volume replacement is effective, the serum sodium and osmolality should gradually return to normal and should be maintained at normal levels.

Once exogenous ADH is administered, this replacement fluid administration rate will be tapered as urine volume decreases.

Provision of Exogenous Antidiuretic Hormone
ADH is provided by IV or intranasal route (Table 8-10). A positive response to the ADH includes a decrease in urine volume (to <1 ml/kg/hr), an increase in urine specific gravity (>1.010), and an increase in urine osmolality (200 to 300 mOsm/L). Potential side effects include abdominal cramping.

Table 8-10
Drugs Used in the Treatment of Central Diabetes Insipidus in Children

Drug	Dose	Duration of Action
Hormone replacement		
Aqueous vasopressin	5-10 units SC	3-6 hr
Lysine vasopressin	2-4 units IV	4-6 hr
Vasopressin tannate in oil	1-5 units IM	24-72 hr
DDAVP	5-30 μg IN	12-24 hr
Nonhormonal agents		
Chlorpropamide	1 g/m^2/day	Divided tid

Modified from Yared A, Foose J, Ichikawa I: Disorders of osmoregulation. In Ichikawa I, editor: *Pediatric textbook of fluids and electrolytes*, Baltimore, 1990, Williams & Wilkins.

- *Intravenous ADH:* Dilute 20 U/ml aqueous solution to a concentration of 2 mU/ml. Administer a 15 mU/hr infusion or a single IV dose of the 20 U/ml solution (0.5 to 1 ml/day). Response should be apparent within 15 minutes and will last approximately 2 to 6 hours. If there is no response, double and then triple the infusion or repeat the single dose (with a physician's order).
- *Intranasal ADH (l-deamino-8-D-arginine-vasopressin or DDAVP):* Administer a dose of 0.05 to 0.3 ml (5 to 30 μg) of 0.01% solution (100 μg/ml) divided into 1 to 2 doses into the posterior nasal area (rather than the posterior nasal pharynx). Response (decrease in urine volume and increase in urine concentration) should be apparent within 8 to 20 hours but will last approximately 6 to 24 hours.

Brain Death and Organ Donation
Etiology/Pathophysiology

Brain death is the *total and irreversible cessation* of brain stem and cortical brain function. Potential causes include trauma, anoxia, metabolic conditions, or the end result of a compromise in cerebral perfusion or cerebral herniation.

Brain death is as irreversible a form of death as when the heart stops beating and fails to respond to resuscitation. However, following brain death, a perfusing cardiac rhythm may continue, and mechanical ventilation may maintain oxygenation of the blood, so that the patient appears to be alive. However, mechanical ventilatory support is not "life support," since the child has died. The ventilator is merely oxygenating the blood; it is not keeping the child alive.

Brain death pronouncement and family consent are required if the child's vascular (solid) organs are to be obtained for donation following death. Brain death pronouncement requires very specific examination, as well as documentation in the chart of the examination and pronouncement. Federal legislation requires notification of the local federally funded organ procurement agency of a potential organ donor, and notification of the potential donor's family about the option of organ and tissue donation. This notification must be recorded in the patient's chart.

Every state recognizes cessation of brain function as a legal definition of death. Every hospital receiving Medicaid reimbursement is required to have protocols in place for the identification of potential organ donors.

Criteria for Pronouncement of Brain Death

Two conditions must be present for pronouncement of brain death: (1) complete cessation of clinical evidence of brain function and (2) irreversibility of the condition. The cause of brain death should be known. Most clinical criteria used for brain death pronouncement in children are consistent, although some criteria differ in terms of recommendations for confirmatory tests (Box 8-9).

The cessation of brain function must be irreversible (e.g., devastating head injury or anoxic insult) rather than due to conditions such as hypotension, hypoglycemia, or hypothermia, which may cause temporary depression of neurologic function. In the past, if the patient had received barbiturates or narcotics, documentation of subtherapeutic levels of these drugs was required, to ensure that these drugs were not depressing the patient's response. Subtherapeutic levels of sedatives are required if an EEG is used as a confirmatory test. However, if cerebral perfusion studies are used as a confirmatory test, the barbiturates or narcotics may be detectable in serum samples (they do not affect perfusion studies).

Box 8-9

Criteria for Pediatric Brain Death Determination

Irreversible Condition

Requires observation over time (length of observation time increases during infancy)
Absence of complicating factors
Adequate resuscitation provided

Absence of Brain Function

Flaccid paralysis (no posturing, no response to *central* pain stimulus)
Absence of brain stem and cranial nerve function
  No pupil response to light
  No corneal (blink) reflex
  No oculocephalic reflex (doll's eyes)
  Absence of eye movements
  No oculovestibular reflex (cold water calorics)
  No cough or gag reflex
  Apnea despite documented $Paco_2$ >55-60 mm Hg

Possible Confirmatory Tests

EEG (requires special electrode placement, amplitude, absence of sedative drug levels, normothermia)
Radionuclide angiogram
Carotid arteriogram
Additional tests, including cold xenon blood flow study, brain stem evoked potentials, and Doppler cerebral blood flow studies, are under investigation

From Hazinski MF: *Nursing care of the critically ill child,* ed 2, St Louis, 1992, Mosby.

Observation Period   Brain death pronouncement requires observation over time. Repeat clinical examinations separated by an observation period help ensure that irreversible cessation of brain function has occurred. The younger the child, the longer the suggested interval between examinations. Some centers adhere to these criteria very strictly, whereas other centers use cerebral perfusion studies to shorten the observation time. Be familiar with your hospital protocol and ensure that that protocol is followed exactly. The following are the

1987 recommendations from the Task Force for Brain Death Pronouncement in Children, which may be modified by the hospital:

- *Infants 7 days to 2 months:* Two examinations separated by at least 48 hours. Confirmation is also recommended using two EEGs separated by at least 48 hours.
- *Age 2 months to 1 year:* Two examinations separated by 24 hours. One negative EEG is recommended, and a cerebral radionuclide angiographic study may substitute for the second EEG.
- *Beyond 1 year of age:* The Task Force recommends two examinations separated by at least 12 hours. A 24-hour observation period is suggested if the cause of death is a hypoxic-ischemic insult. Confirmatory tests are not suggested.

Physical Examination to Document Absence of Brain Stem Function The child must be absolutely unresponsive to external stimuli, with absence of *voluntary* movement and speech. No brain stem or cranial nerve function can be present. The pupils must be dilated (cannot be constricted) and fixed in midposition, and apnea must be present. Flaccid paralysis must be present. The oculocephalic and oculovestibular reflexes should be *absent.*

Oculocephalic Reflex ("Doll's Eyes") The oculocephalic reflex is tested by turning the head from midline to the side while holding the eyelids open to observe eye movement.

- *Intact oculocephalic reflex:* The eyes will turn consensually in the sockets in the direction opposite head rotation (i.e., if the head is turned from midline to the right, the eyes will rotate toward the left).
- *Absent oculocephalic reflex:* The eyes will remain fixed in their sockets despite rotation of the head.

Oculovestibular Reflex ("Cold Water Calorics") The oculovestibular reflex tests brain stem pathways involved in movement of the eyes. This test should only be performed if the tympanic membrane is intact. The head is elevated 30 degrees, and the ear canal is flushed with ice water (so that the ice water comes into contact with the tympanic membrane).

- *Intact oculovestibular reflex:* Cranial nerves III and VI are stimulated, and slow horizontal movement toward the stimulus is followed by rapid nystagmus away from the stimulus.
- *Absent oculovestibular reflex:* The eyes will remain fixed in midposition.

Cranial Nerve III Cranial nerve III produces pupil constriction in response to light and an automatic blink when any object approaches the eye. When brain stem function is absent, the pupils will be fixed and unresponsive to light. Although the pupils are typically fully dilated, they may be midsize. In addition, the cornea can be lightly stroked with a cotton-tipped applicator and a blink will not be observed.

Cranial Nerves IX and X Cranial nerves IX and X are evaluated simultaneously through an attempt to stimulate a cough and gag reflex. A suction catheter is inserted into the back of the pharynx; no cough or gag will be observed if brain stem function is absent.

Apnea Apnea must be documented (Box 8-10) by observing absence of spontaneous ventilation despite an arterial carbon dioxide tension that is sufficiently high to stimulate ventilation (exceeding 55 to 60 mm Hg). Since patients with head injury generally receive mechanical ventilatory support to maintain a normal $PaCO_2$, ventilatory support is withdrawn, and oxygenation is maintained during the apnea test.

Oxygen must be provided during the apnea test, to prevent the development of hypoxemia; adequate oxygenation is confirmed using pulse oximetry. This oxygen can usually be effectively delivered by a T-connector at the end of the endotracheal tube. Alternatively, the oxygen may be administered through a suction catheter joined to oxygen tubing; the suction catheter is inserted into the endotracheal tube. If hypoxemia (decrease in hemoglobin saturation) develops during the test, it may be necessary to interrupt the test and return the child to mechanical ventilatory support (this is especially likely if acute respiratory distress syndrome [ARDS] is present).

Obtain an arterial blood gas sample at the beginning of the study to document normocarbia and to predict the length of the apnea test. During apnea

---

Box 8-10

Apnea Test for Brain Death Determination

1. Adjust ventilatory support to ensure normal oxygenation and normocarbia (Paco$_2$ 35-45 mm Hg). Utilize pulse oximetry and end-tidal carbon dioxide monitoring if possible; obtain arterial blood gases before study.
2. Preoxygenate patient for 5 minutes before study using 100% oxygen.
3. Remove patient from ventilator and provide passive oxygenation with 100% oxygen (6 L/min or twice the minute ventilation appropriate for child's weight) delivered to endotracheal tube (using "blow-by" tubing) or via suction catheter (joined to green oxygen tubing) inserted into endotracheal tube.
4. Closely observe patient during 5- to 10-minute duration of study; no chest movements or respiratory effort will be present if brain function has ceased. Abort study if cardiovascular deterioration occurs.
5. Monitor pulse oximetry during trial; adjust oxygen delivery as needed to ensure effective oxygenation. Monitor transcutaneous carbon dioxide tension if possible during study. Draw arterial blood gas sample at conclusion of study. Paco$_2$ will rise approximately 4-5 mm Hg/min during apnea.
6. In order to confirm apnea, no respiratory effort can be noted and Paco$_2$ at end of study should exceed 55 mm Hg.

From Hazinski MF: *Nursing care of the critically ill child,* ed 2, St Louis, 1992, Mosby.

---

the Paco$_2$ will rise approximately 4 to 5 mm Hg for each minute of apnea. Therefore it will require approximately 5 minutes of apnea to raise the Paco$_2$ from 40 mm Hg to 55 to 60 mm Hg. By comparison, if the apnea test is begun with the child's Paco$_2$ at 30 mm Hg, 6 to 8 minutes of apnea will be required to raise the Paco$_2$ to 55 to 60 mm Hg.

Throughout the apnea test, the nurse must remain at the bedside, watching the child closely for any evidence of respiratory effort. In addition, the nurse must monitor the child's heart rate and systemic perfusion. At the end of a 5- or 10-minute observation period, an arterial blood gas sample is drawn, and mechanical ventilatory support is resumed.

Confirmatory Tests   Confirmatory tests are not required for children older than 1 year of age when the cause of brain death has been established and all clinical criteria have been met. Sedative and barbiturate levels must be subtherapeutic, and the body temperature and serum electrolytes must be normal, however, if brain death pronouncement is to be based on clinical criteria alone. These patients may be examined twice (examinations separated by 6 to 24 hours) and pronounced brain dead at the time of the second examination.

In 1987 the Task Force on Brain Death Determination in Children recommended the EEG as the confirmation test of choice for young children less than 1 year of age and for those with hypoxic-ischemic cerebral insult. However, a "technically satisfactory radionuclide angiogram" was also noted by the Task Force to be acceptable.

If the EEG is performed to confirm brain death, levels of sedative drugs, including barbiturates, must be subtherapeutic, the child's temperature must be >32° C, and electrolyte concentrations must be normal; in addition, the EEG technique must be modified for a "brain death" study. The electrodes are placed farther apart than for a normal EEG, the voltage is increased, and a long, uninterrupted recording is made at the end of the study to document 30 minutes of electrocerebral silence.

Slow activity has been documented on the EEG in as many as 25% of adults and in many children with clinical signs of brain death that are confirmed by perfusion studies. Alternatively, a case study report documented return of cerebral activity following a flat EEG during the neonatal period. When these false positives are considered in light of the multiple requirements that must be met before the EEG can even be performed, other confirmatory tests may be more practical and reliable for brain death pronouncement in the pediatric intensive care unit (PICU).

Cerebral angiography or radionuclide CT scans may be used to confirm brain death by absence of cerebral perfusion. These blood flow studies are not influenced by the presence of electrolyte imbalance, barbiturates, or other sedative drugs.

Pronouncement of brain death in the neonate requires application of neonatal-specific criteria. In neonates irreversible cessation of brain function may be difficult to establish because the cause of the neurologic dysfunction is often unknown. In addition, isolated reports of survival in neonates with flat EEGs and absence of clinical evidence of neurologic function have raised questions regarding the accuracy of clinical brain death pronouncement.

In general, the pronouncement of newborn brain death is performed in a manner similar to that described above, although it is not recommended to occur before the newborn is 7 days of age. The cause of brain death is determined, and the timing of cessation of brain function is established (if possible). Repeat examinations are performed, and confirmatory studies are nearly always performed, although the EEG may be positive despite the absence of CBF. Unfortunately, experience is limited with CBF studies performed during the first days of life. Longitudinal studies will be required to establish universal neonatal criteria for brain death pronouncement.

Management: Organ Donation

Contact the local organ procurement agency *as soon as* a potential organ donor is identified. The agency coordinator will review the child's history and chart to determine if there are any absolute or relative contraindications to organ donation. Such contraindications are few, but they should be ruled out so that the family does not become excited about organ donation that is not feasible.

Sequence of Donation It is extremely helpful for the parents to talk with an organ donation coordinator. This individual is skilled in talking with parents during an extremely stressful time and can provide the parents with specific information. This coordinator will also write to the family later and inform them (in general terms) of the disposition of their child's organs. Parents often find this information extremely gratifying. Parents should be aware that there is no cost to them for the organ donation and that the process will not delay or alter standard funeral arrangements. The process may, however, take approximately 4 to 12 hours to finalize, because surgical teams from the transplant centers

that will receive the organs generally assemble and fly to the child to recover the organs.

The organ procurement agency assumes all financial responsibility for the care of the body once the child is pronounced brain dead and the parents agree to organ donation. If any diagnostic studies are obtained before the pronouncement that will contribute to the donation process, those costs are also assumed by the organ procurement agency. Once pronouncement has occurred, the donor coordinator supervises support of systemic and organ perfusion until donation actually occurs.

Once the parents sign the consent for organ donation, the child's age, weight, blood type, and available organs are listed on a national computer. If the organs are compatible with several potential recipients, priority is given to the most severely ill recipient. Organs are generally distributed at a regional level before they are available at a national level. It is very important that both donor and recipient families realize that these organs are distributed fairly.

Support of the Family The death of a child is always tragic. During the child's critical illness, the parents may be constantly at the bedside; thus they are often physically and emotionally exhausted when death is pronounced. Any delay in confirmation of brain death can be particularly stressful. Presumably, brain death pronouncement is attempted to enable donation of the child's organs. Therefore it is very important that the parents be approached in a sensitive and compassionate manner about this issue (see also Chapter 4).

The nurse is typically the member of the health care team who is closest to the family of the dying child. Although it is necessary to offer hope to parents of dying children, the nurse is often the best individual to help that family prepare for the death of the child. If the parents are allowed to remain with their child as the child's condition deteriorates, they will see that everything possible is done for the child. If, on the other hand, the parents are separated from the child for most of the child's final hours, it may be difficult for the parents to trust that all possible therapy has been exhausted and that nothing more can be offered.

If the family introduces the subject of organ donation, the discussion can evolve naturally around their questions. The nurse will be aware of the best time to discuss potential organ donation with the family. This discussion must be compassionate and accurate. The parents should not be approached about organ donation unless the likelihood of the child's survival is low. The family can be understandably confused by contradictory or inconsistent statements from members of the health care team. When a child is brain dead, oxygenation, ventilation, and perfusion can be maintained, but the ventilator does not "keep the child alive" and should not be referred to as "life support." The parents must be aware that the diagnosis of brain death is made according to established protocols so that there is *no possibility for error.*

The parents should be allowed to remain with the child as much as possible during the time preceding the child's death, and they should be asked if they would like to visit the child immediately before or after the brain death studies are performed. The family may also wish to see the child again after pronouncement but before organ donation has occurred.

It is estimated that one third of children awaiting organ transplantation will die before a donor is located; thus organ donation is clearly beneficial for the recipient. However, organ donation can benefit the family of the donor, too. Parents have expressed gratitude that something positive could come out of the tragic death of their child, enabling a part of their child to survive through the gift of organ donation. Approximately 75% to 100% of parents approached about donation of their child's organs will agree to organ donation; unfortunately, only approximately half of all families of potential organ donors are approached.

The family's decision about organ donation may be influenced by religious or cultural beliefs. However, it is most often influenced by the family's relationship to the staff and the manner in which the subject of organ donation is introduced.

Support of the Vascular (Solid) Organ Donor

Maintenance of the cadaveric donor until actual organ donation requires expert critical care to ensure that perfusion to solid organs remains excellent. This care is provided by the bedside nurse, physicians, and the organ donation coordinator. Often, if medications are prescribed, the recipient transplant surgeon is consulted. Since several transplant teams may be coming to obtain organs from the same donor, the transplant coordinator is often responsible for integrating the orders of teams from two or more different hospitals, and the nurse is responsible for implementing the orders. This requires skill and patience.

Hypotension is a common problem during donor maintenance. It often results from hypovolemia and expansion of the vascular space associated with loss of brain stem regulation of vascular tone. Most organ donors are relatively hypovolemic because fluid restriction and osmotic diuretics were part of therapy for increased ICP. In addition, approximately one third of pediatric organ donors demonstrate DI; unreplaced urine fluid losses can result in rapid development of hypovolemia and compromise of organ perfusion. Fluid administration with frequent bolus therapy of isotonic fluid (20 ml/kg) is usually required.

If DI is present, replace urine volume losses with an equal volume of 2.5% dextrose and 0.2% NaCl (see Diabetes Insipidus). If urine losses are excessive, exogenous ADH is often administered, most commonly in the form of DDAVP (see Diabetes Insipidus). DDAVP is thought to produce less splanchnic (hepatic and renal) vasoconstriction than vasopressin, and administration of the drug is usually preferable to the fluid and electrolyte imbalances that can accompany urine loss and attempted replacement.

Cardiovascular dysfunction is common in the pediatric donor. Arrhythmias and hypotension are encountered in more than half of the donors; the most common arrhythmias observed include bradycardia and ventricular arrhythmias. Electrolyte imbalances, including hypokalemia, hypernatremia, and hyperglycemia, are also encountered frequently.

Blood pressure and systemic perfusion are maintained through volume administration, if possible. If it is necessary to administer an inotropic or vasoactive medication, a low dose of dopamine (<10 μg/kg/minute) is administered. If large doses of vasoactive medications are required to maintain systemic perfusion, myocardial injury may be present. Higher doses of vasopressors may be required but are used with caution, since they may increase myocardial afterload and oxygen consumption and may compromise hepatic and renal blood flow.

Maintain the donor's temperature carefully. Hypothermia should be prevented, since it may further depress myocardial function. An overbed warmer or heating lamps are usually required, since the hypothalamus is no longer functional.

Levels of thyroid hormones, particularly tri-iodothyronine (T_3), are decreased in many organ donors. The cause is unknown but may be related to pituitary impairment. For this reason, T_3 (dose: 100 μg/500 ml NaCl, @ 50 ml/hour × 1 hour, then 25 ml/hr; reduce dose for tachycardia or hypertension) or T_4 may be administered to donors to increase blood pressure and/or enable weaning of inotropic agents.

Support of the Nurse It is extremely difficult to care for a dying child and to support the family. At the very time that the child requires the most attentive physical care, the family requires the most sensitive emotional support. The bedside nurse should ask for help in order to be able to spend time with the family.

When a nurse is closely involved with the child and family, the nurse must have the opportunity to grieve for the child. Before that nurse begins to care for the organ donor, the nurse should have the opportunity to think about the child and family and be assured that they were given the best support possible.

Care of the organ donor is extremely hectic and can be extremely rewarding. Many nurses have voiced satisfaction in participation in the donor process, because they could see something wonderful come from tragedy. For further information about care of the dying child and family, see Chapter 4.

Postoperative Care of the Pediatric Neurosurgical Patient

Care of the child following neurosurgery requires maintenance of vital functions, assessment of neurologic function, recognition and treatment of potential complications of the craniotomy, mainte-nance of fluid and electrolyte balance, management of pain, nutritional support, and provision of psychosocial support to the child and family.

Postoperative assessment is facilitated by information obtained during a thorough *pre*operative examination of the child. Knowledge of the child's baseline or preoperative condition enables prompt recognition of changes in the child's neurologic function. For this reason, this section begins with the preoperative assessment.

Preoperative Assessment

Obtain as much information as possible about the child's behavior from the parents or primary caretaker. If the child is transported to the hospital by medical personnel, obtain information from the health care team previously involved in the child's care and from the parents (by telephone, if necessary).

If possible, record the child's normal psychosocial skills, achievement of developmental milestones and motor activity, self-comforting measures, communication style, sleep patterns, feeding preferences, and behavior when frightened or angry. Record the names of family members, special friends, pets, and favorite activities.

Neurologic Function

Note the presence and severity of any preexistent neurologic symptoms such as seizures, coma, blindness, cranial nerve palsies, delayed developmental milestones, abnormal posturing or motor activity, or abnormal or absent reflexes. Obtain and record the head circumference of the infant or toddler.

Level of Consciousness Use terms that describe rather than classify behavior. The older, verbal child can be asked about his or her name, age, birthday, and normal home activities. Alert, accurate answers are normal, and confused answers and lack of response to voice or painful stimulus are abnormal. The infant's LOC is evaluated by observing the infant's cry and response to auditory and tactile stimuli, and feeding and sleeping behavior. A high-pitched, breathless cry is abnormal. Excessive irritability or lethargy is abnormal in the child of any age, and *a decreased response to painful stimuli is worrisome.*

Motor Activity and Ability to Follow Commands
Record head control, grasp, strength of extremities, and symmetric withdrawal of the arms and legs following a painful stimulus. The older child should demonstrate ability to follow commands by holding up two fingers, sticking out his or her tongue, or wiggling toes on request. Evaluate antigravity muscles by asking the child to close his or her eyes and hold arms extended; discrepancies of arm strength can be appreciated if one arm drifts down. Ask the cooperative child to lift arms and legs against resistance. Strength of grasp bilaterally should also be evaluated. If possible, observe the child's gait and note any irregularities.

Reflexes   Inspect the child's pupil size and response to light. Evaluate the child's cranial nerve function during the course of normal activities. The complexity and extent of the evaluation will be determined by the child's clinical condition.

Cardiorespiratory Function

Airway, Oxygenation, and Ventilation   Note the respiratory rate and pattern. Determine the presence of a cough and gag reflex. Hypoxemia or hypercapnia should be corrected preoperatively, and the child's baseline arterial blood gases should be recorded if they are obtained.

Systemic Perfusion   The skin should be warm with brisk capillary refill if the ambient temperature is warm. Pulses should all be strong. The heart rate and blood pressure should be appropriate for age and clinical condition (see inside front cover for normal vital signs).

Fluid and Electrolyte Balance and Nutrition

Record the child's general level of nutrition and hydration. Determine if any electrolyte imbalances are present preoperatively. If SIADH or DI is present preoperatively, it should be recorded along with any drug therapy (including dosage) required. Note the child's normal feeding behavior, food preferences, and sleep patterns.

Psychosocial Preparation

Ideally, the surgery is planned on an elective basis, and the child's parents or primary caretakers will participate in the preparation of the child. The child may wish to visit the postoperative unit, but this visit should be carefully planned, and the things the child sees must be carefully controlled.

If the child is admitted to the critical care unit following trauma or an acute medical emergency, the child will require time during the postoperative period to come to terms with the hospital admission and surgery.

Parents must also be prepared for the child's likely appearance postoperatively. They should know to expect a bulky head dressing and facial edema. If time allows, the parents should be given the opportunity to view anticipated postoperative monitoring equipment during the preoperative preparation.

Preparation for Postoperative Care (Setup)

Assemble all equipment at or near the bedside and ensure that it is in working order. Prepare all monitoring systems (e.g., arterial and ICP monitoring) and fluids. A pediatric mechanical ventilator should be prepared for use at the bedside, with a hand ventilator (bag), mask, and appropriate suction equipment. A spare endotracheal tube should be readily available with reintubation equipment.

Drugs used in the treatment of increased ICP, including mannitol, vasopressors, or furosemide, should be readily available, as should drugs used for pharmacologic paralysis, sedation, and analgesia. An emergency drug sheet or Broselow Resuscitation Tape (Armstrong) will assist in preparation for administration of drugs. The Broselow tape will also enable selection of appropriate emergency equipment sizes (see inside back cover).

Initial Postoperative Evaluation

Cardiorespiratory Function

Airway, Oxygenation, and Ventilation   Assess the child's airway and ventilation while receiving reports from the anesthesiologist/anesthetist and neurosurgeon. Position the child so that the neck is extended and suction the airway if necessary. The respiratory rate should be appropriate for age and clinical condition. *At all times during postoperative care, be prepared to protect the airway and ensure effective ventilation.* Insertion of an oropharyngeal or nasopharyngeal airway or intubation may be required to maintain a patent airway, particularly if the child is obtunded or unconscious.

Evidence of respiratory distress includes tachypnea or an inappropriately slow respiratory rate, retractions, nasal flaring, grunting, stridor, apnea, gasping, or deterioration in color. Inadequate ventilation can produce hypoxemia and hypercapnia, which in turn can contribute to increased CBF and increased ICP. Evaluate pulse oximetry, end-tidal carbon dioxide, and arterial blood gases. Hypoxemia is treated with supplemental oxygen, and hypercarbia and severe hypoxemia unresponsive to oxygen administration require mechanical ventilatory support. If increased ICP is present, the $PaCO_2$ is maintained at approximately 32 to 34 mm Hg.

If severe respiratory distress or inadequate ventilation is detected, provide ventilation with a bag and mask while the airway is assessed; assist with intubation and initiation of mechanical ventilation if they are not already provided. Causes of acute deterioration or inadequate ventilation in the *intubated* child include tube displacement, tube obstruction, pneumothorax, and equipment failure.

Systemic Perfusion   Evaluate the child's systemic perfusion; the heart rate should be appropriate for age and clinical condition. Bradycardia is ominous and may indicate increased ICP or hypoxemia—both should be ruled out. Tachycardia is often a nonspecific sign of distress and may be an early indication of cardiorespiratory distress, fever, pain, or fear.

Extremities should be warm with brisk capillary refill if the ambient temperature is warm. Peripheral pulses should be strong, and blood pressure should be appropriate for age (see also table on inside front cover):

- *Median systolic pressure beyond 1 year of age:* 90 mm Hg + (2 × age in years)
- *Systolic hypotension beyond 1 year of age:* <70 mm Hg + (2 × age in years)

Hypotension or hypertension should be investigated and treated immediately. Hypotension may result from blood loss or hypovolemia and requires volume therapy. Hypertension may indicate increased ICP.

Oxygen Supply-Demand Ratio   If the child is critically ill or injured, with evidence of respiratory failure, shock, or increased ICP, systemic oxygen delivery should be maximized while oxygen demand is minimized. Oxygen delivery is determined by the hemoglobin concentration and its saturation and by the cardiac output. Therefore support cardiorespiratory function and consider transfusion if significant anemia is present.

Minimize oxygen demand: treat fever while keeping the child warm, provide analgesia, look for and promptly treat signs of infection, and consider sedation or pharmacologic paralysis with analgesia to reduce the work of breathing. If therapeutic hypothermia is used, prevent shivering. Report seizures and treat SE immediately.

Neurologic Function

Assess the neurologic status quickly, thoroughly, and frequently. Evaluate the child's *level of consciousness* in light of the child's age and baseline condition, and notify a physician of any deterioration.

Any one of several neurologic scoring tools may be used to monitor the child's neurologic status, provided that it is *consistently* used by all members of the health care team; modified versions of the GCS are the most popular. Evaluate the child's *ability to follow commands* (hold up two fingers, wiggle the toes, or stick out the tongue). If the child is obtunded or unconsciousness, evaluate the child's *response to painful stimuli,* using both central and peripheral stimuli. To evaluate localization of pain, provide a truncal painful stimulus above the nipple line and determine if the child reaches for the stimulus. To evaluate withdrawal from pain, pinch the medial aspect of each extremity and determine if each extremity abducts (withdraws) from the stimulus. Purposeful responses include localization and withdrawal. Nonpurposeful movements include vague movement or decorticate or decerebrate posturing in response to pain.

Evaluate *pupil size and response to light;* report pupil dilation and sluggish response to light immediately. Most cranial nerve functions, such as cough and gag reflexes, can be evaluated during routine nursing care activities; however, be sure that these are consistently evaluated and report loss of these reflexes to a physician immediately.

Monitor for evidence of seizure activity, such as tonic-clonic movements or lateral eye deviation. If pharmacologic paralyzing agents are provided, seizures may not be apparent without an EEG. Signs of subclinical seizures include pupil dilation, fluctuations in vital signs (including tachycardia or bradycardia and hypotension or hypertension), and compromise in systemic perfusion.

If an ICP monitoring catheter is in place, join it to an appropriately zeroed and calibrated monitoring system (see Increased Intracranial Pressure, p. 383 under Common Clinical Conditions, p. 388). Obtain specific orders for actions to be taken if the ICP rises above 20 to 25 mm Hg (e.g., hyperventilate, administer diuretics, open the ventricular drain). Notify a physician of ICP spikes above 20 to 25 mm Hg and any associated clinical change.

Fluid and Electrolyte Balance and Nutrition

Evaluate fluid balance on an hourly basis for the first several hours following surgery and be alert for the development of inadequate or excessive urine output. Insert a nasogastric tube if the child is intubated or if respiratory distress or gastric distension is present.

If intravascular volume and systemic perfusion are adequate, most children receive approximately 50% to 75% of maintenance fluid requirements in the form of 5% to 10% glucose and 0.45% NaCl. Aggressive fluid administration is avoided unless it is necessary to restore or maintain systemic perfusion. Hypotonic fluids should *not* be administered, since they may contribute to an abrupt drop in serum sodium and osmolality, with a corresponding extravascular fluid shift.

Monitor the child's serum electrolytes, particularly the serum sodium concentration. Signs of SIADH must be detected immediately; these signs include a decrease in urine volume, an increase in urine sodium and osmolality, and a decrease in serum sodium concentration. Treatment includes limitation of fluid intake (see p. 409).

Monitor for signs of DI, including an increase in urine volume and a decrease in urine specific gravity (<1.005) and osmolality. If DI develops,

urine fluid losses must be replaced by IV route every 15 to 20 minutes, and ADH must be administered in the form of vasopressin or DDAVP (see p. 411).

Postoperative Complications

Postoperative complications can include signs of increased ICP and neurologic deterioration, or they may include signs of cardiorespiratory deterioration, endocrine or fluid and electrolyte problems, incisional pain or inflammation, or spinal cord complications. Signs of potential postoperative complications or need for further medical evaluation are listed in Table 8-11.

Increased Intracranial Pressure

Increased ICP results from an uncompensated increase in the volume of brain, blood, or CSF within the skull. Increased ICP may result from cerebral edema caused by an extravascular free water shift, such as occurs if the serum sodium concentration decreases abruptly. The CBV can increase as a result of an increase in CBF, intracranial hemor-

Table 8-11
Clinical Signs Suggestive of Postoperative Complications and Need for Further Medical Evaluation

System	Clinical Sign
Neurologic	Severe headache, waves of headache
	Pupil changes
	Decreased level of consciousness
	Increased focal neurologic deficit
	Seizures
	Bradycardia and hypertension
	Recurrent vomiting, vomiting without nausea
Endocrine	Increased or decreased urine output
	Hypotension
Systemic	Low or high blood pressure
	Changes in ventilation
	Increases in temperature
Local incision	Bleeding
	Severe local pain
	Wound dehiscence
Spinal	Changes in sensory or motor level

rhage, or obstruction to cerebral venous return. Any of these conditions can develop during the postoperative period.

Clinical Presentation General signs and symptoms of increased ICP are reviewed earlier in the chapter (see Box 8-5). They include a decrease in LOC (confusion, irritability or lethargy, inability to follow commands, decreased response to painful stimuli), and pupil dilation with sluggish response to light. Late signs of increased ICP can include hypertension, bradycardia, and apnea, but these signs generally occur late in the clinical course, when herniation is imminent. If an ICP monitor is in place, it will enable quantification of the ICP and calculation of the CPP.

Clinical signs of neurologic deterioration will also be affected by the site of surgery. Potential indicators of postoperative deterioration based on the operative region are listed in Table 8-12.

Management The treatment of increased ICP requires determination of the cause of the problem and elimination of that cause. Establishment of effective oxygenation and ventilation is the first treatment of increased ICP because it can control the CBF and CBV and may produce a decrease in ICP, particularly if complicated by hypoxemia or hypoventilation (see also Management, p. 394).

Increased Cerebral Blood Flow/Volume Establish adequate ventilation and oxygenation via bag-valve-mask and ultimately through intubation and mechanical ventilation to maintain $PaCO_2$ at 32 to 34 mm Hg and PaO_2 80 to 100 mm Hg. If systemic perfusion and arterial pressure are adequate, elevate the head of the bed 30 degrees to enhance cerebral venous return.

Cerebral Edema Administer mannitol, glycerol, or another hypertonic agent to promote intravascular fluid shift and diuresis. Furosemide may be administered to produce a more rapid diuresis. Avoid acute decrease in serum sodium concentration, which will contribute to further extravascular fluid shift and cerebral edema.

Increased Cerebrospinal Fluid A ventricular drain may be inserted to drain CSF intermittently or continuously, particularly if CSF pathways are obstructed (e.g., caused by blood in the ventricular system) or if CSF reabsorption is compromised (e.g., by diffuse subarachnoid hemorrhage).

Seizures A single seizure does not necessarily require treatment. However, SE must be treated immediately, since it will increase the cerebral oxygen demand and can contribute to a mismatch between cerebral perfusion and cerebral oxygen demand, resulting in ischemia (see Status Epilepticus under Common Clinical Conditions). Consider seizures/SE as a potential cause of increased ICP, particularly if it is associated with pupil dilation and tachycardia or bradycardia.

Syndrome of Inappropriate Antidiuretic Hormone Secretion SIADH can complicate neurologic injury or surgery. Clinical signs include a decrease in serum sodium concentration, a decrease in

Table 8-12
Postoperative "Red Flags" According to Operative Region

Operative Region	Red Flag Symptom	Pathology
Posterior fossa	Waves of severe headaches	Acute hydrocephalus
	Bradycardia and hypertension	Bleeding and/or swelling
	Deteriorating consciousness	Bleeding and/or swelling
	Altered reflexes	Edema, ischemia, clot
Supratentorial	Increased headache	Bleeding, edema
	Increased focal deficit	Edema, hemorrhage, ischemia
	Seizures	Edema, ischemia
Intraventricular	Increased headache	Acute hydrocephalus
	Decreased consciousness	Hydrocephalus, hemorrhage
	Focal deficit	Subdural or epidural hemorrhage

urine volume, and an inappropriately high urine sodium concentration. Treatment includes reduction in fluid intake to 30% to 70% of calculated maintenance fluid requirements. If neurologic symptoms (seizures or evidence of increased ICP) develop, 3% saline (3 to 5 ml/kg) may be administered (see Syndrome of Inappropriate Antidiuretic Hormone Secretion under Common Clinical Conditions, p. 409).

Diabetes Insipidus DI most commonly complicates neurosurgery near the pituitary gland (e.g., resection of a craniopharyngioma). Clinical signs include a large quantity of very dilute urine (specific gravity <1.005). If urine volume losses are not replaced, hemoconcentration and hypovolemia will rapidly result. Treatment includes intravenous replacement of all urine fluid/volume losses (milliliter for milliliter) at approximately 10- to 20-minute intervals) and administration of ADH in the form of vasopressin or DDAVP (see Diabetes Insipidus under Common Clinical Conditions, p. 411).

General Supportive Care

General supportive care requires monitoring and support of cardiorespiratory function, maintenance of fluid and electrolyte balance, nutritional support, and analgesia (Box 8-11).

Fluid and Electrolyte Balance and Nutrition

Ensure that intravascular volume is adequate, and monitor serum electrolytes. Prevent an acute decrease in the serum sodium concentration (e.g., from administration of hypotonic fluids or development of SIADH). Monitor serum osmolality—it can be estimated from the serum sodium and glucose concentrations and the BUN (see Box 8-8). Typically, the osmolality is maintained at approximately 300 to 310 mOsm/L.

Nutritional requirements cannot be provided with 5% to 10% glucose solutions and must be ensured via parenteral or enteral feedings. Enteral feeding should be instituted as soon as possible postoperatively.

Analgesia

Assess and treat pain. Certainly, if the child is comatose or receiving pentobarbital, pain may not be perceived. However, as the child's LOC improves, pain must be anticipated and treated (see Chapter 3). IV narcotics are often used while the child is mechanically ventilated, but codeine via suppository or elixir may be the analgesic of choice when the child is breathing spontaneously, since it will not depress respirations.

Infection Control

Although prophylactic antibiotics are administered perioperatively, infection may complicate any ICU stay or surgery. The risk of infection is particularly high if surgery was performed to repair a compound skull fracture, cerebral contusion, or skull penetration by a foreign object, or if the child develops a CSF leak. The risk of infection is reduced with good handwashing technique and maintenance of appropriate aseptic or sterile technique during catheter insertion and IV tubing and dressing changes. Monitor the child's temperature and white blood cell (WBC) count and differential closely (see discussion of septic shock, p. 140, and discussion of neutropenia, p. 563). Treat fever with antipyretics (acetaminophen, 10 mg/kg/dose orally or rectally; maximum: 650 mg every 4 hours) or a cooling blanket, and attempt to identify the source of infection. If antibiotics are prescribed, administer them on time and monitor peak-and-trough aminoglycoside levels.

Complications of Immobility

The comatose or paralyzed child can develop so-called hazards of immobility (including atelectasis, skin breakdown, decreased muscle tone, and contractures). If the child is unconscious for several days, obtain a consultation from physical and occupational therapists.

Psychosocial Support

Neurosurgery will be frightening for both the child and the parents. Postoperative support may be most effective if the nurse meets with the parents preoperatively and determines the family's perceptions of and concerns about the surgery and postoperative care. During surgery, periodic reports of progress in the operating room (transmitted if the surgeon agrees) may reduce stress for the family. Such interim reports can break up a long wait into more manageable intervals.

Immediately following surgery, the parents must be prepared for the sight of the child and the

Box 8-11

Postoperative Care of the Pediatric Neurosurgical Patient

1. **Potential inadequate airway, oxygenation, and ventilation,** which may result from increased intracranial pressure (ICP) and hypoventilation, depressed level of consciousness and hypoventilation or airway obstruction, neurologic pulmonary edema, or associated trauma or infection. Assess and support as needed.

2. **Potential inadequate systemic perfusion,** which can be caused by increased ICP, inappropriate intravascular volume (possibly a complication of diuretic therapy or development of diabetes insipidus), electrolyte imbalance, or complications of associated trauma or infection. Assess and support heart rate, intravascular volume relative to the vascular space, myocardial function, and blood pressure.

3. **Potential inadequate cerebral perfusion,** which may be caused by increased intracranial pressure, hypotension, hypoxemia, maldistribution of cerebral blood flow, or brain death. Assess child frequently and carefully, and notify physician of any change immediately.
   a. Assess neurologic function frequently; report any deterioration to physician:
      (1) Evaluate and document level of consciousness.
      (2) Assess using Glasgow Coma Scale (see Table 8-6).
      (3) Evaluate pupil size and response to light.
      (4) Evaluate evidence of cranial nerve function during normal nursing care activities (e.g., evaluate cough and gag during suctioning).
   b. Monitor ICP; ensure that monitoring system is functioning properly. Obtain orders for treatment if ICP >20 mm Hg or >25 mm Hg.
   c. Treat increased ICP if present:
      (1) Assist with intubation and ensure that airway, oxygenation, and ventilation are adequate. Maintain Pao_2 at 90-100 mm Hg, oxyhemoglobin saturation at 98%-100%, and $Paco_2$ at 32-34 mm Hg.
      (2) Ensure that heart rate, blood pressure, and systemic perfusion are adequate. Support as needed.
      (3) If ventricular catheter is in place, drain ventricular fluid per order if ICP rises.
      (4) If arterial blood pressure is adequate, elevate head of bed 30 degrees.
      (5) Keep head in midline.
      (6) Prevent hypovolemia, hypervolemia, hyponatremia, or acute fall in serum sodium or osmolality.
      (7) Ensure that adequate analgesia is provided, consider sedation, anesthesia.
      (8) Monitor for signs of deterioration, including signs of herniation (pupil dilation, tachycardia or bradycardia, hypertension, hypoventilation or apnea, decrease in cranial nerve function), and notify physician immediately.
      (9) Emergency management of increased ICP may include hyperventilation, administration of diuretic (typically mannitol), possibly drainage of ventricular cerebrospinal fluid, and possibly induction of anesthesia or barbiturate coma.
   d. Evaluate and support systemic perfusion.
   e. Ensure that airway, oxygenation, and ventilation are adequate; support as needed.

4. **Potential fluid and electrolyte imbalance,** which may result from limitation of fluid intake, administration of diuretics, or development of syndrome of inappropriate antidiuretic hormone secretion or diabetes insipidus. Monitor fluid intake and output, maintain electrolyte balance and serum osmolality, and notify physician of any change.

5. **Potential pain,** which may be caused by underlying trauma, meningitis, or invasive monitoring catheters. Assess pain and ensure that analgesia is adequate. Monitor for evidence of neurologic deterioration closely if child is sedated.

6. **Potential status epilepticus,** which may result from progression of seizures associated with trauma, meningitis, or stroke. Note that tonic-clonic activity will not be observed if child is receiving pharmacologic paralysis. Signs of seizures may include wide fluctuation in heart rate or vital signs, or lateral eye deviation.

7. **Potential child and parent anxiety,** which may result from child's underlying disease or

Continued

Box 8-11

Postoperative Care of the Pediatric Neurosurgical Patient—cont'd

injury and intensive care unit (ICU) sights and sounds. Assess sources of child's and family's fears; provide information, clarification, and support as needed.

8. **Potential infection,** which may result from underlying disease or injury, invasive catheters, and ICU hospitalization. Monitor for signs of infection; administer antibiotics precisely as ordered. Monitor aminoglycoside peak-and-trough levels. Monitor for signs of sepsis and report to a physician immediately.

9. **Potential compromise in nutrition.** Recognize problem and provide enteral nutrition as

soon as possible; ensure adequate caloric and nutrient intake.

10. **Potential knowledge deficit.** Provide teaching as parents and child are ready.

11. **Potential impaired mobility related to prolonged bed rest.** Obtain physical therapy, occupational therapy consultation. If child is comatose, obtain foot splints, provide passive range-of-motion exercise, position child carefully, and turn frequently.

---

postoperative monitoring equipment. Bring them in to see the child as soon as the child arrives in the ICU so that they can reassure themselves that the child has survived. They may need encouragement to touch and talk to the child, but may also need time to assimilate the child's condition.

Box 8-11 lists potential patient problems and nursing diagnoses that may be used to formulate a nursing care plan.

Specific Diseases

Head Trauma

Etiology/Pathophysiology

Head trauma is responsible for approximately 200,000 pediatric hospitalizations and 4000 deaths annually. Most severe pediatric head injuries are closed head injuries, resulting from blunt trauma, such as motor vehicle–related trauma or child abuse. Penetrating injuries caused by firearms are responsible for an increasing number of head injuries in adults and children.

Children are particularly likely to sustain severe head injury if they are unrestrained in a motor vehicle crash or if they are struck by an automobile while walking or riding a bicycle. Throughout infancy and early childhood, children

are relatively "head heavy"—the head is disproportionately large in relation to the rest of the body. As a result, if the child is propelled unrestrained in a crash, the child will most commonly fly headfirst, and acceleration-deceleration injuries will occur when the head eventually strikes an object.

Diffuse head injury is more likely to result from blunt head trauma, particularly acceleration-deceleration injuries during childhood. This is because the child's brain is more homogenous than the adult's brain; it has a higher water content and less myelinization than the adult's brain. For this reason, acceleration-deceleration forces occurring during trauma are more likely to produce global injury and shear hemorrhages in the child than in the adult.

The head injury causes a primary insult that cannot be reversed. However, secondary insults, such as hypoxemia, hypercarbia, hypotension, hyponatremia, and SE, can complicate the injury and must be prevented. Hypoxemia and hypotension can be particularly damaging to the injured brain and can increase both morbidity and mortality if they occur during the first days after the initial trauma. This is because head trauma causes a mismatch between CBF and metabolic requirements for oxygen. This mismatch is created by mediators that alter cerebrovascular tone, permeability, and reactivity, as well as cerebral metabolism. As a result, some areas of the brain are hyperemic, with excessive blood flow, which may contribute to increased ICP, whereas other areas of the brain are characterized by inadequate blood flow and ischemia. These ischemic areas can be devastated by hypoxemia or hypotension. Respiratory insufficiency at the scene, or unrecognized or inadequately treated hemorrhagic shock may cause these early secondary insults.

The most common types of cerebral injuries are concussions, contusions, skull fractures, and vascular injuries, including epidural or subdural hematoma or subarachnoid hemorrhage (Figure 8-5). Each of these injuries is presented here. When blunt head trauma occurs, particularly with acceleration-deceleration forces, the resulting injury may occur directly under the site of impact (the *coup*) or on the side of the brain opposite the impact (the *countercoup* injury). The countercoup injury probably results when the brain strikes the skull.

Concussion   A concussion is a moderate cerebral injury resulting from a blow or acceleration-deceleration injury that produces no structural brain damage. CSF pressure does rise transiently, and minor changes may be apparent on the EEG.

Contusion   A contusion is a localized brain injury consisting of bruising, hemorrhage, and tissue edema. The severity of the contusion is determined by its size and location. Approximately 10% of children with contusions will develop posttraumatic seizures.

Skull Fracture   A skull fracture is a break in the continuity of the cranial bones that may or may not be associated with displacement of the bone fragments. Complications can result if the bony fragments are displaced into the brain or if underlying structures, such as the brain tissue, meninges, or blood vessels, are damaged.

Epidural Hematoma   An epidural hematoma (EDH) consists of an accumulation of blood (often arterial) between the skull and the dura, which usually results from a low-velocity blow to the skull. It is frequently associated with a skull fracture. The most common form of EDH occurs when a temporal fossa injury and skull fracture are asso-ciated with a tear in the middle meningeal artery. When sufficient blood accumulation occurs, the ICP may rise dramatically and rapidly. EDHs should be diagnosed by a CT scan before clinical deterioration. They should also be suspected as a cause of sudden clinical deterioration during the first hours after a head injury.

Subdural Hematoma   A subdural hematoma (SDH) is present when bridging veins are torn and blood accumulates between the dura and the arachnoid membranes. *SDHs are often present bilaterally and often result from child abuse.*

SDH may be characterized as acute, subacute, or chronic based on the time between injury and clinical detection. An *acute SDH* follows a severe head injury, and blood accumulation and clinical signs develop within hours of the injury. A suba-cute SDH develops soon after a less severe contusion and is associated with loss of consciousness and an increase in ICP. A *chronic SDH* develops weeks or months after a minor head injury.

Subarachnoid Hemorrhage   A subarachnoid hemorrhage (SAH) results from a severe head injury and tearing of the subarachnoid vessels. Seizures or increased ICP can rapidly develop. SAHs are frequently seen following child abuse, motor vehicle–related trauma, or falls from very high places. A large SAH can result in the development of communicating hydrocephalus because the SAH interferes with the reabsorption of CSF by the subarachnoid villi.

Intracerebral/Intraventricular Hemorrhage   An intracerebral hemorrhage is bleeding associated with severe head injury, usually diffuse acceleration-deceleration injuries. It may be observed within the parenchyma of the brain or in the ventricles, and it is often extensive. Blood in the ventricles may cause obstructive hydrocephalus, because the blood cells obstruct narrow CSF passages. This hydrocephalus may develop acutely (within hours of the head trauma) or later (weeks after the injury).

Cerebral Edema or Cerebral Swelling   Cerebral edema is caused by an increase in brain water content. This may be caused by an extravascular fluid shift associated with a sudden fall in the serum

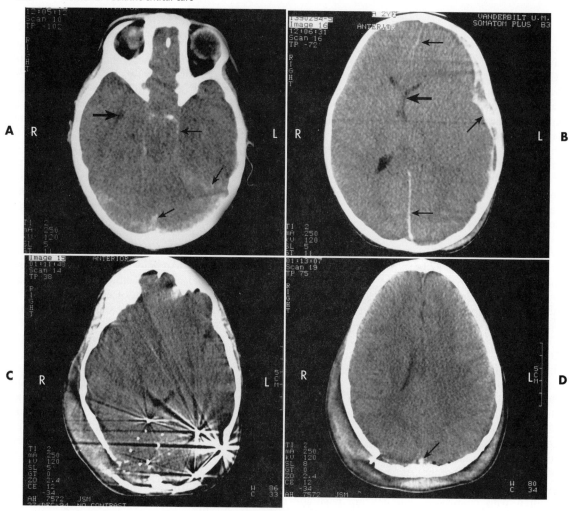

Figure 8-5   Computed tomography (CT) scans of children with head injuries. **A** and **B,** These CT scans were taken from a 22-month-old infant with intentional trauma, with a blunt head injury (patient's left and right sides are labeled). **A,** This view shows no patent third or fourth ventricle (the child was herniating despite aggressive therapy). *Thin arrows* show subarachnoid blood. The *thick arrow* points to the right occipital horn of the right lateral ventricle. The left occipital horn is not visible. The larger right horn suggests that edema on the left side of the brain is greater than on the right side and is causing a midline shift and prevention of drainage of the right ventricle into the third ventricle. This suggestion is confirmed in view *B.* **B,** This view shows several complications of blunt head trauma. There is a loss of the gray-white interface; thus the entire CT scan appears pale—this is consistent with a severe injury and secondary anoxic insult (the child demonstrated agonal respirations on arrival of the paramedics). The three *thin arrows* point to more subarachnoid blood. The edema in the left hemisphere is definitely greater than in the right hemisphere, causing a midline shift (apparent when looking at the blood in the midline). The compressed left lateral ventricle *(thick arrow)* is clearly displaced to the right side. **C** and **D,** These CT scans shows some effects of penetrating head trauma in a 7-year-old who was shot with shotgun pellets. **C,** The pellets and the occipital scull fractures they produced are clearly visible. **D,** The white circle *(arrow)* is depicting a clot in the superior sagittal sinus as it drains down to the torcular Herophili. This clot, obstructing cerebral venous return, complicated the head injury and placed the child at risk for the sudden development of increased ICP due to venous obstruction.

sodium level or osmolality. Cerebral edema may also be caused by an increase in cerebral cell membrane permeability, caused by cerebral ischemia or the formation of free oxygen radicals or other mediators following head injury. The cerebral edema resulting from an extravascular fluid shift develops immediately after the fall in the serum sodium level or osmolality. Hypoxia or shock (ischemia) produce cerebral edema that peaks at approximately 48 to 72 hours or longer after the injury.

Cerebral swelling is the term used to describe an increase in brain volume resulting from the development of regional hyperemia or CBF in excess of metabolic requirements. This increase in brain blood flow is caused by the formation or activation of a variety of mediators, such as tumor necrosis factor or platelet activating factor, which cause vasodilation, increased capillary permeability, and maldistribution of cerebral blood flow. Cerebral swelling peaks at approximately 24 to 48 hours after head trauma.

Clinical Presentation

Clinical signs and symptoms of head injury are most often those resulting from increased ICP. However, clinical signs associated with specific injury are summarized here.

Concussion   A concussion produces loss of consciousness for a variable period. This loss of consciousness may be associated with depressed (but present) reflexes, brief slowing of respirations, bradycardia, and possibly hypotension. After the patient regains consciousness, traumatic amnesia may be present. No signs of further neurologic injury should be present, however. Occasionally patients develop *postconcussion syndrome,* including headache, malaise, vertigo, anxiety, or fatigue.

Contusion   The clinical signs of contusion are determined by the severity of the cranial injury, the volume of bleeding present, and the amount of bleeding that develops. Loss of consciousness may or may not occur. Posttraumatic seizures develop in approximately 10% of children with contusions; thus hospitalization is required.

Skull Fracture   Clinical signs and symptoms of a skull fracture will depend on the location of the fracture and on the extent of the underlying cranial injury. Linear skull fractures are diagnosed by radiographic examination, although a CT scan may be required to diagnose a basilar skull fracture. Depressed or compound skull fractures may be palpable and should be suspected if the contour of the skull is altered. Profuse bleeding may result if the depressed skull fracture is present over the sagittal or lateral sinus.

A basilar skull fracture is often associated with a CSF leak from the nose or ear. Although the CSF leak itself is not harmful, it indicates communication between the subarachnoid space and the ear or upper respiratory tract that creates the risk of meningitis. CSF leaks should be suspected if clear drainage is present from the nose or ear of the child with a basilar skull fracture. Additional signs of basilar skull fracture include bleeding from the nose, mouth, or ear; perimastoid discoloration (so-called Battle's sign); blood behind the eardrum; palsies of cranial nerves I, III, and VIII; or pneumocephaly.

Epidural Hematoma   Approximately one third of children with EDH demonstrate brief loss of consciousness immediately after the injury, then a lucid period for several hours, followed by sudden deterioration as blood accumulates in the skull, producing critical elevation in the ICP. Signs of deterioration include a headache, decreasing LOC, and signs of increased ICP (e.g., pupil dilation, decreased responsiveness). Another one third of children with EDH never lose consciousness, and the final third lose consciousness and do not regain it for several hours or days.

An EDH should be suspected in any child who develops headache, decreased LOC, and unilateral pupil dilation (typically on the side of the injury, although contralateral dilation may result from a countercoup injury) after head injury. A CT scan will confirm the EDH.

Subdural Hematoma   Acute SDH is caused by a severe head injury and typically results in significant signs of neurologic dysfunction. Approximately two thirds of children with acute SDH lose consciousness. Bilateral SDH is often present and may be associated with diffuse injury. Focal signs of injury, including unilateral pupil dilation, focal seizures, or hemiparesis, are often observed. Severe increased ICP can develop rapidly, particularly if associated cerebral lacerations, contusions, or hematomas are present. Diagnosis of the SDH and any associated injuries can be confirmed by a CT scan.

Chronic SDH is often caused by serous exudate and products of blood breakdown. They are rarely seen in children beyond 2 years of age. The child with chronic SDH may develop headache and progressive decreased LOC weeks or months after a mild head injury. Ipsilateral pupil dilation may be observed, as well as papilledema. Hemiparesis can also develop. Retinal hemorrhages are observed in 10% of children with chronic SDH.

Subarachnoid Hemorrhage SAH is often associated with severe head injury and is diagnosed by a CT scan. SAH may result in the development of communicating hydrocephalus days or weeks after a head injury.

Intracerebral/Intraventricular Hemorrhage These hemorrhages are often associated with severe head injury and are diagnosed by a CT scan. Intraventricular hemorrhage can cause acute or late hydrocephalus; thus the child must be monitored closely for signs of sudden deterioration.

Cerebral Edema or Cerebral Swelling Significant cerebral edema or cerebral swelling will produce signs of increased ICP. The timing of these signs will be determined by the cause of the cerebral edema, and the clinical severity of the signs will be determined by the intracranial compliance. If intracranial volume is already increased (e.g., hydrocephalus or intracranial bleeding is present), minimal edema may contribute to a significant rise in ICP and the potential for cerebral herniation.

An increase in brain water content (cerebral edema) is most likely to develop in association with an acute fall in the serum sodium level or osmolality, such as may occur with SIADH. This cerebral edema and potential signs of increased ICP will develop at the time of the fall in the serum sodium level or osmolality.

Cerebral edema may develop following an ischemic insult. This cerebral edema will most likely be maximal 48 to 72 hours or more following the ischemic insult and may cause signs of increased ICP at that time.

Cerebral swelling, caused by a regional increase in brain blood flow in excess of cerebral metabolic requirements, may be most likely to produce signs of increased intracranial volume and increased ICP within the first 24 to 48 hours after a head injury.

"Talk and Die" Phenomenon Occasionally a potentially significant closed head injury (e.g., from a motor vehicle collision or fall) produces no early signs and symptoms such as loss of consciousness but is associated with later, sudden deterioration, cerebral herniation, and death. This clinical picture may develop in the absence of a mass lesion (such as an EDH) and has been called the "talk and die" injury and the "pediatric concussion syndrome."

Initially the child is alert, with a high (9+) GCS score. Several (6 to 50) hours after the injury, the child suddenly becomes restless or irritable, or difficult to arouse, with pupil dilation with decreased response to light. Seizures may also be associated with the deterioration.

The ultimate cause of death is cerebral herniation, probably caused by the rapid development of cerebral swelling. Postmortem examination reveals regional cerebral hyperemia, often associated with multiple cerebral contusions. Although the severity of the head injury may not initially be detectable with clinical examination, it will usually be apparent on a CT scan.

Management

Children with mild head injury are usually admitted to the critical or intermediate care unit for skilled continuous nursing observation. All children with moderate or severe head injury require critical care. A CT scan should be performed whenever the child has a history consistent with a serious head injury (e.g., a fall from a significant height, unrestrained occupant of a severe motor vehicle collision, etc.), even if the child initially appears alert and oriented.

A spinal cord injury should be presumed to be associated with any serious head trauma until it has been definitely ruled out. The cervical spine should be immobilized, and the child should be log-rolled whenever turning is necessary. Evaluate the patient's movement and sensation in all four extremities on a regular basis (see Spinal Cord Injury, p. 431). The *development of a progressive neurologic deficit in the patient with a spinal cord injury is a neurosurgical emergency—notify the neurosurgeon immediately.*

The goals of management of the child with a head injury will be to preserve systemic perfusion and oxygen delivery, to maintain effective cerebral perfusion (this requires control of ICP), to detect early signs of neurologic deterioration, and to prevent secondary insults to the brain.

Airway, Oxygenation, and Ventilation The first priority is establishment and maintenance of an adequate airway, and intubation should be accomplished if needed. Increased ICP may cause apnea. Conversely, hypoventilation can contribute to hypoxemia and hypercapnia, which will contribute to an increase in CBF and ICP. For these reasons, establish and maintain effective oxygenation and ventilation.

Indications for intubation in the child with a head injury include impaired airway clearance or compromise in protective reflexes (weak cough or gag), hypoxemia, hypoventilation, evidence of increased ICP, associated shock or respiratory failure, or need for prolonged imaging studies. If the child is conscious, rapid sequence induction intubation may enable intubation without precipitation of a gag reflex and further increase in ICP (see pp. 65 and 313). However, succinylcholine may increase CBF and the ICP; thus it should be used with caution. Alternatively, anesthetic agents may be used during intubation; the half-life of these agents is longer, but they may not produce the undesirable rise in ICP.

Systemic Perfusion Shock (fluid) resuscitation may be necessary if poor systemic perfusion is present. Signs of inadequate systemic perfusion include inappropriate tachycardia or bradycardia, unusual irritability or lethargy for age, cool extremities with prolonged capillary refill despite a warm ambient temperature, thready or absent peripheral pulses, and urine output <1 ml/kg/hr. Shock may be present despite a normal blood pressure. Hypotension (in children beyond 1 year of age = systolic blood pressure ≤70 mm Hg plus twice the age in years) indicates the presence of *decompensated* shock.

Volume resuscitation includes bolus administration of isotonic crystalloids (20 ml/kg over ≤20 minutes). Blood administration (10 to 20 ml/kg packed red blood cells) may be required (see Figure 12-6, p. 602) in the presence of hemorrhage or coagulopathy, or if the shock persists despite the administration of two to three crystalloid boluses. If shock persists, multiple organ injury and abdominal hemorrhage must be ruled out. A pediatric surgeon should be consulted.

Severe head injury results in the release of tissue thromboplastin, which may produce a coagulopathy. Disseminated intravascular coagulation (DIC) is treated with blood products.

Oxygen Supply-Demand Ratio If the child is critically injured, with evidence of respiratory failure, shock, or increased ICP, attempt to maximize systemic oxygen delivery while minimizing oxygen demand. Oxygen delivery is determined by the hemoglobin concentration and its saturation and by the cardiac output. Therefore support cardiorespiratory function and consider transfusion if significant anemia is present.

Minimize oxygen demand: treat fever while keeping the child warm, provide analgesia, look for and promptly treat signs of infection, and consider sedation or pharmacologic paralysis with analgesia to reduce the work of breathing. If therapeutic hypothermia is used, prevent shivering. Report seizures and treat SE immediately.

Neurologic Function Perform careful neurologic assessment and notify a physician of any deterioration. Signs of deterioration include:

- Decrease in responsiveness and LOC, including inability to follow commands
- Decreased response to painful stimulus (e.g., decorticate posturing in child who previously localized pain, or absent response in child who previously demonstrated decerebrate posturing)
- Pupil dilation with decreased constrictive response to light (note that *consensual* pupil constriction should be present)

- Loss of cranial nerve or motor or sensory function
- Late signs of increased ICP (and imminent brain stem herniation): hypertension, bradycardia, and apnea

Report any seizures to a physician. Lateral, consensual eye deviation should be presumed to represent seizure activity until this possibility has been ruled out. Seizures may be impossible to detect in the child receiving paralytic agents but should be suspected if pupil dilation or unexplained fluctuations in the heart rate, blood pressure, or systemic perfusion are observed. Risk of posttraumatic seizures is most likely in children with severe head injury, diffuse cerebral edema, acute subdural hematoma, or an open depressed skull fracture with parenchymal damage. Note that SE must be treated promptly in children with head injury because SE results in an increase in CBF and the metabolic rate of oxygen consumption and may contribute to a rise in ICP or cerebral ischemia. Prophylactic anticonvulsant therapy remains controversial.

The child with increased ICP should be intubated, oxygenated, and ventilated ($PaCO_2$ of 32 to 34 mm Hg). Hypovolemia and hypervolemia are avoided, as is a rapid decrease in the serum sodium concentration. Children with head injury may develop SIADH, and unrestricted fluid intake may result in acute hyponatremia and resultant cerebral edema.

A CT scan is usually performed on admission. It may be electively repeated approximately 5 to 7 days after the injury or on an urgent basis if any deterioration occurs. *Indications for urgent surgical intervention in the child with head injury include significant neurologic deterioration in a child with an expanding epidural or (occasionally) a subdural or (rarely) an intracerebral hematoma.*

Poor prognostic findings following head injury include cardiovascular instability despite shock resuscitation, absence of spontaneous respirations, fixed pupils, absent (flaccid) response to pain, DI on admission, severe DIC, or a GCS score of 3 to 4. If brain death criteria are met, the family must be consulted about the possibility of organ donation.

Supportive Care Look for other injuries. Monitor function of all organs. Be alert for evidence of unexpected deterioration.

Concussion Concussions are not associated with any abnormalities on the CT scan, but the child is admitted to the hospital for observation. Postconcussion syndrome may produce complaints of headache, dizziness, malaise, and fatigue days or weeks after the concussion.

Contusion Treatment is determined by the extent of the contusion and the severity of secondary injuries (see following discussions of skull fractures, epidural and subdural hematomas, etc.). Posttraumatic seizures are present in approximately 10% of patients.

Skull Fracture Most simple, linear fractures require no treatment. Depressed skull fractures are surgically elevated if the fragment is depressed ≥5 mm or more than the thickness of the skull. They may also be elevated for cosmetic reasons.

Skull fractures located near the sagittal or lateral sinus may be associated with a venous channel tear and external or intracranial bleeding. Shock resuscitation and surgical control of the bleeding site will be required.

Compound (open, depressed) skull fractures require surgical intervention. Debridement and repair of dural tears is performed.

Basilar skull fractures require observation. Prophylactic antibiotic therapy is required if CSF leaks develop. Most CSF leaks will seal spontaneously within a few weeks. Chronic leaks require surgical repair.

If a basilar skull fracture or facial fractures (with dural tears) are present, nasogastric tubes may migrate intracerebrally during insertion. For this reason, nasogastric tubes are not routinely inserted and should be inserted with extreme caution in children with basilar skull fractures or facial fractures. Orogastric tubes may be used for these patients, or a physician may assist with the insertion of the nasogastric tube.

Epidural Hematoma This lesion should be detected by a CT scan, and surgical intervention is required. Intubation and hyperventilation are performed in preparation for surgery. If neurologic deterioration occurs before surgical intervention, morbidity and mortality are increased.

Subdural Hematoma Detection and treatment of increased ICP is required when acute SDH is present. Indications for surgery have not been universally established; surgery may be considered for a large SDH associated with an increase in ICP, although the surgery often does not halt the rise in ICP.

Treatment of chronic SDH remains controversial. The diagnosis is made by a CT scan. Subdural taps may be performed to evaluate the fluid accumulated and may be required to relieve increased ICP. The taps may also eliminate the problem. Surgical intervention is occasionally necessary for treatment of symptomatic fluid reaccumulation.

Subarachnoid Hemorrhage Treatment of SAH is symptomatic. Aggressive medical management of increased ICP may be necessary. If the SAH interferes significantly with CSF reabsorption, communicating hydrocephalus may develop late after the head injury, necessitating insertion of a ventriculoperitoneal shunt.

Intracerebral/Intraventricular Hemorrhage Surgery is performed if a hematoma develops and produces a mass effect and increased ICP. Postoperative management may be complicated by increased ICP, seizures, and motor or sensory deficits.

CSF drainage is required if intraventricular hemorrhage produces acute obstructive hydrocephalus. If the hydrocephalus develops late after the injury, insertion of a ventriculoperitoneal shunt may be required.

Cerebral Edema/Cerebral Swelling Increased ICP caused by brain edema or swelling is presented in detail earlier in this chapter (see Increased Intracranial Pressure under Common Clinical Conditions, p. 394).

Psychosocial Support Both parents and children require a great deal of support. The child may be agitated or disoriented, and the parents may feel guilty or fear for the child's life. If child abuse is suspected, the child abuse team must be notified as quickly as possible so that the child is protected.

Many children demonstrate functional morbidity following head injury. Postinjury sequelae include sleep disturbances, moodiness, discipline problems, and academic difficulties. Rehabilitation and long-term follow-up are often required (see also Chapter 12).

Spinal Cord Injury

Etiology/Pathophysiology

Spinal cord injury (SCI) during childhood most often results from motor vehicle crashes or falls. In adolescents, motor vehicle crashes (including motorcycle injuries) and sports and diving injuries are the most common causes of SCI.

SCI is less common in pediatric than in adult trauma for several reasons. The child's spine is more elastic and mobile than the adult's spine. Although the soft pediatric vertebrae are less likely to fracture than adult vertebrae, there are several reasons why the pediatric spine is vulnerable to injury when it is subjected to acceleration-deceleration forces. These are reviewed briefly here.

The young child's head is larger and heavier in proportion to the remainder of the body than the adult's head. Therefore the head is more likely to "lead," with resulting hyperextension or flexion of the neck, if the child is thrown from a motor vehicle or falls.

The ligaments along the young child's cervical vertebrae are relatively lax, and the immature paraspinous muscles allow vertebrae to shift during injury. The facet joints of the cervical vertebrae (particularly C1 to C3) are relatively flat in infants and toddlers; thus they may shift during application of force. High cervical spinal injuries (at the level of the second cervical vertebra) are the most common type of SCI occurring in young children for this reason.

Pediatric SCIs occur when vertebral bodies are fractured or when *subluxation* (partial dislocation) of the vertebrae occurs. Very young children are likely to sustain subluxation injuries without associated fractures. These subluxation injuries will result in anterior-posterior malalignment of contiguous vertebrae and compression of the spinal canal. Commonly, SCI can occur in children without radiographic abnormality (SCIWORA), a form of pediatric SCI present in 20% to 60% of victims. An MRI scan may reveal the injury, but this scan may be impractical if the child is unstable.

The neurologic dysfunction resulting from SCI can occur at the time of the primary injury or from compromise of spinal cord perfusion, and edema and necrosis. Secondary injury to the spinal cord may also result from movement of the neck during transport or initial resuscitation if the spine is inadequately immobilized. Herniation of a disk and development of a subdural hematoma are unusual causes of progressive neurologic dysfunction following an SCI. Vasospasm and thrombosis in spinal cord vessels may contribute to ischemia and dysfunction.

Clinical Presentation

Clinical Evaluation   The clinical consequences of the SCI are determined by the level and severity of the SCI (Table 8-13). If the SCI is mild or moderate, complete recovery of neurologic function is possible, even if complete neurologic deficit is present on admission. However, if the initial insult is severe (particularly if severe subluxation occurred) or is associated with the development of edema, loss of function and sensation below the level of injury can be permanent and complete. Secondary injury (e.g., neck extension during intubation) may also result in progression of the injury.

Approximately half of all children with SCI demonstrate some neurologic deficit on initial examination, most commonly a loss of some or all movement and sensation below the level of injury. The degree of the deficit is characterized as follows:

1. *Complete injury:* Complete absence of *all* movement and sensation below the area of injury. Rectal sphincter tone is absent.
2. *Incomplete (partial) injury:* Transient weakness or paresthesia. Several specific types of incomplete injuries may be observed:
   a. *Anterior cord syndrome:* Absent motor function and pain sensation but preservation of position and vibratory sensation caused by anterior spinal artery injury.
   b. *Central cord syndrome:* Bilateral arm weakness but intact lower extremity and perianal function caused by injury to the central portion of the cord.
3. *Spinal shock:* Transient loss of all motor, sensory, and segmental reflex function below the level of injury, which mimics complete cord transection. Function and sensation usually return within 24 hours (to

Table 8-13
Clinical Signs Associated With Level of Spinal Cord Injury

Lost Function, Sensation, Reflex	Level of Injury
Spontaneous respirations	C3-C4 or above (NOTE: Patients with C5-C6 lesions maintain diaphragm innervation, so diaphragmatic breathing is observed.)
Sensation in top of shoulder	At or above C4
Elevation, extension of arms	Above C5-C7
Biceps reflex	Above C5-C6
Sensation in thumb	At or above C6
Sensation to middle, ring fingers	At or above C7
Opening, closing of hand	Above C7-T1
Sensation at nipple line	At or above T4
Sensation at umbilicus	At or above T10
Abdominal reflex	Above T7-T12
Elevation of legs	Above L2-L4
Quadriceps reflex	Above L2-L4
Ability to wiggle toes	Above L3-S1
Sensation in big toe	At or above L4
Achilles' reflex	Above L5-S3
Sensation at top of little toe	At or above S1
Plantar reflex	Above S1-S2
Ability to tighten anus	Above S3-S5

distinguish from complete injury), when the extent of the deficit becomes apparent.

Careful, repeat clinical examination of movement and sensation in all extremities must be performed until definitive studies are completed, since many children demonstrate delayed onset of symptoms and some children may demonstrate progression of injury.

Diagnostic Studies   Many SCIs can be detected by good-quality cervical and thoracic anteroposterior and radiographic x-ray films. A lateral radiograph should be obtained that includes the first cervical vertebra to the first thoracic vertebra. If the radiographs are equivocal or nonvisualized SCI is suspected, flexion-extension radiographs are obtained after the child is stable.

The definitive diagnostic study of SCI is MRI, although this study is impractical if the child is unstable. A CT scan will allow good visualization of the upper cervical spinal column, soft tissue, and vertebrae. This examination should be part of the CT scan performed for every child with a severe closed head injury.

If the child is awake and responsive, the child should be asked about pain in the neck and shoulders and along the vertebral column. The presence of pain is a significant indication of possible vertebral/spinal cord injury.

Management

Management of the child with SCI is designed to minimize the potential for further injury while supporting recovery of spinal cord function. In general, the spinal cord is immobilized until the child is stable; then definitive therapy is provided.

Immobilization   SCI should be suspected in any child who has sustained severe or multisystem organ trauma or has a mechanism of injury that may have resulted in SCI. *The spine should be immobilized until SCI has been ruled out.* Children should be restrained properly on spine boards with cervical collars. However, it is essential that these devices "fit" properly. The occipital portion of the skull is often prominent in the infant and toddler; if the child is placed supine, resting on the occipital area of the skull, neck flexion can occur. If the

spine board has a pediatric head well, this problem is eliminated. If the spine board does not have a pediatric well, the torso should be elevated with a folded blanket or sheet to maintain neutral position of the head and neck. The child's torso should be restrained on the spine board using straps or tape.

The cervical collar should be fitted so that neck flexion or extension is prevented. If the collar is too large, neck flexion and airway obstruction can occur.

If intubation is required, at least one rescuer will be required to immobilize the head and neck during the intubation attempt. The child's torso should also be immobilized with straps or restraints. During the intubation attempt, the rescuer responsible for the cervical spine immobilization should prevent head and neck flexion, extension, or other movement but should not attempt to place traction on the cervical spine.

Resuscitation   SCI may produce significant vasodilation that may persist for 24 to 48 hours following the injury. Fluid administration will be required to ensure adequate intravascular volume relative to this expanded vascular space. This fluid is usually provided in the form of boluses of isotonic crystalloids. Hypotonic fluids should not be used for volume resuscitation and are generally avoided in the patient with multisystem trauma and head injury. The fluid is titrated to maintain effective systemic perfusion and urine output. Vasopressors may be needed to ensure that blood pressure is adequate.

Steroids   Steroid administration within the first 8 hours after injury is now advocated to prevent secondary spinal cord edema and inflammation. Large-dose methylprednisolone administration (bolus of 30 mg/kg, then continuous infusion of 5.4 mg/kg/hr for 23 hours) may increase functional recovery in adult patients with SCI. Although similar results have not been documented in children, this form of steroid administration has become standard.

Tongs and Traction   Cervical spinal injury is often stabilized with Gardner-Wells tongs or halo traction until spinal fusion is accomplished electively several weeks after the injury. Weight is added to the traction device until the vertebral bodies are aligned. Provide analgesia if the child is awake and responsive, since weight addition will cause discomfort. Monitor movement and sensation closely to ensure that all function and sensation is preserved as traction is added, and notify a physician immediately of any deterioration. Once the vertebral bodies are aligned, the traction is maintained for several weeks, although use of a halo vest will enable limited ambulation.

Indications for Urgent Surgery Indications for urgent surgical intervention in the child with SCI include:

- Neurologic deterioration (ascending paralysis or sensory loss)
- Extremely unstable vertebral injury (particularly likely in children <3 years of age)
- Spine that cannot be aligned with traction (or alignment does not persist)

Intracranial Tumors

Etiology/Pathophysiology

Primary brain tumors are the most common form of cancer in children and adolescents, accounting for approximately 20% of all childhood neoplasms. Improved survival among children with intracranial tumors has been achieved within the past decade as a result of cooperative group trials of therapeutic protocols.

Tumors can arise from any tissue in the body, but most tumors of childhood arise from the inappropriate development of primitive neuroepithelial cells. Although the cause is unknown, the role of genetic predisposition and environmental factors continues to be explored.

Intracranial tumors produce an increase in intracranial volume, and increased ICP develops unless the skull can expand commensurately. Expansion into and compression of adjacent brain tissue can also compromise cerebral functions. Tumors are classified by location (supratentorial vs. infratentorial), by cell type, and by degree of malignancy (Box 8-12). It is important to note that tumors can be malignant by either cell type or position.

Supratentorial Tumors The two most common supratentorial tumors in children are astrocytomas

and craniopharyngiomas. *Astrocytomas* arise from abnormal proliferation of cerebral astrocytes. They can develop in the frontal, temporal, and central parietal areas of the cerebral hemispheres, or they can invade the brain stem or third ventricle, causing hydrocephalus. Astrocytomas can be slow or fast growing and are graded on a scale of 1 to 4 based on the degree of cell differentiation present in the tumor.

Craniopharyngiomas result from the growth of displaced neuroepithelial cells and develop within or just above the sella turcica or within the third ventricle. Growth of the craniopharyngioma can obstruct the foramen of Monro, the optic chiasm, the pituitary gland, or the hypothalamus.

Infratentorial Tumors Infratentorial tumors are usually detected early in their development, since clinical signs develop when they compress vital structures.

Medulloblastomas are the most malignant of the posterior fossa tumors because they grow rapidly and tend to recur after surgical excision. They are diagnosed most commonly in children 1 to 5 years of age. They arise from neuroepithelial cells and extend from the medulla into the fourth ventricle, subarachnoid space, third ventricle, or spinal column along CSF pathways.

Astrocytomas are a relatively common type of brain tumor. They are located either in the cerebellum, where they are usually benign and operable, or confined to the pons, where they are usually malignant and fatal. The mean age at diagnosis is 7 years.

Ependymomas arise from neuroepithelial cells and most frequently grow into and obstruct the fourth ventricle.

Clinical Presentation

Intracranial tumors may grow to a large size without producing symptoms until they invade vital brain tissue or cause increased ICP. In children up to 12 years of age, the skull may expand to accommodate a gradual increase in intracranial volume.

General signs of intracranial tumor during childhood include signs of increased ICP, headache, emesis, anorexia, ataxia, cranial nerve palsies, nystagmus, paresis, seizure activity, and hydrocephalus. Specific signs of increased ICP caused by an intracranial tumor include papilledema, an altered LOC, visual disturbances (diplopia and blurring of

Box 8-12

Pediatric Central Nervous System Tumors Classified by Location and Clinical Signs

Classification of Central Nervous System Tumors by Location

Supratentorial tumors
- Hemispheres: astrocytoma, sarcoma, meningioma
- Midline tumors: craniopharyngioma, optic glioma, pinealoma, ependymoma

Infratentorial tumors
- Cerebellar and fourth ventricle: astrocytoma, medulloblastoma, ependymoma
- Brain stem: brain stem glioma

Spinal cord tumors: ependymoma, astrocytoma

Generalized disease with brain tumor components: von Recklinghausen disease, tuberous sclerosis, Sturge-Weber disease, von Hippel-Lindau disease, ataxia telangiectasia, nevoid basal cell carcinoma syndrome

Metastatic tumors

Brain Tumor Localization and Associated Clinical Changes

Frontal lobe tumors
- Often asymptomatic until late
- Symptoms of increased intracranial pressure (ICP) or generalized or focal seizures may appear
- Personality changes, behavioral problems
- Gait problems, paresis, urinary incontinence, speech disorders
- Altered reflexes: tonic plantar reflex, grasp reflex, Babinski's sign

Parietal Lobe Tumors
- Tend to be symptomatic before frontal lobe tumors
- Symptoms of increased ICP
- Visual disturbances, papilledema
- Loss of memory or spatial disorientation
- Altered reflexes: Babinski's sign

Temporal lobe tumors
- Speech disorders likely if tumor involves left hemisphere
- Hearing disorders and tinnitus
- Loss of smell
- Hallucinations, dreams, space perception disturbances
- Altered reflexes: contralateral to tumor

Occipital tumors
- Loss of vision, nystagmus
- Seizures
- Tingling or (later) weakness
- Somatosensory disturbances, visual phenomena
- Altered reflexes: uncommon until late

Modified from Van Eys J: Malignant tumors of the central nervous system. In Sutow WW, Fernbach OJ, Vietti TJ, editors: *Clinical pediatric oncology*, ed 3, St Louis, 1984; Nelson DF et al: Central nervous system tumors. In Rubin P, editor: *Clinical oncology: a multidisciplinary approach for physicians and students*, ed 7, Philadelphia, 1993, WB Saunders; and Hazinski MF: *Nursing care of the critically ill child*, ed 2, St Louis, 1992, Mosby.

---

vision), headache, and emesis. The headache is characteristically intermittent but progressive. It tends to be present on awakening and is often associated with vomiting but not nausea. Infants with intracranial tumors will develop a bulging anterior fontanelle, and torticollis or nuchal rigidity may be present.

Some clinical signs may enable localization of the tumor in the intracranial vault. These localizing signs include:

- *Strabismus, diplopia, or blurring of vision:* Compression of cranial nerve VI or lateral brain herniation

- *Ataxia or nystagmus:* Compression or erosion of the cerebellum
- *Paresis:* Compression of the brain stem or pyramidal tract
- *Hydrocephalus:* Obstruction of a CSF pathway
- *Seizures:* Rarely an early sign of an intracranial tumor but can develop late

Signs of the tumor may be apparent on physical examination, particularly if cranial nerve function and visual fields are carefully evaluated and evidence of increased ICP (including papilledema) is recognized. The MRI has become the diagnostic tool of choice for detection and localization of brain tumors in the brain stem, posterior fossa, and spinal cord. CT scans complement the information obtained by MRI. Plain skull radiographs are usually not helpful, although they occasionally demonstrate characteristic changes associated with some tumors (e.g., calcification near the sella turcica by a craniopharyngioma). Arteriography may be used to further define the tumor.

Management

Care of the child with an intracranial tumor requires treatment of intracranial hypertension, surgical resection, if possible, and antineoplastic therapy (including radiation and chemotherapy). Critical care is usually required following neurosurgery or for management of sepsis or other complications of chemotherapy-induced immunosuppression (see Chapter 11).

The child and family require long-term physical and emotional support. Two excellent texts are cited in the Suggested Readings for more detailed review of the pathophysiology, treatment, and prognosis of these childhood cancers (Fochtman and Foley, 1995; Schwartz et al, 1993).

Meningitis

Etiology/Pathophysiology

Meningitis is an acute inflammation of the meninges and CSF. It may result from progression of an upper respiratory tract infection, otitis media, or bacteremia. It may also complicate a neurosurgical procedure or skull fracture with a dural tear or perforation. Neonatal meningitis typically results from transmission of maternal gastrointestinal or genital tract infection or from transmission from caregivers (including hospital personnel).

The infection is associated with development of a purulent exudate over the surface of the brain. Cerebrovascular endothelial damage can produce cerebral vasculitis, thrombosis, or infarction. Cerebral microthrombi and vasculitis can compromise cortical blood flow and produce extravascular fluid movement, contributing to cerebral edema and possibly to subdural effusion. Edema or scarring of the outlet of the third ventricle produces stenosis of the

Sylvian aqueduct and results in obstruction to CSF flow and hydrocephalus.

Clinical Presentation

The history and physical examination in *infants,* particularly those younger than 3 to 6 months of age, are often nonspecific. Unusual irritability or lethargy is often reported and may be associated with poor feeding, vomiting, fever, and seizures. Infants may demonstrate a high-pitched cry. If the ICP is high, the anterior fontanelle is full. The presence of nuchal rigidity (stiff neck) provides an index of suspicion but is often absent.

Children with meningitis often demonstrate signs of meningeal irritation, including complaints of headache, sore neck, and photophobia, and caregivers may notice increased irritability or lethargy. Nonprojectile vomiting, altered respiratory pattern (including apnea), Kernig's sign (pain with leg extension), and Brudzinski's sign (flexion of the neck stimulates flexion of the knees and hips) may also be present.

The condition of the infant or child with meningitis may deteriorate rapidly, progressing from fever and irritability to seizures, decreased LOC, and coma. Bacteremia or sepsis and septic shock may complicate the clinical picture (see discussion of shock, p. 140); thus appropriate cultures and therapy will be required.

The lumbar puncture is the definitive diagnostic test for meningitis (Table 8-14). A serum complete blood count (CBC) and glucose concentration are obtained before the lumbar puncture. CSF characteristics may enable differentiation of the various causes of meningitis:

- *Bacterial meningitis:* CSF is often cloudy, with low CSF glucose concentration (<50% serum glucose), high protein concentration, and >100 white blood cells/mm^3 (particularly neutrophils). Culture is positive. Gram stain is positive.
- *Viral or fungal meningitis:* CSF glucose concentration is normal, and CSF protein is only slightly elevated.
- *Aseptic meningitis:* Moderate or large number of cells (especially polymorphonuclear leukocytes early and lymphocytes late). Gram stain is negative. Viral culture may be positive.

Table 8-14

Cerebrospinal Fluid Analysis in Bacterial and Viral Meningitis

	Normal				
	Preterm	**Term**	**>6 Mo**	**Bacterial**	**Viral**
Cell Count (WBC/mm^3)*					
Mean	9	8	0	>500	<500
Range	0-25	0-22	0-4		
Predominant cell type	Lymph	Lymph	Lymph	80% PMN leukocyte	PMN leukocyte initially; lymphocyte later
Glucose (mg/dl)					
Mean	50	52	>40	<40	>40
Range	24-63	34-119			
Protein (mg/dl)					
Mean	115	90	<40	>100	<100
Range	65-150	20-170			
CSF/blood glucose (%)					
Mean	74	81	50	<40	>40
Range	55-150	44-248	40-60		
Tests					
Gram stain	Negative	Negative	Negative	Positive†	Negative
Bacterial culture	Negative	Negative	Negative	Positive‡	Negative

From Barkin RM, Rosen P: *Emergency pediatrics: a guide to ambulatory care,* ed 3, St Louis, 1990, Mosby.

*Total WBC/mm^3 by age in the normal child can be further delineated as follows (mean $\pm$ 2 SD): <6 wk: 3.7 $\pm$ 6.8; 6 wk-3 mo: 2.9 $\pm$ 5.7; 3-6 mo: 1.9 $\pm$ 4.0; 6-12 mo: 2.6 $\pm$ 4.9; > 12 mo: 1.9 $\pm$ 5.4.

†If Gram stain is negative, a methylene blue stain may distinguish intracellular bacteria from nuclear material.

‡85% of partially treated patients will have a positive Gram stain and >95% will have positive cultures. Counterimmunoelectrophoresis may be helpful if the culture is negative.

Management

If the infant or child is critically ill, support of the airway, ventilation, and perfusion is essential. *Eradication of bacterial meningitis, however, requires prompt initiation and uninterrupted administration of appropriate IV antimicrobial agents.* Quickly establish and carefully maintain IV access. Broad-spectrum antibiotics are administered until results of Gram stain and cultures and sensitivities are obtained; the antibiotics are then modified accordingly (Table 8-15).

Evaluation of systemic perfusion and neurologic function should be performed frequently until the child is stable. Report any deterioration in either systemic perfusion or neurologic function immediately to a physician. If septic shock complicates the meningitis, it will require aggressive fluid resuscitation (using isotonic crystalloids), as well as vasopressor and possibly inotropic therapy. Oxygenation and ventilation must also be supported, and it may be necessary to sedate the patient and take over the work of breathing. Fever should be treated with antipyretics.

Antibiotic therapy is essential for successful treatment of bacterial meningitis and should begin immediately. If the antibiotics are effectively treating the meningitis, the child's neurologic function should improve. Deterioration in neurologic func-

Table 8-15
Antibiotic Management of Bacterial Meningitis

<2 mo

Unknown etiology	Ampicillin 100-200 mg/kg/24 hr q4-6h IV *and* cefotaxime (or equivalent) 100-150 mg/kg/24 hr q8-12h IV; or ampicillin *and* gentamicin 5-7.5 mg/kg/24 hr q8-12h IV (or tobramycin 4-6 mg/kg/24 hr q8-12h IV)
E. coli	Chloramphenicol 50-100 mg/kg/24 hr q6h IV or cefotaxime, as above; treat 21 days or longer
Group B streptococci	Penicillin G 150,000-250,000 units/kg/24 hr q4-6h IV *and* gentamicin, as above; treat 14 days or longer
L. monocytogenes	Ampicillin, as above; treat 14 days or longer

2 mo-9 yr

Unknown etiology	Cefotaxime 200 mg/kg/24 hr q6h IV (or ceftriaxone 100 mg/kg/24 hr q12h IV or cefuroxime 200 mg/kg/24 hr q6h IV); or ampicillin 200-400 mg/kg/24 hr q4h IV *and* chloramphenicol 100 mg/kg/24 hr q6h IV (rarely used)
H. influenzae	Cefotaxime 200 mg/kg/24 hr q6h IV (or ceftriaxone 100 mg/kg/24 hr q12h IV or cefuroxime 200 mg/kg/24 hr q6h IV or ceftizoxime 200 mg/kg/24 hr q6-8h IV); or ampicillin 200-400 mg/kg/24 hr q4h IV *and* chloramphenicol 100 mg/kg/24 hr q6h IV (rarely used); treat 10 days
S. pneumoniae†	Penicillin G 250,000 units/kg/24 hr q4h IV; treat 10 days
N. meningitidis	Penicillin G 250,000 units/kg/24 hr q4h IV: treat 7-10 days

>9 yr

Unknown etiology	Penicillin G 250,000 units/kg/24 hr q4h IV*
S. pneumoniae†	Penicillin G 250,000 units/kg/24hr q4h IV*; treat 10 days
N. meningitidis	Penicillin G 250,000 units/kg/24 hr q4h IV*; treat 7-10 days

From Barkin RM: Meningitis, bacterial. In Barkin RM, editor: *Pediatric emergency medicine: concepts and clinical practice,* ed 2, St Louis, 1997, Mosby.
Serum concentration of chloramphenicol should be maintained at 10-25 μg/ml.
Duration of therapy in uncomplicated cases in children <2 mo of age is generally 14-21 days or longer. Older children may generally be treated for 10 days, depending on the response to therapy and the pathogen. Patients with complicated cases require longer duration.
*Adult: 10 million-20 million units/24 hr q4h IV.
†If resistance suspected, initiate vancomycin 40-60 mg/kg/24hr q6h IV.

tion suggests the development of increased ICP and additional complications of the meningitis, such as subdural effusions or cerebral edema. Increased ICP is treated with intubation and mechanical ventilation, support of oxygenation, maintenance of $PaCO_2$ at approximately 32 to 34 mm Hg, and osmotic diuresis (e.g., mannitol). For further information, see Increased Intracranial Pressure under Common Clinical Conditions, p. 394.

The incidence of *Haemophilus influenzae* meningitis has decreased dramatically following the introduction of an *H. influenzae* vaccine. However, the disease still occurs in nonimmunized children. Corticosteroid administration during the treatment of *H. influenzae* meningitis is thought to reduce the incidence of subsequent hearing loss. Dexamethasone (0.6 mg/kg/day) is usually admin-istered intravenously every 6 hours for the first 4 days of therapy, beginning shortly before or at the time of commencement of antibiotic therapy. The nurse should be alert for signs of gastrointestinal hemorrhage or secondary infection, which may complicate steroid administration. Use of dexamethasone in association with the treatment of other forms of (non-*H. influenzae*) meningitis is controversial (American Academy of Pediatrics, 1997).

The need for prophylactic antibiotic therapy for day care contacts of the child with *H. influenzae* infection is controversial and is left to the discretion of the child's physician. The day care management should instruct all parents to seek prompt medical attention if signs of meningitis develop in other children attending the day care program. The risk of *H. influenzae* type B infection is increased for any children less than 4 years of age living in the same home as the patient. Therefore, if any children do live in the home, Rifampin prophylaxis (for children >1 year, 20 mg/kg/day; maximum: 600 mg/dose) for 4 days is recommended by the American Academy of Pediatrics for all household contacts (including adults).

Prophylactic antibiotic administration is recommended for household, day care, and nursery school contacts of the patient with *Neisseria meningitidis* infection. These contacts should begin antibiotics within 24 hours of the patient's diagnosis. Prophylaxis is also recommended for anyone with intimate contact with the patient (including baby-sitters who may have kissed the child).

Encephalitis

Etiology/Pathophysiology

Encephalitis is an inflammation of the brain. It is often associated with other infections such as viral illness (most often herpes simplex), but it may be caused by arboviruses carried by arthropods (e.g., eastern or western equine encephalitis). These forms of encephalitis often occur in outbreaks during the summer and fall and most commonly affect children 5 to 14 years of age (see Arboviruses section in American Academy of Pediatrics: *Red Book*). Encephalitis may occasionally follow vaccination.

The term *encephalitis* is used to refer to an infectious or inflammatory cerebral disorder. The term *encephalopathy* is used to refer to any neurologic disorder of unknown or noninfectious cause associated with a change in level of consciousness, irritability, seizures, and motor or sensory deficit. This section refers to encephalitis alone. For hepatic encephalopathy, see p. 518.

The entrance of toxic or infectious agents into the brain produce an inflammatory response that is associated with cerebral edema, cellular damage, and transient neurologic dysfunction. The encephalitis may be present in association with meningitis.

Clinical Presentation

The child with encephalitis develops symptoms during or immediately after an acute viral illness or following exposure to a toxic or inflammatory agent. The child usually complains of a headache and photophobia and may demonstrate irritability, lethargy, a change in level of consciousness, or nuchal rigidity. Visual, auditory, or speech disturbances; seizures; or loss of consciousness may also develop. Seizures may be a presenting sign or may present several days (or even weeks or months) after diagnosis. High fever is not common.

Newborns with herpes encephalitis typically present at 9 to 11 days after birth and may present with sepsis or associated meningitis. Skin lesions may be present.

A lumbar puncture is usually performed to rule out a bacterial cause of the symptoms. It usually reveals a normal CSF pressure, normal or increased cell count, normal or slightly increased protein concentration, and normal glucose concentration. The CSF culture and Gram stain will yield no bacterial growth, but serologic studies may aid in the diagnosis of a viral agent, and detection of virus-specific IgM antibody in the CSF is diagnostic. An EEG (if performed) will reveal diffuse cortical inflammation, and a CT will fail to demonstrate a localized area of infection.

Management

Management of encephalitis is largely supportive. Children are usually admitted to the PICU for diagnostic studies and monitoring for 24 to 48 hours or until stable. The child is monitored closely for signs of neurologic deterioration, and analgesics may be prescribed to relieve persistent or severe headache. If at all possible, the child should be kept in a quiet room with reduced light.

If the encephalitis is secondary to a bacterial or fungal infection, it is treated with appropriate antimicrobial agents. Herpes or varicella encephalitis may be treated with antiviral agents (e.g., acyclovir: 45 mg/kg/day). For information about Lyme disease (a tick-borne infectious disease that may cause encephalitis) and sepsis and septic shock, see pp. 158 and 282.

Near-Drowning

Etiology/Pathophysiology

Each year, an estimated 4000 children die annually as a result of submersion. Many more times that number are left permanently neurologically devastated. Most pediatric near-drowning episodes are preventable, since most occur in the home while the child is under the supervision of an adult.

The pulmonary complications of submersion are summarized in Chapter 6. The following discussion addresses only the potential neurologic complications of submersion.

Within 3 minutes of submersion in warm water, most patients will develop sufficient hypoxia and cerebral ischemia to produce loss of consciousness. If submersion continues, CNS dysfunction develops, and the EEG eventually becomes flat. Further ischemia and hypoxia may produce brain death.

The hypoxia during submersion may not be sufficient to produce brain death at the time of submersion. However, it may be sufficient to result in profound cerebral cellular damage, which will result in later development of cytotoxic cerebral edema. This edema typically produces signs of increased ICP approximately 48 to 72 hours after the submersion episode.

The severity of neurologic sequelae following near-drowning is dependent on the duration of submersion, the temperature of the water, and the time that elapses before effective cardiopulmonary resuscitation (CPR) is provided. The time of submersion as reported by bystanders is notoriously unreliable, however; thus it is often impossible to guess the duration of cardiopulmonary arrest.

When very small children are submerged in very cold water, the diving reflex may be stimulated. This reflex results in initial apnea, loss of consciousness, bradycardia, hypertension, and shunting of blood to vital organs (and away from the skin and splanchnic vascular beds). This reflex may slow the metabolic rate and redistribute blood flow sufficiently to prevent profound neurologic injury. However, such "protection" can not be assured, and intact survival has been reported only occasionally in very small children submerged in icy ($<5°$ C) water.

Clinical Presentation

If the duration of submersion is extremely brief, the child may regain spontaneous respirations when pulled from the water. The stimulation of rescue and initial resuscitation maneuvers (shaking to determine responsiveness, opening the airway) may also result in return of spontaneous respirations. If submersion has lasted longer than 1 to 4 minutes,

however, most children will be apneic and flaccid when pulled from the water. If skilled CPR is immediately initiated, some of these children will demonstrate a perfusing cardiac rhythm and spontaneous respirations on arrival in the emergency department, and these children will usually recover. The presence of any spontaneous movement or posturing by the time of arrival in the first emergency department is also consistent with neurologic recovery.

However, if skilled resuscitation has been performed at the scene and during transport, and the *normothermic* child demonstrates *pulseless cardiac arrest on arrival in the emergency department,* it is extremely unlikely that neurologic recovery will occur. In the near-drowning literature, virtually all normothermic children who are asystolic on arrival in the emergency department die or survive in a persistent vegetative condition. Additional poor prognostic indicators include the presence of flaccid paralysis and absence of pupil response to light. If such children receive aggressive resuscitation in the emergency department and hospital, systemic perfusion may be restored, but the child is likely to remain in a persistent vegetative state. Therefore the need for aggressive or prolonged resuscitation should be carefully considered and recommendations made to the family. The family's wishes should also be ascertained.

Management

If the near-drowning victim is awake and responsive following resuscitation, further neurologic support is not required. The child should be closely monitored, and aggressive respiratory support may be required for the treatment of pulmonary complications (see Chapter 6).

If the child with severe neurologic injury is vigorously supported during the first hours after the near-drowning episode, some gasping respirations are likely to be observed within 12 to 24 hours. These respirations indicate perfusion of a portion of the brain stem but are not indicative of a good outcome. If these respirations are present, brain death pronouncement (and organ donation) is not possible.

Signs of increased ICP may develop within hours following submersion or may not develop for 48 to 72 hours after submersion. When results of ICP monitoring have been reported following near-drowning, virtually all children who demonstrated an ICP above 20 mm Hg died or survived with profound neurologic impairment. Aggressive therapy for the intracranial hypertension following submersion does not appear to change the outcome.

The parents of the near-drowning victim will need a great deal of compassionate support. If the child develops brain death, the parents should be offered the option of organ donation (see Brain Death and Organ Donation under Common Clinical Conditions, p. 411). Support of the parents is reviewed in Chapter 4.

Critical Illness Polyneuropathy

Etiology/Pathophysiology

Polyneuropathy and myopathy have been described in both adults and children following critical illness. This complication is described as a syndrome of muscle weakness that may include tetraplegia or prolonged dependence on mechanical ventilation. Electrophysiologic testing, when performed, has documented distal axonal nerve degeneration and denervation, and muscle atrophy. Once this syndrome develops, intensive physical therapy is required, and recovery, if it occurs, may require a year or longer.

The precise etiology of this problem is unclear. Although initially described in association with prolonged mechanical ventilation and sepsis, this syndrome has been reported in association with many conditions requiring critical care and prolonged mechanical ventilation. Most patients who develop this neuromyopathy have required prolonged bed rest, have received neuromuscular blockade (most often vecuronium), and have, in many cases, received additional drugs that may exert synergistic effects on the neuromuscular junction. Many—but not all—have developed sepsis in the course of their critical illness.

High-dose steroids have been shown to cause severe muscle atrophy and thus may contribute to the development of a neuromyopathy associated with neuromuscular blockade, particularly when the blockade is induced with aminosteroids such as pancuronium and vecuronium. Aminoglycoside antibiotics may potentiate the effects of neuromuscular blockade and contribute to the development of a neuromyopathy, because these antibiotics have intrinsic neuromuscular blocking effects of their own. Drugs such as furosemide and the benzodiazepines (midazolam and diazepam) also act synergistically with the neuromuscular blocking agents. Reduced renal clearance may contribute to the problem, reducing drug clearance. It is likely that an initial insult (e.g., trauma, surgery, infection) causes release of cytokines and alters perfusion to the neuromuscular junction, rendering this unit more susceptible to the effects of drugs such as steroids or aminoglycosides.

Management

The best way to treat this neuromyopathy of critical illness is to prevent it. If administration of neuromuscular blockade is anticipated, all medications the child is receiving should be reviewed, and, if possible, additional drugs likely to contribute to the neuromyopathy should be avoided. Although it may not be practical to avoid *all* drugs, modification of drug selection or the dosing regimen may be attempted. If concurrent steroid administration will be required (e.g., for a child with asthma or chronic lung disease), aminosteroid neuromuscular blocking agents (specifically pancuronium and vecuronium) should probably not be used, and agents such as doxacurium or atracurium, which do not contain steroids, should be considered instead. Paralyzing agents should be titrated to patient response, and peripheral nerve stimulators and the "train of four" response (see Chapter 3) should be used to prevent excessive administration of neuromuscular blockade. Passive range-of-motion exercises should be performed during periods of pharmacologic paralysis, and active range-of-motion exercises should be begun as soon as the patient is awake. It is important to note that this neuromyopathy of critical care may develop despite all attempts to prevent it. Aggressive physical therapy should be initiated as soon as the diagnosis is suspected.

Common Diagnostic Tests

One of the best methods of evaluating neurologic function is the clinical examination. However, the critically ill or injured child is often comatose, negating the value of much of the clinical examination. ICP monitoring may be helpful at these times (this form of monitoring is discussed on p. 383,

Intracranial Pressure and Volume Relationships, under Essential Anatomy and Physiology). In addition, a few diagnostic studies can provide important information about the child's diagnosis, clinical status, and prognosis.

Before any of these procedures is performed, the procedure should be explained to the child in age-appropriate terms. The child should receive analgesia appropriate for the procedure and the child's clinical condition, and the child must be closely monitored throughout the procedure.

Lumbar Puncture

Definition and Purpose

A lumbar puncture (LP) or spinal tap includes introduction of a needle into the subarachnoid space of the lumbar spinal cord. The needle is inserted with a stylet into the interspace between the third and fourth lumbar vertebrae.

The LP may be performed to measure CSF pressure, to examine the CSF, or to introduce medication, air, or radiopaque contrast material into the subarachnoid space. The LP will aid in the diagnosis of intracranial or intraventricular hemorrhage if blood is present in the CSF. The CSF can be sent for a Gram stain, cell count, and glucose and protein content to aid in the diagnosis of CNS infection or inflammation. In addition, anesthesia or antibiotics may be introduced into the subarachnoid space to reduce pain or treat infection. Finally, injected air or contrast material can be used to outline subarachnoid structures or identify CSF obstructions or leaks. In the PICU an LP is used most often to confirm the diagnosis of a CNS infection.

Procedure

Before the procedure the child is examined for signs of increased ICP. If increased ICP is present in the *infant,* the LP may proceed with caution if a CSF sample is absolutely necessary to treat the child's CNS disease. If signs of increased ICP are present in the *older child,* the LP may be postponed, because the sudden release of CSF and pressure that occurs during the LP may result in herniation of the brain stem through the foramen magnum.

The child is placed in the knee-chest position, usually lying on a side. The child must be held firmly to prevent excessive movement during the procedure. The back is draped, and the puncture area is identified and scrubbed with a surgical preparation. The remainder of the procedure is accomplished using sterile technique.

Lidocaine is instilled intradermally around the area of anticipated puncture, to provide analgesia. The needle and stylet are inserted firmly into the subarachnoid space; frequently the puncture of the dura is audible. Once the dura is pierced, the stylet is withdrawn. The opening CSF pressure (if obtained) is obtained at this time using a manometer.

CSF samples are obtained after a few drops of CSF are allowed to drain passively from the needle hub. CSF for microbiology is generally obtained in three tubes as follows:

- Tube 1: Culture and Gram stain analysis
- Tube 2: Protein and sugar analysis
- Tube 3: Cell count

Additional tubes are collected as needed for viral cultures or other studies.

A closing pressure may be obtained after the CSF has been collected.

The appearance of the CSF and the opening and closing pressures should be recorded on the patient's chart. The CSF may appear bloody as a result of a traumatic tap or as a result of intracranial or intraventricular hemorrhage. If the blood resulted from a traumatic tap, the CSF collected will be initially bloody and then should become progressively clearer as it is collected. If, however, the CSF is bloody as a result of an intracranial or intraventricular hemorrhage, the final CSF collected will still be bloody in appearance. Normal CSF content is listed in Table 8-4. CSF findings in meningitis are listed in Table 8-14.

Potential Complications

The most serious (although uncommon) complication of an LP is brain stem herniation. Therefore, during and after the LP, the child's neurologic status should be closely monitored. New signs of increased ICP or signs of deterioration in responsiveness should be reported to a physician immediately. Additional complications of an LP include severe headache and bleeding from the puncture site. Many physicians request that the child be kept in a reclining position for 4 to 6 hours after the procedure to reduce the risk of headache. Analgesics should be administered as needed.

Electroencephalography

Definition and Purpose

The electroencephalogram (EEG) is a recording of the electrical potentials that arise from the brain. These potentials can be quantified, localized, and compared with established normal EEGs for the patient's age to aid in the diagnosis of seizure activity or CNS injury or dysfunction. An isoelectric EEG in the absence of hypothermia or sedation is one of the criteria used to confirm brain death.

Procedure

The EEG is recorded by placement of approximately 17 to 21 electrodes on the surface of the scalp. The electrodes are fixed to the scalp with an acetone-soluble paste. A unique electrode placement is required if the EEG is performed to confirm brain death; thus the technician must be notified in advance if this form of EEG study will be required.

The EEG is performed when the patient is reclining and still. EEGs for critically ill patients are generally performed in the ICU. If the child is alert, sedation may be required.

The EEG is typically recorded continuously for 20 minutes; longer recordings will be necessary if additional studies (such as measurement of brain stem evoked potentials) are required. Extraneous or sudden noise or lights can stimulate cranial nerve activity; thus they should be minimized during the recording.

Potential Complications

There are no complications of the EEG procedure itself. The nurse must avoid touching the patient if possible. However, required nursing care activities always take priority, and the technician should be notified when the patient is touched.

Computed Tomography

Definition and Purpose

Computed tomography (CT), or computerized axial tomography (CAT), consists of a series of skull radiographs analyzed and reconstructed by a computer to form a pictorial image of the intracranial contents. The scan uses an x-ray beam in motion that obtains a series of radiographic films in a predetermined plane. These films are converted to images similar to those that would be produced if radiographs could be obtained of separate layers of the brain.

The CT scan is a noninvasive method of visualizing a variety of neurologic disorders, including space-occupying lesions, hematoma, hemorrhage, hydrocephalus, brain abscess, and cortical atrophy.

Procedure

The patient must be brought to the CT scanner, which is usually located in the radiology or emergency department. The child is positioned supine on a mobile platform that is then moved toward the scanner so that the child's head ultimately is positioned within the scanner. A portion of the scanner will move around the child's head so that the x-ray beam is directed at many different angles; hundreds of radiographs are obtained and reconstructed during the scan. The entire scan takes 20 to 30 minutes. Occasionally, contrast agents are administered intravenously immediately before the scan to enable better visualization of intracranial structures.

During the procedure, the nurse and x-ray technicians must be positioned behind a lead screen to minimize stray radiation exposure. This makes monitoring of the child's cardiorespiratory status difficult. If the child is extremely unstable, a heart rate monitor with alarms (and possibly ICP and pulse oximetry monitors) should be used.

Potential Complications

There are no complications associated with the CT scan itself. If contrast material is used, it carries the risk of sensitivity reaction. Extravasation of the contrast will produce a tissue burn.

Magnetic Resonance Imaging

Definition and Purpose

Magnetic resonance imaging (MRI) is the application of a strong external magnetic field around the patient. This magnetic field causes rotation of the cell nuclei in a predictable direction at a predictable speed. The result of the rotation of the nuclei is a resonant image that is extremely well defined and will enable visualization of soft tissues better than any other noninvasive device.

The patient is placed on a movable gurney and is slid into the tube. The MRI moves around the patient. The patient must remain still during the procedure, and sedation may be required.

Procedure

The MRI scanner is usually located well away from critical care units. At present, scanning can only be performed on relatively stable patients because no metal-constructed mechanical devices may be placed in proximity to the magnetic field. Totally plastic mechanical ventilators are available for use in the MRI scanner, but monitoring systems cannot be used. Thus the MRI is most often used for children recovering from critical illness or injury.

Potential Complications

The MRI does not use any radiation; thus there are no complications related to radiation exposure or to the MRI itself. The most challenging aspect of care is the monitoring of the patient during the scan.

Cerebral Angiography

Definition and Purpose

Cerebral angiography uses an injected radiopaque contrast agent to visualize the cerebral circulation. The progress of the contrast material through the cerebral circulation is recorded with radiographs for further study.

Procedure

Contrast material is injected into a selected cerebral vessel—usually into the internal carotid artery. The sequential radiographs are obtained in the radiology department.

Potential Complications

A reaction to the contrast agent can occur following angiography; this can produce fever, a rash, and hypotension similar to signs of anaphylaxis. If an active cerebral hemorrhage is present or develops during the procedure, the contrast agent can enter cerebral tissue, producing a cerebrovascular accident (stroke), seizures, increased ICP, cerebral arterial thrombosis, dysphagia, or visual disturbances.

In addition, injection of the contrast material directly into the internal carotid artery may stimulate the carotid baroreceptors, causing compensatory bradycardia and hypotension.

Quantitative Cerebral Blood Flow Studies

Definition and Purpose

Cerebral blood flow (CBF) may be quantified using cold xenon to enhance a CT scan, enabling evaluation of regional and global CBF. This technique is most useful to evaluate trends in regional blood flow with changes in the patient's condition or therapy.

CBF may also be calculated through continuous monitoring of cerebral venous oxyhemoglobin saturation. This continuous monitoring may be accomplished using a fiberoptic catheter. The fiberoptics in the catheter transmit light and capture light that is reflected from hemoglobin molecules. A microprocessor calculates the hemoglobin saturation based on differences in light reflection between oxygenated hemoglobin and nonoxygenated hemoglobin. A decrease in cerebral venous oxygen saturation will result from a decrease in cerebral oxygen delivery or an increase in cerebral oxygen consumption. Cerebral oxygen delivery decreases if the arterial oxygen content or CBF decreases. If arterial oxygen content is unchanged and cerebral oxygen consumption is presumed to be stable, a decrease in cerebral venous oxygen saturation is thought to indicate a decrease in CBF. A cerebral venous oxygen saturation below 50% has been linked with a poor prognosis in some adult studies.

Procedure

Cold xenon tomography requires inhalation of cold xenon and performance of a CT scan. The xenon is distributed rapidly and disappears within a few minutes.

The calculation of cerebral venous oxygen saturation requires insertion of a fiberoptic catheter into the jugular venous bulb. The fiberoptic must be calibrated before insertion.

Potential Complications

There have been no significant complications associated with cold xenon blood flow analysis. The xenon may have a sedative effect on the patient; therefore the patient's airway and ventilation must be monitored closely. The xenon may also affect cerebrovascular resistance and blood flow, although such effects are usually minimal.

Complications of fiberoptic monitoring of cerebral venous oxygen saturation are those of central venous catheterization.

Suggested Readings

American Academy of Pediatrics Committee on Infectious Diseases: *1997 Red Book: Report of the Committee on Infectious Diseases,* ed 24, Elk Grove, Ill, 1997, American Academy of Pediatrics.

Bernard SA, Jones BMacC, Horne MK: Clinical trial of induced hypothermia in comatose survivors of out-of-hospital cardiac arrest, *Ann Emerg Med* 30:146-153, 1997.

Bolton CF: Sepsis and the systemic inflammatory response syndrome: neuromuscular manifestations, *Crit Care Med* 24:1408-1416, 1996.

Chestnut RM, Prough DS: Critical care of severe head injury, *New Horizons* 3(3):365-593, 1995.

Deresiewicz RL et al: Clinical and neuroradiographic manifestations of eastern equine encephalitis, *N Engl J Med* 336:1867-1874, 1997.

Fochtman D, Foley GV, editors: *Nursing care of the child with cancer,* ed 3, Philadelphia, 1995, Saunders.

Gaskill SJ, Marlin AE: *Handbook of pediatric neurology and neurosurgery,* Boston, 1993, Little, Brown.

Hund EF et al: Critical illness polyneuropathy: clinical findings and outcomes of a frequent cause of neuromuscular weaning failure, *Crit Care Med* 24:1328-1333, 1996.

Lang DA et al: Diffuse brain swelling after head injury: more often malignant in adults than children? *J Neurosurg* 80:675-680, 1994.

Marion DW et al: The use of moderate therapeutic hypothermia for patients with severe head injuries: a preliminary report, *J Neurosurg* 79:354-362, 1993.

Muckart DJJ, Bhagwanjee S: American College of Chest Physicians/Society of Critical Care Medicine Consensus definitions of the systemic inflammatory response syndrome and allied disorders in relation to critically injured patients, *Crit Care Med* 25:1789-1795, 1997.

Schutzman SA et al: Epidural hematomas in children, *Ann Emerg Med* 22:535-541, 1993.

Schwartz CL et al: *Pediatric solid tumors.* In Rubin P, editor: Clinical oncology: a multidisciplinary approach for physicians and students, ed 7, Philadelphia, 1993, Saunders.

Sheinberg M et al: Continuous monitoring of jugular venous oxygen saturation in head-injured patients, *J Neurosurg* 76:212-217, 1992.

Shiozaki T et al: Effect of mild hypothermia on uncontrollable intracranial hypertension after severe head injury, *J Neurosurg* 79:363-368, 1993.

Simma B et al: A prospective randomized and controlled study of fluid management in children with severe head injury: lactated Ringer's solution versus hypertonic saline, *Crit Care Med* 26:1265-1270, 1998.

Steingrub JS, Mundt DJ: Blood glucose and neurologic outcome with global brain ischemia, *Crit Care Med* 24:802-806, 1996.

9 Renal Disorders

Cathy Headrick, Mary Fran Hazinski,
Jeannette Kennedy Alexander

Pearls

◆ The normal volume of hourly urine output in children is small, and a small compromise in urine volume may indicate a significant compromise in renal perfusion or function.

◆ Urine output will decrease if cardiac output and renal blood flow are compromised.

◆ Renal failure may be present in a child with a low, "normal," or high volume of urine output.

◆ Accurate measurement of urine volume and composition provide fundamental data on which clinical decisions are made.

◆ Renal replacement therapies differ significantly in their ability to eliminate excess intravascular fluid, restore electrolyte imbalance, and eliminate toxins. In addition, these therapies differ in potential complications. The nurse must be aware of the differences between and among these therapies.

Additional Helpful Chapters

Chapter 5: Cardiovascular Vascular Disorders (Shock)
Chapter 6: Respiratory Disorders (Acid-Base Disorders)
Chapter 10: Gastrointestinal Disorders (Dehydration and Fluid Balance)

Introduction

The kidney is the organ most responsible for maintaining fluid and electrolyte homeostasis. It continuously adjusts extracellular fluid volume, solute concentration, and pH. It secretes organic acids, bases, and most ingested food additives and chemicals. It participates in maintaining calcium-phosphorus-parathormone balance, participates in erythropoietin and red blood cell synthesis, and contributes to a variety of feedback systems. These functions are performed simultaneously, and interactions among these various renal functions often occur.

Essential Anatomy and Physiology

Kidney Structure and Gross Anatomy

The kidneys lie anterior and lateral to the twelfth thoracic and first, second, and third lumbar vertebrae. The kidneys are located behind the abdominal peritoneum; thus they are retroperitoneal structures. The left kidney usually is slightly higher than the right kidney. A longitudinal section of the kidney shows the three general areas of renal structure: the cortex, the medulla, and the pelvis. The *cortex* contains all of the glomeruli, the proximal and distal convoluted tubules, and the first portions of the loop of Henle and the collecting ducts. The renal *medulla* is composed of collecting ducts that grow progressively larger as they approach the renal pelvis. The renal *pelvis* is the expanded upper end of the ureter; it subdivides to form the major and minor calyces. These calyces receive urine that will flow from the kidney via the ureter to the bladder. The functioning unit of the kidney is the nephron, which consists of a vascular component, a tubular component, and the collecting ducts (Figure 9-1).

Vascular Component

The renal arteries branch from the aorta at the level of the second and third lumbar vertebrae; together they receive 20% of the total cardiac output. These vessels divide into arterioles, which either deliver nutrients to the renal medulla, cortical tissue, and capsule or enter the glomerular capsule. These glomerular arterioles contribute to formation of urine.

The afferent arteriole enters the glomerular capsule and divides to form the *glomerulus,* a tuft of capillaries that allows filtration through the capillary membranes. The glomerular capillaries reform into a second arteriole called the efferent arteriole (Figure 9-2). Constriction or dilation of the afferent or efferent arterioles will alter the resistance to flow through the glomerular capillaries and thus will regulate glomerular filtration.

After leaving the glomerulus, the efferent arterioles form a network of capillaries that surround the convoluted tubules and loop of Henle. These peritubular capillaries then converge into venules that return renal venous blood to the systemic circulation via the inferior vena cava.

Tubular Component

Filtered fluid from the glomerulus will enter the tubules at Bowman's capsule (see Figure 9-1), a single layer of flat epithelial cells in the renal cortex that surrounds the glomerulus. From Bowman's capsule the fluid flows through the proximal convoluted tubule (PCT), the loop of Henle, and the distal convoluted tubule (DCT).

Collecting Ducts

Small collecting ducts carry filtrate to the renal medulla, where they join other small ducts to form larger ducts, which in turn drain into a minor calyx in the renal pelvis. Ultimately, fluid from the renal pelvis will flow into the ureter and will enter the bladder.

Glomerular Function

Net filtration pressure (NFP) within the nephron is the difference between forces *favoring* filtration (largely resulting from capillary hydrostatic pressure) and forces *opposing* filtration (caused by intravascular colloid osmotic pressure and the hydrostatic pressure within Bowman's capsule).

NFP = Forces favoring filtration −
        Forces opposing filtration

NFP = Capillary hydrostatic pressure −
  Intravascular colloid osmotic pressure and
  Bowman's capsule hydrostatic pressure

In the kidney, vascular resistance changes to maintain a relatively constant blood flow and pres-

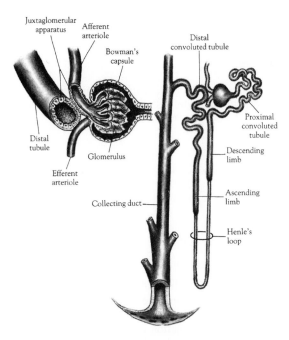

Figure 9-1 Components of the nephron. (From Thompson JM et al: *Mosby's manual of clinical nursing,* ed 3, St Louis, 1993, Mosby.)

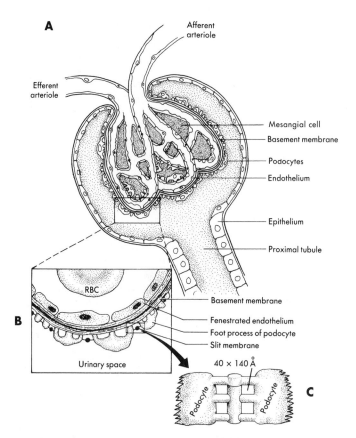

Figure 9-2   **A,** Anatomy of the glomerulus. **B,** Cross section through the glomerulus showing glomerular capillaries, endothelium, basement membrane, and podocytes of the epithelium. **C,** Enlarged view of the filtration membrane. (From Berne RM, Levy MN: *Physiology,* ed 2, St Louis, 1982, Mosby.)

sure through the kidneys across a range of arterial pressures and blood flows. When mean arterial pressure increases, the afferent arterioles constrict; this constriction restricts renal blood flow and prevents transmission of the entire increase in arterial pressure to the glomerulus. When arterial pressure falls, the sympathetic innervation to the afferent and efferent arterioles increases arterial tone and the resistance to flow into and out of the glomerulus. This change in arterial resistance can maintain the glomerular filtration rate at near-normal levels despite a fall in renal blood flow.

The ability to respond to changes in flow into and out of the glomerulus allows the kidney to maintain solute and volume regulation at relatively constant levels despite changes in systemic arterial blood pressure and renal blood flow; this ability is termed "autoregulation." When arterial pressure is extremely high or low, however, autoregulation will fail and renal blood flow becomes simply proportional to arterial pressure.

Glomerular Filtration Rate

Renal function can be evaluated by calculating the glomerular filtration rate (GFR). The GFR is roughly equivalent to the creatinine clearance, provided that renal function is not severely impaired. Creatinine clearance is calculated using simultaneous measurements of the concentration of creatinine in the plasma and in the urine. The relationship between the plasma and urine concentrations of creatinine (Cr), the urine volume formed per unit of time, and the GFR is expressed as follows:

$$GFR = \frac{Urine\ (Cr) \times Volume\ of\ urine\ per\ minute}{Plasma\ (Cr)}$$

There are several factors that can affect the relationship of urine creatinine, serum creatinine, and urine volume. For example, the relationship is not valid in the presence of severe renal dysfunction. In addition, laboratory determination of serum creatinine concentration may be affected by some cephalosporin antibiotics. For this reason, the serum creatinine level should be drawn when drug levels are at their lowest.

The GFR is expressed in milliliters per minute per square meter of body surface area (BSA). This enables direct comparison of the renal function of children and adults, despite a difference in size. The child's GFR is approximately 55 to 65 ml/min/m^2 and will approach adult values (120 ml/min/1.73 m^2) by 3 years of age.

Tubular Function

Solute Reabsorption and Secretion

If kidney function were limited to plasma ultrafiltration, urine formation would deplete the body of vital solutes and water. To modify the volume and content of the ultrafiltrate before it is eliminated, the tubules selectively reabsorb and secrete substances.

Substances are both actively and passively reabsorbed from the renal tubular fluid, through the tubular luminal cell membrane, into the interstitial fluid. These substances then pass into the adjacent peritubular capillaries for return to the systemic venous circulation. Reabsorbed substances include sodium, chloride, bicarbonate, and water.

Reabsorption of many substances from the renal tubules is limited to a maximum quantity over time; this *transport maximum* can be influenced by hormones or drugs. The active reabsorption of some substances is limited by the capacity of the active transport tubular carriers. The *renal threshold* of a substance is the serum or plasma and filtrate concentration at which some of the active transport tubular carriers become saturated with the substance, so that some of that substance begins to appear in the urine. For example, under normal conditions, all glucose is reabsorbed by the tubules and returned to the blood, and no glucose is present in urine. However, once the serum glucose concentration exceeds approximately 180 mg/dl (the renal threshold for glucose), some glucose tubular carriers will be saturated, and glucose will begin to appear in the urine.

The *proximal tubule* is largely responsible for the reabsorption of water and electrolytes; it neither concentrates nor dilutes the urine. The proximal tubule reabsorbs 65% of the filtered sodium and water, almost 100% of the filtered glucose and amino acids, 65% of the filtered potassium, and 90% of the bicarbonate and phosphate.

Although most substances enter the tubules through filtration at the glomerulus, other substances can actually be *secreted* into the urine by the tubules. Substances dissolved in the serum of the peritubular capillaries cross into the tubular cell and are actively or passively transported into the tubular lumen to be excreted in the urine. Substances commonly secreted by the tubules include organic acids and bases, food additives, and many drugs and chemicals.

Water Balance and Urine Concentration

The function of the loop of Henle is to remove additional solute and water from the ultrafiltrate. Using a countercurrent mechanism, the loop of Henle adjusts the filtrate osmolality. The distal tubule is the site for final adjustments in the urine sodium and potassium content for urine concentration. The final urine concentration is determined in the distal tubule and collecting ducts. Urine concentration depends on the active transport of sodium out of the distal tubule and the relative permeability of the collecting ducts to water.

The transport of sodium in the distal tubule is dependent on the volume and character of the fluid from the loop of Henle. It is also influenced by the hormones renin, aldosterone, and antidiuretic hormone (ADH). Aldosterone is responsible for reabsorption of a small but significant portion of the sodium filtrate; increased aldosterone levels increase the active reabsorption of sodium, which produces water reabsorption. Increased aldosterone levels also decrease potassium reabsorption.

ADH is produced in the hypothalamus, chiefly in response to an increase in serum osmolality. In the presence of ADH, the distal tubules and collecting ducts become highly permeable to water; water is reabsorbed and urine volume is reduced and concentration is increased. The reabsorption of water will reduce the serum osmolality and should then reduce ADH secretion. Low ADH levels (neurogenic diabetes insipidus) or decreased renal response to ADH (nephrogenic diabetes insipidus) will decrease water reabsorption and result in the secretion of large quantities of dilute urine (Figure 9-3) and progressive hemoconcentration.

Electrolyte Balance

The kidneys regulate the serum concentrations of sodium, potassium, phosphate, calcium, and magnesium through alterations in the reabsorption of these electrolytes from the filtrate or secretion of these electrolytes into the urine (Table 9-1). The renal capacity to regulate electrolyte balance is compromised by a reduction in GFR and changes in volume status.

Acid-Base Balance

The kidneys regulate plasma pH and HCO_3^- concentration through hydrogen ion secretion, as well as bicarbonate reabsorption and reclamation in the proximal tubule. The kidneys can compensate for an acidotic or alkalotic condition, correcting the serum pH to near-normal levels. However, this compensation takes several hours to begin and will not be fully effective for several days (Box 9-1). In addition, *this compensation will never "overcorrect" the pH;* the stimulus for the compensation is eliminated once the pH approaches normal.

Table 9-1
Renal Response to Electrolyte Imbalances

Solute	Alteration	Renal Response
Potassium	Increase in intracellular potassium	Stimulates increased secretion and excretion of potassium
	Increase in plasma potassium	Stimulates adrenal cortex to secrete aldosterone, which promotes secretion and excretion of potassium
	Acidosis	Decreases potassium excretion; potassium shifts from cells into plasma
	Alkalosis	Increases potassium excretion; potassium shifts into cells
Phosphate	Decreased renal function	Decreases renal excretion of phosphates
	Increased tubular reabsorption of sodium	Decreases tubular reabsorption of phosphate
		Stimulates active absorption of phosphate (and calcium) by intestine
		Converts vitamin D to its active form (some conversion also occurs in the liver), which stimulates renal tubular reabsorption of phosphate and calcium
		Stimulates release of parathormone (PTH), which enhances intestinal absorption of calcium and phosphate
Calcium	Decreased plasma concentration	Stimulates release of PTH, which decreases renal excretion of calcium and increases urinary excretion of sodium
	Increased plasma concentration	Inhibits release of PTH
Magnesium	Increased extracellular fluid volume	Stimulates increased magnesium excretion
	Decreased extracellular fluid volume	Inhibits magnesium excretion

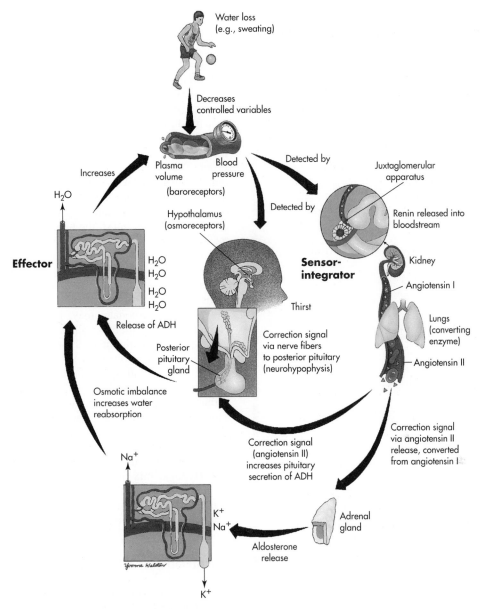

Figure 9-3 Cooperative roles of antidiuretic hormone (ADH) and aldosterone in regulating urine and plasma volume. A drop in blood pressure or plasma volume (e.g., dehydration) or a rise in serum osmolality triggers the hypothalamus to rapidly release ADH from the posterior pituitary gland. ADH increases water reabsorption by the kidney by increasing permeability of the distal tubules and collecting ducts to water. Hypotension is also detected by each nephron's juxtaglomerular apparatus, which responds by secreting renin. Renin triggers the formation of angiotensin II, which stimulates release of aldosterone from the adrenal cortex. Aldosterone then slowly boosts water reabsorption by the kidneys by increasing reabsorption of sodium. Because angiotensin II also stimulates secretion of ADH, it serves as an additional link between the ADH and aldosterone mechanisms. (From Thibodeau GA, Patton KT: *Anatomy and physiology,* ed 3, St Louis, 1996, Mosby.)

Rules for Assessment of Respiratory and Renal Compensatory Responses in Acid-Base Disturbances

Compensatory mechanisms bring pH *toward* but not *to* normal level.

If *respiratory* compensation is intact in metabolic disturbances:

1. $(HCO_3^-) + 15 = $ Last 2 digits of pH, or
2. $Paco_2 = $ Last 2 digits of pH

If *metabolic* compensation is intact in respiratory disturbances:

In *acute* respiratory *acidosis:*

$$\Delta(HCO_3^-) = 0.1 \times \Delta Paco_2$$

In *chronic* respiratory *acidosis:*

$$\Delta(HCO_3^-) = 0.35 \times \Delta Paco_2$$

In *acute* respiratory *alkalosis:*

$$\Delta(HCO_3^-) = 0.2 \times \Delta Paco_2$$

In *chronic* respiratory *alkalosis:*

$$\Delta(HCO_3^-) = 0.5 \times \Delta Paco_2$$

where Δ indicates the degree of deviation from normal value.

Renal Response in Acidosis

Potassium excretion increases
Chloride is reabsorbed with sodium
Excretion of bicarbonate

Renal Response in Alkalosis

Potassium excretion increases
Bicarbonate is reabsorbed with sodium
Chloride is excreted
Bicarbonate diffuses into plasma
Hydrogen ions are reabsorbed
Excretion of acids (e.g., ammonium) increases

From Ichikawa I, Narins RG, Harris HW Jr: Regulation of acid-base homeostasis. In Ichikawa I, editor: *Pediatric textbook of fluids and electrolytes,* Baltimore, 1990, Williams & Wilkins.

As metabolic acidosis develops, there is an increase in the hydrogen ion concentration in the proximal tubule. This is a major stimulus for increased bicarbonate reabsorption or reclamation in the proximal tubule. The hydrogen ion is secreted into the proximal tubule in exchange for a sodium ion. Inside the tubule the hydrogen ion combines with filtered bicarbonate to form carbonic acid and then quickly dissociates into carbon dioxide and water. The carbon dioxide diffuses back into the renal tubular cell, where it recombines with water to form carbonic anhydrase and then quickly dissociates into a hydrogen ion and bicarbonate. The bicarbonate diffuses out of the tubular cell, and ultimately into the plasma, while the hydrogen ion is again secreted into the renal tubule. This method of reclaiming bicarbonate ions results in a net reabsorption of filtered bicarbonate ions without a net reabsorption of hydrogen ions.

"New" bicarbonate may be formed when carbon dioxide combines with water, yielding carbonic acid. The carbonic acid then dissociates into hydrogen ions and bicarbonate. The hydrogen ion can be bound to phosphate buffers or ammonia to form hydrogen phosphate or ammonium, nonresorbable substances that are eliminated in the urine. This mechanism results in the formation of titratable acids.

Changes in serum potassium and chloride concentrations may also affect bicarbonate reabsorption. Hypokalemia and hypochloremia increase hydrogen ion concentration in the renal tubular cells; thus hydrogen ion secretion and bicarbonate reabsorption in the renal tubule are enhanced. This can produce hypokalemic or hypochloremic alkalosis.

Interpretation of Arterial Blood Gases   Interpretation of acid-base balance from arterial blood gas values requires evaluation of the pH in light of the arterial carbon dioxide tension ($Paco_2$), the base excess or deficit, and the serum bicarbonate concentration. If the pH is <7.35, acidosis is present; if it is >7.45, alkalosis is present. Although respiratory or renal compensation for acidosis or alkalosis may restore the pH to near-normal levels, it will not completely correct the pH, and compensatory mechanisms will never "overcorrect" the pH.

If an alteration in pH is present, the role of carbon dioxide tension in the pH alteration should be evaluated. This requires calculation of the predicted pH based on the existing $Paco_2$. For every uncompensated torr unit (or millimeter of mercury) rise in the $Paco_2$ above 45, the pH should fall 0.008 below 7.35. For every uncompensated torr unit fall in the $Paco_2$ below 35, the pH should rise 0.008 above 7.45. For ease of calculation, a normal pH of 7.4 and a normal $Paco_2$ of 40 mm Hg can be used (Box 9-2). If the actual pH is higher than that predicted from the $Paco_2$, metabolic alkalosis is present; if the actual pH is lower than that predicted from the $Paco_2$, metabolic acidosis is present. This calculation does not, however, enable distinction of the primary change from the compensatory change.

The base deficit or excess is a calculated value that normally ranges from -2 to $+2$. A base deficit more negative than -2 indicates the presence of metabolic acidosis or metabolic compensation for respiratory alkalosis. A base excess more positive than $+2$ indicates the presence of metabolic alkalosis or metabolic compensation for respiratory acidosis.

Evaluation of the Serum Bicarbonate Level The serum bicarbonate level is normally approximately 24 to 28 mmol/L. A serum bicarbonate level >28 mmol/L indicates metabolic alkalosis or metabolic compensation for respiratory acidosis. A serum bicarbonate level <24 mmol/L indicates metabolic acidosis or (less commonly) metabolic compensation for respiratory alkalosis.

Calculation and Evaluation of the Anion Gap The anion gap is the difference between the positively charged ions (cations, chiefly sodium and

---

Box 9-2

Systematic Arterial Blood Gas Analysis

1. Determine if the pH is acidotic, alkalotic, or normal. For simplicity, a normal pH of 7.4 is used (acidosis = pH < 7.4; alkalosis = pH > 7.4).
2. Determine if hypocarbia or hypercarbia is present. For simplicity, a normal $Paco_2$ of 40 mm Hg is used (hypercarbia = $Paco_2$ >40 mm Hg; hypocarbia = $Paco_2$ <40 mm Hg).
3. *If hypercarbia is present,* evaluate the contribution of the $Paco_2$ to the change in pH:
   a. Subtract 40 from the patient's $Paco_2$.
   b. Multiply the number obtained in *a* by 0.008.
   c. Subtract the number obtained in *b* from 7.4; the resulting number is the pH predicted from the $Paco_2$.
      (1) If the patient's pH is *lower* than the predicted pH, metabolic acidosis is complicating the hypercarbia.
      (2) If the patient's pH is *higher* than the predicted pH, metabolic alkalosis (or renal compensation for respiratory acidosis) must be present.
4. *If hypocarbia is present,* evaluate the contribution of the $Paco_2$ to the pH:
   a. Subtract the patient's $Paco_2$ from 40.
   b. Multiply the number obtained in *a* by 0.008.
   c. Add the product obtained in *c* to 7.4; the resulting number is the pH predicted from the $Paco_2$.

   (1) If the patient's pH is *higher* than the predicted pH, metabolic alkalosis must be associated with the hypocarbia.
   (2) If the patient's pH is *lower* than the predicted pH, metabolic acidosis must be associated with the hypocarbia.
5. *Calculate the base deficit:*
   a. If the patient's pH is lower than the pH predicted from the $Paco_2$, metabolic acidosis must be present:
      (1) Subtract the predicted pH from the patient's pH (a negative number will result).
      (2) Multiply the product of *(1)* by 66. This negative number (more negative than -2) indicates metabolic acidosis.
   b. If the patient's pH is *higher* than the pH predicted from the $Paco_2$, metabolic alkalosis must be present.
      (1) Subtract the predicted pH from the patient's pH (a positive number will result).
      (2) Multiply the product of *(1)* by 66. This positive number (more positive than $+2$) indicates metabolic alkalosis.

potassium) and the negatively charged ions (anions, chiefly chloride and bicarbonate). Normally the concentration of anions and cations is approximately equal—the difference is no greater than 10 to 12 mEq/L. Calculation of the anion gap attempts to quantify substances that are not measured in common laboratory tests (e.g., sulfate, phosphate, lactate, ketoacids, and albumin). It can be estimated by the following formula:

$$\text{Anion gap} = (\text{Serum Na}^+ + \text{Serum K}^+) \\ - (\text{Serum Cl}^- + \text{Serum HCO}_3-)$$

For example:

$$\text{Anion gap} = (140 + 4) - +(105 + 27)$$

Normal anion gap is approximately 10 to 12 mEq/L.

Lactic acidosis caused by shock is associated with an increased anion gap, reflecting a fall in the serum bicarbonate level that is not balanced by a rise in serum chloride ion concentration. Occasionally acidosis may be termed a normal anion gap acidosis if the fall in serum bicarbonate is balanced by a rise in serum chloride (e.g., hyperchloremic metabolic acidosis).

For further information regarding interpretation of acid-base balance and arterial blood gas values, see Chapter 6, p. 300.

Composition and Distribution of Body Water

Normal Free Water Distribution

Body water is divided into the extracellular and intracellular compartments. Beyond approximately 6 weeks of age, intracellular water constitutes approximately 67% of total body water, and extracellular water constitutes approximately 33% of total body water (Figure 9-4). During the first weeks of life, a larger proportion of the body water is extracellular, and approximately one half of the infant's extracellular fluid is exchanged daily. As a result, the infant is particularly vulnerable to the development of dehydration if there is any compromise in fluid intake or any increase in fluid loss.

Serum Osmolality

Normal serum osmolality is approximately 272 to 300 mOsm/L (also recorded in milliosmoles per kilogram). Sodium is the major intravascular ion that influences serum osmolality. However, if the serum glucose concentration or blood urea nitrogen (BUN) is extremely high (e.g., in diabetic ketoacidosis), these electrolytes can also influence serum osmolality. Serum osmolality can be estimated using the following formula:

$$2 \times \text{Sodium concentration (mEq/L)} = A \\ + \frac{\text{Glucose concentration (mg/dl)}}{18} = B \\ + \frac{\text{BUN (mg/dl)}}{2.8} = C$$

$$A + B + C = \text{Total approximate} \\ \text{serum osmolality (mOsm/L)}$$

If the serum glucose concentration and BUN are not elevated, serum osmolality can be quickly estimated by doubling the serum sodium concentration and adding 20. Calculations using this method do *not* account for changes in serum osmolality secondary to administration of hypertonic agents such as mannitol or glycerol. In addition, this formula can be inaccurate in the presence of hyperlipidemia.

Factors Influencing Water Movement

Under normal conditions, free water, electrolytes, and osmolality are equilibrated across the vascular membrane between the intravascular and interstitial spaces. Acute changes in the osmolality of the cellular, vascular, or interstitial fluid compartment will result in an acute free water shift until osmolality is equalized. The most compelling fluid shifts will occur to restore equal osmolality across the *vascular* membrane, between the intravascular and interstitial spaces (Table 9-2).

Any condition that produces an acute change in serum osmolality will create an acute osmotic gradient across the vascular membrane, and free water will shift from the compartment of lower osmolality to the compartment of higher osmolality until osmolality is equalized. It is important to note that these changes occur with *any* acute rise or fall in serum osmolality, whether these changes result from a disorder (e.g., di-

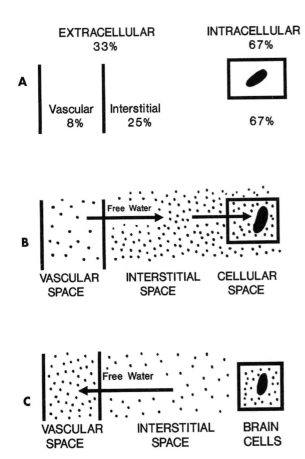

Figure 9-4   A, Distribution of total body water. Beyond the first 6 weeks of life, two thirds of total body water is located in the cellular space, and one third of total body water is located in the extracellular space. One fourth of the extracellular water (this constitutes one twelfth, or 8%, of *total* body water) is located in the vascular space, and three fourths of the extracellular water (approximately one fourth, or 25%, of *total* body water) is located in the interstitial space. **B,** Extravascular fluid shift resulting from an *acute* fall in serum osmolality. If intravascular osmolality falls *acutely* (e.g., when the serum sodium concentration falls abruptly), an acute osmotic gradient will be created between the intravascular and interstitial spaces, and free water will move from the vascular to the interstitial (and possibly cellular) spaces. **C,** Intravascular fluid shift resulting from an *acute* increase in serum osmolality. If the serum osmolality rises *acutely* (e.g., from an abrupt rise in the serum sodium concentration), an acute osmotic gradient will be created between the intravascular and interstitial space. Free water will move from the interstitial space into the vascular space. Free water can also shift from the cellular space and ultimately into the vascular space. However, cells within the brain excrete idiogenic osmoles, which maintain intracellular osmolality and enable the cells of the brain to hold onto free water. These idiogenic osmoles, then, protect the brain cells from acute extracellular fluid shifts. However, when rehydration occurs, they may contribute to free water uptake by the brain cells. (From Hazinski MF: *Nursing care of the critically ill child,* ed 2, St Louis, 1992, Mosby.)

abetic ketoacidosis) or its treatment. Therefore the serum sodium and osmolality should be monitored, and changes should be made gradually.

If intravascular *osmolality acutely decreases* (e.g., the serum sodium concentration falls acutely or hyperglycemia is rapidly corrected), *free water will shift out of the vascular space* to the interstitial space until osmolality in these two compartments is again equal. Fluid shifts into the interstitial space may result in cerebral edema (see Figure 9-4, *B*).

If intravascular *osmolality acutely increases* (e.g., the serum sodium concentration rises acutely or the serum glucose concentration increases to very high levels), *free water will shift into the vascular space* from the interstitial space. Significant fluid shifts from the interstitial to the vascular space may produce intracranial hemorrhage (see Figure 9-4, *C*).

As a rule, acute changes in serum osmolality should be avoided. Any acute shifts into or out of brain tissue may result in tearing of cerebral bridging veins, producing intracranial hemorrhage or a neurologic condition known as acute pontine myelinolysis. In addition, fluid shifts out of the vascular space may produce cerebral edema. The brain tissue contains no lymphatics to carry edema fluid back into circulation; thus cerebral edema may produce increased intracranial pressure (ICP).

Postoperative Water Distribution and Balance

Body fluid composition and distribution is altered postoperatively, secondary to secretion of ADH and aldosterone. ADH and aldosterone are secreted in response to stimuli such as catecholamine

Table 9-2

Factors Influencing Free Water Movement Into and Out of the Vascular Space

Factor	Effect on Water Balance
Acute change in compartment osmolality	Free water movement across vascular and cellular membrane
Acute change in serum sodium	
Acute decrease	Intravascular → interstitial water movement can produce cerebral edema
Acute increase	Interstitial → intravascular water movement can produce intracranial hemorrhage
Response during critical illness	
Increased ADH secretion, increased intravascular volume	Decreased intravascular osmolality
Increased aldosterone secretion	Decreased intravascular osmolality

release, hypotension, and pain. As a result, there may be a decrease in urine output and an increase in urine concentration with fluid retention and hemodilution. Since the newborn kidney is immature and has limited ability to concentrate urine, the neonate may have a decreased urine output but only moderately increased urine concentration.

Postoperative fluid administration should be determined by the type of fluid lost and the adjustments in sodium and water balance necessary (Table 9-3):

- Gastrointestinal fluids are replaced with 0.45% NaCl.
- Urine and insensible losses are replaced with 5% or 10% dextrose solutions containing 0.2% or 0.45% NaCl.

Dextrose-and-water solutions are generally avoided during the postoperative period, since the postoperative patient may be prone to stress and ADH or aldosterone secretion, as well as sodium and water retention. Dextrose-and-water solutions are occasionally used following cardiovascular surgery if limitation of sodium intake is desired.

Urine output should be closely monitored. If fluid administration is adequate, urine volume should exceed 1 ml/kg/hr. Fluid administration may be limited in the presence of respiratory, cardiac, or renal failure or if the child is at risk for the development of increased ICP or the syndrome of inappropriate antidiuretic hormone secretion (SIADH). In

Table 9-3

Fluid Replacement for the Postoperative Patient

Fluid Loss	Replacement Solution
Urine losses	0.45% NaCl
Insensible losses (skin, respiratory)	0.2% NaCl
Gastrointestinal losses	0.45% NaCl

these situations (when fluid intake is limited), a urine output of 0.5 to 1 ml/kg/hr may be acceptable.

Urine osmolality is a better indicator of renal function than urine specific gravity. Normal urine osmolality is approximately 300 mOsm/L (or mOsm/kg). If renal function is good, the urine-plasma osmolality ratio should be 1.1:1 or higher. Urine osmolality should always be higher than plasma osmolality. If renal function is poor, urine and plasma osmolality are often equal.

Diuretics

Diuretics increase urine volume. They work primarily to decrease tubular reabsorption of sodium and chloride, which indirectly decreases water reabsorption from the tubules, so that water loss in the urine is increased. Commonly used diuretics can be divided into the following main categories according to their site of action and their chemical groups: loop diuretics, osmotic diuretic agents, thiazide diuretics, and potassium-sparing diuretics (Table 9-4).

Loop diuretics, including furosemide (Lasix) and ethacrynic acid (Edecrin), are the most potent of the diuretics used in the care of critically ill children. They inhibit sodium chloride transport in the ascending limbs of the loop of Henle, so that natriuresis and diuresis result. Loop diuresis also results in increased potassium, hydrogen, and calcium ion loss. These drugs are very useful in the treatment of the child with marginal renal function, although both have also been associated with ototoxicity.

Osmotic diuretics, including mannitol, urea, and glucose, exert their effects as a result of their high osmolality. Once these agents are filtered through the glomerulus, they pull additional free water into the filtrate, increasing urine volume. Although these drugs are not the diuretics of choice for routine diuresis, they can be useful in promoting diuresis in children with marginal renal function. These drugs can cause hemoconcentration; therefore they should be used with caution in dehydrated or hypernatremic patients.

Thiazide diuretics, such as hydrochlorothiazide, block reabsorption of sodium and chloride in the cortical segment of the distal tubule. All produce significant potassium and calcium loss in the urine and can depress the GFR.

Potassium-sparing diuretics also inhibit sodium reabsorption in the distal tubule. These drugs, including spironolactone, result in sodium and water excretion and potassium reabsorption. Spironolactone is an aldosterone antagonist and does not depress the GFR. Because these drugs are not as potent as other diuretics, they are often administered in conjunction with other agents. The potassium-sparing diuretics have a long half-life.

Common Clinical Conditions

Dehydration

Etiology/Pathophysiology

Dehydration occurs when the total output of all fluids and electrolytes exceeds the total fluid and electrolyte intake. This may result from inadequate fluid intake or excess fluid loss. Dehydra-

tion produces a deficiency in both fluids and electrolytes.

Dehydration caused by inadequate fluid intake can result from inadequate intravenous (IV) fluid therapy or inadequate fluid intake in the infant with a gastrointestinal virus. It may also result from excessive fluid losses, including losses caused by vomiting and diarrhea, losses caused by diabetes insipidus, or inadequate replacement of gastric fluid suction. Vomiting and diarrhea not only produce large fluid loss, but they also produce a significant loss of sodium, chloride, hydrogen, and bicarbonate ions.

The physiologic consequences of dehydration are caused predominantly by the depletion of intravascular volume and by changes in the serum sodium concentration. The more significant the loss of intravascular volume, the more likely the child is to develop a compromise in systemic perfusion (shock). Acute changes in serum sodium associated with dehydration will cause free water shifts into and out of the vascular space, which will influence the severity of the intravascular volume deficit. Finally, as the dehydration is treated, persistent shock, free water shifts, and electrolyte imbalances can further complicate the clinical course.

Clinical Presentation

Dehydration is classified in two ways: by the severity of the fluid deficit and by the serum osmolality. Initially the severity of the dehydration is estimated from the patient's clinical appearance. Then, when the serum sodium concentration is available from the laboratory, the dehydration is classified by osmolality, and adjustment is made, if needed, in the estimation of dehydration severity.

Initial Estimation of Clinical Severity Clinical severity is determined initially by the effect of the dehydration on clinical appearance and cardiovascular function (Table 9-5). The serum sodium concentration is assumed to be normal.

- *Mild clinical isotonic dehydration:* Cardiovascular function is not compromised, but the child's skin and mucous membranes are dry.
- *Moderate clinical isotonic dehydration:* Signs of peripheral circulatory failure are present; thus some evidence of adrenergic re-

Table 9-4
Diuretic Therapy for Children

Drug (Trade Name)	Peak Effect	Action	Dosage	Effect on Serum Potassium
Acetazolamide (Diamox) Amiloride (Midamor)*	2 hr 3-4 hr PO	Carbonic anhydrase inhibitor Inhibits sodium reabsorption in distal convoluted tubule, cortical collecting tubule, and collecting duct	5 mg/kg/24hr per day or every other day 0.3-0.45 mg/kg/24 hr with hydrochloro-thiazide	↓↓ K$^+$ is "saved"
Bumetanide (Bumex)	15-30 min IV, 1-2 hr PO	Inhibits Na$^+$ reabsorption in loop of Henle; also blocks Cl$^-$ reabsorption	0.25-0.5 mg/dose q6-12h IV; 0.02-1 mg/dose PO	↓↓
Chlorothiazide (Diuril)	2-4 hr	Inhibits tubular reabsorption of Na$^+$ in distal tubule and loop of Henle; also inhibits water reabsorption in loop	20-40 mg/kg/day PO divided bid	↓↓
Ethacrynic acid (Edecrin)	5-10 min IV, 0.5-8 hr PO	Same as furosemide (see below)	0.5-2 mg/kg/IV dose; 2-3 mg/kg/PO dose	↓↓↓
Furosemide (Lasix)	5-20 min IV, 1-2 hr PO	Inhibits NaCl transport in loop of Henle and proximal and distal tubules	1-2 mg/kg/IV dose; 1-4 mg/kg/PO dose	↓↓↓
Hydrochlorothiazide (Esidrix, HydroDiuril, Oretic)	2-4 hr	Inhibits Na$^+$ reabsorption in distal tubule and loop of Henle and inhibits water reabsorption in loop	2-3 mg/kg/day PO in 2 divided doses (every 12 hr)	↓↓
Hydrochlorothiazide plus spironolactone (Aldactazide)	2-4 hr (prolonged effects)	Hydrochlorothiazide functions as above; spironolactone functions as aldosterone antagonist and inhibits exchange of Na$^+$ for K$^+$ in distal tubule	1-2 mg/kg/24 hr; <6 mo: 2-3 mg/kg/24 hr	Approximately unchanged
Mannitol	5-10 min IV	Osmotic diuretic; inhibits tubular reabsorption of water and electrolytes	0.75 mg/kg/dose over 20-25 min	Approximately unchanged
Metolazone (Zaroxolyn)	2 hr (prolonged effects)	Inhibits Na$^+$ reabsorption at cortical diluting site and in proximal convoluted tubule; results in approximately equal Na$^+$ and Cl$^-$ excretion; may increase K$^+$ excretion (increased delivery of Na$^+$ to distal tubule and Na$^+$/K$^+$ exchange)	0.2-2.5 mg/day PO given in divided doses (every 12 hr)	↓↓
Spironolactone (Aldactone)	1-4 days (prolonged effects)	Aldosterone antagonist; inhibits exchange of Na$^+$ for K$^+$ in distal tubule; typically administered in combination with other diuretics	1.3-3.3 mg/kg/day PO	K$^+$ is "saved"
Torsemide (Demadox)*	10 min IV, 1 hr PO	Inhibits Na$^+$/K$^+$/Cl$^-$ transport carrier system in loop of Henle	0.1-0.3 mg/kg/day IV or PO	↓↓
Triamterene (Dyrenium)	2-4 hr PO	Increases urinary excretion of Na$^+$, Cl$^-$, and water; does not alter GFR	4-6 mg/kg/24 hr, divided bid, tid, or qid	K$^+$ is "saved"

*Experience in children is limited.

Table 9-5
Effects of Isotonic, Hypotonic, and Hypertonic Dehydration on Clinical Appearance and Cardiovascular Function

Clinical Parameters*	Mild	Moderate	Severe
Isotonic Dehydration			
Body weight loss			
Infant	5% (50 ml/kg)	10% (100 ml/kg)	15% (150 ml/kg)
Adult	3% (30 ml/kg)	6% (60 ml/kg)	9% (90 ml/kg)
Skin turgor	Slightly ↓	↓↓	↓↓↓
Fontanelle	May be flat or depressed	Depressed	Significantly depressed
Mucous membranes	Dry	Very dry	Parched
Skin perfusion	Warm, normal, color	Extremities cool Pale color	Extremities cold Mottled or gray color
Heart rate	Mild tachycardia	Moderate tachycardia	Extreme tachycardia
Peripheral pulses	Normal	Diminished	Absent
Blood pressure	Normal	Normal	Reduced
Sensorium	Normal or irritable	Irritable or lethargic	Unresponsive
Urine output	Slightly ↓	Mild oliguria	Marked oliguria or anuria
Azotemia	Absent	Present	Present and severe
Modification of Assessment Based on Serum Sodium and Osmolality			
Hypotonic dehydration (serum sodium concentration <130 mEq/L)		These above signs are associated with mild hypotonic (hyponatremic) dehydration and mild volume deficit (50 ml/kg in infants)	These signs are associated with moderate hypotonic (hyponatremic) dehydration and moderate volume deficit (100 ml/kg in infants)
Hypertonic dehydration (serum sodium concentration >150 mEq/L)	These signs are associated with moderate hypertonic (hypernatremic) dehydration and moderate volume deficit (100 ml/kg in infants)	These signs are associated with severe hypertonic (hypernatremic) dehydration and severe volume deficit (150 ml/kg in infants)	

Modified from Hazinski MF: *Nursing care of the critically ill child,* ed 2, St Louis, 1992, Mosby.
*The interpretation of the assessments must be appropriately modified for age and for *type* of dehydration (hypotonic or hypertonic dehydration).

distribution of blood volume is apparent, although the blood pressure is normal.

- *Severe clinical isotonic dehydration:* Decompensated shock (with hypotension) is present.

Isotonic dehydration will compromise intravascular volume and systemic perfusion once the infant or child loses the equivalent of 7% to 10% of body weight. The adolescent may demonstrate compromise of systemic perfusion with a 5% to 7%

weight loss. In an attempt to compensate for changes in intravascular volume and systemic perfusion, adrenergic compensatory mechanisms are activated to maintain cardiac output and to redistribute intravascular volume to maintain essential systemic perfusion. Clinical signs of adrenergic stimulation include tachycardia, peripheral vasoconstriction, and decreased urine output. If systemic perfusion is severely compromised, metabolic acidosis and multisystem organ failure may develop.

Determination of the Type of Dehydration by Serum Sodium Concentration Dehydration is also classified according to the resulting serum sodium concentration:

- *Isotonic dehydration:* Serum sodium concentration is approximately 130 to 150 mEq/L. Loss of fluid is proportional to the loss of sodium; thus the serum sodium concentration is normal, and fluid loss from all body compartments is proportional.
- *Hyponatremic dehydration:* Serum sodium concentration is <130 mEq/L. Loss of sodium is greater than the net loss of fluid; as a result, the serum sodium concentration is low. When acute hyponatremia develops, the serum osmolality falls, producing an acute extravascular fluid shift. Free water moves from the lower osmolality intravascular space to the higher osmolality interstitial space until equilibration is restored. Because fluid loss is predominantly from the intravascular space, systemic perfusion will be compromised even at a relatively small volume deficit. Clinical signs will be severe at only a moderate fluid volume deficit, and moderate at only a mild fluid volume deficit.
- *Hypernatremic dehydration:* Serum sodium concentration is >150 mEq/L. Because fluid loss exceeds sodium or solute loss, the serum sodium concentration rises. In this case intravascular volume may be maintained by the intravascular free water shift that occurs. Free water moves from the lower osmolality interstitial space into the higher osmolality intravascular space until equilibration is restored. As a result, clinical signs are mild at a moderate fluid volume deficit, and moderate at a severe fluid volume deficit.

Estimation of Fluid Deficit Initially, when the child presents with dehydration, the severity of the dehydration is estimated based on the child's clinical presentation. During that estimate, the child's serum sodium concentration is unknown and is thus assumed to be normal (i.e., dehydration is assumed to be isotonic). Before fluid replacement therapy is calculated and initiated, shock resuscita-

tion is provided. Then, once the serum sodium concentration is determined, the dehydration is classified by osmolality as isotonic, hypertonic, or hypotonic, and the initial estimated severity of dehydration and estimated fluid volume deficit are revised accordingly. *Revise the severity of the dehydration in the same direction as the serum sodium is altered.* For example, if the serum sodium concentration is *high, increase* your initial impression or estimate of the severity of the dehydration by one level.

- *Isotonic dehydration:* The clinical signs are as predicted; thus no adjustment in dehydration severity is required.
- *Hypotonic dehydration:* The fluid deficit will be *less severe* than the clinical signs suggest (because most fluid lost is from the intravascular compartment). As a result, the severity of the dehydration should be *decreased* one level from that estimated by clinical appearance (revise estimate from severe to moderate or from moderate to mild).
- *Hypertonic dehydration:* The fluid deficit will be *more severe* than the clinical signs suggest (because intravascular volume is maintained by the high serum osmolality). As a result, the severity of the dehydration should be *increased* one level from that estimated by clinical appearance (revise estimate from mild to moderate or from moderate to severe).

The final fluid deficit can now be estimated (see Table 9-5) as follows:

- *Mild dehydration:* Deficit of approximately 50 ml/kg (or the equivalent of 5% of body weight in children and 3% of body weight in adolescents; 1-kg weight loss is equivalent to a 1-L fluid deficit)
- *Moderate dehydration:* Deficit of approximately 100 ml/kg (or the equivalent of 5% to 10% of body weight in children and 3% to 7% of body weight in adolescents)
- *Severe dehydration:* Deficit of approximately 150 ml/kg (or the equivalent of >10% of body weight in children and >7% of body weight in adolescents)

Management

General Guidelines   The goals of treatment of dehydration include:

- Restoration and maintenance of intravascular volume and systemic perfusion
- Replacement of the volume and electrolyte deficit, as well as any ongoing losses
- Provision of maintenance fluid requirements

Treatment should include prevention of secondary insults such as the development of electrolyte imbalances, cerebral edema, or intracranial hemorrhage (Table 9-6).

Regardless of the type of dehydration present, once the dehydration is moderate or severe, establishment of IV access will be required. Assess the child's systemic perfusion carefully and provide resuscitation if shock is present. *Throughout therapy, constantly assess the child's clinical status and response to therapy,* including systemic perfusion, urine output, neurologic function, and electrolyte balance. If therapy is successful, the child's perfusion, urine output, and mental status should all improve; *failure to improve or deterioration despite therapy is a "red flag" and may indicate the presence of complications.*

Intravenous Access   At least one and preferably two large-bore venous catheters should be inserted and maintained. If shock is present and IV access cannot be achieved rapidly in children less than 6 years of age, an intraosseous catheter should be inserted to provide vascular access. If neither peripheral vascular nor intraosseous access can be achieved in a child with shock due to dehydration, a venous cutdown must be performed.

Some form of vascular access must be established immediately to enable volume resuscitation for the child in shock due to dehydration. If the child must be transported, vascular access should be established and secured, and some volume resuscitation accomplished before transport. Delays can be life threatening for the child in shock.

Table 9-6
Management of Dehydration

Goal	Actions	Outcomes
Shock resuscitation	Adequate IV, intraosseous (IO) access Adequate fluid therapy	Improved level of consciousness Appropriate heart rate Adequate blood pressure Appropriate urine output (>1 ml/kg/hr once perfusion is restored) Lactic acidosis corrected
	Maintain electrolyte balance	Normal serum sodium concentration restored and maintained
Supportive care	Assess ventilatory function	Adequate oxygenation and CO_2 elimination
	Assess neurologic function	Stable or improving neurologic status
	Correct hypoglycemia	Normal serum glucose
	Monitor body temperature	Normothermia

PALS Guidelines for Shock Resuscitation

IV access	Two large-bore IV catheters are preferred; if unsuccessful after 3 attempts or 90 sec, proceed with IO access (in children less than 6 years of age) or central venous access (in children over 6 years of age)	
Fluid therapy	Isotonic fluids (normal saline or lactated Ringer's) for initial fluid therapy; 20 ml/kg should be repeated, if necessary, until adequate perfusion	

Shock Resuscitation   If shock is present, volume resuscitation is provided with normal saline or lactated Ringer's solution in boluses of 20 ml/kg until systemic perfusion is adequate. Bolus fluid administration is definitely indicated if shock is present, but it should not be continued once systemic perfusion has been restored. This is particularly true in the presence of hypertonic dehydration, because repeat bolus administration of fluid can contribute to a rapid decrease in the serum sodium concentration (see below). Once systemic perfusion is adequate, the fluid volume deficit is calculated and replaced over the appropriate time period (typically 24 to 48 hours; see Hypotonic and Hypertonic Dehydration in following paragraphs), while maintenance fluid requirements are provided and ongoing fluid losses are replaced.

Supportive Therapy   Supportive therapy during treatment of dehydration includes assessment and support of cardiovascular, neurologic, and respiratory status; evaluation and support of electrolyte and acid-base balance; maintenance of temperature; and monitoring of weight. The infant's heel stick and serum glucose concentration should be monitored throughout therapy, and a continuous source of glucose intake provided if hypoglycemia is detected. Glucose infusion is preferable to repeated bolus administration of hypertonic glucose, since the latter method of glucose correction will result in wide fluctuations in the serum glucose concentration and serum osmolality.

Hypotonic Dehydration   When *hypotonic* dehydration is present, fluid loss has occurred predominantly from the *intravascular* space; thus clinical signs will be significant even at a relatively small fluid volume deficit. Remember that the severity of volume deficit estimated from initial clinical evaluation should be reduced one level or degree (from severe to moderate or from moderate to mild) if the serum sodium concentration is <130 mEq/L.

  Goals of Therapy   Restoration of systemic perfusion and intravascular volume is the priority.

- *Bolus fluid therapy:* Isotonic crystalloid (20 ml/kg) bolus is repeated until systemic perfusion is adequate.

- *Estimated volume deficit replacement:* Replacement is 50% within the initial 8 hours, with the remaining 50% replaced within the next 16 hours.

Replacement fluids are provided *in addition to* calculated maintenance fluid requirements and replacement of any ongoing losses. The replacement fluid of choice is usually 0.9% sodium chloride (contains 154 mEq/L Na^+) or 0.45% NaCl (contains 77 mEq/L Na^+).

Sodium content to be provided in the replacement fluid is determined by the sodium deficit. Half of the sodium deficit should be replaced in the first 8 hours of therapy, and the remaining deficit should be replaced in the next 16 hours. The sodium deficit is calculated as follows:

$$Na^+ \text{ deficit (in mEq)} = (135 \text{ mEq/L} - \text{Patient's serum } Na^+) \times (0.55 \times \text{Weight in kg})$$

The child's serum sodium concentration should rise no faster than 1 to 2 mEq/L/hr to prevent neurologic complications. Note that a rapid *fall* in serum sodium may cause seizures and cerebral edema, whereas a rapid *rise* in serum sodium may cause intracranial hemorrhage or other complications.

If neurologic symptoms of hyponatremia develop (seizures, decreased level of consciousness, evidence of cerebral edema, and increased ICP) or the serum sodium concentration is <120 mEq/L, administer 3% saline (provides 0.513 mEq Na^+/ml), 3 to 5 ml/kg.

This dose of 3% saline will provide 1.5 to 2.5 mEq/kg of NaCl and should raise the serum sodium 3.5 to 4.5 mEq/L. Repeat administration of the hypertonic saline should be administered if neurologic symptoms persist or deficit is severe.

  Indications of Improvement   If the child becomes more alert and systemic perfusion and urine output improve while electrolyte and acid-base balance are maintained or restored, therapy has been effective.

Hypertonic Dehydration   When *hypertonic* dehydration is present, fluid loss has occurred predominantly from the *extravascular* space. The increase in serum sodium produces an intravascular fluid shift, so that the intravascular volume is maintained. As a result, clinical signs will be mild despite a moderate fluid volume deficit, and will be moderate at a severe fluid volume deficit. Remember that the volume deficit estimated from the initial clinical evaluation should be *increased* one level or degree (from mild to moderate or from moderate to severe) if the serum sodium concentration is >150 mEq/L.

Goals of Therapy Major goals of therapy are restoration of adequate perfusion and prevention of a precipitous fall in the serum sodium concentration. Bolus fluid therapy is administered if needed to restore systemic perfusion. CAUTION: Aggressive fluid administration beyond that needed to restore systemic perfusion can result in a precipitous fall in the serum sodium concentration.

- *Bolus fluid therapy:* Isotonic crystalloid (20 ml/kg) is provided as a bolus and repeated as needed to restore systemic perfusion.
- *Estimated volume deficit replacement:* Replacement is gradual over 48 hours, with 50% replaced within the initial 24 hours and the remaining 50% replaced within the next 24 hours.
- *Estimate of water deficit:*

50 ml/kg if serum $Na^+ = 150$ mEq/L

90 ml/kg if serum $Na^+ = 160$ mEq/L

140 ml/kg if serum $Na^+ = 170$ mEq/L

Replacement fluids usually consist of 5% dextrose and 0.45%NaCl (77 mEq/L Na^+). Replacement fluids are provided *in addition to* calculated maintenance fluid requirements and replacement of any ongoing losses.

Monitor neurologic status closely during rehydration: cerebral edema secondary to water intoxication most often occurs within the first 4 to 24 hours after initiation of fluid therapy and is more likely to occur if the sodium level is decreased too rapidly (>1 to 2 mEq/L/hr or >10 to 15 mEq/24 hr). If seizures or a change in level of consciousness develop, notify a physician immediately.

IV administration of hypertonic (3%) saline or mannitol can increase intravascular osmolality and stop the fluid shift from the vascular to the interstitial and cellular spaces. If there is no response to this therapy, cerebral hemorrhage or increased ICP may be present (see Chapter 8).

Monitor the serum sodium concentration to ensure gradual reduction during therapy:

- If serum sodium concentration is >175 mEq/L, decrease the concentration by 15 mEq/L during the first 24 hours. *Dialysis may be necessary for severe hypernatremia (serum sodium concentration >180 mEq/L).*
- If serum sodium concentration is <175 mEq/L, correct the concentration by approximately 50% during the first 24 hours (to approximately 160 mEq/L).

Indications of Improvement A positive response to rehydration will include improvement in systemic perfusion, including an increased urine output and improved level of consciousness.

Hyponatremia/Syndrome of Inappropriate Antidiuretic Hormone Secretion/Water Intoxication

Etiology

Hyponatremia is a low serum sodium concentration, typically <130 mEq/L. It can result from excess intravascular water or inadequate serum sodium. It may be caused by increased sodium losses, free water gain (such as occurs with the syndrome of inappropriate antidiuretic hormone secretion [SIADH]), inadequate intake of sodium, adrenal insufficiency, aggressive diuretic therapy, and insufficient sodium administration.

SIADH, one cause of hyponatremia, can develop in virtually any critically ill or injured child. SIADH has been reported in postoperative patients, especially if hemorrhage, trauma, or significant fluid loss has occurred. SIADH may complicate meningitis, encephalitis, hydrocephalus, increased ICP, head trauma, subarachnoid hemorrhage, brain tumor, or coma. It is important to identify patients at risk for the development of SIADH and monitor the serum sodium concentration accordingly to recognize SIADH as soon as it develops.

Pathophysiology

Sodium is the major intravascular ion that determines serum osmolality. Acute alterations in serum sodium are not desirable, since they can be associated with acute changes in serum osmolality and acute fluid shifts into and out of the vascular space.

If true hyponatremia develops, serum osmolality will decrease. If the serum sodium concentration and osmolality fall *gradually,* small fluid shifts will occur until the osmolalities equilibrate between the intravascular and interstitial spaces. These small shifts are well tolerated. On the other hand, if the serum sodium concentration and osmolality fall *acutely,* an acute fluid shift from the intravascular space to the interstitial space will occur, and cerebral edema may result.

A laboratory report of low serum sodium may be misleading. The "pseudohyponatremic state" may represent sodium dilution associated with significant hyperlipidemia, hyperproteinemia, or hyperglycemia. The absolute quantity of intravascular sodium may be normal, but the *concentration* per liter of plasma is diluted when these conditions cause an intravascular fluid shift. A fall in the concentration of sodium alone may not affect the serum osmolality if it is associated with a rise in one of the other particles that influence serum osmolality (including glucose or BUN). If the serum osmolality is unchanged or changes gradually, significant fluid shifts and their associated complications will not occur.

If hyponatremia is associated with hyperglycemia, the hyponatremia should be proportional to the hyperglycemia in order for the serum osmolality to be maintained. In general, *the serum sodium concentration is expected to decrease approximately 2 mEq/L below 135 mEq/L for every 100 mg/dl rise in the serum glucose concentration above 100 mg/dl.* As the serum glucose concentration falls or is reduced toward normal, however, the serum sodium concentration should increase proportionately. The serum sodium concentration should rise approximately 2 mEq/L for every 100 mg/dl fall in serum glucose).

Syndrome of Inappropriate Antidiuretic Hormone Secretion SIADH develops when ADH is secreted in the absence of a physiologic stimulus. In fact, ADH secretion continues despite a fall in serum sodium and osmolality. As a result, water retention produces a progressive fall in serum sodium and osmolality, whereas the urine sodium concentration is high.

Clinical Presentation

Symptomatic hyponatremia may develop with a serum sodium concentration of <130 mEq/L if the drop in serum sodium has been acute. If the serum sodium concentration falls gradually (e.g., with the development of adrenal insufficiency), symptoms may not develop despite a very low serum sodium concentration.

Clinical signs of hyponatremia include seizures, abdominal cramps, anorexia, nausea, and diarrhea. Clinical signs of hyponatremia with a low serum osmolality include neurologic symptoms, including seizures, cerebral edema, and increased ICP.

Clinical signs of SIADH include serum hyponatremia, a low serum osmolality, high urine excretion of sodium and high urine osmolality, normal renal function, normal adrenal function, and decreased urine output (the urine volume is variable). Urine sodium and osmolality are measured and compared with the serum sodium and osmolality. If the kidneys are functioning normally in the patient with hyponatremia and hypoosmolality, the urine sodium and osmolality should not be higher than the serum sodium and osmolality, because the kidneys should be excreting free water to correct the low serum sodium and osmolality. Therefore a urine sodium and osmolality *higher than* the serum sodium and osmolality in the presence of hyponatremia and hypoosmolality confirms the diagnosis of SIADH. *SIADH should be suspected in patients at risk, and the nurse should be alert for its development, particularly following head injury, meningitis, and neurosurgery.*

Management

The major treatment for hyponatremia is treatment of the cause and supportive care. Elimination of excess intravascular water or increased sodium administration is generally required. If *neurologic symptoms* develop, the serum sodium must be increased immediately as follows:

- *Saline administration:* Hypertonic (3%) NaCl (3 to 5 ml/kg will provide approximately 1.5 to 2.5 mEq sodium/kg). To raise the serum sodium concentration 5 mEq/L, a total dose of approximately 6 ml/kg will be required.

- *Diuresis:* Furosemide, 1 to 2 mg/kg

Treatment of SIADH requires restriction of fluid intake to 30% to 70% of the calculated normal total intake. Typically, this results in gradual but consistent correction of the serum sodium concentration. If neurologic symptoms develop, hypertonic saline and furosemide are administered as indicated earlier in this paragraph. Monitor serum electrolytes, serum osmolality, and urine osmolality, and monitor for evidence of neurologic deterioration, which may indicate persistent hyponatremia or cerebral bleeding. Document all sources of fluid intake and output, and evaluate the appropriateness of the IV fluid solution.

Diabetes Insipidus

Etiology

Diabetes insipidus (DI) is caused by inadequate secretion of ADH (central or neurogenic DI) or inadequate renal response to ADH (nephrogenic DI). As a result, the kidney is unable to concentrate urine, and large amounts of water are lost in the urine. Neurogenic DI most often complicates surgery near the pituitary gland, severe head injury, central nervous system infections, intraventricular hemorrhage, or hypoxic encephalopathy. It also appears in patients who are pronounced brain dead and thus should be anticipated during support of the vascular organ donor.

Nephrogenic DI can result from a hereditary, sex-linked recessive trait. Therefore it is present from birth.

Pathophysiology

The pituitary gland and the kidney regulate serum osmolality through adjustment in the permeability of the collecting duct and distal tubule to water. When serum osmolality increases, osmoreceptors stimulate vasopressin secretion by the hypothalamus. This alters the permeability of the renal distal tubule and collecting duct to water. Water is reabsorbed, and a more concentrated urine is excreted.

This reabsorption/retention of water produces a fall in serum osmolality, which eliminates the stimulus for vasopressin secretion by the hypothalamus.

If vasopressin is absent or the kidney does not appropriately respond to vasopressin, water will be lost into the urine instead of being reabsorbed. Urinary water loss produces hemoconcentration and may result in profound hypernatremia. The rise in serum osmolality draws interstitial and intracellular water into the vascular space. That fluid is also filtered by the glomerulus and lost in the urine. Volume-sensitive receptors respond to the decrease in circulating volume. This causes an increase in aldosterone secretion and an increase in sodium and water reabsorption by the proximal tubule. However, this water reabsorption can't compensate for the tremendous water losses in the urine. The serum sodium concentration continues to climb.

Water loss in the urine can be extremely high, resulting in the rapid development of hypovolemia. If the child is unable to independently take fluid by mouth and urinary fluid losses are not replaced, hypovolemic shock can quickly develop.

Clinical Presentation

The presentation of the child with DI is determined by the fluid balance maintained during the DI. If fluid losses are replaced, intravascular volume will be maintained and symptoms may be minimal. If fluid losses are not replaced, hypovolemic shock, hypertonic dehydration, and their complications can quickly develop.

Signs of DI in the critically ill child include an extremely high urine output with a low urine specific gravity (<1.005) and low urine osmolality (<280 mOsm/L). The presence of a low urine sodium concentration and low urine osmolality distinguish DI from acute tubular necrosis. Urine output may exceed 1 L/hr. If excessive urine losses are not immediately replaced, signs of hypovolemic shock will develop, including tachycardia and peripheral vasoconstriction. Hemoconcentration and hypernatremia will also develop.

The infant with nephrogenic DI typically presents with hypernatremic dehydration and may also present with seizures or "failure to thrive," which may erroneously be attributed to gastroenteritis. Continued polyuria is inconsistent with the diagnosis of simple dehydration, however, and should prompt investigation. Signs of DI in the ambulatory patient include polydipsia and polyuria. The polyuria is associated with a low urine osmolality in the presence of high serum osmolality.

It is extremely important to evaluate the child's fluid balance frequently. If excessive urine losses are not replaced, hypovolemic shock will quickly develop.

Management

Acute management of DI is focused on the replacement of urinary fluid and electrolyte losses, and on management of the related symptoms while maintenance fluid requirements are delivered. In addition, exogenous vasopressin (Pitressin) is administered to those patients with vasopressin-sensitive DI.

Fluid Therapy   Two large-bore venous catheters are inserted if possible. A central venous catheter is useful to monitor CVP and to provide a reliable route of rapid fluid delivery for replacement of urinary losses. The second IV catheter enables uninterrupted delivery of maintenance fluid requirements. If clinically significant hypovolemia is present, a 20 ml/kg bolus of 2.5% glucose and 0.45% NaCl is administered over 15 to 20 minutes and repeated as needed until systemic perfusion improves.

Urine output is measured and replaced several times every hour until exogenous vasopressin administration is effective. Typically, urine output is tallied every 10 or 15 minutes, and that quantity of fluid is replaced over the next 10 to 15 minutes by IV infusion, in addition to maintenance fluid administration. IV fluids used for urine replacement should have a low glucose and sodium concentration, such as 2.5% glucose and 0.2% NaCl.

The effectiveness of the fluid replacement is determined through evaluation of systemic perfusion (neurologic status, skin perfusion) and central venous pressure (CVP), if measured. Simultaneous measurement of urine and serum sodium, potassium, chloride, and osmolalities will enable evaluation of the propriety of the fluid and electrolyte replacement. Urine specific gravity should be followed closely, as frequently as every hour.

Vasopressin Therapy   Exogenous vasopressin is administered to those patients with neurogenic DI

(see Table 8-10). It may also be administered to patients with nephrogenic DI as a test dose.

In the ICU, aqueous vasopressin is typically administered by IV route (2 to 4 U). Although the subcutaneous (5 to 10 U) or intramuscular (1 to 5 U) route may be used, absorption through these routes is less predictable, and the sites may be painful. Intranasal vasopressin (DDAVP) produces fewer systemic effects and more prolonged effects than other forms of vasopressin; thus it is often the route of choice for maintenance vasopressin therapy.

A positive response to vasopressin therapy is demonstrated by a decrease in urine volume (less than or equal to 1 ml/kg/hr), a rise in urine specific gravity ($>$1.010), and a rise in urine osmolality (to 280 to 300 mOsm/L). The reduction in urine volume will enable tapering of the volume and frequency of IV replacement of urine output. Side effects of vasopressin are particularly pronounced with IV administration and include tachycardia, bradycardia, hypertension, hypotension, abdominal cramping, and other signs of hypersensitivity.

Patients with nephrogenic DI are unresponsive to exogenous vasopressin. For these patients, oral replacement of urinary water losses is critical. In addition, a low-sodium and low-protein diet is provided, combined with the use of a thiazide diuretic. The thiazide diuretic may reduce the water requirements significantly. However, complications such as hypokalemia and other fluid and electrolyte disturbances must be avoided.

Hypokalemia

Etiology

Although potassium is the chief *intra*cellular cation, serum concentrations of potassium reflect the extracellular potassium concentration, which is relatively low (3.5 to 4.5 mEq/L). Hypokalemia is present when the serum potassium concentration is $<$3.5 mEq/L. It can result from true potassium losses, dilution of existing intravascular potassium, or a shift of potassium out of the vascular space. Hypoaldosteronism can cause potassium and chloride depletion and a possible metabolic alkalosis.

True potassium losses can be caused by loss of potassium-rich gastrointestinal fluids, such as occurs in vomiting, diarrhea, or unreplaced drainage of gastrointestinal fluids. Renal potassium losses can result from conditions that stimulate potassium excretion in exchange for hydrogen ions, such as in renal tubular acidosis, hypochloremic alkalosis, or diabetic ketoacidosis. Renal excretion of potassium is enhanced by several drugs, including diuretics, amphotericin, and carbenicillin.

Hypokalemia can also result from potassium dilution. Classically, this occurs during administration of large quantities of fluids that contain no potassium chloride.

Hypokalemia can result from a shift of potassium from the vascular to the (intra)cellular space. This can occur with a rise in serum pH, such as occurs with the development of alkalosis or the correction of acidosis.

Pathophysiology

Hypokalemia is present when the serum concentration is <3.5 mEq/L. Since the gradient between the extracellular (or serum) and intracellular potassium concentration determines the excitability of nerve and muscle cells, hypokalemia can affect the electrocardiogram (ECG), as well as nerve and muscle function.

Changes in the acid-base balance can influence the serum potassium concentration. Therefore *the serum potassium concentration should always be interpreted in light of the child's current pH and in light of anticipated changes in the pH in response to therapy.* When the pH increases (with the development of alkalosis or correction of acidosis), potassium ions move from the vascular space into the cells in exchange for hydrogen ions. An abrupt increase in pH by 0.1 unit can reduce serum potassium levels by 0.6 to 0.7 mEq/L. This shift should be anticipated with the correction of acidosis; if the child's serum potassium concentration is normal and the child is acidotic, a decrease in the serum potassium concentration to below normal should be anticipated as the acidosis is corrected. Therefore potassium administration should be planned.

Hypokalemia may perpetuate metabolic alkalosis, as in hypokalemic metabolic alkalosis. This can occur when diuretic therapy is not accompanied by adequate potassium replacement. As the kidney attempts to reabsorb potassium, it excretes hydrogen ions and reabsorbs bicarbonate in the proximal tubule. Treatment of hypokalemia is required to resolve the alkalosis.

Clinical Presentation

Severe hypokalemia can produce nausea and vomiting, paralytic ileus, lethargy, confusion, and cardiac arrhythmias. ECG changes include low-voltage QRS complexes, presence of a U wave, flattened T waves, and a prolonged QT interval.

Mild to moderate hypokalemia produces mild symptoms of muscle weakness and diminished reflexes. A hypokalemic metabolic alkalosis may be noted.

Chronic hypokalemia compromises renal concentrating ability and results in polyuria. At this point, the kidney also loses its ability to conserve potassium.

Management

Remember that the serum potassium concentration should be interpreted in light of the child's current pH and anticipated changes in pH in response to therapy. A normal serum potassium concentration is probably inadequate if the child is acidotic and correction of the acidosis is planned. Alternatively, a low serum potassium concentration may be acceptable if alkalosis is present and will be corrected.

Symptomatic and Moderate to Severe Hypokalemia Hypokalemia associated with arrhythmias, paralytic ileus, or moderate to severe hypokalemia is treated with IV administration of potassium chloride. The child's urine output should be monitored to ensure that renal failure is not complicating the clinical picture.

Administer potassium chloride (0.5 to 1 mEq/kg IV) over 2 to 3 hours. (NOTE: This should *not* be labeled "bolus" therapy—it is a potassium *infusion* over hours, *not* a rapid infusion over minutes.) *Dilute* IV potassium and administer *slowly* over several hours to avoid vascular irritation or burns. If administered through a peripheral IV line, the ideal concentration is 3 to 4 mEq/dl, but greater concentration may be required. If central venous administration is provided or fluid restriction is necessary, concentration may be 1 mEq/10 to 20 ml.

Mild Hypokalemia Asymptomatic mild hypokalemia may be corrected with oral potassium supplementation. Total daily potassium requirements average 20 to 40 mEq/kg/day.

Hypokalemic Metabolic Alkalosis Correction of the hypokalemia can be provided with oral potassium supplements that provide approximately 2 to 4 mEq/kg/day of potassium (higher doses are required if potassium losses are increased). If the hypokalemia is also associated with hypochloremia, administration of ammonium chloride may be indicated. Half of the corrective dose of ammonium chloride is administered, and the child's acid-base balance is then reevaluated. Half of the corrective dose can be calculated as follows:

mEq ammonium chloride for 50% correction
$$= 0.25 \text{ L/kg} \times \text{Weight in kg} \times (HCO_3^- - 24)$$

Respiratory Alkalosis If the hypokalemia is associated with respiratory alkalosis, correction of the alkalosis is the treatment of choice. If the alkalosis will be maintained (e.g., in the treatment of pulmonary hypertension), potassium administration will correct the hypokalemia but must be tapered when the respiratory alkalosis will be discontinued.

Hyperkalemia

Etiology

Hyperkalemia can result from excessive potassium administration, inadequate potassium excretion by the kidneys, or a shift of potassium from the cellular to the vascular space with a fall in serum pH. Hyperkalemia may also result from potassium release from injured cells, which may occur in association with severe dehydration, trauma or burns, shock or sepsis, transfusion reaction, or acute tumor lysis syndrome. Hyperkalemia may be a sign of congenital adrenal cortical hyperplasia.

Pathophysiology

Potassium excess is present when the serum value is >5.5 mEq/L. When the potassium concentration increases, the membrane potential in excitable tissue is affected. A high serum potassium concentration hyperpolarizes membranes but can result in cardiac conduction disturbances and arrhythmias.

Acidosis can be associated with an acute increase in the serum potassium concentration because it produces an intravascular shift of potas-

sium as hydrogen ions move from the vascular space into cells in exchange for potassium. Therefore hyperkalemia in the presence of acidosis should be expected to correct when the acidosis is treated. A rising pH, due to the development of alkalosis or correction of acidosis, produces a fall in the serum potassium level. An abrupt increase in pH (alkalosis) by 0.1 unit may reduce the serum potassium concentration by 0.6 to 0.7 mEq/L. Therefore a serum potassium level that is high despite the presence of alkalosis indicates significant hyperkalemia. If serum potassium is normal in an alkalotic patient, it should be expected to rise further as the alkalosis is corrected.

Clinical Presentation

Remember that the serum potassium concentration should be interpreted in light of the child's current pH and anticipated changes in pH in response to therapy. A normal serum potassium concentration may quickly become a high serum potassium concentration if the child is alkalotic and correction of the alkalosis is planned. Alternatively, a high serum potassium concentration may be acceptable if acidosis is present and will be corrected.

The serum potassium concentration should always be evaluated in light of renal function, and a rise in serum potassium should be anticipated when renal function is compromised. Hypokalemia should be treated with caution in the child with a compromise in renal function, since supplementation may result in "overcorrection" of the potassium and creation of hyperkalemia.

Severe Hyperkalemia *Once the serum potassium concentration is >7 to 8 mEq/L, symptoms of hyperkalemia, particularly cardiac arrhythmias, should be anticipated and treatment should be initiated.* ECG changes are most common, including a prolonged PR interval, absence of a P wave, ventricular arrhythmias or fibrillation, and cardiac arrest.

Mild to Moderate Hyperkalemia Mild increases in serum potassium produce skeletal and smooth muscle weakness, flaccid muscles, and decreased reflexes. ECG changes include peaked T waves, a widening QRS complex, ST segment depression, and decreasing amplitude of the R wave.

Management

Hyperkalemia should be prevented whenever possible by identifying patients at risk and curtailing sources of potassium intake. In addition, the effect of changes in serum pH and renal function on serum potassium should be considered and treatment adjusted accordingly.

Severe, Symptomatic Hyperkalemia Once the serum potassium concentration is >7 to 8 mEq/L or is associated with ECG changes, intravascular potassium must be emergently reduced by one or more of the following methods (Table 9-7):

- *Stabilize myocardial membranes:* Administer calcium gluconate (60 to 100 mg/kg IV) or calcium chloride (20 to 25 mg/kg IV). Administer by slow IV push (no more than 100 mg/min).
- *Shift potassium into cells:* Create serum alkalosis with administration of sodium bicarbonate and administer glucose plus insulin.

- *Prevent ongoing gastrointestinal absorption of potassium:* Administer sodium polystyrene sulfonate (Kayexalate).
- *Remove potassium:* Provide exchange transfusion or dialysis.

Moderate, Asymptomatic Hyperkalemia If the serum potassium concentration is <7 mEq/L and significant symptoms are absent, intravascular potassium is removed by one or a combination of the following methods:

- *Expansion of the extracellular fluid space:* Bolus (20 ml/kg) of potassium-free 0.9% NaCl
- *Excretion of potassium from the body:* Administer sodium polystyrene sulfonate enema (1 g/kg)

Mild, Asymptomatic Hyperkalemia Mild hyperkalemia not associated with symptoms may be treated through elimination of potassium intake,

Table 9-7
Emergency Management of Hyperkalemia

Therapy	Dose	Onset of Effect	Duration of Effect
Stabilize Myocardium			
Calcium gluconate	0.6-1ml/kg of 10% solution (60-100 mg/kg)*	1-3 min	30-60 min
Calcium chloride	0.2-0.25 ml/kg of 10% solution (20-25 mg/kg)*	1-3 min	30-60 min
Shift Into Cells			
Sodium bicarbonate	1 mEq/kg IV bolus	5-10 min	1-2 hr
Insulin plus glucose	Regular insulin (0.1 U/kg IV) plus 2.5% glucose (1-2 ml/kg) 1-2 ml/kg 25% glucose	30 min	4-6 hr
Remove From Body			
Diuresis with furosemide	1-4 mg/kg IV bolus	When diuresis starts	When diuresis ends
Cation-exchange resin (sodium polystyrene sulfonate [Kayexalate])	0.5-1 g/kg plus sorbitol	1-2 hr	4-6 hr
Peritoneal dialysis or hemodialysis	Per institution	As soon as started	Until dialysis is completed

Modified from Hazinski MF, Cummins RO: *The 1997-1999 handbook of emergency cardiovascular care,* Dallas, 1997, American Heart Association.
*Administer by *slow* IV push (no faster than 100 mg/min).

treatment of the underlying cause (e.g., acidosis, dehydration), and dilution (administration of potassium-free fluids to expand the extracellular fluid space and reduce the serum potassium concentration).

Acute Renal Failure

Etiology

Acute Renal Failure (ARF) is the loss of renal capacity for filtration and tubular reabsorption. ARF may be categorized as prerenal, intrarenal (acute tubular necrosis [ATN]), or postrenal. Postrenal failure is usually associated with obstruction at any point in the ureters, bladder, or urethral meatus. ARF secondary to postrenal failure is responsible for a relatively small percentage of ARF and is treated surgically; therefore it is not discussed further here.

Prerenal Failure   Prerenal failure is probably the most common cause of ARF. It results from a decrease in renal perfusion, with a resulting decrease in glomerular perfusion and GFR. Impaired renal blood flow may be secondary to impaired cardiac performance, vasodilation, or intravascular volume depletion (see Shock, p. 130). Vasoconstrictive agents, such as alpha-adrenergic agents and indomethacin, may also decrease renal perfusion. With prompt recognition and restoration of adequate renal blood flow, prerenal ARF has a good prognosis for kidney function.

Intrarenal Failure   Intrarenal failure, or ATN, typically results from an acute insult to the kidneys, such as a drug reaction, acute hemolysis, or administration of high osmotic loads. Nephrotoxic ATN is a result of a toxic insult to the renal tubules, such as occurs with nephrotoxic drugs (e.g., cephalosporins, aminoglycosides, sulfonamides), radiographic contrast dye, organic solvents, or inappropriate levels of hemoglobin or myoglobin. The pathophysiology is similar to ischemic ATN; however, the healing process and prognosis are better.

Ischemic ATN (hemodynamically mediated renal failure) is related to a sudden and sustained decline in renal blood flow and the GFR, with necrosis of tubule cells secondary to nephrotoxic injury. The body attempts to compensate and maintain an adequate renal blood flow and GFR. Renal compensatory and autoregulatory mechanisms are exhausted, renal oxygen delivery is critically impaired, and tubular and cellular damage occurs.

Pathophysiology

The pathophysiology of ATN can be explained by a combination of factors:

- *Vasoactive factors:* Arteriolar vasoconstriction is induced.
- *Tubular factors:* As hydrostatic pressure increases, a back leak occurs from the tubular lumen to the vasa recta. Cellular sloughing and casts cause tubular obstruction.
- *Vascular factors:* In low blood flow states, nephrotoxins are concentrated in the renal tubular cells. Glomerular capillary permeability to protein increases. Hyperkalemia can develop because distal tubular injury impairs potassium secretion. In addition, the decrease in GFR and urine output reduces potassium secretion by the cortical collecting tubules.
- *Metabolic factors:* Damage to the cell membrane and impaired cellular function occur as the calcium flux is altered and oxygen free radicals are formed.

Clinical Presentation

ARF is characterized by a BUN >80 mg/dl and a serum creatinine concentration >1.5 mg/dl. Oliguria is a common but not invariable clinical sign of ARF. Occasionally, nonoliguric renal failure develops, with a normal urine volume or polyuria.

Once ARF develops, the kidney's ability to regulate fluid volume is compromised. Hypervolemia will develop, and this may contribute to the development of congestive heart failure unless fluid administration is curtailed.

Renal regulation of potassium, calcium, and glucose concentrations is seriously impaired. Hyperkalemia may develop and can rise rapidly in the presence of acidosis, hemolysis, infection, gastrointestinal bleeding, or trauma. Hyperphosphatemia develops as a result of the fall in GFR and will contribute to hypocalcemia. Renal activation of vitamin D is also reduced. Hypoglycemia may develop in young infants, particularly if nutrition is compromised.

Regulation of acid-base balance is compromised. Renal tubular acidosis may develop as the kidney's ability to excrete hydrogen ions and form titratable acids is limited. This acidosis can contribute to worsening of the hyperkalemia. Patients with ARF may also develop anemia and coagulopathies and are at risk for development of gastrointestinal hemorrhage and infection. Finally, clinical signs of uremia may be present, including an altered level of consciousness, anorexia, nausea, abnormal platelet function, diminished white blood cell function, and pericarditis.

Once ARF develops, it is important to differentiate between reversible prerenal or postrenal causes and renal failure resulting from parenchymal damage (Table 9-8). The most accurate test to differentiate prerenal failure from ARF caused by renal factors is calculation of the fractional excretion of sodium (FE_{Na}). Note that this test will not yield reliable results if diuretic therapy has recently been provided. The FE_{Na} requires simultaneous collection of a urine and serum sample and is calculated as follows:

$$FE_{Na} = \frac{\dfrac{\text{Urine sodium concentration}}{\text{Serum sodium concentration}}}{\dfrac{\text{Urine creatinine concentration}}{\text{Serum creatinine concentration}}} \times 100$$

Prerenal failure is indicated by an $FE_{Na} < 1\%$ (or 2.5% in neonates). Intrarenal failure is indicated by an $FE_{Na} > 1\%$ to 3%.

Prerenal Failure   The FE_{Na} is low in prerenal failure because a healthy kidney with decreased perfusion will respond by retaining sodium and water and excreting a small volume of concentrated urine. Urine osmolality will typically be >500 mOsm/L with a serum sodium concentration of <300 mOsm/L. The BUN is typically high in proportion to the serum creatinine (ratio >20:1) because the urea is reabsorbed as the kidneys reabsorb sodium and water.

Intrarenal Failure   The FE_{Na} is high when the ARF is due to intrarenal causes because renal function itself is compromised. The urine is typically not concentrated and may contain casts of renal tubular cells. If the urine is positive when tested for blood, hemoglobinuria or myoglobinuria should be suspected.

Radiologic Consultation   Radiologic consultation may be helpful if serum and urine laboratory values are inconclusive. The risk of IV pyelography outweighs its benefit. Ultrasonography can document the presence of one or two kidneys and enable evaluation of renal size, the urine collection system, the renal parenchyma, and the renal vessels. The presence of azotemia and small kidneys indicates underlying chronic renal disease. The presence of enlarged kidneys often indicates hydronephrosis, renal vein thrombosis, nephrotic

Table 9-8
Clinical and Laboratory Differentiation of Prerenal Failure vs. Acute Tubular Necrosis

	Prerenal	ATN
Urine output	Decreased	Decreased or normal
Urine sediment	Normal	Red blood cell casts, cellular debris
Specific gravity	High	Low
Osmolality (urine/plasma)	>1.5 (>1.2 in neonates)	<1.2
Urine sodium	Low	High
Creatinine (urine/plasma)	>15:1	<10:1
FE_{Na} (%)*	<1 (<2.5 in neonates)	>2 (>3 in neonates)
Creatinine	Normal or slowly increasing	High and increasing
BUN	High	High and increasing

*Administration of furosemide (Lasix) may affect results and/or measurement of urine sodium concentration.

Box 9-3

Management of Acute Renal Failure

Plan of Care to Support Renal Function
1. Eliminate the cause of acute renal failure (ARF), if known.
2. Discontinue or alter the dose of potentially nephrotoxic medications.
3. Maintain adequate intravascular volume.
4. Maintain adequate blood pressure.
5. Once adequate blood pressure and hydration are restored, consider medications:
   a. Diuretics (e.g., furosemide)
   b. Low-dose dopamine (1-5 µg/kg/min)
6. Consider renal replacement therapy if unable to support function with above measures:
   a. Hemodialysis
   b. Peritoneal dialysis
   c. Continuous renal replacement therapy

Desire Patient Outcomes
1. Urine output remains adequate.
2. Laboratory values indicate resolving ARF (e.g., stabilized or decreasing BUN and creatinine).
3. Cardiac output remains adequate.
4. Fluid and electrolyte balance is maintained.

Box 9-4

Potential Complications of Acute Renal Failure

Cardiovascular: Arrhythmias, decreased cardiac output, hypertension
Respiratory: Pneumonia, pulmonary edema
Gastrointestinal: Hemorrhage, nausea and vomiting, malnutrition
Neurologic: Altered mental status
Metabolic: Acidosis, hypocalcemia, hyperkalemia, uremia, hypermagnesemia, hyperphosphatemia, hyperuricemia
Hematologic: Anemia, coagulopathy
Infection: Sepsis, pneumonia

---

syndrome, cystic disease, acute glomerulonephritis, or various infiltrative diseases. Radionucleotide scanning documents renal perfusion and function (e.g., urinary tract obstruction, renal vein thrombosis, inflammatory conditions of the kidney, renal artery disease). Renal biopsy should be performed only when there is reasonable belief that the test results will alter therapy, and the benefits of the results outweigh the risks of the procedure.

Management

Management of the child with ARF is highlighted in Box 9-3

Potential Complications of ARF   Potential complications of ARF are listed in Box 9-4. Throughout therapy, these complications should be anticipated, prevented when possible, and treated immediately when detected.

Fluid Balance and Systemic and Renal Perfusion

The goal of treatment of ARF is to maintain fluid balance and adequate renal perfusion without creating fluid overload. CVP measurements can be used to evaluate intravascular fluid volume and to titrate fluid administration and removal. Monitor systemic perfusion closely. Indications of poor perfusion are cool extremities, sluggish capillary refill, and diminished peripheral pulses. Tachycardia or tachypnea, and metabolic acidosis may indicate inadequate cardiac output. Systemic hypotension is a late sign of inadequate cardiac output. A CVP of 2 to 5 mm Hg should be sufficient to maintain cardiac output if myocardial function is normal; higher filling pressures (10 mm Hg or higher) may be required in the presence of myocardial failure.

If significant hypovolemia is present, administer a fluid challenge (20 ml/kg) of a crystalloid solution. If systemic perfusion improves following the bolus but there is no increase in urine output, furosemide (1 to 4 mg/kg/dose) or mannitol (0.2 to 0.5 g/kg) may be prescribed.

Cardiovascular Support   If oliguria is associated with a CVP of 5 to 10 mm Hg, renal failure may be a result of low cardiac output from myocardial (pump) failure. Hypoglycemia, hypocalcemia, and acidosis can all depress cardiac function and should therefore be detected and treated. Once electrolyte balance is restored, administration of a sympathomimetic inotropic agent may be required. The sympathomimetic drug of choice for the oliguric patient with cardiovascular dysfunction is dopamine. Dopamine may produce selective dilation of the renal artery and an increased renal blood flow and GFR when administered in low doses (1 to 5 μg/kg/min). However, higher doses of dopamine (>10 μg/kg/min) should probably be avoided if ARF is present, as they may produce alpha-adrenergic effects, including renal vasoconstriction, decreased renal blood flow, and decreased urine output (see Table 5-13).

Additional sympathomimetic agents, such as dobutamine (1 to 10 μg/kg/min) or isoproterenol (0.05 to 0.2 μg/kg/min), may also be administered if prerenal failure is present. If systemic perfusion remains poor, systemic vasodilators, such as sodium nitroprusside (0.5 to 8 μg/kg/min) or nitroglycerin (0.1 to 10 mg/kg/min), may be considered (see Table 5-14).

Diuretic Therapy   Diuretic therapy may be indicated if the sympathomimetic or vasodilator therapy results in an increase in systemic perfusion and blood pressure without a concurrent rise in urine output. Intravenous furosemide may be administered (1 to 4 mg/kg/dose, although a single dose may be as high as 5 to 10 mg/kg). Mannitol (0.2 to 0.5 g/kg) should be administered with caution because of the potential for creation of intravascular hypervolemia.

A response to diuretic therapy should be demonstrated 1 to 3 hours after dosing. If the urine output does not improve during this time, the child is presumed to have renal failure and renal parenchymal damage. If hypervolemia is compromising cardiovascular function, renal replacement therapy may be indicated.

Fluid Therapy   If *oliguric* renal failure is present, fluid therapy should be limited to that required to maintain intravascular volume and to avoid hypovolemia. Hypervolemia must be prevented. Fluid intake is restricted to a volume equal to the total amount of insensible water loss plus any urine output and other nasogastric or drain output (Box 9-5). Fluid replacement should be calculated based on a strict account of all fluid intake and output. Fluid choice is determined by electrolyte and acid-base balance. Repeated fluid boluses and repeated diuretic dosing in the unresponsive patient should be limited to avoid hypervolemia and changes in serum osmolality.

Box 9-5

Estimation of Insensible Water Losses*

Infants (<10 kg): 35 ml/kg/day or 300 ml/m^2/24 hr

Children (>10 kg): 15-20 ml/kg/day or 300 ml/m^2/24 hr plus urine output

*NOTE: Insensible water losses are increased in the presence of fever or during catabolic states.

Electrolyte and Acid-Base Balance   Electrolyte and acid-base balance must be monitored closely and maintained during all stages of renal failure. Water and salt depletion can develop during *nonoliguric* renal failure as these substances are lost in the urine. Calcium, potassium, and hydrogen ions may be lost with high urine output.

Potassium Balance   Alterations in the serum potassium level often develop during ARF. The serum potassium level should be evaluated frequently. Potassium administration should be limited unless significant hypokalemia is present. Hyperkalemia should be treated promptly (see Hyperkalemia, p. 469).

Phosphorus and Calcium Therapy   Most patients with ARF develop hyperphosphatemia. Hyperphosphatemia should be treated because it usually produces hypocalcemia, which can result in neuromuscular or cardiovascular dysfunction. Significant hyperphosphatemia should be treated in order to avoid symptomatic hypocalcemia. Calcium carbonate tablets may be used to treat mild or moderate asymptomatic hyperphosphatemia. Severe or symptomatic hyperphosphatemia (causing severe hypocalcemia) is treated with a renal replacement therapy such as hemodialysis or continuous venovenous hemofiltration.

Significant hypocalcemia is treated with infusions of 10% calcium gluconate (60 to 100 mg/kg/dose, up to 2 g) or calcium chloride (20 to 50 mg/kg/dose, up to 1 g). Calcium should be administered slowly to prevent bradycardia. The most effective treatment for hypocalcemia under these conditions is the resolution of hyperphosphatemia.

Metabolic Acidosis   Acidosis can depress enzyme and cellular mitochondrial activity and may contribute to nausea, vomiting, hyperkalemia, and cardiovascular dysfunction. Mild acidosis can be treated with hyperventilation. Severe acidosis, unresponsive to changes in ventilation, may require the administration of a buffering agent such as sodium bicarbonate. In the hypercarbic, acidotic patient, other agents such as tris (hydroxymethyl) aminomethane (THAM) may be considered. However, since THAM may produce hyperkalemia and hypoglycemia, it is rarely used in the presence of renal failure.

The typical sodium bicarbonate dose to correct metabolic acidosis is 1 mEq/kg. The dose may also be calculated according to the base deficit (base deficit $\times$ body weight in kilograms $\times$ 0.3 to correct half of the deficit) or the serum bicarbonate or carbon dioxide level ([15 $-$ serum CO_2] $\times$ body weight in kilograms $\times$ 0.3). Sodium bicarbonate is administered in a diluted 1:1 form because of its high osmolality. Because sodium bicarbonate contains sodium, repeated doses may enhance water retention and edema.

Glucose   Serum glucose levels should be monitored frequently, especially in the infant and young child. Treat hypoglycemia promptly with a continuous infusion of a glucose solution (2 to 4 ml/kg/hr of 5% dextrose solution or 1 to 2 ml/kg/hr of 10% dextrose solution). If the serum glucose is severely low, an initial bolus of glucose (25% dextrose, 2 to 4 ml/kg) may be provided. Repeat "bolus" administration of hypertonic glucose is an undesirable way to correct hypoglycemia because it may result in wide fluctuations in the serum osmolality and serum glucose concentrations, producing free water shifts into and out of the vascular space.

Hematologic Complications   ARF can produce anemia and coagulopathies. It is important to monitor for signs of complications, including petechiae, ecchymoses, gastrointestinal bleeding, or other sources of bleeding. The platelet count, prothrombin time (PT), and partial thromboplastin time (PTT) should be monitored regularly. Blood component therapy should be administered as needed.

Infection Control   The child with ARF has an increased risk for infection because of a compro-

mised nutritional state. Any invasive catheters or tubes also increase the risk of infection.

Treatment of Hypertension   Hypertension may occur secondary to hypervolemia or high plasma renin activity. Severe or symptomatic hypertension is treated with antihypertensive agents. Drug dosages should be titrated carefully in the presence of decreased GFR:

- Sodium nitroprusside: 0.5 to 8 μg/kg/min
- Nitroglycerin: 0.1 to 10 μg/kg/min
- Hydralazine: 0.15 mg/kg/dose IV or IM, given up to every 4 hours
- Nifedipine: 0.25 to 0.5 mg/kg PO every 6 to 8 hours

Nutrition   Adequate nutrition will assist in recovery from ARF. Oral or nasogastric feedings are preferred. However, if the child cannot tolerate this route, parenteral alimentation should be initiated as soon as possible. Adjustments should be made in the daily caloric intake to account for catabolism and to limit the accumulation of metabolic waste products.

Adjustment of Medication Dosages   When the child develops ARF, *all medication doses should be reevaluated,* especially doses of drugs that are excreted by the kidneys. Adjustments may be made according to serum drug level monitoring or according to estimated drug clearance rates. If the nonrenal excretion of a specific drug is known and the child's creatinine clearance is known, the daily clearance of a specific drug can be estimated. Modification of drug dosages for the patient with renal failure is presented under Diagnostic Studies and Adjustments of Medications in Renal Failure, Box 9-7, p. 490 and Table 9-11, p. 491.

Psychosocial Support   The potential psychosocial effects of ARF are complicated and multifactorial. This demands focus by every member of the health care team on the educational and psychosocial needs of the child and family.

Indications for Renal Replacement Therapy   If the child in ARF is unresponsive to initial therapy or continues to deteriorate despite aggressive management, renal replacement therapy may be required. The appropriate therapy is often determined by a combination of the following factors: severity of illness, severity of complications, weight of the child, hemodynamic stability, and facility resources available.

Renal Replacement Therapy in Children

Renal replacement therapies for infants and children include peritoneal dialysis, hemodialysis, and continuous renal replacement therapy.

Acute Peritoneal Dialysis

Indications

Indications for peritoneal dialysis (PD) include congenital metabolic disease, ATN, renal cortical necrosis, obstructive uropathy, renal agenesis, bilateral renal dysplasia, and other renal dysfunction requiring long-term, nonemergent therapy. PD is often selected over other renal replacement therapies for infants and children who cannot tolerate anticoagulation or displacement of blood volume. PD may be used to treat either ARF or chronic renal failure.

Technique

PD may be classified as continuous ambulatory PD (CAPD), manual PD, or continuous cycling PD using a cycler computerized mechanical device. Peritoneal access is achieved with placement of a soft catheter into the peritoneal space. Catheter placement may be performed in the operating room or at the bedside.

PD uses the principle of diffusion to move water and solutes across the peritoneal membrane. When dialysate with an osmolality higher than vascular or interstitial osmolality is introduced into the peritoneal cavity, free water and electrolytes will move from the blood vessels supplying the peritoneal membrane across the semipermeable peritoneal membrane into the cavity, where they can be drained through the peritoneal catheter. The rate of removal of water and solutes (ultrafiltrate) is en-

hanced by increasing the dextrose and osmolality of the dialysate solution or by increasing the amount of time the dialysate solution dwells in the peritoneal space.

The amount of dialysate placed into the peritoneal space (inflow volume) is gradually increased as tolerated to a volume of 15 to 50 ml/kg of body weight. Standard dialysate solution contains dextrose, sodium, calcium, magnesium, chloride, and lactate (which is metabolized to produce bicarbonate). Potassium, heparin, antibiotics, or antifungal medications can be added to the peritoneal fluid as needed.

CAPD or manual PD may be required in infants and small children when inflow volumes are <50 ml. Signs of excessive inflow volume include an uncomfortable fullness and pain or discomfort on inflow. Inflow should be reduced if these develop. The dialysate solution must be warmed to or near body temperature to prevent hypothermia.

Manual Peritoneal Dialysis Manual PD requires more nursing time than the cycler method because the nurse must manually instill and drain fluid, time dwell intervals, measure inflow and outflow volumes, calculate net ultrafiltration after each dwell time, and tabulate the cumulative ultrafiltrate. Dialysate is infused by gravity into the peritoneal space through the catheter, and then the inflow tubing is clamped. Buretrols should be placed between the dialysate bags and the patient to prevent unintentional infusion of large volumes of dialysate if the inflow clamp loosens.

Clots, kinks, and catheter position can compromise dialysate inflow. Once the desired volume is instilled, the catheter is clamped, and a timer is set to mark dwell time completion. Dwell times generally range from 15 to 30 minutes. On completion of the dwell time, the catheter is unclamped, and the outflow drains by gravity to a collection bag and is measured. The net ultrafiltrate is calculated (outflow volume minus inflow volume). The inflow-dwell-outflow cycle is repeated at ordered time intervals.

Cycler Peritoneal Dialysis Cycler PD uses a closed system and a programmable, automated mechanism for measurement and delivery of inflow, monitoring of dwell time, drainage, and calculation of ultrafiltrate. This system requires less hands-on nursing time, is associated with a reduced infection rate because the system is closed, and has a built-in mechanism for dialysate warming. Dwell times impact waste removal and fluid removal. Long dwell times may achieve good waste and solute clearance but poor fluid removal. Short dwell times have poor waste and solute clearance but remove a significant amount of fluid.

Variables to Be Recorded   During any form of PD, records of total fluid intake and output must be strictly maintained. The volume of dialysate infused, the dwell time, and the volume of fluid recovered are each recorded. The volume of fluid recovered should always equal or exceed the amount infused. When the volume recovered exceeds that infused, it is recorded as a negative total, since it represents fluid removed from the patient. If the volume recovered is less than the volume infused, a positive balance is recorded When a positive balance develops, mechanical obstruction is the likely cause, and a physician should be notified; this problem must be corrected.

Potential Complications

A major potential complication of PD is peritonitis, which can produce cloudy dialysate, abdominal pain, tenderness, or sepsis. Mechanical and iatrogenic catheter problems can also develop. These problems include leakage at the insertion site, bowel perforation, retroperitoneal hemorrhage, increased intraabdominal pressure due to obstruction of the catheter, and hernia. Bloody dialysate may be observed for the first 24 to 48 hours after catheter insertion but is usually self-limiting.

Fluid and electrolyte imbalances may develop during PD. Hypertonic dehydration and hemoconcentration can develop if too much free water is removed too rapidly. This complication is prevented by beginning with a low osmolality dialysate and increasing it gradually if needed to remove fluid. Other potential systemic complications include impaired pulmonary function related to abdominal distension and fluid overload, decreased cardiac output and stroke volume related to fluid volume overload or loss, hypoproteinemia due to loss of protein in the dialysate, and hyperglycemia related to absorption of dextrose from the dialysate. Hyperglycemia may require treatment with insulin.

Pain is a common complaint during initial dialysis infusions and outflows. It is typically present during inflow as a result of pressure created by volume accumulation in the peritoneum. Pain may be relieved by floating the catheter to another position when the abdomen is filled or by changing the patient's position. Pain may also be caused by extremes of dialysate temperature. Pain during outflow may be minimized by leaving a small volume of dialysate in the peritoneum at the end of every cycle.

Hemodialysis

Indications

Indications for hemodialysis include symptomatic electrolyte imbalance (such as symptomatic hyperkalemia), hypervolemia, pulmonary edema, severe acidosis, anuria that is not responsive to other therapy, severely elevated BUN with elevated creatinine, cardiac failure, tumor lysis syndrome, hepatic failure, and other conditions that require rapid, efficient correction of the abnormality.

Technique

Hemodialysis uses an extracorporeal circuit that carries blood from the child through a filter, an artificial kidney, and back to the child. The artificial kidney has a semipermeable membrane through which water, solutes, and other substances are filtered (ultrafiltrate). Removal of solutes occurs through the filter by diffusion, which is created by the infusion of the dialysate into the filter (the other side of the semipermeable membrane) in a direction opposite the flow of blood. Negative pressure is added to the dialysate side of the circuit to increase fluid and solute removal from the blood. Positive pressure is added to the venous side of the blood circuit, thus increasing resistance to blood flow so excess fluid can be more readily removed. Vascular access may be obtained using one double-lumen central venous catheter, or an arterial catheter and a venous catheter, or via two single-lumen central venous catheters.

It is important to consider the extracorporeal circuit volume in relation to the child's circulating blood volume to prevent hypovolemia. In general, if the extracorporeal circuit volume is greater than 10% of the child's circulating blood volume or if the child weighs less than 10 kg, it is necessary to prime the hemodialysis circuit with a colloid substance. Small-volume filters and circuit sizes have enabled use of hemodialysis for small infants.

Potential Complications

Potential complications of hemodialysis in infants and children include hypovolemia, hypotension, hypervolemia, systemic bleeding, anemia, artificial kidney rupture or circuit disconnection, infection, and transfusion reaction. Fluid shifts and disequilibrium may develop if sodium, urea, or other osmotic particles are removed too quickly from the patient's blood and the patient's serum osmolality falls rapidly.

The dialysis technician or nurse will be responsible for monitoring the dialysis circuit and keeping tract of fluid intake and output through that circuit, but the bedside nurse is responsible for monitoring the patient's vital signs, oxygenation, hemodynamics, fluid status, electrolyte balance, and physiologic response to treatment. The dialysis technician or nurse and bedside nurse should work together to determine the best sites for medication administration and times for blood sampling.

Inadequately treated hypovolemia, rapid electrolyte and pH changes, and hypoxemia can compromise cardiac function and systemic perfusion. Volume expanders such as albumin or colloid products (or both) should be readily available and used as needed. Administration of hyperosmotic agents (mannitol) may increase diuresis.

Hemodialysis removes water-soluble drugs with low molecular weights, along with the solutes, water, and toxins; therefore drug dosing must be adjusted for the patient receiving hemodialysis. A hemodynamically unstable child may not tolerate hemodialysis and may require a more gradual method of fluid removal, such as PD or continuous renal replacement therapy.

Hemoperfusion

Hemoperfusion is useful in removing protein- and lipid-bound substances and may be particularly effective in the removal of some poisons. The vascular access and circuit used for hemoperfusion are identical to those used for hemodialysis with the substitution of a cartridge containing activated charcoal for the artificial kidney, filter, and dialysate.

The hemoperfusion circuit is usually primed with colloid or blood, and anticoagulation must be provided. Rebound toxicity is the most common complication observed following hemoperfusion as the lipid-bound drugs that have been stored in tissues move into the vascular space hours after the hemoperfusion has removed the drugs from the blood.

Continuous Renal Replacement Therapy

Indications

Indications for continuous renal replacement therapy (CRRT) include ARF with hemodynamic instability, azotemia, severe electrolyte imbalance, hypervolemia, and symptomatic metabolic abnormalities. CRRT is appropriate for hemodynamically unstable patients who are unable to tolerate hemodialysis and for patients who are not candidates for PD (e.g., patients with abdominal trauma or surgery who develop ARF). Continuous, extracorporeal renal replacement therapies include slow continuous ultrafiltration (SCUF), continuous arteriovenous ultrafiltration (CAVU), continuous arteriovenous hemodiafiltration (CAVHD), continuous venovenous hemofiltration (CVVH), and continuous venovenous hemodiafiltration (CVVHD). These types of CRRT are compared in Table 9-9.

Technique

Vascular access may be achieved through an arterial catheter and a venous catheter, through a double-lumen venous catheter, or through two single-lumen venous catheters. Continuous therapy using an arteriovenous circuit is described as continuous arteriovenous hemofiltration (CAVH). If dialysate solution is added to the circuit to utilize diffusion to remove solutes and fluid, the therapy is referred to as continuous arteriovenous hemodiafiltration (CAVHD). CRRT using a venovenous circuit is described as continuous venovenous hemofiltration (CVVH). If dialysate solution is added to this circuit to utilize diffusion to remove solutes and fluid, the therapy is referred to as continuous venovenous hemodiafiltration (CVVHD).

The CAVH circuit is dependent on the arterial blood pressure to propel the blood through the tubing and filter. Therefore the blood flow and efficiency of the CAVH circuit is limited by the mean arterial pressure of the patient. In contrast, the

Table 9-9
Comparison of Forms of Continuous Renal Replacement Therapy*

	Access	Equipment Needs	Advantages	Disadvantages
CAVU or	Arteriovenous		Simple	
SCUF	or venovenous		Less costly	
CAVH	Arteriovenous			
CAVHD	Arteriovenous		Better solute clearance	
CVVH	Venovenous	Blood pump required	No arterial access required; independent of mean arterial pressure	
CVVHD	Venovenous	Blood pump required	Better solute clearance	Complex

*See text for abbreviations.

CVVH circuit does not use arterial access and requires a blood pump to propel the blood through the tubing and filter. Although CVVH requires more mechanical devices, it offers an efficient circuit that is driven by a pump instead of the patient's blood pressure. CVVH is becoming a preferred type of CRRT for the hemodynamically unstable patient in many neonatal and pediatric intensive care units.

Methods of Measuring Filtration Capability or Performance of Continuous Venovenous Hemofiltration

Clearance is the removal of solutes from the plasma and is dependent on the device's capability for removing individual molecules, the size of the solute, the solute's protein-binding capacity, and the rate of blood flow through the hemofilter. Negative pull pressure can be added by using an infusion pump to draw ultrafiltrate across the filter. Clearance for a particular molecule can be expressed by the ultrafiltrate-plasma ratio, known as the *sieving coefficient.*

$$\text{Sieving coefficient}$$
$$= \frac{\text{Concentration of ``X'' in ultrafiltrate}}{\text{Concentration of ``X'' in plasma}}$$
$$= \frac{(X)\, Uf}{(X)\, Plasma}$$
$$= 100\% \text{ clearance})$$

Another indicator of the efficiency of the system is the *filtration fraction (FF).* The FF is reflective of the fraction of plasma water that is being removed by ultrafiltration. Optimal FF is a percentage that is sufficiently high to provide adequate solute and fluid removal needs, but not so high that blood viscosity and increased oncotic pressure impact filter performance.

$$FF(\%)$$
$$= \frac{\text{ultrafiltrate rate (ml/min)} \times 100}{\text{Plasma flow rate at inlet (ml/min)}}$$
$$= \frac{Qf}{QP} \times 100$$

Clinical Considerations for the Critically Ill Child on Continuous Venovenous Hemofiltration

Vascular Access   Vascular access is the key to success and the major source of frustration. It is often the limiting factor in CVVH blood pump speed and circuit efficiency. The vascular access catheter may be placed in the femoral or subclavian vein. Large catheters placed in relatively small vessels may require reversal of flow through the distal port in order to achieve adequate blood flow rates.

Circuit Priming   It is important to determine the relationship of circuit blood volume to the patient's circulating blood volume. In general, if the circuit

Table 9-10
Primary Pump Alarms on the Continuous Venovenous Hemofiltration Circuit

Alarm	Etiology	Things to Investigate	Possible Solutions
Low arterial/inflow pressure, (high negative "pull" pressure)	*Low blood flow;* difficulty pulling blood into circuit	? Kink or clot in catheter or arterial tubing; ? catheter wedged against vessel wall	Flush catheter; unkink tubing/catheter; reverse catheter flow
High arterial/inflow pressure	Rare; difficulty pushing blood through hemofilter	? Tubing reversed through roller head; ? kink in tubing from roller head to hemofilter	Trace tubing from patient to filter to ensure proper setup and patency
Low venous/outflow pressure	*Low resistance;* drop in blood flow entering venous side of circuit; decreased resistance required to push blood back to patient	? Loose connection or disconnection (blood or air leak) ? inadequate pump blood flow rate ? filter clotted	Trace tubing from filter to patient to ensure all connections tight; increase pump speed;* assess patency of filter
High venous/outflow pressure	*High resistance;* increased force required to push blood out of circuit to patient	? Tubing or catheter obstruction; ? clot or kink in tubing	Trace tubing (filter to patient) and ensure proper tubing set-up and patency; relieve obstruction in catheter as appropriate
Air detector	Air sensed by detector	? Air bubble; ? blood level in drip chamber is low, and turbulence is high; ? loose connection	Raise level of blood in drip chamber, or decrease pump speed; tighten all connections

*Venous pressure must be greater than 10 mm Hg for pump to operate.

blood volume is greater than 10% of the patient's circulating blood volume, or if the child weighs less than 10 kg, the circuit should be primed with a colloid product, such as reconstituted blood or 5% albumin. Common circuit alarms and their causes are listed in Table 9-10.

Fluid Balance Careful monitoring of intake and output balance is required for any patient in renal failure, but it is particularly important when the patient is receiving renal replacement therapy. If large volumes of filter replacement solution are used, as in high-flow predilution CVVH, the risk and implications of basic fluid calculation errors are high. Ideally, the CVVH blood pump, filter replacement solution pump, dialysate pump, and ultrafiltrate pump are all part of one integrated system.

If the CVVH system is a collection of a blood pump and several infusion pumps that are integrated, the bedside practitioner must strictly measure hourly intake and output for each. In this type of combined setup, an infusion pump is traditionally added to the ultrafiltrate tubing to ensure a constant ultrafiltrate production rate and to regulate fluid removal. It is important to remember that an infusion pump may have as much as a 5% error in measurement. Therefore the amount of filter replacement solution, dialysate, or ultrafiltrate displayed by the infusion pump may be ±5% of the actual volume delivered. In small neonates it may be necessary to measure fluid removal with a graduated cylinder or other more accurate measurement device.

Thermoregulation   A significant amount of heat is lost in the extracorporeal circuit. Recent advances in CVVH systems have decreased the extracorporeal blood volume to less than 80 ml and have reduced the heat loss through the circuit. However, thermoregulation may be necessary depending on the size of the child and the volume of the extracorporeal circuit. If a blood or fluid warmer is not integrated into the CVVH system, a warmer infusion system should be added to the circuit. External heating devices, such as overbed warmers, are inadequate for infants and small children.

Anticoagulation   In an effort to maintain patency of the circuit, a continuous heparin infusion may be necessary. Routine flushes of normal saline, lactated Ringer's, or filter replacement solution through the system have not been demonstrated to be effective in preventing clot formation in the circuit in the clinical setting. If there is no indication of coagulopathy, a heparin bolus is given to the patient at least 3 minutes before initiation of therapy. Then heparin is administered to maintain activated clotting times at 1½ times normal (approximately 180 to 200 seconds). The use of other agents to decrease platelet aggregation is under investigation.

Hemodynamic Support   It is important to observe for hemodynamic changes during initiation of the therapy, as well as during initial and progressive fluid removal. If precautions are taken, hemodynamic instability during initiation of CVVH is rare. Unlike CAVH, CVVH will function regardless of the child's mean arterial pressure and can therefore be used in times of low cardiac output.

During initiation of the therapy, hypotension may be caused by rapid blood administration and citrate-phosphate (blood preservative) binding of serum ionized calcium. If the circuit has been primed with a citrate-phosphate-dextran–preserved blood product, serum ionized calcium levels should be determined before starting the therapy, and concurrent administration of serum ionized calcium considered. Additional calcium replacement should be available at the bedside and may be administered during initiation of the CVVH to prevent hypotension. In addition, because of drug clearance by the hemofilter, it may be necessary to titrate the

infusion of vasopressor just before and/or in the first few minutes after initiation of CVVH.

To prevent hypotension related to hypovolemia, the fluid removal rate should be determined by intravascular fluid status. It may be necessary to begin an ordered zero fluid balance and slowly adjust the balance as the patient tolerates it. Strict recording of fluid intake and output is performed hourly. The formula for determining the hourly filter replacement fluid (FRF) rate is as follows:

$$FRF = \text{Total fluid out} - \text{Total fluid in} + \\ \text{Hourly fluid balance (which may} \\ \text{be negative or positive)}$$

If the child is receiving multiple blood products and/or fluid boluses, determine what is to be included in the formula as fluid to be "taken off" and what is fluid given to maintain intravascular volume. If additional fluid or pharmacologic support is required to maintain hemodynamic stability, reevaluate fluid removal rates and consider the effect of hypovolemia.

Complications

The most common complications associated with renal replacement therapies are fluid balance problems.

Specific Diseases

Nephrotic Syndrome

Etiology

Nephrotic syndrome is an association of clinical signs and biochemical abnormalities that occurs secondary to renal damage. It is characterized by the simultaneous presence of proteinuria (>0.1 g/kg/day or 2 g/m^2/day), hypoproteinemia (especially hypoalbuminemia), and edema. Hyperlipidemia and lipiduria are secondary complications.

Nephrotic syndrome may be classified by etiology or by histologic changes present in the glomerulus. However, the most common form is not associated with systemic disease or causative agent and is classified as primary (idiopathic) nephrotic syndrome.

Secondary nephrotic syndrome can occur as a result of secondary renal involvement associated with systemic disease such as infections, sickle cell disease, Hodgkin's disease, or systemic lupus erythematosus.

Drug or chemically induced nephrotic syndrome can result from aminoglycoside toxicity or effects of amphotericin B. The two main effects of the drug toxicity are renal tubular cell injury (primarily at the distal tubule) and acute afferent arteriolar vasoconstriction. Nephrotoxicity is predictable and usually reversible, and the severity of the effects on the tubules and glomerular filtration is proportional to drug dosage.

Secondary nephrotic syndrome may occasionally develop following administration of radiocontrast agents. The risk of nephrotoxicity with these agents is greatest in patients with preexisting renal dysfunction, diabetes, hypovolemia, proteinuria, or hyperuricemia. The nephrotoxicity generally presents in the first 24 hours after infusion. It may be mild with minimal symptoms or severe with symptoms of oliguria and pathologic changes in the proximal tubule. Protection against nephrotoxicity may be achieved through administration of calcium channel blockers.

Pathophysiology

In most cases nephrotic syndrome is "minimal change nephrotic syndrome," an uncomplicated primary nephrotic syndrome with no glomerular changes apparent under light microscopy. Other forms of nephrotic syndrome are characterized by thickening or sclerosis of the glomeruli.

The common element in all types of nephrotic syndrome is damage to the glomerular basement membrane. This damage results in increased glomerular permeability to protein. The proteinuria causes a fall in serum albumin levels. This results in a decrease in intravascular colloid osmotic pressure. Movement of fluid from the intravascular to the extravascular spaces is enhanced, producing edema and decreased intravascular volume.

The GFR will fall as a result of the fall in intravascular volume, and aldosterone and ADH release will be stimulated. This produces an increase in sodium and water reabsorption with resultant decrease in intravascular osmolality and further movement of fluid into the tissues. The patient may demonstrate a low or high intravascular volume. This is partly determined by the amounts of renin and aldosterone secretion, and the relative amounts of sodium and water retention. However, all patients demonstrate edema. Generalized edema is likely to develop once the serum albumin concentration drops below 2 g/dl.

Clinical Presentation

Children with nephrotic syndrome are generally asymptomatic except for discomfort related to generalized edema. Periorbital edema, dependent edema, and finally ascites develop. Generalized edema may also produce diarrhea, vomiting, or anorexia. Gastrointestinal symptoms and a generalized catabolic state deplete protein stores and are associated with significant malnutrition and loss of muscle mass.

Fluid balance is complicated by free water retention and extravascular fluid shifts. Hypovolemia and a compromise in systemic perfusion can complicate fluid shifts and diuretic therapy.

Oliguria is present. The urine is acidic, containing a large amount of protein, which may give it a foamy appearance. It may be tinted pink as a result of microscopic hematuria, and it may contain granular and cellular casts.

Severe hypoalbuminemia is generally present, with albumin levels of <2.5 g/dl. Electrolyte imbalances are common. Dilutional hyponatremia is secondary to free water retention. Hypokalemia develops secondary to hyperaldosteronism and poor dietary intake. Total serum calcium levels may be falsely low as a result of hypoalbuminemia. Some children will exhibit an increase in serum creatinine and BUN.

Nephrotic syndrome produces hematologic complications. Platelet aggregation and increased levels of beta-thromboglobulin produce hypercoagulopathy and increased risk of thromboembolism.

Management

Goals of Management of Nephrotic Syndrome
Goals of management include restoration or maintenance of:

- Adequate circulating blood volume
- Adequate systemic perfusion
- Fluid and electrolyte balance

In addition, maintenance of optimal renal function (including limitation of glomerular damage) and prevention of infection are necessary.

Restoration of systemic perfusion requires assessment and manipulation of intravascular fluid volume status. If systemic perfusion is compromised, insertion of a central venous monitoring catheter will enable measurement of CVP to evaluate intravascular volume and facilitate titration of fluid therapy. Bolus fluid therapy (10 to 20 ml/kg) of normal saline, lactated Ringer's solution, albumin, or a mixture of saline and albumin (80 ml of saline to every 20 ml of 25% albumin) should restore adequate intravascular volume. Excessive fluid administration should be avoided.

Specific Therapies for Nephrotic Syndrome   Laboratory studies to be monitored on a regular basis include complete blood count, serum electrolytes, calcium, phosphorus, BUN, creatinine, total protein, albumin, cholesterol, triglycerides, complement (C_3), and urinalysis and urine osmolality. Each urine sample should be checked for proteins and urine osmolality. The urine specific gravity will not reflect renal concentrating ability, since it will be falsely elevated when proteinuria is present.

Salt restriction, albumin infusion, or diuretics may reduce edema and lessen symptomatic complaints. However, vigorous diuresis should be avoided, since it may compromise intravascular volume and produce hemoconcentration. Salt-poor albumin may be administered before diuretic therapy to ensure that circulating blood volume is adequate. Potassium supplements will be required unless an aldosterone antagonist diuretic is used.

If the child is between 1 and 7 years of age, with normal complement (C_3) concentration and minimal hematuria, minimal change nephrosis is the likely diagnosis, and steroid therapy is the treatment of choice. A 4-week course of corticosteroid therapy (prednisone, 2 mg/kg/24 hr) abolishes most symptoms, including proteinuria, in most children. The urine should be checked for the presence of protein for several months after initiation of therapy. The steroid dose can be tapered over several months once the child responds. If proteinuria continues despite a 28-day course of continuous prednisone therapy, a renal biopsy is indicated to better differentiate the degree of glomerular in-

volvement. Steroid-resistant nephrotic syndrome or relapsed nephrotic syndrome may require treatment with alkylating agents.

The risk of infection is increased by nutritional compromise and steroid therapy. The child should be monitored for infection and sepsis, but prophylactic antibiotics are not warranted.

Significant edema will make the child uncomfortable and may contribute to skin breakdown. In young children significant ascites may compromise respiratory effort. It is helpful to keep the child as ambulatory as possible to prevent skin breakdown and to prevent hypoventilation and atelectasis.

Acute Glomerulonephritis

Etiology

Glomerulonephritis may be a primary or secondary disease. It is caused by immunologic events within the glomerulus that are triggered by glomerular injury. The most common form of glomerulonephritis in children has been linked to nephritogenic forms of streptococcus. This disease has also been linked to bacterial, viral, parasitic, pharmacologic, and toxic agents.

Pathophysiology

The pathophysiology of glomerulonephritis is not completely understood. Antigen-antibody complexes are thought to play a significant role. The complexes become fixed to the glomerular basement membrane and stimulate the formation and secretion of other mediators that influence glomerular filtration. As glomerular involvement progresses, the area is invaded by white blood cells, which may cause temporary or permanent changes in the glomerular membrane structure and permeability. Glomerular blood flow decreases as a result of arteriolar constriction, capillary obstruction by thrombi, endothelial cell edema, proliferation of endothelial cells, and white blood cell infiltration. The decrease in glomerular blood flow contributes to a reduction in GFR. Hematuria, mild proteinuria, edema, hypertension, and oliguria all result.

Clinical Presentation

The onset of glomerulonephritis is typically abrupt. If it is related to nephritogenic streptococcal infection, symptoms usually develop 8 to 14 days after group A beta-hemolytic streptococcal pharyngitis or 14 to 21 days after streptococcal pyoderma (impetigo). The symptoms are usually self-limiting. One half of children with poststreptococcal glomerulonephritis demonstrate hypertension, which may be severe. For information regarding treatment of hypertension, see Table 5-14, p. 154.

Macroscopic hematuria is a common presenting sign, and urinalysis may reveal red blood cell casts. Symptomatic edema and proteinuria are present, although these symptoms are not as severe as they are with nephrotic syndrome. The child is often oliguric but is rarely anuric. The GFR and FE$_{Na}$ are often reduced, but renal concentrating ability may be normal.

Changes in the serum and urinary electrolytes often resemble those observed with prerenal failure. The creatinine concentration is often normal, but the BUN is typically elevated. Dilutional hyponatremia and anemia are often present, and the serum albumin level may be low. Hyperkalemia may develop and produce changes in the cardiac rhythm.

Hypervolemia may produce signs of congestive heart failure, including tachycardia, hepatomegaly, increased CVP, tachypnea, and increased respiratory effort. For more information about recognition and management of congestive heart failure, see p. 118.

Management

Most children with glomerulonephritis recover completely. Treatment is aimed at preventing complications of the acute renal disease. Treatment of ARF requires limitation of fluid intake and careful regulation of fluid and electrolyte and acid-base balance. Hyperkalemia should be prevented if possible but will require urgent treatment if symptoms develop (see Hyperkalemia under Common Clinical Conditions). If hypervolemia produces complications such as congestive heart failure, diuresis and inotropic and vasodilator agents will often be required (see Chapter 5).

A renal biopsy is indicated to confirm the diagnosis of acute glomerulonephritis. Antibiotic therapy does not influence recovery and is only indicated if the child has positive bacterial cultures.

Systemic Lupus Erythematosus: Renal Involvement

The glomerular lesions in patients with SLE result from the deposition of complexes of anti-DNA antibodies and DNA. Three types of renal involvement in SLE are focal lupus nephritis, diffuse lupus nephritis, and membranous lupus nephritis.

Focal lupus nephritis rarely produces nephrotic syndrome. This form of SLE involvement usually resolves completely with adrenal corticosteroid therapy.

Diffuse lupus nephritis is characterized by severe proteinuria, hypertension, and renal insufficiency. Remissions may occur but are usually incomplete.

Membranous lupus nephritis produces widespread glomerular involvement with many cellular changes and thickening of glomerular capillary walls. Clinical manifestations include proteinuria, occasional hematuria, renal insufficiency, and hypertension. Remission may occur, but proteinuria usually persists.

Hemolytic Uremic Syndrome

Etiology

Hemolytic uremic syndrome (HUS) is the simultaneous occurrence of acute hemolytic anemia, thrombocytopenia, and ARF. HUS is responsible for the majority of cases of ARF in children.

In recent years, several outbreaks of HUS have been linked to episodes of *Escherichia coli* from contaminated food. Coxsackie virus has also been isolated from HUS patients. Typical infectious episodes are characterized by a diarrheal prodromal period. Infectious episodes not related to food contamination occur most commonly in the summer in the northern hemisphere. Atypical HUS may occur sporadically and does not include a diarrheal prodromal period.

Pathophysiology

HUS seems to be related to a localized intravascular coagulation. It is characterized by microangiopathy with platelet aggregation and fibrin deposition in small vessels, including small arterioles in the kidney, gut, and central nervous system. Hemolytic anemia may be severe and rapidly progressive. It is believed to be a result of shearing of red blood cells as they pass through narrowed vessels. Platelets are also damaged in this way, producing thrombocytopenia for 1 to 2 weeks.

HUS is also associated with damage to the glomerular endothelial cells. Renal blood flow and the GFR can be reduced in proportion to the degree of glomerular injury. Children with HUS may demonstrate varying degrees of gastrointestinal distress, from mild gastroenteritis to bloody diarrhea. Neurologic involvement may range from irritability to seizures, abnormal posturing, or coma. Worsening neurologic signs are associated with a poor prognosis.

Clinical Presentation

The presentation of HUS may closely follow or coincide with a case of mild gastroenteritis or other forms of infection. The child may present with bloody stools.

Within a few days of presentation, the child develops pallor, purpura, rectal bleeding, or other signs of hemorrhage. The peripheral blood smear demonstrates fragmented red blood cells (a microangiopathic hemolytic anemia), fibrin split products, and thrombocytopenia. Within a few days of the onset of anemia, the reticulocyte count will be high.

The child may be oliguric or anuric. This may be difficult to appreciate if watery diarrhea is present in the diapers. Urinalysis reveals the presence of fibrin, proteinuria, microscopic or macroscopic hematuria, and urinary cell casts.

Serum levels of creatinine, BUN, phosphate, and potassium are elevated. Hyperkalemia may develop and progress rapidly if gastrointestinal bleeding is present. The serum bilirubin level usually is not elevated, although hepatosplenomegaly is observed. Hypervolemia, congestive heart failure, and pulmonary edema may develop if renal function is severely compromised. Hypertension may be present and severe.

Immunoglobulins and complement studies are normal. There is no evidence of a consumptive coagulopathy.

Management

Management is primarily focused on general supportive care and treatment of complications such as ARF, anemia, central nervous system symptoms, and gastrointestinal dysfunction.

Goals of management include restoration or maintenance of:

- Fluid and electrolyte balance
- Adequate red blood cell volume
- Appropriate cardiovascular function and blood pressure
- Neurologic function

Anemia is treated through red blood cell administration. Renal replacement therapy may be required to treat hypervolemia, hyperkalemia, severe uremia, and complications that are unresponsive to other therapies.

Hypertension is treated with vasodilators. The dosage of these and any drugs administered must be evaluated in light of the child's compromised renal function (see Table 5-14).

The child's neurologic status should be evaluated constantly, and any deterioration reported to a physician immediately. Central nervous system complications are managed symptomatically. Increased ICP is treated with support of oxygenation and ventilation, elevation of the head of the bed, and administration of diuretic agents as needed (see p. 394).

If the gastrointestinal complications are severe, oral intake may be restricted, and it may be necessary to provide parenteral nutrition. Calories must be provided within a limited fluid intake, and those calories should come from glucose rather than from protein in order to minimize the azotemia.

Acute Tumor Lysis Syndrome

Etiology

Acute tumor lysis syndrome (ATLS) consists of several metabolic abnormalities that result from rapid tumor cell breakdown. It usually develops during the initiation of antineoplastic therapy for large, rapidly growing tumors, but it may also develop before therapy. Neoplasms most commonly associated with ATLS include Burkitt's lymphoma, T-cell leukemias or lymphomas, or leukemia with a high white blood cell count.

Pathophysiology

As cells break down, they release intracellular contents, including uric acid, potassium, phosphate, and tissue thromboplastin into the circulation. Massive amounts of these metabolites overwhelm the kidney's ability to excrete them; thus elevated levels of uric acid, potassium, and phosphate develop. The phosphate precipitates with calcium, producing hypocalcemia. Thromboplastin release may precipitate disseminated intravascular coagulation.

Uric acid precipitates in the kidneys, producing tubular obstruction, decreased urine output, and renal failure.

The severity of this syndrome is proportional to the tumor burden. A previous history of renal impairment increases the risk of development of renal failure in association with ATLS.

Clinical Presentation

ATLS is characterized by the following:

- Hyperuricemia and potential renal failure with its complications
- Hyperkalemia (may produce ECG changes)
- Hyperphosphatemia
- Hypocalcemia (may produce tingling, muscle cramps, seizures, and decreased myocardial function)

Management

ATLS should be prevented, if possible. This is accomplished through identification of patients at risk and institution of therapy to avoid accumulation of metabolites of rapid cell breakdown. Initial antineoplastic doses are adjusted to prevent extremely rapid cell breakdown. Monitoring of renal function and electrolytes is required from the time of diagnosis through the first round of therapy.

To prevent uric acid crystal formation, aggressive fluid administration (1.5 to 2 times maintenance fluid requirements) is provided. Urine output is closely monitored. Notify a physician if urine output decreases. Uric acid production is reduced through allopurinol (100 to 300 mg/day) administration. Decreased urine output is treated with diuresis. Renal replacement therapy or hemodialysis may be required.

Severe hyperkalemia will require urgent treatment with calcium, sodium bicarbonate, glucose plus insulin, and sodium polystyrene sulfonate (Kayexalate) enema (see Hyperkalemia).

Hypocalcemia is treated with calcium administration, although this problem will continue as long as hyperphosphatemia persists.

Renal Trauma

Etiology

Renal trauma is the most common genitourinary injury observed in multisystem trauma victims and is responsible for one third to two thirds of all genitourinary injuries. Contusion or laceration comprises most renal injuries. Children have a greater vulnerability than adults to renal trauma, because of the larger size of the child's kidneys in relation to the size of the abdomen, underdevelopment of the child's abdominal wall muscles, and lack of protection from the lower ribs.

Pathophysiology

The most common source of renal trauma is blunt trauma, primarily from motor vehicle–related injuries. The two types of blunt trauma causing most renal injuries are direct compression from external force and deceleration injury. With deceleration injury, laceration of the renal artery may occur. Lumbar scoliosis and fracture of the body or transverse processes of the spine may also transmit significant injury to the retroperitoneal region of the kidney. Acute renal insult may also result from decreased perfusion associated with shock and hemorrhage.

Penetrating trauma has been an uncommon type of renal injury in children in the past. However, this type of injury is becoming more common as a result of the epidemic of gunshot injuries.

Clinical Presentation

Signs and symptoms of genitourinary trauma include blood at the urethral meatus, a high-riding prostate gland, gross hematuria, and labial, scrotal, or perianal ecchymosis or hematoma. These signs and symptoms are contraindications to bladder catheterization and should be reported to a physician.

Hematuria occurs in 90% of patients with renal trauma. If the patient is hypovolemic, hematuria may not be observed until fluid replacement has occurred. There is no correlation between the magnitude of injury and the degree of hematuria.

The child with blunt trauma may be asymptomatic or complain of abdominal or flank pain. Suspicion of injury must be raised by consideration of the mechanism of injury. With penetrating trauma, proximity of the wound to the genitourinary area increases suspicion of renal trauma.

Computed tomography (CT) is the standard imaging study for acute renal trauma in children. Advantages of the CT scan include accurate demonstration of renal injury, visualization of non-vascularized regions, and simultaneous visualization of the intraabdominal area. It is less time consuming and easier than arteriography. Abdominal films or kidney, ureter, and bladder (KUB) films demonstrating obliteration of the renal shadow are suggestive of renal trauma. However, up to 85% of plain abdominal films demonstrate normal findings despite proven renal trauma.

An excretory urogram (intravenous pyelogram) is the standard study for diagnosis of renal injury. Ultrasonography has limited application in evaluation of renal trauma. Doppler-enhanced ultrasound gives information related to renal perfusion and integrity of vascular pedicles of the kidney. Arteriography may assist in planning surgical intervention. A radionuclide renal scan demonstrates renal function, perfusion, and urinary extravasation. It is useful if there is a contraindication to contrast dye. Use of magnetic resonance imaging (MRI) is limited because the amount of information gained is not substantially greater than is provided by other studies.

Management

Most penetrating renal injuries require surgical exploration and potential intervention. The management of blunt trauma is dependent on the stability of the child and the extent of injury. Eighty-five percent of blunt trauma results in minor injury, requiring only observation and bed rest until gross hematuria resolves. If results from initial radiographic studies are abnormal, continued follow-up for a year or more may be necessary.

Management of major renal trauma is controversial when considering an operative vs. a nonoperative approach. Continued hemorrhage, hemody-

namic instability, and devastating renal organ injury are common indications for urgent surgical intervention (see Chapter 12). Long-term follow-up (6 months to 1 year) is important because hypertension is a subtle yet frequent complication of renal vascular trauma.

Chronic Renal Failure

Etiology

Chronic renal failure (CRF) is present when normal concentrations of body substances cannot be maintained by the kidney under normal living conditions. Glomerular nephropathy is the primary cause of CRF. CRF may occur as a result of congenital disorders or malformation of the renal system, renal infections, severe trauma, or glomerular disease. Renal insufficiency with CRF may range from that requiring careful management of fluid and nutritional intake to that requiring dialysis or CRRT.

Pathophysiology

CRF is present when renal function is below 25% to 30% of normal as reflected in a creatinine clearance of 30 to 40 ml/min/m^2. With this level of renal dysfunction and decreased clearance, urea is increased to >20 mg/dl. The serum creatinine concentration is >1.5 mg/dl.

Uremia results from the accumulation of waste products and the fluid imbalances that occur in patients with CRF. Renal dysfunction may cause hypervolemia, electrolyte and acid-base imbalance, anemia, hypertension, renal osteodystrophy, metastatic calcifications, and accumulation of uremic toxins.

If the ability to concentrate urine is impaired, the kidneys produce urine with a fixed osmolality. Acute increases in sodium intake can produce sodium and water retention, whereas severe sodium and water restriction may result in hyponatremia because the kidneys are unable to conserve sodium. Urinary loss of sodium and water may produce volume depletion, further reductions in GFR, and a greater increase in BUN.

In severe CRF a change in serum sodium balance may develop. These patients have a very low GFR that is inadequate to excrete the amounts of sodium and water normally ingested. Retention of sodium and water may produce edema, vascular congestion, hypertension, pulmonary edema, or heart failure. Management of these complications may require renal replacement therapy.

Normal maintenance of a stable serum potassium concentration requires secretion of potassium by the distal tubules. Even when CRF is present, undamaged nephrons may be capable of increasing potassium secretion to compensate for the damaged nephrons. For this reason, it is rarely necessary to restrict potassium intake until the GFR is at very low levels. However, ingestion of large amounts of potassium should be avoided. Hypokalemia occasionally develops as a result of a decreased potassium intake or diuretic therapy.

Patients with CRF generally develop metabolic acidosis as a result of the bicarbonate wasting and decreased distal tubule ability to produce ammonia. Exogenous bicarbonate administration may only increase urinary bicarbonate loss. The rate of ammonia production decreases in proportion to the fall in GFR.

Patients with CRF have reduced intestinal absorption of calcium as a result of decreased renal production of vitamin D. When the GFR falls below 25% of normal, the plasma phosphate concentration begins to rise. The rise in phosphate results in a fall in serum ionized calcium.

Both red blood cell and platelet production may be impaired. The life span of the red blood cell is shortened by uremia. The platelet number may be normal, but platelet function is reduced.

Patients with CRF may develop neurologic complications, including uremic encephalopathy and neuropathy. The cause of encephalopathy and neuropathy is unknown but may be related to fluid and electrolyte imbalance.

Clinical Presentation

Patients with CRF often have vague complaints of fatigue, weakness, anorexia, nausea, abdominal pain, headaches, and failure to grow. Polyuria or oliguria, polydipsia, and mild edema are usually present.

Sodium and potassium concentrations are often normal, although imbalances may be present or produced by diuretic therapy. Typical electrolyte imbalances include high serum phosphate, hypocalcemia, high BUN, high uric acid, and elevated serum creatinine. Metabolic acidosis is common.

Anemia and thrombocytopathia with prolonged bleeding times may be present. Growth failure is common, and renal osteodystrophy is often apparent with metastatic calcifications.

Neurologic complications may include signs of encephalopathy with irritability, lethargy, or increased ICP (see Chapter 8, p. 388). Neuropathy may produce weakness, muscle cramps, tetany, or muscle wasting.

Management

Care of the child with CRF requires manipulation of fluid and dietary intake to maintain fluid and electrolyte balance and control toxin accumulation. Nutritional support is challenging but essential. The sodium and potassium content in fluids and foods must be totaled and regulated.

The child with CRF is susceptible to infections and skin breakdown and therefore requires careful attention to skin integrity and wound healing. Finally, medication dosages must be adjusted in accordance with the level of renal function remaining (see Diagnostic Studies and Adjustments of Medications in Renal Failure, pp. 490-491). If hypervolemia or electrolyte imbalances become severe, CRRT or dialysis will be required.

Hepatorenal Syndrome

Etiology

Hepatorenal syndrome is characterized by advanced liver disease and renal failure with oliguria, and sodium and water retention. It usually occurs in association with fulminate hepatic failure, hepatic malignancy, liver resection, or biliary tract obstruction.

Pathophysiology

Primary renal disease is usually not present, but renal failure is a secondary complication of reduced renal perfusion. Blood flow and perfusion to the kidneys is decreased by hypotension or hypovolemia, which may result from gastrointestinal bleeding or use of diuretics. Hypoperfusion may also be caused by a decrease in cardiac output or a relative hypovolemia caused by portal hypertension and resultant splanchnic sequestration. The liver may fail to remove a variety of vasoactive substances, leading to increased levels of circulating angiotensin, vasopressin, prostaglandins, catecholamines, or vasodilators, which will contribute to either renal vasoconstriction or hypotension.

The renal failure is characterized by renal arteriolar constriction, decreased GFR, and increased sodium and water retention (secondary to hyperaldosteronism).

Clinical Presentation

Clinical signs include those of liver failure, oliguria, and possible hypotension. Nonspecific symptoms include nausea, weakness, and fatigue.

Oliguric renal failure is characterized by an increase in BUN and serum creatinine. Although the urine osmolality may be high, the urine sodium concentration is low. Secondary complications of fluid and electrolyte imbalance, as well as complications of liver failure, will be observed.

Management

Management is similar to that provided for ARF. Extreme care must be taken to support optimal intravascular volume and systemic perfusion while restoring and maintaining fluid and electrolyte balance.

Renal Transplantation

All candidates for renal transplantation must have end-stage renal disease (ESRD) or rapidly approaching ESRD. Common causes of ESRD requiring transplantation include congenital renal disorders, glomerulonephritis, and ESRD secondary to other disease states or treatment. Failure to respond to conservative management is no longer a criterion for transplantation.

Transplantation may now be considered at the time of diagnosis of ESRD. The child must have a normal or repairable bladder and urinary outflow tract and be free of major complications (malignancy, advanced cardiopulmonary disease) and active infection. Nutritional status should be adequate, and psychiatric and socioeconomic parameters should be viewed as appropriate. Infection-free successful transplantation is largely dependent on the recipient's immunologic response to the transplant.

Postoperative care is accomplished via protocol that is transplant center specific. However, for all pa-

tients, strict recording of fluid intake and output must be maintained, and the surgeon should be notified immediately of any decrease in urine output. Typically, a high urine output is maintained, and urine output is generally replaced milliliter for milliliter.

Postoperatively, the risk for infection is minimized with strict adherence to handwashing and other institutional infection control guidelines and the use of aseptic technique with all dressing changes. It is also important to maintain pulmonary toilet, closely monitor urine output, maintain adequate nutritional intake, observe for signs and symptoms of infection, and maintain fluid and electrolyte balance (BUN, creatinine, calcium, phosphate, urinary protein).

Administer the daily immunosuppressive medication regimen as ordered and follow serum levels as appropriate. Potential complications include ATN, rejection, infection, obstruction to urinary flow, hypovolemia, renal artery stenosis, renal vein thrombosis, and ureteral leaks.

Diagnostic Studies and Adjustments of Medications in Renal Failure

Renal Function Studies

The most common calculations used to evaluate renal function are included in Box 9-6. All require collection of a timed urine sample, as well as collection of a serum sample during the urine collection. The timed urine sample begins when the first urine specimen is collected and discarded. Any urine made after that time is collected, and the time from the beginning to the end of the collection period must be precisely recorded.

Modification of Drug Dosages in Renal Failure

When renal function is compromised, all doses of drugs the patient receives should be evaluated and adjusted as needed. Drugs requiring adjustment and methods of adjustment are listed in Box 9-7 and Table 9-11.

Box 9-6

Common Formulas Used in Evaluation of Renal Function

Fractional Excretion of Sodium (FE$_{Na}$)

$$\text{Fractional excretion Na (\%)} = \frac{\dfrac{\text{Urine sodium concentration}}{\text{Serum sodium concentration}}}{\dfrac{\text{Urine creatinine concentration}}{\text{Serum creatinine concentration}}} \times 100$$

Prerenal azotemia is associated with an FE$_{Na}$ <1% (< 2.5% in neonates), and renal failure is associated with an FE$_{Na}$ >2% (>3.5% in neonates). This equation is not valid if recent diuretic therapy has been provided.

Glomerular Filtration Rate (GFR)

$$\text{GFR} = \frac{\text{Urine creatinine concentration} \times \text{Volume of urine/min}}{\text{Plasma creatinine concentration}}$$

This relationship is not valid in the presence of severe renal dysfunction.

Estimation of Serum Osmolality

$$2 \times \text{Sodium concentration (mEq/L)} = \underline{\hspace{1.5cm}}$$

$$+ \frac{\text{Glucose concentration (mg/dl)}}{18} = + \underline{\hspace{1.5cm}}$$

$$+ \frac{\text{Blood urea nitrogen (mg/dl)}}{2.8} = + \underline{\hspace{1.5cm}}$$

$$\text{Total serum osmolality (mOsm/L)} = \underline{\hspace{1.5cm}}$$

$$\text{Normal} = 272\text{-}300 \text{ mOsm/L}$$

Renal Failure Index (RFI)

$$\text{RFI} = \frac{\text{Urine sodium concentration}}{\dfrac{\text{Urine creatinine}}{\text{Serum creatinine}}}$$

Normal RFI is <2.5 in neonates and <1 in infants and children; RFI >2-2.5 is typically associated with renal failure.
This equation will not provide valid reflection of renal failure if recent diuretic therapy has been provided.

Modified from Hazinski MF: *Nursing care of the critically ill child,* ed 2, St Louis, 1992, Mosby.

Box 9-7

Drugs Requiring No Adjustment in Renal Impairment

Amitriptyline
Busulfan
Ceftriaxone*
Choramphenicol
Chlorpheniramine
Chlorpromazine
Clindamycin
Clonidine
Cloxacillin
Cytosine arabinoside
Dexamethasone
Diazepam
Diazoxide*†
Dicloxacillin
Diltiazem
Doxapram
Erythromycin
Esmolol
5-Fluorouracil‡
Furosemide
Haloperdiol
Heparin
Imipramine
Hydrocortisone
Ketoconazole
Metolazone

Miconazole
Nafcillin
Naloxone
Nifedipine
Nitroglycerin
Oxacillin
Prazosin§
Prednisone
Prednisolone
Propranolol
Pyrimethamine
Rifampin
Succinylcholine‡
Theophylline*
Valproic Acid
Vinblastine
Vincristine
Warfarin

From Johns Hopkins Hospital Department of Pediatrics: *The Harriet Lane Handbook,* ed 14, edited by Barone M, St Louis, 1996, Mosby.
*Extra dose for hemodialysis recommended.
†Extra dose for peritoneal dialysis recommended.
‡In end-stage renal failure, acute hyperkalemia may develop.
§Patients may respond to low doses.

Table 9-11
Modification of Drug Dosages in Renal Failure

Drug	Route of Excretion	Normal T$_{1/2}$ (hr)	Normal Dose Interval	Method	>50	10-50	<10	Supplemental Dose for Dialysis
Antimicrobials Requiring Adjustment in Renal Failure								
Acyclovir	Renal	2.1-3.8	q8h	I	q8h	q12-24h	q48h	Yes (He), no (P)
Amikacin	Renal	2-3	q8-12h	I	q12h	q12-18h	q24-48h	Yes (He,P)
Amoxicillin	Renal (hepatic)	0.9-2.3	q8h	I	q8h	q8-12h	q12-16h	Yes (He), no (P)
Amphotericin B	Nonrenal	24	q24h	I	q24h	q24h	q24-36h	No (He,P)
Ampicillin	Renal (hepatic)	0.8-1.5	q4-6h	I	q6h	q6-12h	q12-16h	Yes (He), no (P)
Aztreonam	Renal (hepatic)	1.3-2.4	q6-8h	D	100%	50%-75%	25%-33%	Yes (He,P)
Carbenicillin[a]	Renal (hepatic)	1.2-1.5	q6h	I	q8-12h	q12-24h	q24-48h	Yes (He), no (P)
Cefaclor	Renal (hepatic)	0.75	q8h	D	100%	50%-100%	33%	Yes (He,P)
Cefadroxil	Renal	1-2	q12h	I	q12h	q12-24h	q24-48h	Yes (He)
Cefamandole	Renal	1	q4-8h	I	q6h	q6-8h	q8-12h	Yes (He)
Cefazolin	Renal	1.4-2.2	q8h	I	q8h	q12h	q24-48h	Yes (He), no (P)
Cefixime	Renal (hepatic)	3-4	q12-24h	D	100%	75%-100%	50%	Yes (He), no (P)
Cefotaxime	Renal (hepatic)	1	q6-8h	I	q6-8h	q8-12h	q12-24h	Yes (He), no (P)
Cefoxitin	Renal	1	q6-8h	I	q8h	q8-12h	q24-48h	Yes (He), no (P)
Ceftazidime	Renal (hepatic)	1.8	q8-12h	I	q8-12h	q12-24h	q24-48h	Yes (He,P)
Cefuroxime (IV)	Renal	1.6-2.2	q6-8h	I	q8-12h	q24-48h	q48-72h	Yes (He), no (P)
Cephalexin	Renal	0.9	q6h	I	q6h	q6-8h	q8-12h	Yes (He), no (P)
Cephalothin[b]	Renal (hepatic)	0.5-1	q6h	I	q6h	q6-8h	q8-12h	Yes (He), no (P)
Codeine	Hepatic (renal)	2.5-3.5	q4-6h	D	100%	75%	50%	?
Ethambutol	Renal	4	q24h	I	q24h	q24-36h	q48h	Yes (He), no (P)

Continued

From John Hopkins Hospital Department of Pediatrics: *The Harriet Lane handbook*, ed 14, edited by Barone M. St Louis, 1996, Mosby.
He, Hemodialysis; *P*, peritoneal dialysis.
[a]May inactivate aminoglycosides in patients with renal impairment.
[b]May add to peritoneal dialysate to obtain adequate serum levels.

Table 9-11
Modification of Drug Dosages in Renal Failure—cont'd

Drug	Route of Excretion	Normal T$_{1/2}$ (hr)	Normal Dose Interval	Method	Adjustments in Renal Failure — Creatinine Clearance (ml/min) >50	10-50	<10	Supplemental Dose for Dialysis
Antimicrobials Requiring Adjustment in Renal Failure—cont'd								
Foscarnet	Renal	3-4.5	q8h	D	See package insert			Yes (He)
Fluconazole[b]	Renal	20-50	q24h	D	100%	25%-50%	25%	Yes (He,P)
Flucytosine	Renal	3-6	q6h	I	q6h	q12-24h	q24-48h	Yes (He,P)
Ganciclovir	Renal	2.5-3.6	q8-12h	DI	100% and q12h	50% and q12h	25% and q24h	Yes (He)
Gentamicin[b]	Renal	2.5-3	q8-12h	I	q8-12h	q12h	q24h	Yes (He,P)
Imipenem/cilastatin	Renal	1-1.4	q6-8h	D	100%	50%	25%	Yes (He)
Isoniazid	Hepatic (renal)	2-4 (slow)[c] 0.5-1.5 (fast)	q24h	D	100%	100%	66%-75%	Yes (He,P)
Kanamycin	Renal	2-3	q8h	I	q8-12h	q12h	q24h	Yes (He,P)
Loracarbef	Renal	0.8-1	q12h	I	q12h	q24h	q72-120h	Yes (He)
Methicillin	Renal	0.5-1	q4-6h	I	q4-6h	q6-8h	q8-12h	No (He,P)
Metronidazole	Hepatic (renal)	6-14	q8h	I	q8h	q8-12h	q12-24h	Yes (He), no (P)
Mezlocillin	Renal (hepatic)	0.5-1	q4-6h	I	q4-6h	q6-8h	q8-12h	No (He,P)
Nitrofurantoin	Nonrenal	1-1.7	q8h	D	100%	100%	Avoid	Yes (He)
Penicillin G	Renal (hepatic)	0.5	q4-6h	I	q6-8h	q8-12h	q12-16h	Yes (He), no (P)
Piperacillin	Renal (hepatic)	0.8-1.5	q4-6h	I	q4-6h	q6-8h	q8h	Yes (He), no (P)
Piperacillin/tazobactam	Renal (hepatic)	Pip:0.8-1.5 Tz:0.7-0.9	q6h	DI	100%	70%	70%	Yes (He)
Sulfamethoxazole	Hepatic (renal)	9-11	q12h	I	q12h	q18h	q24h	No (P)
Ticarcillin[a]	Renal (hepatic)	1-1.5	q4-6h	I	q8-12h	q12-24h	q24-48h	Yes (He), no (P)
Tobramycin[b]	Renal	2.5-3	q8h	I	q8-12h	q12h	q24h	Yes (He,P)
Trimethoprim	Renal (hepatic)	8-15	q12h	I	q12h	q18h	q24h	Yes (He), no (P)
Vancomycin	Renal	6-8	q6-8h	I	q24-72h	q72-240h	q240h	Yes/no (He), no (P)[d]
Zalcitabine	Renal		q8h	I	q8h	q12h	q24h	Yes (He)
Nonantimicrobials Requiring Adjustment in Renal Failure								
Acetaminophen	Hepatic	2	q4h	I	q4h	q6h	q8h	Yes (He) No (P)
Acetylsalicylic acid[e]	Hepatic (renal)	2-19	q4h	I	q4h	q4-6h	Avoid	Yes (He,P)
Adriamycin	Renal (hepatic)	16-30	Single treatment	D	100%	100%	75%	?

Drug	Pharmacokinetics (elimination)	t½ (hr)	Interval	Method	GFR >50	GFR 10-50	GFR <10	Dialysis
Allopurinol[f]	Renal	0.7-1.6	q6-12h	D	100%	50%	10%-25%	Yes (He)
Azathioprine	Hepatic	12.5 min	q12h	D	100%	75%	50%	Yes (He)
Captopril	Renal (hepatic)	1.9	q12h	D	100%	75%	50%	Yes (He)
Carbamazepine	Hepatic (renal)	20-36	q8-12h	D	100%	100%	75%	No (He,P)
Chloral hydrate	Hepatic	7-14	q8h prn	D	100%	Avoid	Avoid	Yes (He)
Cimetidine	Renal (hepatic)	1.5-2	q6h	D	100%	50%	25%	No (He,P)
Digoxin[g]	Renal (GI)	36-44	q24h	—	100%, q24h	25%-75%, q36h	10%-25%, q48h	No (He,P)
Diphenhydramine	Hepatic	4-7	q6h	I	q6h	q6-12h	q12-18h	?
Enalapril	Renal (hepatic)	7	q12-24h	I	100%	75%-100%	50%	Yes (He)
Famotidine	Renal (hepatic)	2.5-4	q12-24h	I	q20-40h	q30-60h	q68-136h	No (He,P)
Fentanyl	Renal (hepatic)	2-4	q1-2h	D	100%	75%	50	?
Hydralazine[h]	Hepatic (GI)	2-4.5	q8h (fast)[i], q12h (slow)	I	q8-12h	q8-12h	q8-16h (fast), q12-24h (slow), 25%-50%	No (He,P)
Insulin (regular)	Hepatic (renal)	9 min	Variable	D	100%	75%	75%	?
Methotrexate	Renal	Triphasic, 0.1, 2.3, 27	Single treatment	D	100%	50%	Avoid	Yes (He), no (P)
Metoclopromide	Renal (hepatic)	4	q6-8h	D	100%	75%	50%	No (He,P)
Midazolam	Renal (hepatic)	1-2	Variable	D	100%	100%	50%	?
Phenobarbital	Hepatic (renal, 30%)	65-150	q8-12h	I	q8-12h	q8-12h	q12-16h	Yes (He,P)
Plicamycin	Renal	1	q24h	D	100%	75%	50%	?
Primidone	Hepatic (renal, 20%)	6-12	q8-12h	I	q8-12h	q8-12h	q12-24h	Yes (He)
Quinidine	Hepatic (renal)	2.5-6.7	q4-6h	D	100%	100%	75%	Yes (He), no (P)
Ranitidine	Renal (hepatic)	1.5-3	q8-12h	D	75%	75%	50%	Yes (He), no (P)
Spironolactone	Renal (hepatic)	10-35	q6h	I	q6-12h	q12-16h	Avoid	?
Thiazides	Renal	1-2	q12h	D	100%	100%	Avoid	?
Triamterene	Hepatic (renal)	2-12	q12h	I	q12h	q12h	Avoid[j]	?

From John Hopkins Hospital Department of Pediatrics: *The Harriet Lane handbook*, ed 14, edited by Barone M. St Louis, 1996, Mosby.

HE, Hemodialysis; P, peritoneal dialysis.

[a] May inactivate aminoglycosides in patients with renal impairment.
[b] May add to peritoneal dialysate to obtain adequate serum levels.
[c] Rate of acetylation of isoniazid.
[d] If using high-flux polysulfone hemodialysis, give supplemental dose after dialysis.
[e] With large doses $T_{1/2}$ prolonged up to 30 hr.
[f] Azathioprine rapidly converted to mercaptopurine, which has a $T_{1/2}$ of 0.5-4 hr.
[g] Decrease loading dose 50% in end-stage renal disease because of decreased volume of distribution.
[h] Dose interval varies for rapid and slow acetylators with normal and impaired renal function.
[i] Rate of acetylation of hydralazine.
[j] Hyperkalemia common with GFR <30 ml/min.

Suggested Readings

Baldwin IC, Elderkin TD: Continuous hemofiltration: nursing perspective in critical care, *New Horizons* 3:738-747, 1995.

Bellomo R et al: Effect of continuous venovenous hemofiltration with dialysis on hormone and catecholamine clearance in critically ill patients in acute renal failure, *Crit Care Med* 22:833-837, 1994.

Bosworth C: SCUF/CAVH/CAVHD: critical differences, *Crit Care Nurs Q* 14:45-55, 1992.

Forni LG, Hilton PJ: Continuous hemofiltration in the treatment of acute renal failure, *N Engl J Med* 18:1303-1309, 1997.

Golper TA, Price J: Continuous venovenous hemofiltration for acute renal failure in the intensive care setting, *ASAIOJ* 936-939, 1994.

Headrick CL, Alexander SR: Continuous venovenous hemofiltration. In Levin DL, Morris FC, editors: *Essentials of pediatric intensive care,* ed 2, New York, 1997, Churchill Livingstone.

Hendrix W: Dialysis therapies in critically ill children, *AACN Clin Issues* 3:605-615, 1992.

Higley RR: Continuous arteriovenous hemofiltration: a case study, *Crit Care Nurs* 16:37-43, 1996.

Macias WL et al: Continuous venovenous hemofiltration: an alternative to continuous arteriovenous hemofiltration and hemodiafiltration in acute renal failure, *Am J Kidney Dis* 18:451-458, 1991.

Mehta RL: Continuous renal replacement therapies in the acute renal failure setting: current concepts, *Adv Renal Replace Ther* 2(suppl 1):81-92, April 1997.

Price C: An update on continuous renal replacement therapies, *AACN Clin Issues Crit Care Nurs* 3:597-604, 1992.

Ronco C et al: Achievements and new directions in continuous renal replacement therapies, *New Horizons* 3:708-716, 1995.

Smoyer W et al: A practical approach to continuous hemofiltration in infants and children, *Dialysis Transplant* 24:633-640, 1995.

Zobel G et al: Five years experience with extracorporeal renal support in pediatric intensive care, *Intensive Care Med* 17:315-319, 1991.

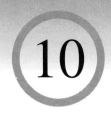

10 Gastrointestinal Disorders

Mary Fran Hazinski, John A. Barnard

Pearls

- Fluid and electrolyte imbalance may develop quickly in children. All sources of fluid intake and output must be closely monitored in the intensive care unit. Replace excessive fluid losses with fluid of appropriate content and volume.
- Signs of inadequate intravascular volume and shock in the child may be subtle. Hypotension is typically only a *late* sign of shock in children; thus the nurse must monitor signs of systemic perfusion (e.g., warmth of extremities, strength of peripheral pulses, evidence of renal and cerebral perfusion) to detect shock before decompensation develops.
- Signs of an acute abdomen (including evidence of gastrointestinal [GI] bleeding or necrotizing enterocolitis) must be detected immediately to maximize the chance of survival.
- Sterile and aseptic technique must be maintained when parenteral alimentation catheters are inserted, and when insertion site dressings, tubing, and solutions are changed, to minimize the risk of infection.
- Enteral feeding should begin as soon as possible. Even small quantities of dilute feedings can be beneficial in reducing the risk of infection and promoting gut healing.

Additional Helpful Chapters

Chapter 3: Analgesia, Sedation, and Neuromuscular Blockade in Pediatric Critical Care
Chapter 5: Shock
Chapter 9: Renal Disorders, Dehydration, Electrolyte imbalances

Essential Anatomy and Physiology

Structures and Functions of Gastrointestinal Organs

The gastrointestinal (GI) tract is designed to convert digested food into nutrients that can be utilized by the cells. This process includes emulsification of the food, mechanical and chemical digestion, and absorption of digested food, as well as fluid secretion and water and electrolyte reabsorp-tion. Wastes are eliminated as stool. This process is summarized briefly here:

1. *Esophagus:* The esophagus is a hollow muscular tube that conducts ingested substances from the mouth to the stomach through peristalsis. The lower esophageal sphincter, located at the junction of the esophagus and stomach, should prevent regurgitation from the stomach. This sphincter may be immature or incompetent during the first months of life, particularly in premature infants,

which may contribute to gastroesophageal reflux.

2. *Stomach:* Food is agitated and emulsified in the stomach with the addition of hydrochloric acid and pepsin. Gastric emptying is regulated primarily by the volume, osmotic pressure, and chemical composition of gastric contents and is controlled by the pyloric sphincter. Gastric emptying is delayed during sleep and can be delayed by the use of sedatives. The residual volume of fluid remaining in the stomach is influenced by the feeding interval, and a small amount of secretions remain even in the fasted patient.

3. *Small intestine:* The small intestine is the primary site for digestion and absorption of fats, amino acids, sugars, and vitamins. Digestion is continued through the action of pancreatic enzymes, intestinal enzymes, and bile salts from the gallbladder. The surface of the small intestine is lined with fingerlike villi, covered with a specialized surface membrane called the brush border; this combination of surfaces tremendously increases the absorptive surface. Nutrient, water, and electrolytes (particularly sodium, glucose, and potassium) are absorbed at the tip of the villus while fluid is secreted at the base of the villus. Most of the water entering the gut daily is absorbed in the small intestine.

4. *Large intestine:* The large intestine consists of the cecum, the appendix, the colon, the rectum, and the anal canal. The colon consists of the ascending, the transverse, the descending, and the sigmoid colon and serves to reabsorb water and electrolytes and propel feces to the anal canal.

5. *Accessory organs of digestion:* These organs consist of the liver, the gallbladder, and the pancreas. These organs all secrete substances needed for digestion and absorption of nutrients in the gut.

   a. *Liver:* The liver is divided into two lobes and is covered by a fibroelastic capsule called Glisson's capsule. The liver is perfused with blood from the hepatic artery, receiving approximately 25% of the cardiac output. The portal vein provides approximately 75% of the blood flow to the liver. The portal vein carries some oxygen but predominantly carries nutrients from the digestive tract (blood flows from the inferior and superior mesenteric veins and the splenic vein) to and through the liver before this blood enters the systemic circulation. The liver serves a wide variety of functions, including formation of bile, formation of clotting factors, formation of plasma proteins, metabolism and storage of nutrients, and metabolism or deactivation for waste products and drugs. The liver also stores vitamins and minerals, and Kupffer's cells destroy intestinal bacteria and foreign particles, which may be carried by the portal vein.

   b. *Biliary tree and gallbladder:* The liver forms and secretes bile, which is conjugated with amino acids in the liver to form bile salts. Bilirubin, formed from aged red blood cells, is also conjugated (joined with glucuronic acid) in the liver, so that it becomes a water-soluble substance and can be excreted in bile. Bile is stored and concentrated in the gallbladder between meals.

   c. *Pancreas:* The pancreas secretes enzymes responsible for the digestion and absorption of fats, carbohydrates, and proteins. The endocrine pancreas synthesizes and secretes insulin.

Gastrointestinal Tract Fluids and Electrolytes

Large volumes of water, electrolytes, and various solutes such as proteins and bile salts are secreted and reabsorbed across the mucosa of the entire GI tract. These processes occur simultaneously with digestion and absorption of the ingested dietary fluids and solids. As a result, there is normally a massive flux of fluids and electrolytes within the GI tract in healthy children on a daily basis (Table 10-1).

Table 10-1
Approximate Compositions of Gastrointestinal Secretions*

Fluid	Fasting				Fed			
	Newborn	Infant	Child	Adult	Newborn	Infant	Child	Adult
Gastric								
pH	2.5	3.2	3.2	1.0	6.8	7.0	7.0	5.0
Na^+	80-100	80-100	80-100	80-100	20-30	20-30	20-30	20-30
Cl^-	100-130	100-130	100-130	100-130	120-150	120-150	120-150	120-150
K^+	5-15	5-15	5-15	5-15	5-15	5-15	5-15	5-15
HCO_3^-	0	0	0	0	0	0	0	0
Biliary								
pH	7.2	7.2	7.2	7.2	7.8	7.8	7.8	7.8
$Na+$	140-180	140-180	140-180	140-180	140-180	140-180	140-180	140-180
Cl^-	60-80	60-80	60-80	60-80	90-120	90-120	90-120	90-120
K^+	3-12	3-12	3-12	3-12	3-12	3-12	3-12	3-12
HCO_3^-	20-30	20-30	20-30	20-30	40-50	40-50	40-50	40-50
Pancreatic								
pH	8.0	8.0	8.0	8.0	8.0	8.0	8.0	8.0
Na^+	125-135	125-135	135-150	135-150	125-135	125-135	135-150	135-150
Cl^-	90-110	90-110	85-95	85-95	20-40	20-40	20-40	20-40
K^+	7-15	7-15	3-8	3-8	7-15	7-15	3-8	3-8
HCO_3^-	25-60	25-60	25-60	25-60	110-130	110-130	110-130	110-130
Jejunal								
pH	7.5	7.5	7.5	7.5	7.5	7.5	7.5	7.5
Na^+	125-135	125-135	135-150	135-150	125-135	125-135	135-150	135-150
Cl^-	120-145	120-145	120-145	120-145	120-145	120-145	120-145	120-145
K^+	7-15	7-15	3-8	3-8	7-15	7-15	3-8	3-8
HCO_3^-	20	20	20	20	20	20	20	20
Ileal								
pH	8.0	8.0	8.0	8.0	8.0	8.0	8.0	8.0
Na^+	125-135	125-135	135-150	135-150	125-135	125-135	135-150	135-150
Cl^-	70-85	70-85	70-85	70-85	70-85	70-85	70-85	70-85
K^+	7-15	7-15	3-8	3-8	7-15	7-15	3-8	3-8
HCO_3^-	40	40	40	40	40	40	40	40

Modified from Hazinski MF: *Nursing care of the critically ill child,* ed 2, St Louis, 1992, Mosby.
*Electrolyte values are in mEq/L.

A variety of diseases and therapeutic interventions may result in excessive losses of fluid and/or electrolytes from the GI tract. Throughout the child's stay in the intensive care unit (ICU), record the volume and appearance of any sources of fluid output to enable calculation of the composition of any necessary replacement fluids and electrolytes. In addition, monitor the child for potential fluid and electrolyte imbalances or complications (Table 10-2). Plan to replace excessive fluid losses with fluid identical in volume and composition to the fluid lost.

Table 10-2
Causes and Symptoms of Common Electrolyte Imbalances

Imbalance	Cause	Symptoms	Diagnostic Tests
Sodium deficit (hyponatremia)	Excessive diaphoresis (e.g., cystic fibrosis), gastrointestinal suction or vomiting, water enemas and irrigations, ileostomy drainage, GI fistula, biliary drainage, potent diuretics, obstruction, peritonitis, pancreatitis, diarrhea NOTE: Hyperglycemia may result in an artificially reduced serum sodium value that reverses as serum glucose is reduced	Apprehension, abdominal cramps, seizures, oliguria or anuria, diarrhea, muscle twitching, salivation, increased deep tendon reflexes, lethargy or confusion, vasomotor collapse: hypotension, tachycardia, cold, clammy skin, cyanosis	Decreased serum sodium, decreased serum chloride, decreased urine specific gravity, increased Hct, increased serum proteins, BUN, and creatinine
Sodium excess (hypernatremia)	Excessive ingestion of salt, watery diarrhea NOTE: With severe dehydration, serum sodium values may be elevated because of hemoconcentration; as patient is rehydrated, serum sodium values may decrease	Dry, sticky mucous membranes, flushed skin, intense thirst, rough and dry tongue, oliguria or anuria, increase in temperature, firm tissue turgor, pitting edema, elevated blood pressure, weight gain (if fluid intake is normal), excitement, mania, seizures	Increased serum sodium, increased serum chloride, increased urine specific gravity, increased RBC, Hct
Potassium deficit (hypokalemia)	Potent diuretics, vomiting, ulcerative colitis, diarrhea, fistulas of small intestine or colon, starvation or wasting disease, low-sodium diet, GI suction, hemorrhage, chronic laxative use, water enema, peritonitis, pancreatitis, prolonged parenteral nutrition, acid-base imbalance	Thirst, malaise or muscle weakness, apathy or drowsiness, tremors, diminished reflexes, flaccid paralysis, tachycardia, hypotension, vomiting, diminished or absent bowel sounds, shallow respirations, anorexia, myocardial irritability	Decreased serum potassium, decreased serum chloride, increased serum HCO_3, acidic urine, ECG changes, cardiac arrhythmias: heart block, cardiac arrest, prolonged QT interval, ventricular irritability
Calcium deficit (hypocalcemia)	Acute pancreatitis, generalized peritonitis, infusion of citrated blood, sprue, fistulas of pancreas or small intestine, malabsorption, diarrhea	Tingling of fingers and toes, tetany, abdominal cramps, ing, carpalpedal spasm, convulsions	Decreased serum calcium, ECG changes
Magnesium deficit	Malabsorption syndrome, diarrhea, bowel resection, alcoholism, hypercalcemia, diuretic therapy, diabetic acidosis, prolonged nasogastric suction	Insomnia, twitching, tremors, seizures, muscle weakness, leg or foot cramps, hypotension, arrhythmias, disorientation, seizures	Decreased serum magnesium, normal serum calcium

Modified from Hazinski MF: *Nursing care of the critically ill child,* ed 2, St Louis, 1992, Mosby; and Given B, Simmons S: *Gastroenterology in clinical nursing,* ed 4, St Louis, 1984, Mosby.

Fluid, Electrolyte, and Energy Requirements

Children require adequate caloric or energy intake to support their rapid growth and development during childhood. The critically ill child typically requires additional calories to heal injuries or wounds or to fight infection, even when that child receives neuromuscular blockade to prevent movement. Typically, fever increases energy requirements 12% per day for each degree Celsius elevation in temperature above 37° C. Pain, burns, and severe trauma and cold stress (in neonates) can increase energy requirements by 40% to 100%.

Nutritional requirements for infants and children can be estimated using Tables 10-3 and 10-4. Note that only 20% of these calories is required for activity; thus 80% of the requirements will be needed even if the child is not moving. Caloric requirements are typically much higher than the estimated value when the child is critically ill or injured.

Fluid and electrolyte requirements also vary as a function of age and clinical condition. Normal requirements are listed in Table 10-5. Note that any

Table 10-3
Nutritional Requirements for Infants and Children

Age	Calories/kg/24 hr
Up to 6 mo	120
6-12 mo	100
12-36 mo	90-95
4 yr-10 yr	80
>10 yr; male	45
>10 yr, female	38

Nutrient	Percent of Total Calories	
Carbohydrates	40%-45%	
Fat	40%	Combined 85%-88%
Protein	20%	

From Hazinski MF: *Nursing care of the critically ill child,* ed 2, St Louis, 1992, Mosby.

Table 10-4
Distribution of Energy Requirements for Infants and Children

	Percent of Caloric Requirements*	
	Infant	Child
Basal metabolic rate (BMR)	50%	50%
Activity	20%	Combined 48%†
Growth	25%	
Loss in stools	5%	2%

From Hazinski MF: *Nursing care of the critically ill child,* ed 2, St Louis, 1992, Mosby.
*An additional 12% is added to BMR for each degree Celsius elevation of body temperature.
†Fluctuates with age and activity level.

Table 10-5
Calculation of Daily Maintenance Fluid and Electrolyte Requirements for Children

Child's Weight	Kilogram Body Weight Formula (Provides Generous Allotment)
Fluids	
Newborn (up to 72 hr after birth)	60-100 ml/kg
Up to 10 kg	100 ml/kg (may increase up to 150 ml/kg to provide caloric requirements if renal and cardiac function adequate)
11-20 kg	1000 ml for the first 10 kg + 50 ml/kg for each kg over 10 kg
21-30 kg	1500 ml for the first 20 kg + 25 ml/kg for each kg over 20 kg

Body Surface Area (BSA) Formula
1500 ml/m^2 BSA/day

Insensible Water Losses
300 ml/m^2 BSA/day

Electrolytes

Sodium (Na$^+$)	3-4 mEq/kg/24 hr
Potassium (K$^+$)	2-3 mEq/kg/24 hr
Calcium (Ca$^+$)	50-100 mg/kg/24 hr
Magnesium (Mg^{++})	0.4-0.9 mEq/kg/day

Modified from Hazinski MF: *Nursing care of the critically ill child,* ed 2, St Louis, 1992, Mosby.

calculation of "maintenance" fluid requirements should use the formulas only as a baseline; the actual volume of fluid administered to the patient must be tailored individually according to the child's clinical condition, fluid balance, and insensible water losses. Fever, use of overbed warmers, and use of phototherapy will increase insensible water losses. Insensible water losses can be estimated at 300 ml/m^2 body surface area (BSA)/day. (BSA can be determined using the BSA nomogram on the inside back cover.)

As a rule, once the child is euvolemic (i.e., has sufficient intravascular volume to maintain effective systemic perfusion), *fluid intake is often limited to less than calculated "maintenance" values in the presence of congestive heart failure, respiratory failure, head injury or increased intracranial pressure (ICP), or renal failure.*

Common Clinical Conditions

Dehydration

Etiology

Dehydration occurs when the total output of all fluids and electrolytes exceeds the patient's total intake. This may result from either inadequate fluid intake or excessive fluid losses. The dehydrated patient demonstrates a deficiency in both fluids and electrolytes, and the deficiency can be classified by the severity of the fluid deficit, as well as by its effect on serum sodium. Hypernatremic, or hypertonic, dehydration is characterized by a high serum sodium concentration, whereas hyponatremic, or hypotonic, dehydration is characterized by a low serum sodium concentration.

Infants and children may develop dehydration more rapidly than adults. Dehydration is often a result of acute viral or bacterial diarrhea, which may be part of a more complex disease, such as hemolytic-uremic syndrome (see Chapter 9, pp. 457 and 483).

Hyponatremic dehydration can develop during hospitalization following administration of hypotonic fluids or following vomiting, diarrhea, or drainage replaced with hypotonic fluids. Hypernatremic dehydration most commonly results from gastroenteritis with vomiting and diarrhea but may complicate burns, fever, diabetes insipidus, aggressive diuresis, and diabetic ketoacidosis.

Pathophysiology and Clinical Presentation

The degree or severity of dehydration is typically expressed as a percentage of total body weight loss. The child's precise normal weight before the illness is often unobtainable; therefore the fluid/weight deficit is estimated from the clinical appearance. This estimation assumes that the serum sodium concentration is normal; if the serum sodium concentration is later found to be high or low, adjustments must then be made in the estimated severity of dehydration and in the estimated severity of the fluid deficit.

The severity of dehydration is classified as mild, moderate, or severe, based on clinical signs, as follows (Table 10-6, see Table 9-5):

- *Mild dehydration:* Loss of up to 5% of body weight in infants or 3% of body weight in children and adolescents. This corresponds to a fluid deficit of approximately 50 ml/kg of normal body weight in the infant and 30 ml/kg of normal body weight in the child or adolescent. The child characteristically looks ill and is irritable and tachycardic, but the blood pressure and respiratory rate are normal.
- *Moderate dehydration:* Loss of up to 10% of body weight in infants or 5% to 7% of body weight in older children and adolescents. This corresponds to a fluid deficit of approximately 100 ml/kg of normal body weight in the infant and 60 ml/kg of normal body weight in the child or adolescent. The child characteristically has signs of peripheral circulatory failure, including cool skin, weak peripheral pulses, prolonged capillary refill, and some mottling or pallor in color. However, blood pressure is normal.
- *Severe dehydration:* Loss of up to 15% of body weight in infants or 7% to 9% of body weight in children and adolescents. This corresponds to a fluid deficit of approximately 150 ml/kg of normal body weight in the infant and 90 ml/kg of normal body weight in the child or adolescent. The child is severely

Table 10-6
Correlation of Clinical Signs of Isotonic Dehydration With Severity of Dehydration*

	Magnitude of Dehydration		
	Mild	**Moderate**	**Severe**
Body weight	5% loss	10% loss	15% loss
Skin turgor	↓	↓↓	↓↓↓
Mucous membranes	Dry	Very dry	Parched
Skin color	Pale	Gray	Mottled
Urine	Slight oliguria	Oliguria	Marked oliguria and azotemia
Blood pressure	Normal	± Normal	Reduced
Pulse	±↑	↑	↑↑

From Winters R: *The body fluids in pediatrics,* Boston, 1973, Little, Brown.
*NOTE: Clinical signs are used to initially estimate severity of dehydration, and serum sodium is assumed to be normal. If, after estimation of severity of deficit, serum sodium is high (>150 mEq/L), *increase severity of dehydration by one level (from mild to moderate or from moderate to severe).* If serum sodium is low (<130mEq/L), decrease severity of hydration by one level (from severe to moderate or from moderate to mild).

ill, with signs of decompensated shock (hypotension), as well as signs of poor perfusion.

Severe dehydration can ultimately compromise intravascular volume and systemic perfusion. Once systemic perfusion is compromised, compensatory mechanisms are activated to redistribute intravascular volume and to maintain essential organ and tissue perfusion. At this point, hypovolemic shock is present (see Chapter 5), and the child characteristically demonstrates peripheral vasoconstriction and decreased urine output. If systemic perfusion is severely compromised, metabolic acidosis will be present. Hypotension indicates the development of decompensated shock, and multisystem organ failure or death may result if the compromise in perfusion is severe or prolonged (see p. 137).

The type of dehydration present—hypotonic, isotonic, or hypertonic—is determined by the serum sodium concentration, as follows:

- *Hypotonic dehydration:* The loss of body sodium is proportionately greater than the loss of body water; thus the serum sodium concentration is <130 mEq/L. An abrupt fall in the serum sodium concentration creates an acute difference between intravascular and interstitial osmolality and will promote an acute free water shift *out of* the vascular

space. As a result, when hypotonic dehydration is present, the fluid deficit is compounded by an extravascular fluid shift. This causes a more severe reduction in intravascular volume at a given fluid deficit and will make clinical signs of hypovolemia more severe than the signs resulting if the absolute fluid deficit volume developed with a normal serum sodium. Thus, *with hypotonic dehydration, the fluid deficit is predominantly from the intravascular space,* making clinical signs more severe at only moderate deficits. Once it is clear that hypotonic dehydration is present, the dehydration volume deficit is reduced one level from that which was estimated from the clinical appearance. The severity of the dehydration and the fluid deficit initially estimated to be severe are reduced to a moderate level, and the severity of the dehydration and fluid deficit initially estimated to be moderate are reduced to a mild level.

- *Hypertonic dehydration:* The loss of fluid is proportionately greater than the loss of water. As a result, the serum sodium rises to >150 mEq/L; this creates an acute difference in osmolality between the intravascular and interstitial space and results in an acute shift of free water into the vascular space. When hypertonic dehydration is present, the fluid loss is predominantly from the interstitial space; the intravascular volume may be maintained despite fluid deficit by this intravascular fluid shift (from the interstitial space). Clinical signs of dehydration with hypertonic dehydration will be milder for the volume of fluid deficit than would occur with either hypotonic or isotonic dehydration. Once it is clear that hypertonic dehydration is present, the severity of the dehydration and the deficit volume is increased one level from that which was estimated from the clinical appearance. Dehydration and fluid deficit originally estimated to be mild are increased to a moderate level, and dehydration and fluid deficit originally estimated to be moderate are increased to a severe level.

Management

Goals of Treatment The goals of treatment for the symptomatic child with dehydration include:

- Restore intravascular volume and effective systemic perfusion (treat shock).
- Replace volume and electrolyte deficit.
- Provide maintenance fluid and electrolyte requirements.
- Replace ongoing losses.

Regardless of the type of dehydration present, you must assess the child's systemic perfusion, establish reliable intravenous (IV) access, provide volume resuscitation, and constantly assess the child's response to therapy.

Treatment of Shock If there is a compromise in systemic perfusion, immediate volume resuscitation is indicated, using isotonic crystalloid. Reliable IV access should be established with one or two large catheters. In children less than 6 years of age, an intraosseous needle can be used for access to the venous system.

Bolus fluid therapy of normal saline or lactated Ringer's solution is provided in amounts of 20 ml/kg and repeated as needed until systemic perfusion is acceptable. Colloids may be added later during resuscitation if needed.

The child's clinical condition should improve if fluid resuscitation is successful. A positive response to fluid administration will include improvement in systemic perfusion, associated with a warming of the skin and extremities, brisk capillary refill, and increase in urine output. The child should become progressively more alert. Acidosis and hypotension should be corrected immediately. If the child does not improve during resuscitation, complicating factors (e.g., the presence of sepsis or intracranial hemorrhage) should be considered and ruled out.

Correction of Fluid and Electrolyte Deficit

Once shock is corrected, the serum sodium concentration should be available; the fluid and electrolyte deficit is calculated, and plans are made to correct the deficit. The fluid deficit is estimated from the child's clinical presentation and is then adjusted based on the serum sodium concentration. The adjustment in dehydration severity required by abnormalities in the serum sodium concentration occurs as follows: the dehydration volume deficit should be adjusted in the same direction as the serum sodium is altered. If the serum sodium concentration is high, *increase* the severity of the dehydration and fluid deficit by one level from that estimated from the clinical appearance. If the serum sodium is low, *decrease* the severity of the dehydration and fluid deficit by one level from that estimated from the clinical appearance.

Example: If the child presents with dehydration and signs of peripheral circulatory failure but normal blood pressure, you would initially classify the child's dehydration as moderate with an estimated fluid deficit of 100 ml/kg. If the child is *hyponatremic* (serum sodium concentration <130 mEq/L), you would adjust the severity of dehydration downward (in the same direction as the sodium is altered) to mild and the estimated fluid deficit to 50 ml/kg. Remember, children with hyponatremic dehydration have lost fluid predominantly from the intravascular space; clinical signs will be more severe than the volume deficit would suggest.

If the child presents with identical clinical signs (signs of peripheral circulatory failure but normal blood pressure) but has *hypernatremia* (serum sodium >150 mEq/L), you would increase the severity of dehydration from moderate to severe (this changes the severity in the same direction as the alteration in serum sodium concentration) and the estimated fluid deficit from 100 ml/kg to 150 ml/kg. Remember, fluid loss in children with hypernatremia will be predominantly from the interstitial space; thus clinical signs will be less severe at greater fluid deficits.

Once the deficit is quantified, plans are made to correct that deficit over a 24- to 48-hour period. If *isotonic or hypotonic* dehydration is present, 50% of the estimated deficit is replaced over the first 8 hours of therapy and the final 50% of the deficit is replaced over the next 16 hours of therapy. The replacement fluid is usually 5% dextrose and 0.45% NaCl with 30 mEq/L of potassium chloride and is administered in addition to maintenance fluids.

If *hypertonic* dehydration is present, the fluid deficit is replaced over 48 hours. Although volume resuscitation is required if shock is present, aggressive fluid resuscitation should not be provided once systemic perfusion is adequate, because even normal saline (0.9% NaCl) is hypotonic to the child's serum; thus bolus administration of isotonic crystalloids can cause the serum sodium concentration to fall abruptly. If the serum sodium concentration falls too rapidly, cerebral edema can develop in association with a fluid shift from the vascular to the interstitial and cellular spaces. *The serum sodium concentration should not fall more rapidly than 10 to 15 mEq/L over a 24-hour period, or more rapidly than 1 to 2 mEq/L in any 1 hour.* The child's neurologic function should be monitored closely; it should improve as fluid resuscitation is accomplished. Any neurologic deterioration should be reported to a physician immediately.

The replacement fluid for hypernatremic dehydration is typically 5% dextrose and normal saline (0.9% NaCl) or 5% dextrose and 0.45% NaCl with 30 mEq/L of potassium chloride. The sodium chloride content of the replacement fluid is selected and adjusted based on the child's serum sodium concentration during therapy.

Young infants have high glucose needs and low glycogen stores and thus may become hypoglycemic during episodes of dehydration. A rapid bedside glucose test should be performed when the young infant presents with dehydration; if hypo-glycemia is present, a small bolus of glucose followed by a glucose infusion should be provided.

General Supportive Care   Maintenance of the IV catheters is essential to enable correction of the fluid volume deficit. The child's clinical response, including urine output and systemic perfusion, should be closely recorded, and the child's electrolyte balance maintained. An accurate weight should be obtained as soon as possible after admission and every morning on the same scale at the same time of day. Ongoing fluid losses should be measured and replaced with fluids of appropriate volume and electrolyte content (Table 10-7). Monitor the child's core body temperature and be alert for signs of infection and sepsis.

Hyperbilirubinemia

Etiology

Bilirubin is the major by-product of hemoglobin. Hyperbilirubinemia is an elevation in the serum levels of bilirubin. Potential causes include:

- *Hemolytic:* Caused by increased red blood cell breakdown
- *Nonhemolytic:* Caused by impairment in bilirubin excretion (e.g., liver disease)

Hyperbilirubinemia can result from elevation in either conjugated or unconjugated bilirubin. Elevated *conjugated* bilirubin is *direct* hyperbilirubinemia, and it most commonly results from biliary tree obstruction, liver disease, or bowel obstruction, although it also may occur with metabolic disorders, sepsis, drug reactions, pyelonephritis, meningitis, or gram-negative infection. Neonatal hepatitis may cause hepatocellular damage and increased conjugated bilirubin.

Elevation of *unconjugated* bilirubin levels is known as *indirect* hyperbilirubinemia. It most commonly occurs as a result of excessive breakdown of red blood cells (hemolytic diseases or extensive bruising) or as a result of impaired transport of bilirubin caused by hypoxia or acidosis or as the result of the administration of albumin-binding drugs that displace bilirubin from albumin. Indirect hyperbilirubinemia is common among premature neonates.

Table 10-7
Practical Approach to Correction of Fluid and Electrolyte Deficits

Type	Component	Deficit 5%	Deficit 10%
Isotonic	Water	50 ml/kg	100 ml/kg
	Na^+	4-5 mmol/kg	8-10 mmol/kg
	K^+	2-3 mmol/kg	4-5 mmol/kg
	Suggested solution*: 5% dextrose and 0.45% NaCl with 20 mmol/L KCl		
Hypotonic	Water	50 ml/kg	100 ml/kg
	Na^+	5-6 mmol/kg	10-12 mmol/kg
	K^+	3 mmol/kg	5 mmol/kg
	Suggested solution*: 5% dextrose and 0.45% NaCl with 20 mmol/L KCl		
Hypertonic	Water	50 ml/kg	100 ml/kg
	Na^+	2-4 mmol/kg	2-4 mmol/kg
	K^+	2-4 mmol/kg	2-4 mmol/kg
	Suggested solution*: 5% dextrose and 0.2% NaCl with 40 mmol KCl/L, or 5% dextrose and 0.45% NaCl with 40 mmol/L KCl (once urine output established) and adjust based on serum sodium		

From Dipchand A: *The HSC handbook of pediatrics,* ed 9, St Louis, 1997, Mosby, p 103.
*Suggested solutions most closely approximate ideal solution to correct both fluid and electrolyte deficits; can also be calculated.

Pathophysiology

Red blood cells are normally sequestered and destroyed in the spleen at the end of their life span. When they are destroyed, the heme portion of the hemoglobin molecule is oxidized, and bilirubin is formed. Bilirubin is bound to albumin in the plasma, and in the liver it is *conjugated,* or combined with a sugar residue called glucuronide. Conjugated bilirubin is water soluble and normally is excreted in bile. Free, or *unconjugated,* bilirubin is lipid soluble, rather than water soluble, and will diffuse freely into the brain and other tissues.

Conjugated, or direct, hyperbilirubinemia is present when ≥15% of the total plasma bilirubin level is conjugated or when the conjugated bilirubin level is >1.5 mg/dl. Physiologic hyperbilirubinemia in the newborn is caused by both a deficiency in bilirubin conjugation and an increase in bilirubin production during the first week of life. *Unconjugated* bilirubin levels >5 mg/dl in an infant less than 24 hours of age or the persistence of unconjugated bilirubin levels >12 mg/dl after

24 hours of age is consistent with *indirect hyperbilirubinemia* and should be investigated.

Kernicterus is the yellow staining of the basal ganglia of the brain of neonates with high concentrations of unconjugated bilirubin (indirect hyperbilirubinemia). Kernicterus causes encephalopathy and permanent brain damage. Acidosis, neuronal dysfunction and alteration in the blood-brain barrier, hypercarbia, and vasculitis are thought to contribute to kernicterus.

Clinical Presentation

Jaundice is characterized by the accumulation of yellow pigment in the skin and other tissues when the bilirubin levels are high. Jaundice can usually be detected when the serum level of total bilirubin is >5 mg/dl (normally it is <1.5 mg/dl).

Jaundice is most easily detected in the sclera and soft palate, but it may be visible on the skin. The urine color may become brown as conjugated bilirubin is excreted in the urine. The stools may become gray or clay colored, indicating absence of

Table 10-8
Diagnostic Tests Used in Differential Diagnosis of Jaundice

	Normal	Hemolytic	Liver Disease	Biliary Tract Obstruction Secondary to Atresia or Stone
Serum Tests				
Alkaline phosphatase	4.0-13.0 King-Armstrong units	Normal	Increase 1 to 3 times; urine dark (late); skin yellow, orange, green	Increased three to eight times; urine dark yellow; skin orange or green
Bilirubin				
Total	0.5-1.4 mg/dl	5-20 mg/dl	Over 15 mg/dl	Normal or increased
Direct	0.2-0.4 mg/dl	Normal or increased	Decreased	Increased
Indirect	0.4-0.8 mg/dl	Increased	Increased	Increased
Cholesterol (total)	150-250 mg/dl	Normal	Normal or decreased	Increased
SGOT	12-36 U	Normal	300-5000 U	300 U or less
SGPT	6-25 U	Normal	300-5000 U	300 U or less
Protein				
Total	6.0-7.8 g/dl	Decreased	Decreased	Normal or slight increase
Albumin	3.9-4.6 g/dl	Decreased	Decreased	Normal or slight increase
Globulin	2.3-3.5 g/dl	Normal	Moderate increase	Normal or slight increase
Prothrombin time	11.0-17.0 sec	Normal	Often abnormal despite vitamin K administration	Normal or returns to normal following vitamin K administration
Urine Tests				
Bilirubin	0	0	Positive	Positive
Urobilinogen	1.4 mg/24 hr	Increased	Increased	Normal
Stool Tests				
Urobilinogen	40-280 mg/24 hr	Over 250 mg/24 hr; normal color	Normal or decreased; normal color	Acholic (0-5 mg/24 hr); clay-colored stool

From Given BA, Simmons SJ: *Gastroenterology in clinical nursing,* ed 4, St Louis, 1984, Mosby; modified from Jaundice-Biochemical Differential Diagnosis, Warner-Teed Pharmaceuticals, Inc., Columbus, Ohio, 1970.

normal fecal elimination of bilirubin. Pruritus, caused by bile salt deposition, develops with direct hyperbilirubinemia.

Total and direct bilirubin levels are measured in the laboratory, and the level of indirect, or unconjugated, bilirubin is the difference between the total and direct bilirubin. *The higher the amount of indirect, or unconjugated, bilirubin in the serum, the greater may be the neonate's risk of kernicterus.*

The relative levels of direct and indirect bilirubin and the liver enzyme concentrations can provide information about the cause of the hyperbilirubinemia (Table 10-8):

- Elevation in total and direct bilirubin levels will be observed when the child has hepatobiliary disease. The indirect bilirubin level may also be slightly elevated.
- Elevation in total and indirect bilirubin levels will be observed in the child with hemolytic disease or hepatic disease. In the presence of liver disease, however, elevation in serum liver enzymes will be observed.

An abdominal ultrasound and radioisotope scan can be used to evaluate bile excretion in the child with hepatobiliary disease. If liver disease is apparent, a liver biopsy may be performed to identify it. Cholangiography with surgical exploration of the biliary tree will confirm the diagnosis of biliary atresia.

Management

Management of hyperbilirubinemia is determined by the cause of the elevated bilirubin. If *direct or conjugated* hyperbilirubinemia is present, the child will require supportive care, as well as monitoring for and treatment of complications of liver failure. Ultimately, creation of a surgical shunt or transplantation may be necessary. Support of nutrition and adequate hydration will be required for all patients with hyperbilirubinemia.

Coagulopathies, anemia, and thrombocytopenia necessitate monitoring for signs of bleeding and will often require blood component therapy. Alteration in medication dosages will be required if hepatic function is severely impaired (see Hepatic Failure). The child with direct hyperbilirubinemia must be kept well hydrated because dehydration will reduce excretion of conjugated bilirubin.

Indirect hyperbilirubinemia is observed most often during the neonatal period, and it is often treated with phototherapy, exchange transfusion, and, occasionally, pharmacologic agents (Figure 10-1). Drugs that bind to serum albumin (including diazepam, furosemide, sodium oxacillin, hydrocortisone, gentamicin, and digoxin) are avoided, if possible, because they may displace serum bilirubin from albumin, thereby increasing the concentration of free bilirubin and the risk of bilirubin diffusion into brain tissue (kernicterus).

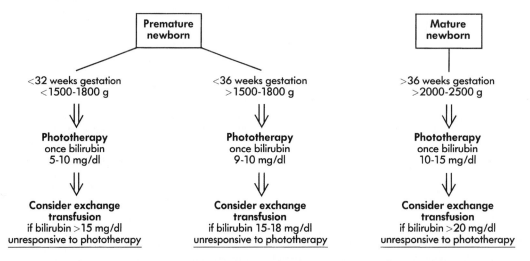

Whenever jaundice is observed, the etiology should be investigated to rule out hemolytic disease and possible G-6-PD deficiency (blood type should be determined for the mother, and blood type and Coombs test performed on the infant's blood sample). If hemolytic hyperbilirubinemia is present, phototherapy is usually effective if it is utilized correctly. Exchange transfusion is *rarely* necessary, and is usually only considered if the bilirubin is high and rising rapidly (faster than 0.5 mg/dl/hr or 10 mg/dl/day) *despite* phototherapy.

Figure 10-1 Suggested guidelines for the management of neonatal hyperbilirubinemia. (From Avery MI, First LR: *Pediatric medicine,* Baltimore, 1988, Williams & Wilkins; and Fanaroff AA, Martin RJ: Jaundice and liver disease. In Fanaroff AA, Martin RJ, editors: *Neonatal-perinatal medicine: diseases of the fetus and infant,* ed 5, St Louis, 1991, Mosby.)

Ascites

Etiology

Ascites is the accumulation of free fluid in the peritoneal cavity. It may result from diffuse inflammation of the peritoneal surface (peritonitis), or it may be associated with increased portal capillary pressure resulting from cirrhosis, severe congestive heart failure, or other obstructive vascular conditions. Ascites may also be associated with diseases that result in sodium and water retention with decreased plasma colloid osmotic pressure (e.g., nephrotic syndrome).

Pathophysiology

Ascites results from the exudation of fluid from the surface of the liver, bowel, or peritoneum. This fluid enters the abdominal cavity instead of the mesenteric or portal venous system for one of the following reasons:

- There is obstruction to flow between the mesenteric or portal vein and the superior vena cava.
- There is an extremely high central venous pressure (CVP).
- Serum albumin content is low.
- Proteinaceous fluid is present in the peritoneal cavity.

When hepatic and portal venous blood flow is obstructed (e.g., with cirrhosis of the liver or systemic congestion as part of congestive heart failure), venous capillary and hepatic sinusoidal pressures rise. Initially, the veins and sinusoids expand to accommodate larger quantities of blood, and hepatomegaly can be documented. Eventually, however, as the capillary hydrostatic pressure rises, fluid begins to exude from the surface of the liver and into the peritoneal cavity. Ascites can also be caused by a very low plasma oncotic pressure, which may be present in nephrotic syndrome or other diseases characterized by hypoproteinemia.

Clinical Presentation

The development of ascites may not be noticed by the child or parents until the fit of clothing is altered. Superficial abdominal veins may be distended and visible on the surface of the abdomen.

The abdomen will be full and is generally dull to percussion, although the dull areas may change with changes in patient position. The girth should be measured every 2 to 4 hours until stable measurements are obtained. A fluid wave may be elicited if the child is cooperative and two observers are present. The first observer places a hand on the midline of the abdomen. The second observer sharply taps the side of the child's abdomen, and this should create a "wave" of fluid that elevates the first observer's hand.

Significant ascites will compromise diaphragm excursion and can lead to respiratory distress. Accumulation of large amounts of ascitic fluid may also eventually cause a hydrothorax. For these reasons, the child's respiratory status must be closely monitored.

Management

Ascites is managed symptomatically. Fluid intake and output, and daily or twice-daily weights are recorded. Abdominal girth is measured every 2 to 4 hours in severe cases (make a mark on the abdomen to indicate where the measuring tape should be placed).

Strict limitation of fluid and sodium intake may be required. At the same time, the child's circulating blood volume and systemic perfusion must be monitored and supported. A CVP catheter may be extremely useful in evaluating circulating blood volume, but the tip should be beyond any area of blood flow obstruction near the liver. Signs of inadequate blood volume include tachycardia, peripheral vasoconstriction, low CVP, decreased or absent urine output, and high urine specific gravity.

Nutrition is extremely important, and efforts must be made to make meals palatable. Mealtime should not be interrupted, if at all possible.

The child's respiratory status must be closely monitored. The child should be positioned, with the head of the bed elevated, in a position that facilitates spontaneous respiratory effort. If the child develops signs of increased respiratory effort, a hydrothorax should be ruled out. Hydrothorax is treated with thoracentesis and possible chest tube insertion if found. Oxygen administration or intubation with mechanical ventilation is occasionally necessary.

The child with ascites is at high risk for infection; thus careful monitoring for signs of infection or sepsis is required. The child will require excellent skin care.

Acute Abdomen

Etiology

The term *acute abdomen* is used to describe any abdominal condition for which urgent surgical intervention must be considered. An acute abdomen usually results from abdominal inflammation (such as appendicitis), obstruction, perforation, hemorrhage, or blunt trauma. In infants an acute abdomen may result from GI perforation because of intestinal obstruction, ischemia, gangrenous volvulus, necrotizing enterocolitis, or iatrogenic perforations. Because peritonitis and abscess formation may cause or complicate the development of an acute abdomen, the need for urgent surgical intervention is always considered.

An acute abdomen may be caused by blunt or penetrating trauma. Blunt trauma can produce visceral perforation or hemorrhage, but signs and symptoms may be masked or delayed for several hours or days. An acute abdomen is particularly difficult to diagnose in the infant or child with a compromise in neurologic condition or in a child receiving steroid therapy.

Pathophysiology

GI perforation will result in leakage of hydrochloric acid, digestive enzymes, and bile, causing chemical irritation of the peritoneum, and chemical peritonitis may follow. Leakage of fecal material from the lower GI tract not only releases aerobic and anaerobic bacteria into the peritoneum, but may also release endotoxin from the cell walls of aerobic gram-negative bacteria, creating endotoxemia and sepsis.

Hemoperitoneum from blunt or penetrating injury may not produce peritonitis until the red blood cells lyse. However, unless the source of bleeding ceases (which can happen with blunt liver or splenic injury), hemorrhagic shock can develop. Undetected abdominal hemorrhage is a leading cause of trauma mortality (see Chapter 12).

Peritoneal contamination or irritation produces increased blood flow to and capillary permeability in the affected areas. The result is transudation of fluid into the peritoneal cavity, so-called third spacing of fluid into the peritoneum. Volume administration may be necessary to maintain systemic perfusion.

Clinical Presentation

The most common symptom of an acute abdomen is pain. Respirations may be rapid and shallow; and voluntary and then involuntary abdominal wall contraction (guarding) may be noted when the abdomen is approached. Rebound tenderness may be noted when pressure on the abdomen is released. Bowel sounds may be decreased or absent, and anorexia, nausea, and vomiting may develop.

In very young children visceral perforation causes signs and symptoms of an acute illness and third spacing of fluids. If a large extravascular shift of fluids occurs, signs of poor systemic perfusion will be associated with an increase in abdominal girth.

Free air may be present on abdominal radiographs if bowel perforation has occurred. Ultrasonography or abdominal computed tomography (CT) scanning will enable the definitive imaging of the abdominal solid organs.

Management

Medical management of the child with an acute abdomen begins with restoration of the intravascular volume to correct hypovolemia and shock. A nasogastric tube may be required to decompress the stomach, and any drainage obtained is checked for the presence of blood. A urinary catheter also is inserted to check for hematuria and to enable the accurate measurement of urine output. If significant bleeding or clinical deterioration is present, urgent surgical intervention is necessary.

If the child is admitted for skilled observation, the nurse is responsible for documenting and reporting the presence and any progression of the following signs:

- Signs of peritonitis, including fever; abdominal tenderness, rigidity, and distension; and nausea and vomiting
- Signs of third spacing of fluid, including increasing abdominal girth, electrolyte imbalances, and evidence of a decrease in intravascular volume

- Persistent pain
- Signs of abdominal obstruction, including abdominal distension, projectile vomiting or vomiting of bile or fecal material, and absence of bowel sounds
- Signs of GI hemorrhage
- Signs of respiratory compromise secondary to increased abdominal tenderness and decreased diaphragm excursion

Report any clinical deterioration to a physician immediately. Indications for surgical intervention include persistent abdominal pain with involuntary guarding and rebound tenderness, evidence of localized peritonitis, or the appearance of free air on the abdominal radiograph. Monitor for signs of respiratory distress and be prepared to support oxygenation and ventilation as needed. The child should receive nothing by mouth.

Portal Hypertension

Etiology

Portal hypertension is an increase in the portal venous pressure above 5 to 10 mm Hg. It is caused by obstruction to the normal flow of blood through the portal venous system, the liver sinusoids, or the hepatic vein. The obstruction to blood flow may be in one of three major locations:

- The portal vein or its tributaries (extrahepatic portal hypertension), caused by congenital or acquired thrombosis of the portal vein
- The liver (intrahepatic portal hypertension), caused by fibrosis from chronic liver disease
- The venous outflow into the inferior vena cava (suprahepatic portal hypertension), caused by inferior vena caval obstruction or hepatic vein occlusion or thrombosis

Pathophysiology

Three major physiologic complications of portal hypertension are congestion of the splenic and mesenteric circulation, the development of collateral vessels, and the sequestration of blood in the splanchnic circulation (the blood vessels from the gut and spleen that normally drain into the portal vein).

When portal vein pressure increases, blood flow from the splanchnic circulation is impeded, and blood pools in the splanchnic circulation. Mesenteric vein thrombosis or mesenteric infarction may develop. Splenic congestion and stasis of blood in the spleen cause hypersplenism and damage to the formed elements of the blood, producing anemia, thrombocytopenia, and neutropenia.

Impedance to portal blood flow and hypertension in the portal and splanchnic circulation promote the formation of collateral vessels between the systemic and portal circulations and the inferior vena cava or other major central veins. These collateral vessels often form around the stomach, the esophagus, and the anus. The vessels in the esophagus may dilate and become esophageal varices. These varices may be a source of sudden hemorrhage (see Gastrointestinal Bleeding, p. 510).

Clinical Presentation

Splenomegaly is one of the first clinical signs of portal hypertension in children. The presence of hemorrhoids, dilated abdominal veins, esophageal varices, and dilated superficial abdominal veins (caput medusae) are highly suggestive of portal hypertension.

Children with portal hypertension and splanchnic sequestration have hypoalbuminemia, and hypersplenism is associated with anemia, thrombocytopenia, and leukopenia. If cirrhosis is present, the child will often appear emaciated.

The diagnosis of portal hypertension can be confirmed with splenic or hepatic vein pressure measurements. Liver function tests and a liver biopsy may be performed to determine the cause or the extent of the primary disease. A barium swallow or esophagoscopy may confirm the presence of varices.

If esophageal varices are present, sudden severe esophageal and GI bleeding may occur without warning, with the onset of hematemesis, melena, or rectal bleeding. Bleeding episodes are often precipitated by a febrile illness (such as an upper respiratory tract infection) and the administration of aspirin, which can depress platelet function.

Management

Emergent Therapy Bleeding from esophageal varices is the most serious acute complication of portal hypertension and requires urgent volume resuscitation and treatment with saline lavage, suppression of hydrochloric acid secretion, gastric cytoprotection, and possible use of vasoconstrictors. These therapies are presented under Gastrointestinal Bleeding.

Supportive Therapy   Supportive therapy for the child with portal hypertension includes monitoring for the development of bleeding, avoidance of factors that may contribute to bleeding episodes, and maintenance of supplies (including blood and blood products) needed for resuscitation. Rectal temperature measurement, prolonged and vigorous crying episodes, constipation, and factors that increase abdominal pressure should be avoided.

Endoscopic Variceal Sclerosis and Variceal Banding   Endoscopic variceal sclerosis can be performed at the bedside with the injection of a sclerosing agent, such as morrhuate sodium, into or around bleeding esophageal varices. With sclerotherapy, esophageal varices can be obliterated completely with repeated injections every 2 to 4 weeks. Complications of this procedure include esophageal stricture, esophageal perforation, and the exacerbation of bleeding.

A promising new technique for obliteration of varices, which may be safer than sclerosis, involves obliteration of varices by endoscopic banding. This procedure may soon be widely available for use in children (Price et al., 1996).

Surgical and Nonoperative Shunts and Devascularization   Indications for urgent surgical exploration for any patient with GI hemorrhage include the development of intestinal perforation or severe hemorrhage unresponsive to medical therapy.

A portosystemic shunt may be created nonoperatively. This procedure, a transjugular intrahepatic portosystemic shunt (TIPS), creates a side-to-side portacaval shunt within the liver. These shunts are being used frequently in adults and occasionally have been performed in children. This technique may be especially useful in children awaiting liver transplantation. A needle is inserted from the right internal jugular vein and is advanced into the hepatic vein, then through the liver parenchyma, and into a branch of the portal vein, creating a tract. A catheter

is then inserted into this tract, and the tract is dilated. An expandable, metallic stent is inserted across the tract to support the shunt (Heymann et al., 1997). This procedure may be complicated by a hemoperitoneum; thus the patient must be monitored closely for evidence of bleeding or an acute abdomen. Shunt occlusion may develop and result in recurrence of signs of esophageal varices.

Surgical intervention for portal hypertension and esophageal varices includes the creation of a shunt or devascularization of the esophagus. Corrective surgery for intrahepatic portal hypertension is liver transplantation.

Palliative surgery for portal hypertension includes the creation of a portasystemic shunt. This procedure consists of diversion (shunting) of portal blood flow directly into the inferior vena cava, bypassing the scarred liver or the obstructed portal vein. A major potential complication of the shunting procedure is thrombosis of the anastomotic vessel and resultant recurrence of the portal hypertension. GI bleeding may also occur postoperatively. Finally, creation of the bypass will enable some blood to bypass the liver; thus detoxification of some drugs and elimination of endogenous wastes such as ammonia will be compromised.

Balloon Tamponade   Balloon tamponade may be effective in the management of bleeding due to esophageal varices, but it can produce complications such as perforation and aspiration (see Gastrointestinal Bleeding). A lubricated pediatric Sengstaken-Blakemore tube is inserted through the nose into the stomach, and the gastric tube is inflated. Once proper tube insertion depth is confirmed, the balloon remaining in the distal esophagus is inflated to a pressure of 20 to 40 mm Hg. The balloon is deflated every 12 to 24 hours, and distal ports are aspirated on a regular basis to check for bleeding. New advances in the use of sclerotherapy and banding have greatly reduced the demand for the use of tamponade therapy.

Gastrointestinal Bleeding

Etiology

GI bleeding in children may result from inflammation of the intestine, congenital or acquired visceral or vascular anomalies, trauma, esophageal varices secondary to portal hypertension, or coagulopathies (see the following paragraph). Microscopic bleeding may not cause symptoms and may be detectable only through analysis of GI secretions or feces.

Pathophysiology

The pathophysiologic response to GI bleeding depends on the rate and duration of blood loss and on the patient's individual capacity to respond to volume depletion. The most striking physiologic response follows acute, massive GI bleeding, with loss of >15% of the patient's intravascular volume within a few minutes or hours. When this occurs, adrenergic compensatory responses divert blood flow from the skin, kidneys, and gut to maintain perfusion of the heart and brain. Blood pressure may be maintained until acute blood loss totals approximately 20% to 25% of total circulating blood volume. Metabolic acidosis indicates inadequate tissue perfusion (see Shock, p. 130).

Clinical Presentation

The appearance of the child with GI bleeding varies considerably, depending on the amount and rapidity of blood loss. The child may be brought to the physician or emergency department after vomiting blood, passing black or tarry stools (melena), or passing bright red blood per the rectum (hematochezia). Bright red vomitus indicates recent or ongoing upper GI hemorrhage, whereas "coffee ground" vomitus indicates that there has been partial digestion of the blood.

The child with gradual hemorrhage may experience weakness and faintness. However, if the GI hemorrhage is sudden and significant, the child may develop signs of hypovolemic shock: tachycardia, thready pulses, agitation, and possible hypotension. Metabolic acidosis will develop when systemic perfusion is inadequate.

All GI fluids and stools of patients at risk should be tested for the presence of blood. The color and source of blood-tinged fluid and the age of the patient will aid in identification of the bleeding source (Table 10-9). Bright red vomitus usually results from esophageal or gastric bleeding, and bright red blood in the stool typically results from rectal bleeding. Maroon, black, or tarry stool often indicates the presence of upper GI bleeding that has been partially digested during passage through the bowel. Digested blood has a specific odor that may be noted on the patient's breath or in feces. Clinical studies indicated for a variety of causes of GI bleeding in children are listed in Table 10-9.

Esophagogastroduodenoscopy (EGD) is an examination of the esophagus, stomach, and upper duodenum and is the most useful diagnostic test for upper GI bleeding. This procedure can be performed in the pediatric intensive care unit (PICU). Flexible sigmoidoscopy or colonoscopy can identify the cause of lower intestinal bleeding. If the findings are negative, a scan to detect bleeding using technetium-labeled sulfur colloid or red blood cells may be performed but can only detect an active bleeding site of >0.5 to 1 ml/min (Splawski, 1997). Air contrast studies are used to diagnose intussusception, and an upper GI series can confirm malrotation with midgut volvulus. An abdominal ultrasound or CT is useful in the diagnosis of abdominal trauma.

Management

The three phases of critical management of the child with GI bleeding are:

- Resuscitation
- Specific diagnosis
- Specific treatment

Resuscitation To enable resuscitation, one or two large-bore IV catheters are inserted and must be carefully maintained. Systemic perfusion is constantly monitored. If shock is present or bleeding is significant, or if organ failure is present, a monitoring CVP line and a urinary catheter are inserted (see discussion of shock in Chapter 5, p. 140).

Isotonic crystalloid is administered in boluses of 20 ml/kg until systemic perfusion is restored. Whole blood is administered to replace ongoing bleeding, and packed red blood cells are administered to replace blood lost. Blood should be warmed before administration to young infants, and calcium supplementation will be required if the blood is preserved with citrate-phosphate-dextran. The hematocrit is monitored every 2 to 4 hours until bleeding is controlled. A physician should be notified if the hematocrit falls.

Effectiveness of the volume resuscitation is determined through assessment of the child's sys-

Table 10-9
Diagnosis of Gastrointestinal Bleeding by Age

Causes	Signs and Symptoms	Tests
Neonate		
Upper GI		
Swallowed maternal blood	First 24 hours	Kleihauer-Betke, Apt
Hemorrhagic disease of the newborn	Oozing from multiple foci	PT and PTT, platelet count
Gastritis, stress ulcer	Difficult delivery, CNS injury, sepsis Irritability, respiratory disease, poor feeding	Chest radiography, KUB, EGD
Esophagitis	Occurs at end of first month of life	Upper GI, pH probe, EGD
Lower GI		
Anal fissure	Bright red blood on outside of stool	Inspection, anoscopy
Colitis	Small, frequent, loose stools with blood mixed in stool	Stool smear for white blood cell count; proctoscopy
Infection	Associated with fever, vomiting	Culture, *Clostridium difficile* toxin, Rotazyme, ova and parasites
Cow milk or soy protein intolerance	Occurs at end of first month	Withdrawal of protein
Hirschsprung's disease	Failure to pass meconium, abdominal distension, sepsis	KUB, barium contrast study, rectal biopsy
Necrotizing enterocolitis	History of compromised infant; occurs in first week of life; vomiting, abdominal distension	Serial KUBs for free air, air in bowel wall or biliary tree
Malrotation with volvulus	Bile-stained vomitus, shock	KUB, emergency upper GI series
Toddler		
Meckel's diverticulum	Painless passage of maroon to melanotic stools	Meckel scan
Duplications	Mass, crampy abdominal pain	Meckel scan, barium contrast studies
Intussusception	Acute onset of abdominal pain, right lower quadrant mass, currant jelly stools, coma	KUB, air contrast study
Preschool-Age Child		
Juvenile polyps	Painless rectal bleeding after bowel movement	Proctoscopy, air contrast studies, colonscopy
Henoch-Schölein purpura	Purpuric rash on lower extremities and buttocks, abdominal pain, vomiting, hematuria, hypertension	Ultrasound, barium contrast studies
Hemolytic-uremic syndrome	Antecedent diarrhea, pallor, petechiae, oliguria	CBC with differential, BUN, sigmoidoscopy, stool culture (*Escherichia coli* 0157)
Esophageal varices	Massive hematemesis, associated ascites, splenomegaly, chronic liver disease	EGD

From Splawski JB: Gastrointestinal bleeding. In Levin DL, Morriss FC, editors: *Essentials of pediatric intensive care,* ed 2, New York, 1997, Churchill Livingstone and Quality Medical Publishing.

Table 10-9
Diagnosis of Gastrointestinal Bleeding by Age—cont'd

Causes	Signs and Symptoms	Tests
School-Age Child		
Peptic ulcer disease	Abdominal pain and vomiting, occult blood to melanotic stools	Hb, Hct, reticulocyte count, EGD
Inflammatory bowel disease	Crampy abdominal pain, weight loss, poor growth, occult to moderate blood	Fecal leukocytes, CBC with differential, ESR, endoscopy with biopsy, barium contrast studies
Any-Age Child		
Swallowed blood	Oral, pharyngeal, or pulmonary lesion, usually bright red	Ear, nose, and throat examination; chest radiography
Mallory-Weiss tear	Nonbloody emesis followed by bloody emesis	History, EGD
Stress ulcers	Sick patient, burn, head injury, sepsis steroid drugs	EGD
Gastritis, esophagitis	Chest and/or abdominal pain, vomiting	EGD
Vascular malformations	Associated cutaneous lesions, Turner's syndrome, hemihypertrophy	CBC with differential, endoscopy, bleeding scans, angiography
Trauma, ingestion, foreign body	History	Chest radiography, KUB, ultrasound, EGD, proctoscopy, CT

temic perfusion. The heart rate should decrease slightly (although bradycardia should not develop), and the skin should become warm with brisk capillary refill and strong peripheral pulses. Urine output should average 1 ml/kg/hr once systemic perfusion is adequate. The child should become more alert as volume resuscitation is performed. If the skin is mottled and cool with delayed capillary refill and weak peripheral pulses, additional volume administration is probably required (see discussion of shock in Chapter 5, pp. 142-144).

Oxygenation and ventilation must be supported. Endotracheal intubation is recommended if shock is present or the child is obtunded.

Neurologic function, urine output, and serum pH are closely monitored, and any deterioration is reported to a physician immediately. Coagulopathies should be ruled out or treated if discovered. Sepsis may be a cause or a complication of GI bleeding and should thus be ruled out.

Specific Diagnosis The diagnosis of GI bleeding is summarized under Clinical Presentation.

Specific Treatment GI bleeding can be treated with saline lavage, reduction of gastric acidity, increasing gastric mucosal protection, and vasoconstriction (Table 10-10).

Room-temperature normal saline lavage is provided through the largest-bore nasogastric or orogastric tube that can be inserted comfortably. Approximately 20 to 50 ml is instilled and then drained by gravity until the return is clear. Saline lavage reduces bleeding and also removes clotted blood and gastric secretions, which will enable better visualization of bleeding sites should endoscopy and sclerotherapy be required. Iced saline does not appear to offer any therapeutic advantage and may contribute to temperature instability in the infant.

Antacids are administered every hour to maintain the gastric pH at >4. If enteral antacid administration is not possible (e.g., an upper endoscopy is planned), parenteral H_2 receptor antagonists, including cimetidine, famotidine, or ranitidine, can be used. Continuous infusion of these drugs may be more effective than intermittent dosing. Oral omeprazole is a long-acting inhibitor of the proton

Table 10-10
Pharmacologic Management of Acute Upper Gastrointestinal Bleeding

Drug	Dosage	Warning	Indications
Acid Neutralization			
Aluminum hydroxide and magnesium hydrochloride (Maalox)	Susp.: $Al(OH)_3$, 225 mg, and $Mg(OH)_2$, 200 mg/5 ml 0.5 ml/kg/dose PO q2-4h Maximum dose: 30 ml	Aluminum and magnesium toxicity in patients with renal impairment	Prevention of stress ulcers, gastritis, esophagitis
Calcium carbonate	Susp.: 1250 mg/5 ml: 500 mg elemental calcium Dosage by elemental calcium <6 mo: 360 mg/day 6-12 mo: 540 mg/day 1-10 yr: 800 mg/day 10-18 yr: 1200 mg/day	CHF, constipation, hyperglycemia, hyperphosphatemia, high sodium content	Antacid used for renal patients
Acid Suppression			
Cimetidine	30-40 mg/kg/day PO or IV divided q6h Maximum dose: 1200 mg/day	Altered mental status Decreased clearance of phenytoin, diazepam, and theophylline	Therapy for stress ulcer, gastritis, esophagitis, peptic ulcers
Ranitidine	2 mg/kg/dose IV or PO q8h IV infusion: 0.10-0.25 mg/kg/hr Adults: 50 mg IV q8h	Dosage adjustment necessary in renal disease Creatinine clearance <50 ml/min, decrease dose to q12h	Same as for cimetidine
Omeprazole	<3 yr: 10 mg PO qd >3 yr: 20 mg PO qd	Microencapsulated beads: cannot be chewed, suspend in weak acid (e.g., apple juice); delayed onset of action	Bleeding that fails to respond to cimetidine or ranitidine
Cytoprotective Agents			
Sucralfate	Children: 500 mg PO or NG qid; suspension: 1 g/10 ml Adults: 1 g PO or NG qid	Constipation	Prevention of stress ulcers, gastritis, esophagitis, peptic ulcers
Vasoconstrictors			
Octreotide	SQ: 1-10 μg/kg/day IV: 0.5-5 μg/kg/day IV infusion: 10-25 μg/hr	Glucose intolerance, hypothyroidism, cholestasis, renal disease Creatinine clearance <10 ml/min, decrease dose by half	Uncontrolled GI bleeding, esophageal or gastric variceal bleeding
Vasopressin	Bolus: 0.3 U/kg (maximum dose: 20 U) in 2 ml/kg of D_5W IV over 10-20 min IV infusion: 0.2-0.4 $U/1.73 \ m^2/min$ for 12-24 hr; decrease dose	Hypotension, myocardial ischemia, arrhythmia, decreased cardiac output, increased BP, peripheral ischemia, hyponatremia Consider nitroglycerin 0.25 to 0.50 μg/kg/min IV and titrate usual dose (1 to 3 μg/kg/min, maximum: 5 μg/kg/min IV) for treatment of systemic side effects	Same as for octreotide; octreotide is the treatment of choice

From Levin DC, Morriss FC, editors: *Essentials of pediatric intensive care,* ed 2, New York, 1997, Churchill Livingstone and Quality Medical Publishing.

Table 10-10
Pharmacologic Management of Acute Upper Gastrointestinal Bleeding—cont'd

Drug	Dosage	Warning	Indications
β-Adrenergic Blocker			
Propranolol	0.5-1/kg/day PO divided q6h Maximum daily dose: 60 mg	Asthma, bronchospasm, heart block, sinus bradycardia, metabolic acidosis, hypoglycemia; not studied in children	Prevention of re-bleeding from varices

pump and may be administered if the H_2 receptor antagonists fail. Omeprazole must be taken orally and may require several days to become effective.

Drugs such as sucralfate form a protective barrier in the stomach and also reduce secretion of prostaglandins and pepsin. This drug may be dissolved in water and administered through a nasogastric tube.

Octreotide may be the drug of choice for the treatment of upper GI bleeding that does not respond to conventional therapy, and it is the treatment of choice for treatment of bleeding due to esophageal varices. Octreotide is a somatostatin analog and can stop or decrease GI bleeding by decreasing splanchnic blood flow so that definitive diagnostic studies and therapy can be accomplished (Splawski, 1997).

Vasopressin may be administered to control GI bleeding, particularly that caused by portal hypertension, because it is a potent vasoconstrictor. It reduces portal venous pressure and bleeding, but it may also produce systemic constriction and a compromise in gut and renal blood flow. Complications of vasopressin may include hypertension, cardiac arrhythmias, hyponatremia, and bradycardia. Urine output will decrease, and abdominal cramping may develop. Concomitant administration of a systemic vasodilator may be indicated to modulate the systemic effects of the vasopressin.

Balloon tamponade may be effective in the management of bleeding due to esophageal varices, but it can produce complications such as perforation and aspiration. Esophageal varices may be obliterated surgically by banding or through the injection of sclerosing agents (this may be performed at the bedside). For further information regarding

the management of esophageal varices, see Portal Hypertension.

Intestinal Failure

Etiology/Pathophysiology

Intestinal failure is the inability to ingest, digest, or absorb adequate nutrition to prevent fluid and electrolyte imbalances and dehydration. As a result of this inability, the patient is totally dependent on parenteral nutrition to survive.

The most common cause of intestinal failure in patients of all ages is short bowel syndrome (SBS). SBS is defined as an inadequate bowel functional area. SBS may develop following extensive small bowel resection during surgical treatment of volvulus, trauma, or inflammation (such as necrotizing enterocolitis).

Clinical Presentation

The child with inadequate intestinal function regardless of cause is likely to demonstrate one or more of the following characteristic signs:

- Vomiting
- Significant diarrhea with malabsorption, fluid and electrolyte losses, and inability to maintain fluid and electrolyte balance and nutrition without parenteral nutrition; weight loss or failure to gain weight in infants
- Pain
- Protein-losing enteropathy

Gastrointestinal bleeding may also be present. Intestinal failure should be suspected in any patient at risk who develops severe and continuous diarrhea following trauma or surgery.

The child's fluid balance and hematocrit should be evaluated carefully. Dehydration, hypovolemic shock, or anemia may be present. Protein-losing enteropathy will be associated with hypoalbuminemia and edema.

Laboratory tests include evaluation of the content of vomitus or stool, including testing for the presence of blood. Vomitus is evaluated for the presence of bile or fecal material.

Stool is tested for the presence of reducing substances by performing a test for glucose on a suspension of stool in water. In normal stool no glucose is present; the presence of glucose indicates nonabsorption or malabsorption of the carbohydrates. Stool should also be tested for the presence of nonabsorbed fats by staining the stool sample for fats.

The diarrhea may be characterized as malabsorption diarrhea, secretory diarrhea, or inflammatory diarrhea. A fourth type of diarrhea, antibiotic-induced diarrhea, should also be ruled out.

- *Malabsorption* diarrhea will cease if oral intake is halted.
- *Secretory* diarrhea is large in volume and will continue despite a lack of oral intake. In secretory diarrhea, the osmolality of the diarrhea is equal to the osmolality created by the stool sodium and potassium contents ($[Na^+ + K^+] \times 2$).
- *Inflammatory* diarrhea will contain white blood cells (or pus), blood, and mucus.

If intestinal failure or SBS develops following surgical resection of the bowel, three phases of intestinal dysfunction or recovery may be observed. All phases are characterized by diarrhea and the risk of fluid and electrolyte imbalance, but as the patient progresses through the phases, more evidence of intestinal function can be identified:

- *Phase 1:* Characterized by diarrhea, fluid and electrolyte loss, and need for provision of fluid and electrolyte requirements and nutritional needs through parenteral nutrition. This phase may last approximately 2 months.
- *Phase 2:* Characterized by a decrease in the volume and frequency of diarrhea, and

demonstration of tolerance of some oral intake. Major nutritional requirements are administered by the parenteral route with gradual transition to the enteral route. This phase may last from 2 months to as long as 1 to 2 years after bowel resection.
- *Phase 3:* Characterized by achievement of enteral function and ability to wean from parenteral nutrition. Some patients never achieve this phase.

Management

Management of the patient with intestinal failure has two phases:

- Stabilization and diagnostic phase
- Recuperative phase

Stabilization and Diagnostic Phase Treatment of hypovolemic shock is a priority. Any existing fluid and electrolyte deficits and anemia are corrected, and GI bleeding is treated, if needed. The cause of the intestinal failure is identified, and reversible causes are corrected, if possible. However, even if the cause of the failure cannot be identified, the failure is treated symptomatically.

Once the child's systemic perfusion is adequate, parenteral alimentation is initiated. This form of alimentation must deliver all fluid, electrolyte, and nutritional requirements until enteral alimentation is possible. Vomiting is treated with insertion of a nasogastric tube and gastric decompression. Fluid lost through gastric suction must be replaced in volume and electrolyte content through the parenteral route. When vomiting ceases, the gastric tube may be clamped for increasing periods to evaluate patient tolerance.

Recuperative Phase Once the patient is stable, supportive therapy is initiated. The goal of this recuperative phase is to assist in reducing the volume of the diarrhea and malabsorption to reduce dependence on parenteral nutrition and to facilitate survival with enteral nutrition (Byrne, Nompleggi, and Wilmore, 1996). The optimal diet for children with intestinal failure has not been determined. Possible types of diets include:

- Elemental diets provide nutrients in predigested forms. These may be easily absorbed, but their high osmolality may contribute to diarrhea in some patients.

- Peptide-based formulas have a lower osmolality than elemental diets and may be absorbed more efficiently than elemental diets.
- Polymeric diets may work "just fine" for many patients, provided that they are started slowly in dilute forms in small quantities and advanced in concentration or volume very slowly.
- For patients with a functioning colon, high-calorie, low-fat diets may reduce fecal loss of calories more than isocaloric high-fat, low-carbohydrate diets.

Supplementation of calcium, magnesium, zinc, and other trace elements is also required. Simple sugar intake is limited, and electrolytes are provided as needed to maintain balance.

Total parenteral nutrition is provided (TPN) unless or until enteral nutrition can replace it.

Advances in Management Two newer approaches to management of intestinal failure include bowel rehabilitation and intestinal transplantation. Bowel rehabilitation is accomplished through one or more of the following:

- Administration of specific growth factors (e.g., growth hormone) or insulin-like growth factor-1 (IGF-1) to enhance mucosal hyperplasia following intestinal resection and to increase colonic mass and biomechanical strength (this may improve peristalsis). Growth hormone also increases sodium and water transport in the small intestine and colon of small animals and may increase amino acid transport in the jejunum.
- Administration of bowel-specific nutrients (such as glutamine or short-chain fatty acids). Glutamine is a major fuel source of GI cells, and it may stimulate cell proliferation and improve absorption in the gut, as well as possibly prevent bacterial translocation.
- Administration of nonnutritive components of the diet (such as soluble fiber) to increase bowel transit and increase stool solidity and colonic water absorption.
- Intestinal transplantation is accomplished much like transplantation of any organ. Im-

munosuppression will be required postoperatively. Signs of failure of the transplanted organ include the signs of intestinal failure: vomiting, diarrhea and malabsorption, bleeding, pain, and possible protein-losing enteropathy.

Hepatic Failure

Etiology

Liver failure is observed most often in children with chronic liver disease. However, it may also result from acute massive necrosis of a previously normal liver (fulminant hepatic failure). Fulminant hepatic failure is defined as liver failure that results in encephalopathy within 8 weeks of the first symptoms of illness or within 2 weeks of the onset of jaundice (Sussman and Lake, 1996). This more acute form of liver failure often results from a viral illness and is associated with an extremely high mortality.

Additional causes of liver failure in previously normal children include idiosyncratic reactions to anesthetics, antibiotics, and chemotherapeutic agents. Accidental ingestion of drugs or toxins such as acetaminophen, pesticides, cleaning compounds, or some plant alkaloids also may produce acute hepatic failure. Shock/ischemic injury and some inherited metabolic disorders can also produce liver failure.

Acetaminophen ingestion/overdose is known to produce liver failure. Recently, acetaminophen-induced liver failure has also been reported in association with intentional administration of the drug in doses only slightly higher than appropriate for age and weight. Parents may administer toxic doses of the drug by administering an inappropriate dose for concentration. For example, administration of the elixir dose (elixir dose = 160 mg/5 ml or 32 mg/ml) when the drop concentration (80 mg/0.8 ml or 100 mg/ml) is used will result in administration of three times the appropriate dose for age).

Liver failure not only produces clinical and biochemical evidence of failing liver function but can also result in the development of hepatic encephalopathy. This will be associated with a decreased level of consciousness and possible signs of increased ICP (see p. 388).

Pathophysiology

Liver failure produces both an accumulation of substances normally removed by the liver and a lack of substances normally manufactured by the liver. Hepatic encephalopathy is a reversible alteration in level of consciousness resulting from metabolic disorders associated with liver failure, such as hyperammonemia.

Hepatic Encephalopathy   Hepatic encephalopathy in children with chronic liver failure is often precipitated by GI bleeding, large ingestion of protein, excessive use of diuretics, sepsis, or the administration of sedatives. As noted above, it may also develop following the creation of portacaval shunts.

Often, the child's serum ammonia levels are inversely related to the child's level of consciousness during the development of hepatic encephalopathy. Ammonia is formed in the GI tract from amino acids following bacterial and enzymatic breakdown of proteins, including blood. If a portacaval shunt has been created, ammonia and other amines absorbed from the GI tract are able to pass directly from the splanchnic circulation to the inferior vena cava. Thus liver failure or liver bypass may result in the accumulation of toxic substances that may impair cerebral function.

Fluid and Electrolyte Imbalances   Children with end-stage cirrhosis, severe hepatic failure, or ascites refractory to diuretic therapy may develop hepatorenal syndrome, a progressive functional renal failure of unknown cause (see p. 487).

With liver failure, electrolyte imbalances may develop. The child's serum glucose level can drop rapidly because gluconeogenesis is no longer completed by the liver. Ascites and hepatorenal syndrome may contribute to abnormalities in serum sodium, chloride, and potassium concentrations, and acid-base imbalances.

Coagulopathies   The child with liver failure will also demonstrate coagulopathies, because the liver will not produce normal amounts of prothrombin, and it will not remove activated clotting factors from the circulation. If portal hypertension is associated with the liver failure, hypersplenism will be associated with thrombocytopenia, which can further increase the child's risk of hemorrhage, particularly if esophageal varices are present. Anemia and leukopenia may also develop.

The pathophysiology of liver failure and resulting clinical signs and symptoms are further depicted in Figure 10-2.

Clinical Presentation

Hepatic Encephalopathy   The development of hepatic encephalopathy is heralded by a decreased level of consciousness. Additional signs include tremors, lack of coordination, muscle twitching, and violent movements. The classic early symptom of hepatic encephalopathy is a peculiar flapping tremor known as *asterixis.* It can be elicited by asking the cooperative child to outstretch the arms and dorsiflex the hand. The child will be unable to maintain the hands in a hyperextended position, and a burst of coarse twitching movements will appear at the wrist.

The staging of hepatic encephalopathy has been described based on the clinical condition, presence of asterixis, and electroencephalogram (EEG). These stages reliably correlate with the outcome:

- *Stage 1:* Slowness of mentation but appropriate responses; periods of lethargy, sleep disturbances. Mild asterixis may be elicited. The EEG has minimal changes.
- *Stage 2:* Increased drowsiness, confusion, inappropriate behavior, disorientation, and mood swings, with generalized slowing of EEG rhythm. Asterixis is easily elicited.
- *Stage 3:* Stuporous; sleeping most of the time but arousable. Marked confusion and incoherent speech are noted. Asterixis can be elicited if the patient is cooperative. The EEG has grossly abnormal slowing.
- *Stage 4:* Comatose; may not respond to noxious stimuli. The EEG shows grossly abnormal slowing with the appearance of delta waves and decreased amplitude.

Fluid and Electrolyte Imbalances   The child with liver failure may have a wide variety of fluid, electrolyte, and acid-base disturbances. Hyperammonemia develops because ammonia that is formed in the GI tract following bacterial and enzy-

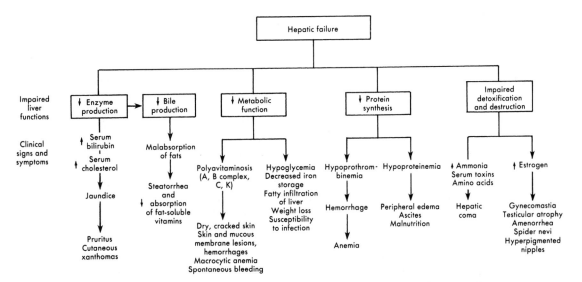

Figure 10-2   Pathophysiology of hepatic failure. (Modified from Whaley LF, Wong DL: *Nursing care of infants and children,* ed 2, St Louis, 1983, Mosby.)

matic breakdown of protein, including blood, is not eliminated by the failing liver. Chronic hyperaldosteronism increases potassium and magnesium loss in the urine, and more hydrogen ion is excreted (in exchange for retained sodium). The children may demonstrate a mild metabolic alkalosis as a result, which may increase the renal potassium losses and hypokalemia. Vomiting and diarrhea can complicate potassium loss and pH imbalances.

Hypoglycemia can develop because gluconeogenesis is no longer completed by the liver. Glucose transport may be depressed by associated pancreatitis and reduced insulin production.

The child with liver failure may demonstrate intravascular volume depletion as a result of ascites or splanchnic sequestration. Congestive heart failure may also be present. Fluid balance must be carefully assessed, and intravascular fluid volume carefully supported.

Hepatorenal Syndrome   Liver failure may be associated with *hepatorenal syndrome,* a progressive renal failure of unknown origin. This is associated with a decrease in glomerular filtration rate, oliguria, and azotemia, which often develops without apparent precipitating factors. Urinalysis is normal, but serum hyponatremia, hypokalemia, and azotemia are present. Note that the serum sodium concentration falls despite the renal retention of sodium, as a result of dilution from the relatively greater absorption of water. The serum creatinine concentration will rise and the urine creatinine concentration will fall if renal function is significantly impaired.

Coagulopathies   Signs of bleeding disorders may be manifested by ecchymosis or petechiae and increased bleeding from puncture sites or mucosal irritation.

Pulmonary Complications   Some children with liver failure demonstrate intrapulmonary shunting of blood with resultant hypoxemia and cyanosis. If shunting develops, arterial oxygen desaturation will be noted by pulse oximetry and will be corrected with oxygen administration.

Chronic Disease   Signs of chronic liver disease include ascites with dilation of superficial abdominal veins (caput medusae), xanthoma formation, clubbing of the nails, gynecomastia, skin ecchymosis, palmar erythema, and spider angiomas. Jaundice is often present. The child frequently appears malnourished, and ascites may be present.

Laboratory Studies If the cause of the liver failure is unknown, a variety of diagnostic studies will be performed, including toxicology screening, liver function studies, liver-spleen scanning, and possibly angiography or liver biopsy. The liver biopsy cannot be performed in the presence of significant coagulopathy; a coagulation profile should be obtained before a biopsy is planned. Viral, bacteriologic, and fungal blood cultures also may be ordered.

Management

The child with liver failure requires simultaneous evaluation and support of all body systems. Careful monitoring for evidence of sepsis or infection and assessment of cardiac, respiratory, neurologic, and renal function is often more important than monitoring the child's liver function. Priorities of management are summarized in Box 10-1 and include:

- Treatment of hypovolemic shock and maintenance of appropriate intravascular volume and systemic perfusion (see Shock, p. 130).
- Support of oxygenation and ventilation. Elective intubation may be required.
- Monitoring for signs of increased ICP and treatment of increased ICP. This may include intubation, oxygenation, support of normal arterial oxygen and carbon dioxide levels, and diuresis. For further information about treatment of increased ICP, see p. 394.
- Correction of electrolyte and acid-base imbalances and support of fluid balance. Administer glucose intravenously as needed to maintain serum glucose in the normal range.
- Detection and treatment of bleeding, including GI bleeding, and correction of significant coagulopathies. Blood component therapy is provided to correct significant coagulopathies, and plasmapheresis may be used (see Gastrointestinal Bleeding).
- Support of renal function. Renal replacement therapies with continuous venoarterial or venovenous hemofiltration may be required (see p. 475).
- Nutritional support.

Support of Liver Function Until liver function returns, treatment of the child with liver failure is primarily supportive. During the acute phase the most important goal of therapy is prevention of major complications such as increased ICP, hemorrhage, fluid and electrolyte imbalances, and renal failure.

Liver transplantation has become the standard of care for the treatment of acute and chronic liver failure. At present, techniques for "liver dialysis" are under investigation and are only available at selected centers (Sussman and Lake, 1996; Sussman and Kelly, 1997). These may ultimately be attractive approaches to maintaining a satisfactory lifestyle in patients with chronic liver failure or as a bridge to transplantation or permanent recovery in children with acute liver injury.

Specific medical treatment for liver failure is not often available. However, promising results have been reported for certain metabolic liver diseases, particularly those causing neonatal liver failure (Schneider, 1996). Hemophagocytic lymphohistiocytosis may be treated with chemotherapy or bone marrow transplantation. Primary bile metabolism disorders may be treated with primary bile acid replacement therapy. Galactosemia and fructosemia are treated with dietary restrictions. Tyrosinemia may be partially responsive to dietary intervention, and promising results have been obtained with the use of a tyrosine metabolism pathway inhibitor. Neonatal hemochromatosis may be treated with iron chelation, antioxidants, and cytoprotection.

Hepatic Encephalopathy The child with liver failure may develop encephalopathy and resultant increased ICP. As a result, it is imperative that the nurse be able to detect early signs of neurologic compromise. A brief but careful neurologic evaluation should be performed when vital signs are measured:

- Pupil size and constriction to light should be noted, and any pupil sluggishness or inequality should be reported to a physician.
- The child's voluntary movements should be observed, and any decreased movement, decreased sensation, abnormal posturing, asterixis, or seizure activity should be reported immediately.
- Assessment of level of consciousness and ability to follow commands is extremely important.

Box 10-1

Nursing Care of the Child With Hepatic Failure

1. **Possible depressed level of consciousness,** which may be a result of increased intracranial pressure (ICP) associated with hepatic encephalopathy. The risk of encephalopathy is particularly high during episodes of infection, hyperammonemia, or high-protein catabolism. Assess level of consciousness and neurologic function frequently, and report any deterioration to a physician immediately. Treat increased ICP if present:
    a. Assist with intubation and ensure that the airway, oxygenation, and ventilation are adequate. Maintain Pao_2 at 80-100 mm Hg, oxyhemoglobin saturation at 98%-100%, and $Paco_2$ at 32-34 mm Hg.
    b. Ensure that heart rate, blood pressure, and systemic perfusion are adequate. Support as needed.
    c. If ventricular catheter is in place, drain ventricular fluid per order if ICP rises.
    d. If arterial blood pressure is adequate, elevate head of bed 30 degrees.
    e. Keep head in midline.
    f. Prevent hypovolemia, hypervolemia, hyponatremia, or acute fall in serum sodium or osmolality.
    g. Ensure that adequate analgesia is provided; consider sedation, anesthesia.
    h. Monitor for signs of deterioration, including signs of herniation (pupil dilation, tachycardia or bradycardia, hypertension, hypoventilation or apnea, decrease in cranial nerve function), and notify a physician immediately.
    i. Emergency management of increased ICP may include hyperventilation, administration of diuretic (typically mannitol), possible drainage of ventricular cerebrospinal fluid (CSF), and possible induction of anesthesia or barbiturate coma.
2. **Potential compromise in airway, oxygenation, and ventilation,** which may result from decreased level of consciousness and hypoventilation. Assess the airway, oxygenation and ventilation, and support as needed.
3. **Potential alteration in systemic perfusion,** which may result from sequestration of fluid, hemorrhage, or extravascular fluid shift. Assess systemic perfusion frequently and support as needed. Support intravascular volume relative to the vascular space, oxygenation, and arterial pressure. Monitor for evidence of bleeding or coagulopathy. Administer blood as needed. Monitor for hyperammonemia following transfusion.
4. **Potential bleeding,** which may be caused by esophageal varices, coagulopathies, or possible sepsis. Monitor for signs of bleeding and be prepared to support systemic perfusion and administer blood products as needed.
5. **Potential alteration in fluid and electrolyte balance,** which may be caused by sequestration of fluid or diuretic therapy. Assess intravascular volume relative to the vascular space; administer fluid therapy or diuretics as needed.
6. **Potential infection or sepsis,** which may result from compromise in immune function associated with liver disease, invasive catheters, or hospital-acquired infection. Monitor for signs of infection, administer antimicrobials, and monitor aminoglycoside peak-and-trough levels. Monitor for signs of sepsis and be prepared to administer fluid and support blood pressure and oxygen delivery.
7. **Potential compromise in nutrition,** which may be caused by impaired liver function, inadequate protein and caloric intake, increased metabolic requirements, and impaired gastrointestinal absorption of nutrients. Calculate caloric intake and develop a plan to deliver adequate nutrition.
8. **Potential pain or discomfort** related to liver failure and ascites and their complications. Assess presence and location of pain and provide adequate analgesia, but consider potential alteration in drug metabolism resulting from liver failure.
9. **Potential worsening of liver failure** caused by progression of disease or infection. Provide supportive care; evaluate child's potential as a transplant candidate.
10. **Potential knowledge deficit** of the child and parents about the child's disease, therapy, and prognosis. Assess the knowledge of the child and family, and provide information and support as needed.
11. **Possible child or family anxiety** related to the child's condition and prognosis. Support the child and family.

- Presence of unusual irritability or lethargy may indicate the development of increased ICP.
- If the child does develop encephalopathy, management will be supportive. Intubation should be performed electively whenever there is any question of the child's ability to maintain a patent airway or if hypoventilation or signs of increased ICP develop. The child's arterial oxygen tension should be maintained at 80 to 100 mm Hg, and the arterial carbon dioxide tension should be maintained at approximately 32 to 34 mm Hg. Hypoxemia, hypercarbia, and hypotension should all be prevented, since they can contribute to a compromise in cerebral perfusion or oxygen delivery.

Fluid and Electrolyte Balance The child with hepatic failure can develop fluid shifts and fluid imbalances related to hyperaldosteronism (and increased sodium and water retention), hypoalbuminemia, portal hypertension, and resultant splanchnic sequestration (see Portal Hypertension) or hepatorenal syndrome.

All sources of fluid intake and output must be measured, and imbalances reported to a physician. The child's fluid balance should be assessed constantly, and adequacy of intravascular volume assured. If ascites is developing, the child's intravascular volume must be closely monitored and supported as needed. If ascites is severe, a hydrothorax may develop and cause hypoventilation and respiratory distress. The hydrothorax is treated with thoracentesis or chest tube insertion.

The child's urine volume must be closely monitored. If urine volume is <0.5 to 1 ml/kg/hr, a physician should be notified. While a decrease in urine output may be appropriate in the face of ascites and decreased intravascular volume, oliguria accompanied by azotemia usually indicates the development of renal failure p. 470.

Electrolyte imbalance may result from fluid shifts, hyperaldosteronism, or diuretic therapy. Serum electrolyte concentrations should be checked frequently, and electrolyte replacement therapy often will be required. Hypoglycemia can develop rapidly, especially in infants; thus the child's serum glucose concentration should be

checked frequently (or rapid bedside glucose testing should be done), and supplemental glucose administered as needed. Glucose infusion is preferable to intermittent bolus glucose administration to correct the serum glucose.

Because the high serum ammonia concentration may contribute to encephalopathy, attempts are made to reduce ammonia production and absorption. The child's protein intake is reduced to 0.5 to 1 g/kg/day. If gastric bleeding develops, the blood should be drained to prevent absorption and further ammonia production.

Nonabsorbable antibiotics (e.g., neomycin, 0.5 to 2 g/m^2/day) are administered via nasogastric tube to eliminate gastrointestinal bacteria. Lactulose (1 mg/kg/dose, three to six times daily) is administered to acidify colonic content, promoting ammonium ion excretion.

Coagulopathies If the child has any clinical evidence of coagulopathies, blood components are administered. Blood and blood components should be available (typed and crossmatched) in the blood bank for use during sudden bleeding episodes. All efforts must be made to prevent oral, tracheal, and GI trauma during intubation, suctioning, and mouth care.

Nutritional Support Nutritional compromise can develop rapidly when the child has hepatic failure. Parenteral nutrition will be required if the child is unable to tolerate oral or tube feedings. The child's daily caloric requirements should be calculated and delivered through a combination of enteral and parenteral feedings, although the enteral route is optimal. Fish and vegetable proteins are generally tolerated better than animal proteins. Administration of vitamin and mineral supplements (especially A, B complex, C, D, E, K, and zinc) is usually necessary (Gecelter and Comer, 1995).

If the child is receiving any medications normally metabolized by the liver, the dosages of these medications should be reviewed and adjusted as needed.

Additional Supportive Care Steroids may be prescribed, particularly if the cause of hepatic failure is thought to be inflammatory but not infectious. Hemodialysis or exchange transfusion may be ordered to reduce serum ammonia levels and eliminate some accumulated toxins.

Postoperative Care: Abdominal Surgery, Liver Transplantation, and Parenteral Nutrition

Postoperative Complications

Abdominal surgery in children is indicated to explore the cause of an acute abdomen or the source of a major GI hemorrhage. It is also indicated for the correction of known anomalies, including mechanical obstructions and deformities, organ malfunction, inflammation, or malignancies. Potential postoperative complications of abdominal surgery include dehydration, third spacing of extracellular fluid, electrolyte imbalance, hemorrhage, paralytic ileus, bowel obstruction, diarrhea, malnutrition, respiratory complications, and infection.

Potential Fluid and Electrolyte Imbalances

Dehydration can occur postoperatively if perioperative fluid losses are not replaced. Adequate provision of maintenance fluids and electrolytes is also required.

Major shifts of fluid from intracellular and intravascular spaces may occur after abdominal surgery. This shift of fluids into nonfunctional compartments is known as *third spacing* of fluids. This third spacing is more likely to occur following injury or inflammation and is thought to be caused by increased capillary permeability and diffusion of plasma proteins and fluids into the peritoneum and bowel wall. Third spacing may cause signs of decreased intravascular volume, including tachycardia, peripheral vasoconstriction, decreased urine output, and a low CVP. Treatment of third spacing requires fluid administration (typically with a combination of crystalloids and colloids) until capillary integrity is restored. As injured or inflamed areas heal and capillary permeability decreases, fluid will shift back into the vascular space; it may be necessary to reduce other sources of fluid administration at this time to prevent the development of hypervolemia.

Vomiting, diarrhea, third spacing of fluids, and gastric suction can all contribute to electrolyte imbalances during the postoperative period. Hydrogen, chloride, and potassium ions are lost in vomitus and nasogastric aspirate; bicarbonate and potassium ions are lost when diarrhea occurs (see Table 10-1). Gastric losses are replaced with 0.45% NaCl with potassium chloride supplement, and intestinal secretions are replaced with lactated Ringer's solution and potassium chloride supplement. Excessive fluid loss from diarrhea is replaced with 0.45% NaCl or lactated Ringer's solution and potassium chloride supplement. Potassium chloride supplement is provided at 20 to 40 mEq/L.

Hemorrhage

Bleeding can develop from the breakdown or rupture of the GI anastomoses or from the development of disseminated intravascular coagulation (DIC). Bleeding must be detected immediately, and volume replacement is required. Reoperation may be necessary. DIC requires supportive care and elimination of the cause of the DIC (see p. 561).

Abdominal/Intestinal Complications

A paralytic ileus often develops following surgery. Oral feedings are initially withheld, and a nasogastric tube is inserted to remove air and gastric secretions. The return of normal bowel activity will produce active bowel sounds, and the child will begin to pass flatus and stool. If enteral feedings will not be provided for several days, parenteral nutrition is required. It is now clear, however, that *enteral* alimentation has many advantages over parenteral forms of nutrition; thus the gut should be used for feeding as soon as possible. The presence of diminished bowel sounds is not a reason to withhold feedings. Small quantities of clear liquids and then dilute elemental formula can be instituted via tube feedings, with careful monitoring of the child's tolerance.

Stool should be tested for blood, and the presence of blood should be reported to a physician. Once feedings are resumed, the stool is tested for the presence of reducing substances (a glucose reagent test is performed on a suspension of stool in water; the presence of glucose indicates the presence of reducing substances), which will indicate malabsorption of carbohydrates. This finding should also be reported to a physician.

Diarrhea may develop in the immediate postoperative period. Once enteral feedings are resumed, diarrhea and malabsorption are often observed. If diarrhea is severe following initiation of enteral feedings, the volume or osmolality (or both) of the feeding should be reduced. Postoperative lactose intolerance should be anticipated, and a lactose- and sucrose-free diet should be considered. Elemental diets, including medium-chain triglycerides and amino acids, may be offered. The addition of glutamine and other substances to the feeding may improve intestinal absorption (see Intestinal Failure under Common Clinical Conditions).

Healing of any surgical anastomoses may produce scarring, constriction, and ultimate obstruction of the intestinal lumen. Also, perioperative infection or inflammation can produce adhesions, which may also cause bowel obstruction. Signs of obstruction include nausea, abdominal distension, rigidity, tenderness, an increase in nasogastric aspirate or residual feedings, or vomiting. The vomitus may include bilious material.

Infection

Infection may be present at the time of the surgery or may develop postoperatively. If bowel perforation was present, the risk of postoperative gram-negative sepsis is significant.

Signs of infection can include fever and redness or tenderness of the abdomen. These signs may not be present in the neutropenic patient, however. Signs of sepsis may include temperature instability, tachycardia, tachypnea with respiratory alkalosis (if the patient is breathing spontaneously), and leukocytosis or leukopenia. Signs of organ failure, including DIC, may include thrombocytopenia, change in level of consciousness, oliguria, or metabolic acidosis (see discussion of septic shock, p. 140).

Postoperative Care

All procedures and treatments should be carefully explained to the child and family, and they should be given the opportunity to discuss their responses to therapy. Because incisions may be particularly threatening to the child, the nurse should provide reassurances that the child's body is intact and will heal. Parents should be encouraged to participate in comforting the child.

Postoperative care of the child recovering from abdominal surgery requires assessment and support of cardiorespiratory function and prevention of complications, meticulous attention to the child's fluid and electrolyte balance and nutrition, and prevention of infection.

During the immediate postoperative period, respiratory compromise must be prevented. Abdominal distension or ascites can compromise diaphragm excursion and produce hypoventilation. Mechanical ventilation may be planned postoperatively, particularly if trauma, sepsis, or other conditions are present. The head of the bed should be elevated 30 degrees to promote diaphragm excursion.

Cardiovascular assessment includes evaluation of the child's intravascular volume and systemic perfusion. Fluid administration will be required if significant third spacing of fluid or bleeding develop. Significant bleeding will require blood component therapy and may indicate the need for surgical reexploration.

Accurate records of all sources of fluid intake and output must be maintained. If excessive fluid intake or output is present, a physician should be notified.

A nasogastric tube is typically inserted during surgery to prevent abdominal distension and discomfort. Nasogastric tubes should be irrigated and aspirated every 2 to 4 hours (or per hospital routine or physician's order). All nasogastric drainage should be measured every 4 to 8 hours. This drainage volume is typically replaced milliliter for milliliter with 0.45% NaCl or lactated Ringer's solution—the fluid type will be determined by the physician's order. If gastric drainage is not replaced, metabolic alkalosis or hypokalemia may result.

The nurse should auscultate bowel sounds every time vital signs are taken. Initially bowel sounds will be absent, but they should gradually return, and the child should begin to pass flatus or stool. The nasogastric tube is generally left in place until bowel sounds return; it may be clamped for several hours before removal. Enteral feedings may be resumed when bowel sounds are diminished, but the patient's tolerance should be monitored closely. Abdominal girth and gastric residuals should be measured, and an increase in either should be reported to a physician. All stool should be tested for blood and the presence of reducing substances, and positive findings should be reported to a physician.

Analgesia should be provided postoperatively. Note that most narcotics will decrease GI motility.

IV antibiotics will be administered if peritonitis is present. If abdominal drains are placed intra-operatively, wound and skin isolation will be required. The amount, consistency, odor, and color of wound drainage should be monitored closely, and wound and blood cultures will be ordered if wound drainage becomes purulent, if the patient becomes febrile, or if other signs of infection or sepsis develop.

Nursing Care Following Liver Transplantation

When the child arrives in the ICU following liver transplantation, assessment of the airway, ventilation, and perfusion have priority. The child's level of consciousness and responsiveness should be evaluated as the child recovers from anesthesia. If the child's neurologic status was compromised preoperatively, the child may not be alert and responsive during the initial postoperative period.

Airway, Breathing, and Circulation

Throughout the child's care, the nurse should evaluate airway patency and effectiveness of oxygenation and ventilation. Mechanical ventilatory support may be required for the first day or days postoperatively, but the child will be weaned from this support as soon as possible.

Systemic perfusion should be monitored continuously. Poor systemic perfusion may indicate hemorrhage, hypoxemia, or sepsis. If coagulopathies were present preoperatively, postoperative bleeding should be anticipated. Heparin should not be added routinely to the flush solutions of invasive intravascular monitoring lines for this reason. If excessive bleeding is noted from any wound or drain, a physician should be notified immediately. A coagulation panel should be obtained to differentiate "surgical" bleeding from a coagulopathy.

Hypertension may develop postoperatively. It typically results from aggressive fluid administration, particularly if cyclosporine (Cyclosporin A) is

administered (this drug decreases urine volume). Treatment may include diuresis or the administration of vasodilators.

Neurologic Function

Monitor the child's neurologic function closely. Record the child's pupil response to light and the Glasgow Coma Scale (GCS) score (spontaneous eye opening, spontaneous verbalization, and motor response to stimuli), and report any deterioration to a physician immediately. If the child is unconscious, the most important portion of the GCS will be evaluation of motor function:

- *GCS motor score of 6:* The child can follow commands (ask the child to hold up two fingers, wiggle the toes, or stick out the tongue).
- *GCS motor score of 5:* The child can localize pain (the child will grab toward your hand as you rub the sternum).
- *GCS motor score of 4:* The child will withdraw from a painful stimulus (the child should abduct each extremity when you pinch the medial aspect of each extremity).
- *GCS motor score of 3:* Decorticate posturing.
- *GCS motor score of 2:* Decerebrate posturing.
- *GCS motor score of 1:* Flaccid response is no response.

The best indication of good function of the transplanted liver will be an improvement in the child's neurologic function (see p. 388).

Hepatic Function

Some liver dysfunction is expected immediately after transplantation. The child's liver enzymes will be monitored closely, and a physician should be notified of any elevation in enzymes or bilirubin.

Low-dose dopamine or dobutamine therapy may be administered to improve splanchnic blood flow following transplantation. These drugs should be titrated to maximize therapeutic effects (i.e., improve urine output and systemic perfusion) and minimize side and toxic effects (i.e., tachycardia or hypotension).

Rejection of the transplanted liver may occur in the immediate postoperative period but is most likely between the fourth and tenth postoperative days. Rejection will produce signs of hepatic failure, with an elevation in liver enzymes, electrolyte imbalances (especially hypoglycemia), and the development of coagulopathies. In addition, the patient often develops fever and right upper quadrant or flank pain or tenderness. Jaundice may also be observed (see Hepatic Failure under Common Clinical Conditions).

Fluid and Electrolyte Balance and Renal Function

The child's fluid balance is monitored closely following transplantation. Oliguria typically is observed immediately after the transplantation, particularly if hepatorenal syndrome was present before the transplantation. Diuresis should occur within the first postoperative days. Low-dose dopamine or dobutamine may be prescribed to increase renal blood flow. IV diuretic therapy (furosemide, 1 to 2 mg/kg/dose) may be required to increase urine volume. Occasionally, hemofiltration may be required to remove excessive fluid (see p. 475). The child's blood urea nitrogen (BUN) and creatinine should be monitored on a daily basis. Daily or twice-daily weights should be measured on the same scale at the same time of day.

A nasogastric tube will be placed at the time of surgery, and any gastric drainage is replaced with 0.45% NaCl. Antacids are administered through the nasogastric tube to keep the gastric pH above 4. Type 2 histamine blockers may be provided (see Stress Ulcers under Specific Diseases).

Nutritional Support

Bowel function typically returns within the first few postoperative days, and feeding can be resumed gradually. Many children with liver failure are anorexic; thus a combination of nasogastric feedings and appetizing oral fluids usually enables provision of maintenance calories.

Immunosuppression

Steroids are administered in the operating room and then postoperatively in decreasing doses (typically, methylprednisolone sodium succinate is administered intravenously and then orally) or per hospital transplant policy.

IV cyclosporine is administered in the operating room, and administration is continued postoperatively at a dose of approximately 2 mg/kg/IV dose every 8 hours. Alternatively, FK-506 may be administered. As soon as bowel function returns, oral cyclosporine administration begins (20 mg/kg/day) and IV cyclosporine is tapered. Oral cyclosporine should be diluted at least 10:1 in milk or juice and can only be given in a *glass* container.

The child's urine output and renal function must be monitored closely during cyclosporine therapy, and a physician should be notified if urine output decreases. Trough cyclosporine levels should be evaluated daily, and the dose adjusted accordingly.

Additional immunosuppressive agents will be administered according to the experience of the transplant team.

Parenteral Nutrition

Parenteral nutrition is defined as the administration of nutrients by the intravascular route. This form of nutrition does not provide greater nutrition than enteral feedings, but it can provide nutritional support until enteral nutrition is possible.

Indications for the use of TPN in the neonatal period include congenital anomalies requiring major resection of the small bowel, intestinal obstruction, gastroschisis, necrotizing enterocolitis, and intractable diarrhea. Beyond infancy, pediatric patients typically require TPN for severe malnutrition, preoperative weight loss, inadequate postoperative nutrition, intestinal failure, liver failure, refractory anorexia nervosa, and malignancy. Parenteral nutrition may be used over a long period of time to allow an inflamed or diseased GI tract to rest while healing is enhanced by maintenance of good nutrition.

Routes of Administration

Central Venous Administration   Direct catheterization of the subclavian or other large veins allows the infusion of high-osmolarity solutions into a high-flow venous system. These catheters are typically made of polyethylene or polyurethane. They may be inserted into the superior vena cava through the subclavian vein, innominate vein, jugular vein, or axillary vein. They may be inserted with a percutaneous or a cutdown technique. Long catheters may enable access to the central venous system from virtually any peripheral catheter. These percutaneous indwelling catheters (PICs) may be inserted at the bedside. Long-term central venous catheters, which are inserted in the operating room, include Broviac, Hickman, and Groshong catheters. These catheters all are made of material such as Dacron, which adheres to scar tissue and reduces the risk of dislodgment. Some have a cuff that is positioned around the catheter under the skin to anchor the catheter. These catheters do exit the skin; thus they still introduce a risk of infection.

Long-dwelling central venous catheters may also be totally implanted. Implanted catheters (intradermal venous access devices) consist of a reservoir with a diaphragm that is placed under the skin surface (e.g., a Portacath). Vascular access is achieved by piercing the skin over the diaphragm and then entering the reservoir. These catheters must be heparinized, but they do enable maintenance of skin integrity; thus the risk of infection is reduced.

Peripheral Venous Administration   Parenteral nutrition may be provided peripherally for a limited time, but this does not enable provision of maintenance caloric intake. The maximum concentration of glucose that can be infused into peripheral veins is limited to 10% to 15%. If this solution infiltrates into surrounding tissues, a burn can result.

Parenteral Nutrition Solutions

Parenteral nutrition solutions consist primarily of glucose (as a source of calories) and amino acids (as a source of nitrogen for protein synthesis). Electrolytes, vitamins, minerals, and trace elements also are added to these solutions to meet all of the child's nutritional energy requirements. Fat emulsions may be administered as a separate solution to provide a major source of calories and to prevent essential fatty acid deficiency states.

Nursing Responsibilities

The TPN system should be set up and changed using aseptic technique and according to hospital protocol. If a fat emulsion solution is infused with the TPN, it is typically "piggy-backed" into the TPN tubing at the last connector before catheter entrance to the patient. This reduces the time the TPN amino acids are in contact with the lipids; thus it may reduce emulsification of the lipids.

Fluid and Electrolyte Balance   The nurse should document the quantity and content of the child's fluid intake and output, and evaluate the child's fluid and electrolyte status. Most hospitals have developed guidelines for use of specific tests to monitor patient status during TPN, and these should be followed.

Before each new TPN bag is hung, and when the nurse assumes responsibility for patient care, the nurse should confirm that the appropriate solution is hanging at the bedside. The solution content should be checked against the physician's order.

When TPN is begun, the glucose concentration and the rate of solution infusion is begun at low levels and gradually increased so that the child's insulin production can accommodate the increased glucose load. The child's serum glucose is monitored at the bedside (and also by the laboratory), and urine is checked for the presence of glucose until a stable TPN infusion is achieved. Glucosuria may indicate the presence of high serum glucose levels or infection.

Once the TPN is begun, it should be infused at a constant rate. An abrupt increase or decrease in glucose administration may produce hyperglycemia or hypoglycemia. If the TPN catheter becomes obstructed or cannot function, TPN administration must continue through another catheter to avoid an abrupt reduction in glucose intake. The child should be monitored closely for evidence of hypoglycemia if there is any interruption in the glucose infusion.

Acidosis occasionally develops in the premature infant or the child with renal failure when large protein loads are administered. The development of acidosis may indicate the need to reduce protein intake. It may also indicate the development of sepsis.

Complications   Potential complications of TPN therapy include complications from the catheter and its insertion (hemothorax, hydrothorax, or pneumothorax; bleeding; or infection), fluid and electrolyte imbalances (including hyperglycemia or hypoglycemia), acidosis, hypomagnesemia, hyperlipidemia, copper deficiency, zinc deficiency, cardiac arrhythmias, venous thromboses, air embolus, and skin sloughing.

Potential complications of fat emulsion therapy include ventilation-perfusion abnormalities, eosinophilia, and bilirubin displacement from albumin. Some children develop reactions to lipid infusion, including dyspnea, flushing, nausea, headache, dizziness, or chest and back pain. A physician should be notified immediately if respiratory distress develops, and an arterial blood gas measurement should be obtained to rule out ventilation-perfusion abnormalities.

Because lipid binds with albumin, it will displace bilirubin from albumin. In the presence of newborn hyperbilirubinemia, this could increase the risk of kernicterus. Therefore lipids should not be administered to neonates with jaundice or to children with significant liver disease.

If the TPN IV solution infiltrates, it may produce a chemical burn and tissue sloughing. When infiltration is discovered, the infusion at that site is discontinued (it must be restarted elsewhere). Some physicians order injection of hyaluronidase into the area of infiltration to promote dispersion and absorption of the solution.

Liver dysfunction may be related to TPN administration. Elevation of liver enzymes or cholestatic jaundice may develop. Cholestatic jaundice will produce an elevation in serum conjugated bilirubin, alkaline phosphatase, serum glutamate pyruvate transaminase (SGPT), and serum glutamic-oxaloacetic transaminase (SGOT). These findings typically revert to normal when the TPN is discontinued.

Infection Control   TPN contains a high glucose content and as such provides an excellent medium for bacterial growth. Strict aseptic technique must be used when changing bags, and the catheter system tubing should only be entered when absolutely necessary. The bag and tubing are typically changed every 24 hours (or according to hospital protocol.

The dressing over the catheter insertion site should be changed according to hospital protocol. If an occlusive dressing is applied with sterile technique, it may remain in place as long as it is occlusive and there is no evidence of inflammation. The nurse should assess the insertion site for evidence of inflammation or exudate and report any abnormalities to a physician. The child's temperature should be monitored, and fever reported to a physician.

If infection is suspected, blood cultures are ordered. One set is obtained from the central line, and one set is obtained through a separate venipuncture. If only the cultures obtained through the catheter produce microorganism growth, the catheter stopcock or the catheter itself may be colonized. If both sets of cultures produce microorganism growth and contain the same microorganism, it is presumed that that organism is growing in the blood (e.g., producing a bacteremia, fungemia, or a yeast or rickettsial bloodstream infection). The central venous catheter is presumed to be colonized and is usually removed (per physician's order or hospital policy) once another reliable route of vascular access is obtained.

Specific Diseases

Congenital Gastrointestinal Abnormalities

The most important aspects of the management of neonatal congenital anomalies are early diagnosis, adequate surgical repair, and prevention or treatment of postoperative complications.

Early signs of congenital GI anomalies include:

- Maternal polyhydramnios, the presence of excessive amniotic fluid during pregnancy (Intestinal block prevents the normal passage and reabsorption of amniotic fluid in the fetus; thus the volume of amniotic fluid increases.)
- Failure of air to pass through the newborn's GI tract immediately after birth (air is not present on abdominal radiographs within 12 hours after birth)
- Failure to pass meconium within the first 24 hours of life

Congenital anomalies of the GI tract are presented in Table 10-11.

Table 10-11

Congenital Gastrointestinal Anomalies

Disease	Etiology	Pathophysiology	Clinical Signs and Symptoms	Nursing Interventions
Congenital Gastrointestinal Anomalies Associated With Respiratory Distress				
Diaphragm hernia	Incomplete fusion of diaphragm at 10 weeks of gestation; usually left side is involved	Abnormal opening between abdomen and thorax; allows stomach and intestines to enter chest; left lung fails to develop and is hypoplastic; heart is displaced to right thorax	Abdomen appears flat; severe respiratory distress develops, including severe respiratory acidosis; heart sounds shifted; R→L shunt is present through patent ductus arteriosus or foramen ovale, since pulmonary vascular resistance is high	Insert NG tube to decompress stomach Position on right side to increase perfusion of right lung Provide skilled respiratory support Monitor ABG If R→L shunt exists, attempt to dilate pulmonary bed (see p. 211) Prepare for surgical correction
Tracheoesophageal fistula	Abnormal separation of esophagus from trachea (develops after 24 days of gestation)	Upper segment of esophagus ends in blind pouch above bifurcation of trachea; fistula to stomach is present	Respiratory distress Dysphagia Excessive salivation Abdominal distension Inability to pass NG tube X-ray film reveals no air in stomach, intestines, and upper mediastinal pouch if esophageal atresia is present	Elevate head of bed 45 degrees IV fluids NPO Respiratory support Prepare for surgical correction or palliative procedure and insertion of gastrostomy tube
Congential Gastrointestinal Anomalies Associated with Obstructive or Bleeding Symptoms				
Malrotation with volvulus	Abnormal movement of intestines around superior mesenteric artery during week 10 of gestation	Malrotation obstructs duodenum in various degrees; strangulation of superior mesenteric artery results from volvulus of small intestine	Vomiting bilious material after first 24-48 hr of life Abdominal distension Visible peristalsis Melena or currant jelly stools Barium x-ray: abnormal rotation of bowel	Measure abdominal girth q4h; notify physician if girth increases 1-2 cm IV fluids NPO Prepare for surgical correction

From Hazinski MF: *Nursing care of the critically ill child,* ed 2, St Louis, 1992, Mosby.

Continued

Table 10-11—cont'd
Congenital Gastrointestinal Anomalies

Disease	Etiology	Pathophysiology	Clinical Signs and Symptoms	Nursing Interventions
Congenital Gastrointestinal Anomalies Associated with Obstructive or Bleeding Symptoms—cont'd				
Hirschsprung's disease	Failure of innervation of GI tract at 5-12 weeks of gestation	With this interruption of peristalsis in lower GI tract, fecal contents are not eliminated; internal sphincter fails to relax	Newborn: failure to pass meconium within 24-48 hr after birth; bilious vomiting; abdominal distension; explosive diarrhea; enterocolitis	Newborn IV fluids NG tube Prepare for surgical reanastomosis, pull-through, and temporary colostomy
			Child: constipation; ribbonlike, foul-smelling stool; abdominal distension; visible peristalsis; malnutrition; anemia; malabsorption Barium x-ray— transition zone of aganglionic segment	Child Low-residue, high calorie, high-protein diet Enemas when needed or stool softeners Prepare for surgical correction; pull-through primary consideration
Imperforate anus and intestinal atresia	Abnormal partitioning between cloaca and urorectal septum at 8 weeks of gestation	Single membrane covering anus or anal agenesis or atresia or intestinal atresia; lack of patency of any segment of bowel because of poor vascular supply to that area of bowel	Abdominal distension; vomiting *High atresia* X-ray—shows lack of progression of air through bowel May pass meconium *Low atresia* Abdominal distension; lack of stools; vomiting X-ray—obstructed pattern with dilated, air-filled bowel	Measure abdominal girth q4h; notify physician if girth increases 1-2 cm Note absence or presence of meconium or stools Note color of vomitus IV fluids NG tube Prepare for surgical correction

From Hazinski MF: *Nursing care of the critically ill child*, ed 2, St Louis, 1992, Mosby.

Table 10-11—cont'd
Congenital Gastrointestinal Anomalies

Disease	Etiology	Pathophysiology	Clinical Signs and Symptoms	Nursing Interventions
Congenital Gastrointestinal Anomalies Associated With Abdominal Wall Defect				
Omphalocele	Failure of GI tract to return to abdominal cavity by 10-11 weeks of gestation; high incidence of other anomalies	Abdominal organs herniate into umbilicus and are covered by a protective sac; defect is variable in size	Temperature instability; dehydration from free water loss; protein loss; hypoglycemia from ↑ caloric expenditure; respiratory distress; all leading to shock	NPO Insert NG tube and attach to low suction Provide IV fluids or TPN Calculate caloric intake and discuss with physician if inadequate Provide neutral thermal environment Keep sac covered with moist sterile gauze preoperatively Dextrostix q4-6h Prepare for surgical correction
Gastroschisis	Failure of mesoderm to completely invade embryonic abdominal wall at week 5 of gestation	Abdominal wall defect of 1-2 inches in diameter; usually located to right of umbilical cord; without a protective sac, abdominal organs herniate	Temperature instability; dehydration; protein loss; hypoglycemia from ↑ caloric expenditure; respiratory distress; all leading to shock	NPO Insert NG tube and attach to low suction Provide IV fluids or TPN Calculate caloric intake and discuss with physician if inadequate Provide neutral thermal environment Cover sac with warm sterile saline sponges and cover with plastic bag or wrap Dextrostix q4-6h Prepare for surgical correction

Inborn Errors of Metabolism

Etiology/Pathophysiology

An inborn error of metabolism is a disorder that results from a genetic inability to produce a protein in its normal configuration. The defect produces a disorder of carbohydrate metabolism, a disorder of fatty acid oxidation, lactic acidosis, a urea cycle enzyme defect, or organic aciduria.

Clinical Presentation

If the child with an inborn error of metabolism presents with a critical illness, the most significant problems include hypoglycemia, metabolic acidosis, and hyperammonemia. Additional critical problems include seizures and jaundice. For a list of errors of metabolism sorted by presenting problem, see Box 10-2.

Management

When the child presents with an inborn error of metabolism, urgent therapy focuses on elimination of the life-threatening complications, including hypoglycemia, metabolic acidosis, or hyperammonemia. However, successful therapy requires identification of the cause of the error and institution of appropriate therapy for the disorder.

Box 10-2

Common Clinical Presentations of Inborn Errors of Metabolism

Inborn Errors of Metabolism Producing Lactic Acidosis

Glycogen storage disease, types I, III
Pyruvate dehydrogenase deficiency
Phosphoenolpyruvate carboxylase deficiency
Leigh's encephalomyelopathy
Organic acidemias
Amino acidemias
Mitochondrial respiratory electron transport chain enzyme deficiencies

Inborn Errors of Metabolism Causing Hyperammonemia

Urea cycle enzyme defects (NOTE: Typically, these are not associated with ketosis or acidosis)
  Ornithine transcarbamylase (OTC)
  Carbamoyl phosphate synthetase (CPS)
  Argininosuccinic acid synthetase (AS)
  Argininosuccinic acid lyase (AL)
The following often present with hyperammonemia and ketosis or acidosis:
  Pyruvate dehydrogenase
  Pyruvate carboxylase
  Propionicacidemia
  Methylmalonicacidemia
  Glutaricaciduria, type II
  HMB-CoA lyase

Inborn Errors of Metabolism Presenting With Seizures

Those producing hypoglycemia

Those producing hypocalcemia
Nonketotic hyperglycinemia
Menkes' syndrome
Medium-chain acyl dehydrogenase deficiency
Multiple acyl dehydrogenase deficiency
Adrenoleukodystrophy
Organic acidemias
Biotinidase deficiency
Tyrosinemia, type I

Inborn Errors of Metabolism Presenting With Neonatal Jaundice

Galactosemia
Fructose intolerance
Tyrosinemia
Galactolytic enzyme deficiencies
Crigler-Najjar syndrome
Alpha-1 antiprotease deficiency
Hemolysis
Wilson's disease

Data from Thornton PS, Berry GT, Stanley CA: Disorders of intermediary metabolism. In Holbrook PR, editor: *Textbook of pediatric critical care,* Philadelphia, 1993, WB Saunders; and Wolff JA, Gilbert-Barness E, Barness LA: Disorders/diseases of inborn errors of metabolism that produce critical illness. In Fuhrman BP, Zimmerman JJ, editors: *Pediatric critical care,* ed 2, St Louis, 1998, Mosby.

When the child arrives in the unit, support of the airway, oxygenation and ventilation, and systemic perfusion will assume priority. In addition, blood samples are drawn to determine the precise defect responsible for the child's condition. A urine and serum sample should be saved during the initial minutes of therapy for later analysis. Initial laboratory tests are determined by the presenting problem and are illustrated in Figure 10-3.

Urgent treatment of hyperammonemia may be accomplished in the following ways (Wolff, Gilbert-Barness, and Barness, 1997):

- Hemodialysis
- Exchange transfusion

- Peritoneal dialysis
- Sodium benzoate: 250 mg/kg/day
- Sodium phenylacetate: 250 mg/kg/day
- Arginine: 300 to 700 mg/kg/day

Once the specific error of metabolism is identified, corrective therapy, if available, may be instituted.

Biliary Atresia

Etiology/Pathophysiology

Biliary atresia is the absence or near-absence of the biliary tree. The atresia may involve isolated segments of the bile duct system or the entire biliary

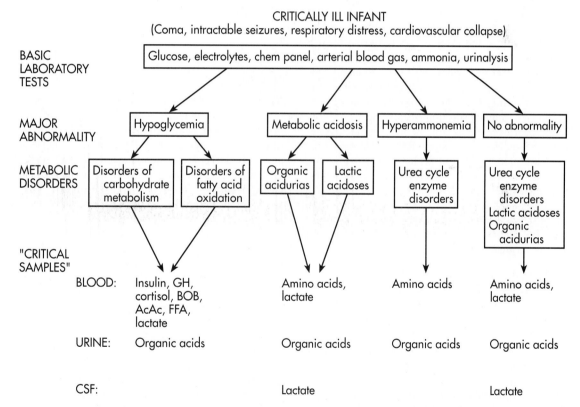

Figure 10-3 Use of routine laboratory tests and "critical" blood and urine specimens to detect disorders of intermediary metabolism in the critically ill infant or child. *GH,* growth hormone; *BOB,* β-hydroxybutyrate; *AcAc,* acetoacetate; *FFA,* free fatty acid: (From Thornton PS, Berry GT, Stanley CA: Disorders of intermediary metabolism. In Holbrook PR, editior: *Textbook of pediatric critical care,* Philadelphia, 1993, WB Saunders.)

tree, including the gallbladder. The cause of the biliary atresia is unknown. Biliary atresia may be associated with the polysplenia syndrome, an association of intracardiac and abdominal rotations and anomalies.

The atresia or obstruction in the biliary tree prevents bile drainage from the liver into the duodenum. The accumulation of bile in the liver causes direct (conjugated) hyperbilirubinemia. If the condition is not diagnosed and surgically corrected before 2 to 3 months of age, cirrhosis of the liver and portal hypertension typically result.

Clinical Presentation

Persistent jaundice and direct (conjugated) hyperbilirubinemia during the first 2 months of life are the first clinical signs observed in infants with biliary atresia. Acholic or gray-colored stools indicate a lack of bile drainage into the GI tract. Bilirubin excretion in the urine colors the urine brown. Pruritus is caused by increased bile salts.

If biliary atresia is not detected or treated, signs of progressive liver disease are evident during the first year of life. These include ascites, poor growth secondary to malabsorption of fats and fat-soluble vitamins, rickets, hypoproteinemia, edema, and petechiae (see Hepatic Failure under Common Clinical Conditions). Signs of portal hypertension may also be present (see Portal Hypertension under Common Clinical Conditions).

Radionuclide scanning and liver biopsy may suggest the diagnosis. An exploratory laparotomy may be performed to confirm the diagnosis and enable surgical palliation.

Management

The specific surgical procedure performed for the infant with biliary atresia is determined by the location and extent of the atretic segment. The prognosis is best when the proximal biliary tree (connected to the liver) is patent and the atretic segment is distal; unfortunately, this combination occurs in few patients.

A modification of the Kasai hepatoportoenterostomy is generally performed as a palliative procedure to provide a route for bile drainage. A successful surgical result will be indicated by satisfactory bile drainage and the resolution of jaundice. However, a large number of children will not have

sufficient bile drainage even after the surgery. Postoperative complications include ascending cholangitis and bleeding, as well as possible complications of underlying liver failure. Cholangitis should be suspected if the infant develops fever postoperatively, and blood cultures should be drawn. A liver biopsy may be necessary to confirm the diagnosis. Aggressive antibiotic therapy is indicated, since cholangitis can extend liver damage.

Drugs such as phenobarbital, bile acids, and bile acid–binding resins may be administered to increase bile drainage. Corticosteroids may be administered to reduce bile duct inflammation. For additional nursing care information see Portal Hypertension and Hepatic Failure under Common Clinical Conditions.

Transplantation is often recommended for the treatment of biliary atresia.

Necrotizing Enterocolitis

Etiology

Necrotizing enterocolitis (NEC) is an acquired disease of unknown origin that develops during the neonatal period. Major risk factors include prematurity, aggressive enteral feedings, infectious agents, and hypoxic-ischemic insults (Figure 10-4).

Prematurity is the primary risk factor; 90% of cases occur in premature infants. Infants <28 weeks of gestation are at greatest risk until they reach a postconceptual age of 35 to 36 weeks. NEC rarely occurs in older children or adults.

NEC occasionally occurs in infants who have never been fed. However, it most often occurs in infants who have been fed, with a history of aggressive advancement of feedings (e.g., >20 Cal/kg/day). Feeding with human milk can reduce the risk of NEC.

It is unclear if infection is a primary or a permissive agent in the pathogenesis of NEC. A variety of bacteria and viruses have been isolated from blood, peritoneal fluid, intestinal tissues, and feces, but no one organism has been implicated.

Decreased bowel perfusion is thought to contribute to NEC, although the link between hypoxic-ischemic insult and NEC has been anecdotal and has not been verified in epidemiologic studies. Neonatal asphyxia and other perinatal insults will

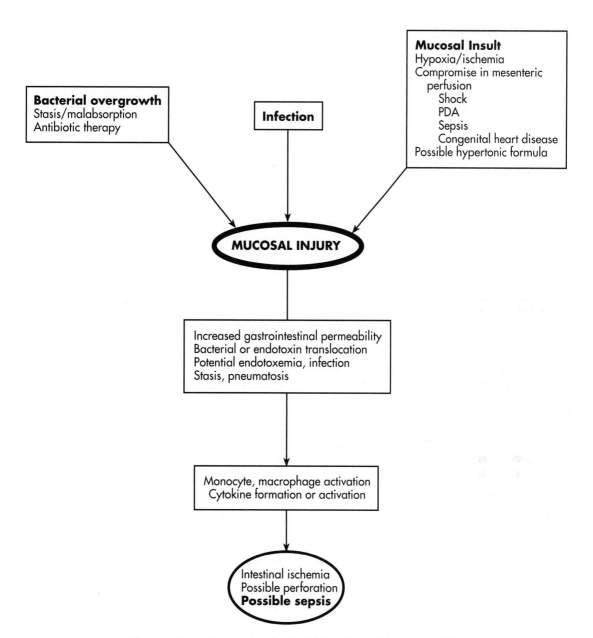

Figure 10-4   Proposed pathophysiology of necrotizing enterocolitis.

cause diversion of blood away from the splanchnic circulation.

Pathophysiology

The GI tract contains gram-negative bacteria, which are normally prevented from passing through the GI mucosa and entering the circulation by a variety of factors. However, the GI tract of the premature neonate is immature in several ways, which can contribute to the translocation of bacteria or endotoxin across the GI mucosa, and to the development of NEC. These factors include decreased immune function, reduced motility and digestive function, and an immature intestinal barrier to bacterial invasion (Neu, 1996).

The neonatal GI tract has diminished immunoglobulin A and G, reduced intestinal lymphocytes, and a poor antibody response. These factors seem to allow bacterial or viral proliferation, particularly in the terminal ileum and colon, where levels of immunoglobulin and lymphocytes are lowest.

The motility of the GI tract of the premature infant is low, with reduced levels of gastric hydrogen ion output and proteolytic enzyme activity. This probably limits the hydrolysis of toxins that may enter the GI tract.

The intestinal epithelial barrier of the premature neonate is more highly permeable than is the intestine of the mature neonate. This facilitates adherence of bacteria to the epithelium and uptake of intact bacteria. If disruption of the mucosal barrier develops (e.g., ischemic insult), translocation of bacteria or endotoxin from gram-negative bacteria will occur.

Inflammatory mediators of the septic cascade contribute to the pathophysiology of NEC. Translocation of gram-negative bacteria or endotoxin from the gram-negative bacteria across the mucosa stimulate the gram-negative septic cascade. Platelet-activating factor, tumor necrosis factor, and some of the interleukins cause vasodilation, increased capillary permeability, platelet aggregation or dysfunction, and maldistribution of blood flow. Free oxygen radical formation also contributes to the inflammatory process and organ dysfunction. These mediators perpetuate the inflammatory process and contribute to hemorrhagic necrosis and ulceration. Perforation of the bowel may occur. As in septic shock, activation of mediators includes activation of the clotting cascade, so DIC may develop (see Septic Shock, p. 131, and DIC, p. 561). Septic shock and multiorgan failure can develop.

Histologic alterations in the bowel of the patient with NEC include mucosal edema, hemorrhage, coagulation necrosis, and mucosal ulceration. These suggest that infection plays a role, but that inflammation and ischemia also contribute to the disease (Neu, 1996).

Clinical Presentation

The classic clinical presentation of the neonate with NEC includes the following group of symptoms:

- Abdominal distension and tenderness
- Pneumatosis intestinalis (gas in the bowel wall, observed on abdominal radiographs)
- Gross or occult blood in the stools
- Complications, including intestinal gangrene, bowel perforation, sepsis, and septic shock

Clinical staging of NEC has been accomplished. Stage 1 is suggestive of the disease (some evidence of blood in stools, abdominal distension, feeding intolerance); stage 2 is definitive (definite distension and tenderness, plus some evidence of metabolic acidosis and pneumatosis intestinalis may be visible on radiographs); and stage 3 is severe (includes signs of shock and organ system failure, pneumoperitoneum).

Signs of clinical deterioration in the newborn with NEC include the development of apnea or bradycardia, lethargy, temperature instability, decreased urine output, and a compromise in systemic perfusion (cool, mottled skin, pallor, decreased intensity of peripheral pulses). Hypotension is a late sign of deterioration. Respiratory and metabolic acidosis and development of DIC indicate the presence of multisystem organ failure.

Management

If NEC is identified in its early stages and treatment is begun promptly, the infant will often improve without surgical intervention. Once the diagnosis of NEC is suspected (stage 1), enteral feedings are discontinued and a nasogastric tube is passed to provide continuous gastric drainage and decompression. Umbilical artery or venous catheters are discontinued. IV fluid therapy and parenteral nutrition are provided. Antibiotics may be administered.

When NEC is suspected, careful observation and support of the neonate is required. Abdominal girths are measured every 1 to 2 hours, and fluid intake and output are closely monitored. All stools are tested for blood and the presence of reducing substances (which will indicate carbohydrate malabsorption). The child's systemic perfusion and respiratory function are closely monitored, and a physician should be notified immediately of any deterioration. Third spacing of fluids and electrolyte imbalances may develop. A surgeon should be notified of the possibility of NEC.

Once the diagnosis of NEC is confirmed (Stage 2 or 3), treatment focuses on support of systemic perfusion and respiratory function, institution of antibiotics (if they have not already been administered), and support of other organ functions. Bolus fluid therapy (using isotonic crystalloids) will probably be required to maintain intravascular volume, and vasoactive agents are often required to optimize perfusion and maintain blood pressure. Blood component therapy may be necessary if DIC develops.

Indications for surgical intervention are listed in Box 10-3. Additional indications may include

---

Box 10-3

Indications for Surgical Intervention in the Treatment of Necrotizing Enterocolitis

1. Free intraperitoneal air
2. Cellulitis of anterior abdominal wall
3. Radiographic evidence of peritonitis
   a. Increased free peritoneal fluid
   b. Increased bowel wall edema
4. Clinical deterioration during medical therapy
   a. Irreversible metabolic acidosis
   b. Shock
   c. Respiratory failure

From Hazinski MF: *Nursing care of the critically ill child*, ed 2, St. Louis, 1992, Mosby.

---

right lower quadrant mass, persistent dilated (and visible) bowel loops, abdominal wall erythema, and thrombocytopenia. Resection of necrotic bowel is necessary, although attempts are made to salvage as much viable intestine as possible. Postoperative complications include temporary malabsorption and the development of intestinal obstruction secondary to the stricture of ischemic portions of the bowel. These infants may develop temporary intestinal failure (see Intestinal Failure under Common Clinical Conditions).

Stress Ulcers

Etiology/Pathophysiology

Stress ulcers occur in all pediatric age groups, including high-risk newborns. Critically ill patients, particularly those with intracranial disease, sepsis, burns, shock, and severe trauma are at highest risk.

The proposed pathophysiology of stress ulceration is shown in Figure 10-5. Hypoxia of the gastric mucosa and the generation of highly injurious oxygen-derived free radicals may be contributing factors.

Clinical Presentation

Nearly all ICU patients develop histologic abnormalities of the gastric mucosa, usually 3 to 7 days following onset of the acute illness or injury and admission to the critical care unit. Initially the only evidence of bleeding may be blood in the nasogastric aspirate or stool. Some patients develop an overtly bloody nasogastric aspirate, and a few patients will develop massive hematemesis with melena and hemorrhagic shock. Abdominal pain is rare.

Upper GI endoscopy, which can be performed at the bedside, is the diagnostic procedure of choice and should be performed when bleeding is significant.

Prevention and Management

Only a limited number of studies on stress ulcer prevention have been reported in children; thus most approaches are derived from experience in adults (Cook et al., 1996; Tryba and Cook, 1997). Stress ulceration can be reduced through the administration of agents that increase the gastric pH

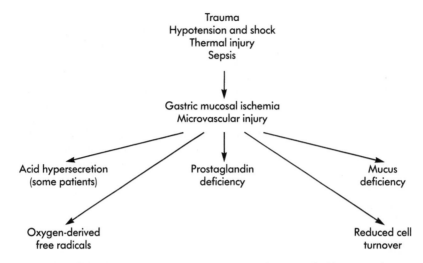

Figure 10-5   Proposed pathophysiology of stress ulcers. (From Hazinski MF: *Nursing care of critically ill children,* ed 2, St Louis, 1992, Mosby.)

Table 10-12 Stress Ulcer Prophylaxis	
Drug	**Dose**
Antacids	2-15 ml PO/NG q1-6h prn, titrated to maintain gastric pH at >4
H₂-blockers	
Cimetidine	Infants (IV/IM/PO): 10-20 mg/kg/24 hr in 4 doses
	Children (IV/IM/PO): 20-40 mg/kg/24 hr in 4 doses
Ranitidine	PO: 4-5 mg/kg/day in 2-3 doses
	IV: 2-4 mg/kg/day in 3-4 doses
Sucralfate	PO: 40-80 mg/kg/24 hr in 4 doses

Data from John Hopkins Hospital Department of Pediatrics: *The Harriet Lane handbook,* ed 14, edited by Barone M, St Louis, 1996, Mosby; and Snyder JD: Gastroenterology. In Graef JW, editor: *Manual of pediatric therapeutics,* ed 5, Boston, 1995, Little, Brown.

(Table 10-12). This includes the use of antacids and H₂-blockers (type 2 histamine receptor blockers). The relative efficacy of antacids and H₂-blockers has been debated, but when all studies are considered together, these agents appear to be equally efficacious. The coating agent, sucralfate, is as effective as H₂-blockers and antacid in the prevention of stress ulceration. Although it has no significant effect on gastric acid secretion, sucralfate is "cytoprotective."

A nasogastric tube should be placed in all critically ill or injured patients, and the gastric pH should be checked at 1- to 2-hour intervals. Antacids should be administered every 1 to 2 hours for pH values of less than 4. This evaluation of gastric pH and antacid therapy is continued even if IV H₂-blockers are provided.

Diabetic Ketoacidosis

Etiology

Diabetes mellitus is a disease of impaired glucose utilization caused by a lack of insulin. Diabetic ketoacidosis (DKA) is a potential complication of diabetes mellitus. DKA results from inadequate insulin to enable use of glucose as an energy store and from complications of hyperglycemia and partial oxidation of lipids as an alternative energy store, including the development of metabolic acidosis and dehydration.

DKA may be precipitated by an infection or a change in the child's feeding behavior, energy requirements, or insulin intake.

Pathophysiology

When glucose is unable to enter the cells to provide substrate for cellular metabolism, lipids are utilized as an alternative source of energy. These lipids are only partially oxidized into free fatty acids and acetoacetic acid. The free fatty acids accumulate, whereas the acetoacetic acid is converted into ketones.

Metabolism of fats and the accumulation of their by-products result in the development of metabolic acidosis. Lipolysis and the development of ketoacidosis are enhanced by the action of other hormones, including epinephrine. Respiratory alkalosis develops to compensate for the metabolic acidosis, and the patient usually demonstrates deep, rapid respirations.

Hyperglycemia is present because intravascular glucose is not utilized, and gluconeogenesis and glycogen breakdown are stimulated by the intracellular lack of glucose. Glucagon, catecholamines, and growth hormones also increase glucose production.

Once the serum glucose concentration exceeds approximately 180 mg/dl, the renal threshold for glucose, glucosuria develops and produces an osmotic diuresis. Urinary excretion of ketoacids enhances urine sodium and potassium losses, although the serum potassium concentration may appear to be within the normal range because acidosis causes a shift of potassium into the intravascular space.

Cerebral edema can complicate DKA. This complication appears to be related to a variety of factors, but particularly to rapid changes in serum osmolality caused by the ketoacidosis and its resuscitation. The development of cerebral edema may be linked to the movement of ketones and hydrogen ions into the brain, the development of intracerebral acidosis, or a rapid reduction in the serum osmolality during correction of the hyperglycemia. Although a dilutional hyponatremia is present during the ketoacidosis, serum osmolality is maintained by the hyperglycemia. However, if the serum sodium fails to rise in proportion to the lowering of the serum glucose during therapy, serum osmolality will fall and the risk of cerebral edema will be high.

Clinical Presentation

The patient with DKA presents with a variety of acid-base and electrolyte imbalances. Hypertonic dehydration with metabolic acidosis is present, and tachypnea results in hypocarbia with partial respiratory compensation. The major biochemical alterations of DKA are listed here:

- Hyperglycemia
- Dehydration
- Ketosis
- Acidosis
- Electrolyte imbalances
- Potential cerebral edema

Acidosis produces an intravascular potassium shift; thus the serum potassium value may appear to be normal or possibly elevated, even though the patient has a *total body deficit of potassium.* Note that as the acidosis is corrected, the serum potassium concentration will fall.

The serum sodium concentration is artificially diluted in the presence of hyperglycemia, because the glucose produces an intravascular fluid shift. To determine if the serum sodium concentration is appropriate for the hyperglycemia, use the following formula:

- For every 100 mg/dl rise in serum glucose concentration above 180 mg/dl, the serum sodium concentration can be expected to fall 1.6 mEq/L below 135 mEq/L.
- For every 100 mg/dl fall in serum glucose concentration during treatment of DKA, the serum sodium concentration should rise 1.6 mEq/L.

Example: For example, if the glucose concentration is 580 mg/dl, this represents a 400 mg/dl rise in glucose above the normal maximum of 180 mg/dl. This hyperglycemia would be expected to depress the serum sodium concentration 4 × 1.6 mEq/L, or 6.4 mEq/L below 135 mEq/L. A serum sodium concentration of 128 to 129 mEq/L can therefore be explained by the hyperglycemia. If the serum sodium concentration is less than 128 to 129 mEq/L, hyponatremia beyond a dilutional effect is present. Note that as the hyperglycemia is corrected, the serum sodium concentration should rise 1.6 mEq/L for every 100 mg/dl fall in the serum glucose concentration.

The child with DKA may be lethargic with a decreased response to stimuli. This lethargy may be explained by the hyperglycemia and the acidosis, but cerebral edema should also be considered as a potential cause. The child's responsiveness should improve as the hyperglycemia and acidosis are treated. Failure to improve during therapy or neurologic deterioration may be caused by cerebral edema. Patients at greatest risk for development of cerebral edema are those with a history of hyperglycemia of several days' duration, moderate or severe acidosis, and relative hyponatremia.

Management

The goals of treatment of DKA include:

- Rehydration and support of systemic perfusion
- Insulin administration
- Restoration, maintenance of serum electrolyte balance
- Prevention of complications
- Supportive care

Admission to an ICU with pediatric expertise is usually indicated for a newly diagnosed diabetic patient with ketoacidosis, or for any patient with significant dehydration and acidosis. The presence of shock requires ICU admission.

Rehydration and Support of Systemic Perfusion and Electrolyte Balance Treatment requires insertion of two large-bore IV catheters. Fluid therapy is required to treat shock, replace the fluid deficit, and provide maintenance fluids:

- *Treatment of shock:* 20 ml/kg of normal saline or lactated Ringer's solution, repeated until systemic perfusion is adequate
- *Deficit replacement:* 0.45% NaCl or normal saline (based on the child's sodium deficit), calculated to replace the fluid deficit over 24 to 48 hours
- *Maintenance requirements:* See Table 10-5

The fluid and electrolyte deficit may be calculated from Table 10-13. The fluid deficit may be estimated at approximately 3500 ml/m^2 BSA/day. This deficit should be replaced over a 24- to 48-hour period *in addition to maintenance fluid requirements.*

Table 10-13
Guidelines for Estimation of Degree of Dehydration in Diabetic Ketoacidosis in Normally Nourished Children

	Mild	Moderate	Severe
Volume of deficit (ml/kg)*			
>2 yr	30	60	90
<2 yr	50	100	150
Clinical measures			
Peripheral perfusion†			
Palpation of peripheral pulses	Full	Full to diminished	Barely palpable to absent
Capillary refill time‡	<2 sec	≤2 sec	>3 sec
Skin temperature	N	N to slightly cool	Cool
Heart rate	N to slightly ↑	↑	↑
Blood pressure	N	N to ↑	↓ N or ↑
Biochemical values: mmol/L (mg/dl)			
Urea nitrogen§	<7 (20)	<10.7(30)	>9 (25)
Predicted Na$^+$	<150	<150	Helpful if ≥150
Glucose	Usually mildly ↑ (e.g., 22 [400])	Usually moderately ↑ (e.g., 33 [600])	Usually greatly ↑ (e.g., 44 [800])

From Harris GD et al: Minimizing the risk of brain herniation during treatment of diabetic ketoacidemia: a retrospective and prospective study, *J Pediatr* 117:28, 1990.
N, normal; ↓, decreased; ↑, increased.
*Actual weight.
†Hypothermia and severe ketonemia may mimic signs of poor peripheral perfusion.
‡Capillary refill time is modified by the hypertonic state. Capillary refill time between 2 and 3 seconds indicates moderate or severe dehydration.
§Values given refer to patients >2 years of age.

The sodium deficit can be estimated once the fluid deficit is determined; the sodium deficit is 150 mEq/L of deficit. This sodium can be delivered using either normal saline or lactated Ringer's solution.

Typically, IV fluids are free of glucose until the serum glucose concentration falls below 300 mg/dl. Then 5% glucose with half-normal or normal saline (0.45% NaCl or 0.9% NaCl is administered.

As fluid resuscitation is accomplished, the child should become more awake, alert, and responsive. In addition, systemic perfusion should improve. If the child fails to improve, a physician should be notified immediately.

Potassium administration will be required once urine output is demonstrated, because the serum potassium concentration will fall as the acidosis is corrected. Once urine output is documented, approximately 40 to 80 mEq/L of potassium chloride will be added to the IV replacement fluids.

The administration of phosphate or buffering agents during the treatment of DKA has been debated, but it is probably unnecessary.

Insulin Administration Exogenous insulin administration is required. IV insulin should be provided to ensure predictable insulin delivery and gradual, consistent lowering of the serum glucose concentration. The child receives 0.1 U/kg of human regular insulin by IV push, followed by a continuous IV infusion of 0.1 U/kg/hr. This infusion can be mixed in three ways:

- Regular insulin (5 U/kg body weight) is placed in 240 ml of normal saline. The solution is infused at a rate of 5 ml/hr to deliver 0.1 U/kg/hr.
- Regular insulin (50 U) can be added to a 250-ml bag of normal saline. An infusion rate of 0.5 times the child's body weight (as milliliters per hour) will deliver 0.1 U/kg/hr.
- Normal saline is mixed with regular insulin to create a solution of 0.5 U/ml, and an infusion rate of 0.2 ml/kg/hr will deliver 0.1 U/kg/hr.

Once the child's serum glucose is <250 mg/dl, subcutaneous insulin is administered (0.25 to 0.5

U/kg). The IV insulin is discontinued when the pH reaches 7.35. From that point, the serum glucose is managed using subcutaneous insulin injections or infusions.

The child's serum glucose should be closely monitored to ensure that it falls no faster than 100 mg/dl/hr. As noted above, the serum sodium should rise 1.6 mEq/L for every 100 mg/dl fall in glucose if serum osmolality is to be maintained.

Restoration and Maintenance of Serum Electrolyte Balance Hyperglycemia should be gradually corrected (at a rate not to exceed 100 mg/dl/hr). The serum sodium concentration should rise in proportion to a fall in the serum glucose concentration. Potassium chloride administration will be required (once urine output is verified) to maintain the serum potassium concentration as the acidosis is corrected. The serum pH should correct as rehydration is accomplished and ketosis resolves.

Prevention of Complications The most severe complication of DKA and its management is the development of cerebral edema. This complication may be prevented with careful attention to fluid and electrolyte balance, but it may develop despite all precautions. Signs of cerebral edema include a deterioration in responsiveness as the hyperglycemia is corrected, possible complaints of a headache, and signs of increased ICP. Mannitol is administered if cerebral edema is suspected. If the child's responsiveness is severely impaired, elective intubation is performed to control oxygenation and carbon dioxide elimination and to protect the airway (see p. 394).

Supportive Care The child receives nothing by mouth until the acidosis is corrected and the hyperglycemia is controlled. Fluid intake and output should be carefully recorded and evaluated. In addition, precipitating factors of the ketoacidosis episode should be identified if possible and treated or prevented. Infection should be ruled out or identified and treated. The child and family may require additional instruction regarding the daily treatment of diabetes mellitus.

Pancreatitis

Etiology/Pathophysiology

The most frequent causes of acute pancreatitis in children are drug therapy (particularly prednisone), blunt abdominal trauma, or mumps. Some cases of pancreatitis are hereditary, but many cases are idiopathic.

Acute pancreatitis results in the escape of pancreatic enzymes from the pancreatic cells into the blood and body fluids. The released enzymes begin an autodigestive process of the pancreas manifested by edema, hemorrhage, or necrosis. The pancreatic enzymes may alter pulmonary and peripheral capillary permeability, resulting in pulmonary edema and respiratory failure, peripheral edema, and third spacing of fluid, leading to a compromise in systemic perfusion.

Clinical Presentation

Abdominal pain is the most consistent symptom produced by acute pancreatitis. Although the pain may vary in onset or intensity, the most intense pain is typically in the epigastrium and may radiate to the back and upper quadrants of the abdomen. The pain is usually constant. Nausea and vomiting are common. In severe cases the patient may be pale and sweaty and complain of dizziness. The patient is usually quiet and prefers to lie on the side with the hips slightly flexed.

In fulminating cases, shock may be present. The child's skin is often pink and warm (as a result of vasodilation and increased capillary permeability resulting from the effects of circulating enzymes), but massive vasodilation produces a relative hypovolemia and maldistribution of blood flow similar to that observed with septic shock. Hypotension may be present.

The abdomen is slightly distended and tender but not rigid, with diminished bowel sounds. A bluish discoloration around the umbilicus (Cullen's sign) or in the flanks (Turner's sign) is indicative of hemorrhagic pancreatitis with ascites. A pleural effusion may be present. Pancreatitis should be suspected in the very young child who complains of vague abdominal pains and presents with unexplained ascites or hemorrhagic pleural effusion.

The serum amylase level is often elevated to more than twice normal, but this value can return to normal within 72 hours of the onset of the pancreatitis. The serum lipase level is elevated and remains elevated longer than the serum amylase level. The white blood cell count may be normal, and the hematocrit may be elevated if intravascular volume depletion is present. Hyperglycemia is common because glucagon is released early in the disease. In fulminant pancreatitis, extensive fat necrosis can produce hypocalcemia, which may be symptomatic.

Management

The prevention, assessment, and treatment of hypovolemic shock is the primary goal of treatment of fulminant pancreatitis. Because capillary permeability is increased, large amounts of fluid can be lost from the vascular space, requiring frequent bolus administration of isotonic fluids, in a manner similar to that required in the treatment of septic shock. As in the treatment of any form of hypovolemia, fluid administration should be titrated to the patient's response (see Shock, p. 140).

Once the diagnosis of acute pancreatitis is made, a central venous line is inserted to enable monitoring of CVP and rapid fluid administration. Isotonic crystalloids are administered in 20 ml/kg boluses and may be alternated with colloid bolus therapy. Fluid therapy is continued as needed to maintain systemic perfusion (as indicated by strong peripheral pulses, adequate blood pressure, good urine output, and improved level of consciousness). Pulmonary edema may develop; thus the need for intubation and mechanical ventilatory support should be anticipated.

Treatment with subcutaneous or IV octreotide in severe cases of acute and chronic pancreatitis may be beneficial. This agent appears to work by markedly reducing pancreatic enzyme secretion, but studies in children are limited. Antioxidant therapy has been used on an investigational basis in adults and children with pancreatitis (Mathew et al., 1996).

Causes of deterioration in the child with acute pancreatitis include the development of progressive hypovolemic shock, pulmonary edema or other forms of respiratory distress or failure, duodenal perforation, GI bleeding, or peritonitis.

The child's fluid and electrolyte balance should be closely monitored, and hypocalcemia corrected if present. The hyperglycemia does not often require treatment. The child receives nothing by mouth, and a nasogastric tube is joined to continuous suction to decompress the stomach. Loss of fluids and electrolytes by this route should be replaced with IV fluids. When oral intake is resumed, a low-fat diet is recommended and supplemental pancreatic enzymes are occasionally administered.

Pancreatitis produces abdominal pain; therefore analgesics should be provided. Morphine and other opiate derivatives should not be used because they increase spasm of the sphincter of Oddi (the opening of the pancreatic duct into the duodenum), causing additional pain.

Viral Hepatitis

Etiology

Viral hepatitis is a primary infection of the liver, most commonly caused by three etiologically and immunologically distinct agents: hepatitis A, hepatitis B and hepatitis C. Additional forms of hepatitis, labeled hepatitis E and G, have also been described in children.

Hepatitis A   Hepatitis A virus (HAV) is present in the blood and feces during the incubation period and can be carried by persons who never develop the disease. Children and young adults are most often infected with this virus, and fecal-oral transmission is the most common method of disease transmission. Classically, food, water, and milk contaminated by the virus are ingested, although outbreaks in day care centers have been reported.

Hepatitis B   Hepatitis B virus (HBV) is transmitted chiefly through blood transfusions or other contact with secretions (including saliva, breast milk, and semen) and serum containing the virus.

Hepatitis C   Hepatitis C virus (HCV) is transmitted in ways that are similar to HBV. Although hepatitis C was formerly the leading cause of blood transfusion–induced hepatitis, advances in the detection of this virus in blood products have greatly reduced the risk by effectively screening contaminated blood products (National Institutes of Health, 1997). Hepatitis rarely causes severe

acute infection but commonly causes chronic hepatitis leading to cirrhosis and the need for liver transplantation.

Hepatitis E and G   Hepatitis E virus (HEV) is transmitted by the fecal-oral route and appears to be rare in the United States. Hepatitis G virus (HGV) is a newly discovered agent that may account for some cases of transfusion-associated hepatitis not due to HBV or HCV. Further study will be required before the full implication of hepatitis G in liver disease is known (Alter et al., 1997). Maternal drug abuse is an important risk factor for hepatitis G and C coinfection (Bortolotti et al., 1997).

Neonatal Hepatitis   Neonatal hepatitis presents during the first 3 months of life. Known causes of neonatal hepatitis include a wide range of metabolic disorders (the most common of which is alpha-1-antitrypsin deficiency) and congenital infections such as rubella and cytomegalovirus.

Pathophysiology

Viral hepatitis causes the destruction of liver cells and results in hepatic inflammation, necrosis, and autolysis. Changes occur diffusely throughout the liver, and liver structure may be distorted. Regeneration of cells does occur; thus there may be recovery with minimal damage. However, chronic hepatitis and cirrhosis may develop, or fulminant hepatitis may occur during the course of the viral illness.

Clinical Presentation

Viral hepatitis is characterized by three stages: the preicteric stage; the icteric stage, and the posticteric stage. Clinical signs of the preicteric stage last approximately 1 week and consist of fever, chills, anorexia, malaise, epigastric distress, abdominal pain, nausea, vomiting, and joint pain. Hepatomegaly and lymphadenopathy are also present.

Weakness, fatigue, pallor, scleral jaundice, darkened urine, and gray-colored stools are the beginning signs of the icteric stage. Influenza-type symptoms, persistent anorexia, pruritus, and palmar erythema may last 2 to 6 weeks.

The posticteric stage is marked by an initial rapid, then gradual disappearance of jaundice, a darkening of stools, and a return of laboratory values to normal. Anorexia and fatigue may continue for several weeks, although this is less likely in children.

Hepatitis A   This form of hepatitis usually begins with an acute illness following an incubation period of 14 to 40 days (average 30 days). Fever is a common symptom early in the disease, whereas jaundice and prodromes of arthritis and rash are uncommon in children.

Hepatitis B   The onset of hepatitis B is usually insidious and occurs after an incubation period of 60 to 180 days.

Hepatitis C   HCV RNA can be detected in the blood within 1 to 3 weeks of exposure. Liver cell injury develops within approximately 50 days. Most patients are asymptomatic with no jaundice, although approximately one fourth will develop nonspecific malaise, weakness, or anorexia, and some will develop jaundice. Fulminant liver failure is rare after this form of the virus. The majority of affected patients fail to clear the virus within 6 months, and approximately 20% develop cirrhosis.

Neonatal Hepatitis   Neonatal hepatitis is manifested by direct hyperbilirubinemia, hepatomegaly, and jaundice. Many of the infants demonstrate resolution of the hepatitis with no residual liver damage. However, in some affected patients, progression of liver damage occurs, and cirrhosis develops.

Laboratory Studies   The ability to identify hepatitis serum markers has made it possible to make a specific diagnosis of types A, B, and C hepatitis. These same markers are used to identify contaminated blood products.

The presence of HBsAg indicates that hepatitis B infection exists and that the patient's blood is infectious. This serum marker is usually present within 1 to 3 weeks of exposure to the virus and is usually undetectable by 4 months following exposure.

The presence of anti-HBs indicates that the patient had a previous infection or previous administration of high-titer hyperimmune B globulin.

This antibody typically is detectable 1 to 4 months after the clearance of serum HBsA and remains present for several years.

Hepatitis C RNA can be detected in the serum of patients within 1 to 3 weeks of exposure. Antibodies to HCV are usually detectable during the course of the illness. As noted above, the majority of patients with HCV fail to clear the virus within 6 months.

Management

Nurses should consistently wear gloves and practice Standard Precautions when handling the blood, feces, urine, and excretions of any patient. Specific precautions necessary to prevent blood-borne infection have been recommended by the Centers for Disease Control and Prevention and are mandated by the Occupational Safety and Health Administration. These are available in every hospital unit.

There is not a well-established treatment for the eradication of viral hepatitis. Hepatitis A is a self-limited infection, and treatment is not necessary. Recent limited success in the treatment of chronic hepatitis B and hepatitis C with gamma-interferon has been achieved. Ongoing research is being conducted with multidrug protocols for eradication of these agents.

A vaccine is now available for hepatitis A, and recommendations for administration are evolving. Hepatitis B vaccine is widely available and should be used by health care workers who come into contact with blood or blood products.

The nurse should monitor the patient with hepatitis closely for the development of signs of fulminant hepatic failure and hepatic encephalitis (see Hepatic Failure under Common Clinical Conditions). Treatment of cirrhosis that may complicate hepatitis is presented below.

Cirrhosis

Etiology/Pathophysiology

Cirrhosis is scarring of the liver that occurs as a secondary complication of liver disease or inflammation. As liver cells are destroyed, they are replaced with new cells and by fibrotic scar tissue. If the disease is limited, hepatic regeneration can occur. With chronic liver damage, however, fibrous tissue develops and the liver assumes an irregular (lobular and nodular) appearance. This fibrous alteration in liver tissue distorts and compresses liver architecture and obstructs blood flow through the liver, causing portal hypertension.

Clinical Presentation

The child with cirrhosis initially demonstrates vague symptoms of GI dysfunction, including lethargy, malaise, irritability, nausea, vomiting, anorexia, fatigue, and diarrhea or constipation. These signs result from disordered protein, glucose, and fat metabolism. The child may complain of epigastric or right upper quadrant pain. The liver ultimately becomes small and atrophied and is usually tender to palpation.

Complications of liver destruction include the metabolic derangements described in the Hepatic Failure section under Common Clinical Conditions. These include disorders of fluid and electrolyte balance, potential hepatorenal syndrome, encephalopathy, and coagulopathies. Ascites and portal hypertension may develop (see sections addressing each of these problems under Common Clinical Conditions). Any drugs or hormones normally metabolized by the liver may be present in abnormally high concentrations. All dosages of drugs should be reviewed in light of the compromise in liver function.

Management

Management of cirrhosis is largely supportive and directed at maintaining fluid and electrolyte balance and nutrition, correcting coagulopathies, and monitoring neurologic status. There is no treatment for cirrhosis. Liver transplantation may be indicated if hepatic destruction is significant.

Inflammatory Bowel Disease/ Toxic Megacolon

Etiology/Pathophysiology

Inflammatory bowel disease is a general descriptive term that includes ulcerative colitis and Crohn's disease. These chronic diseases are not often encountered in the PICU. However, toxic megacolon is one complication of inflammatory bowel disease that may require ICU therapy.

Toxic megacolon is an acute dilation of the colon secondary to severe inflammation of the bowel mucosa. This dilation may be precipitated by manipulation of the bowel during diagnostic tests. The marked dilation of the inflamed bowel causes the colon to lose its tone, and subsequent ileus and microperforations occur.

Clinical Presentation

Spiking fever and acute abdominal pain and distension in a patient at risk are the primary symptoms of toxic megacolon. However, fever may not be present in the child receiving high-dose corticosteroids. The diagnosis is confirmed with a flat-plate radiograph of the abdomen, which reveals marked dilation of the colon.

Management

Medical management includes discontinuation of oral intake and provision of supportive IV fluids, nasogastric suction, and systemic antibiotics. Steroid administration may be continued in patients with severe bowel inflammation. If toxic megacolon does not resolve with supportive medical therapy or if bowel perforation develops, urgent surgical intervention is required.

Management of Poisonings

For treatment of poisonings, see Table 10-14.

Esophageal Burns

Etiology/Pathophysiology

The most frequent cause of esophageal burns in children is the ingestion of caustic agents (e.g., lye or ammonia). The caustic agent produces a chemical burn in the oropharynx, esophagus, or stomach. The intensity of the burn varies from superficial esophagitis (erythema and some edema of the esophageal mucosa) to severe ulceration and necrosis of the esophagus and stomach. With severe burns, esophageal perforation or gastric perforation with peritonitis can occur (see Acute Abdomen under Common Clinical Conditions). A significant burn causes early mucosal ulceration, which is followed by later granulation and then fibrosis of the tissue. The fibrosis may be responsible for the later development of esophageal strictures.

Table 10-14
Commonly Used Agents in Acute Toxicologic Emergencies
This table should be viewed as a resource to rapidly confirm doses and general indications and is not a substitute for more in-depth texts or consultation with a regional poison control center.

Common Toxidromes

The following are symptoms associated with various toxins that may narrow the differential diagnosis while awaiting laboratory confirmation. Not all findings need be present, and mixed ingestions may present with confusing findings.

Narcotics. Pin-point pupils, respiratory depression, hypotension, seizures (with some agents). Symptoms reverse with naloxone.

Anticholinergics (e.g., antihistamines, atropine, phenothiazines). Flushed skin, dilated pupils, hyperreflexia, seizures, tachycardia, dry mucous membranes, decreased bowel sounds, urinary retention, fever, agitation.

Cholinergics (e.g., organophosphate and carbamate insecticides). Salivation, bronchospasm, lacrimation, diarrhea, bradycardia or tachycardia, hypotension, seizures.

Tricyclic antidepressants (e.g., imipramine, amitriptyline). Anticholinergic findings with prolongation of the QRS complex or ventricular tachyarrhythmias.

Sedatives (e.g., benzodiazepines, barbiturates). Coma, hyporeflexia, respiratory depression, hypotension, minimal to no response to naloxone.

Salicylates. Mixed respiratory alkalosis and metabolic acidosis (elevated pH with low bicarbonate).

Methanol/ethylene glycol. Severe metabolic acidosis. Visual disturbances with methanol, oxalate crystals in urine with ethylene glycol. Calculated and measured osmolality (by freezing point method) do not agree (osmolal gap).

Clonidine. Pin-point pupils, bradycardia, variable blood pressure (high or low), hypothermia, widely variable respiratory rate with intermittent apnea, waxing/waning coma. Response to naloxone controversial.

Theophylline/caffeine. Seizures, tachycardia, hypokalemia, metabolic acidosis, nausea and vomiting.

Toxin	Treatment	Dose	Comments
Narcotics	Naloxone (Narcan)	0.1 mg/kg and up as needed	Competitive-increase dose to reverse more serious intoxications
Isoniazid	Pyridoxine (B6)	Same as ingested dose or 2-5 g	May stop seizures—large amounts needed
Organophosphate insecticides	Atropine	0.01 mg/kg and up—no upper limit (minimum dose: 0.1 mg)	Will only block symptoms—pralidoxime also needed
Organophosphate insecticides	Pralidoxime (Protopam)	25-50 mg/kg	Frees the cholinesterase enzyme reversing toxicity
Tricyclic antidepressants	Sodium bicarbonate	1-2 mEq/kg	Reverses arrhythmias
Methanol/ethylene glycol	Ethanol	1 ml/kg of absolute ethanol diluted as needed	Prevents further toxic metabolite formation
Acetaminophen	N-acetylcysteine (Mucomyst)	140 mg/kg PO then 70 mg/kg q 4 hr for 3 days	Need for treatment dictated by serum level—treatment most effective in the first 12 hr after ingestion
Digoxin	Digoxin specific antibody fragments (Digibind)	Dose: 40 mg Fab/0.6mg digoxin total body burden. Calculate body burden: $\dfrac{\text{(Serum digoxin)} \times 5.6 \times \text{kg wt}}{1000}$. To determine the mg dose Fab, divide the result of the above equation by 0.6, then multiply the product by 40 mg—the result is the Digibind dose (see also Table 5-5)	Serum digoxin concentrations will increase after administration. Routine digoxin assays may be inaccurate after Digibind

Modified from Banner W: Appendix D, Poisoning and Antidotes. In Hazinski MF: *Nursing care of the critically ill child,* ed 2, St Louis 1992, Mosby.
BAL, British anti-lewisite.

Table 10-14—cont'd
Commonly Used Agents in Acute Toxicologic Emergencies
This table should be viewed as a resource to rapidly confirm doses and general indications and is not a substitute for more in-depth texts or consultation with a regional poison control center.

Toxin	Treatment	Dose	Comments
Snakebite	Polyvalent crotalidae antivenin (for rattle-snake, copperhead, and mocassin bites)	5-10 vials depending on severity	Dilute with saline (5 vials/250 ml) and administer by infusion over ≈ 2 hr
Coral snake bite	Coral Snake Antivenin	3-5 vials initially	Dilute and give slowly to avoid reactions
Black widow spider bite	Latrodectus Antivenin	Titrate one vial at a time until symptoms abate	Dilute and give slowly
Iron (also aluminum)	Deferoxamine	15 mg/kg/hr as infusion	Rapid infusion associated with hypotension
Lead	BAL (dimercaprol)	50-75 mg/m^2 IM q 4 hr (3-5 mg/kg IM q 4-6 hr)	Given deep IM—very painful and may produce febrile reaction
Lead and other heavy metals	EDTA (Calcium-disodium ethylene diamine tetraacetic acid)	25-50 mg/kg q 12 hr IV	Should not be started without BAL in severe lead intoxication Dosing guidelines vary Dilute and give as a slow infusion over 4-6 hr
Anticholinergics (antihistamines, atropine)	Physostigmine	0.01 mg/kg up to 0.5 mg slowly	May produce bradycardia, wheezing and seizures. Do not use with tricyclic antidepressant toxicity
Methemoglobinemia (from nitrites, chlorates, etc.)	Methylene blue	1 mg/kg as a 1% solution	May be ineffective or produce hemolysis in congenital enzyme defects like G6PD deficiency
Cyanide	Amyl nitrite, sodium nitrite	1 perl 5 mg/kg, repeat with methemoglobin levels known	Produces intentional methemoglobin (<20%) to bind cyanide
	Sodium thiosulfate	250-500 mg/kg	Forms thiocyanate
Insulin, oral hypoglycemic agents	Dextrose	1-2 ml/kg of 25% dextrose	May require extraordinary amounts for prolonged periods of time.

Clinical Presentation

The child usually sips only a small quantity of the caustic agent because intense burning and pain result. The mouth, lips, and larynx become edematous and covered with an exudate. With the ingestion of large quantities of a caustic liquid, similar changes occur in the distal esophagus and stomach. Dysphagia develops immediately but frequently subsides after a few days. Without early treatment, severe strictures can develop, requiring surgery.

Management

The child is not encouraged to vomit the caustic material because this can further damage the esophageal and oropharyngeal mucosa. Instead, antidotes are administered to either neutralize the ingested substance or prevent its absorption. If the pH of the ingested substance is alkaline, large amounts of water diluted with vinegar or citrus juice are administered orally to neutralize the alkali. If the pH of the ingested substance is acidic, milk, soap solutions, or aluminum hydroxide will be used as neutralizers. The hospital or regional poison control center should be consulted about antidotes once the ingested substance is identified.

Children with severe burns require administration of IV fluids. Oral fluids and foods are withheld because the burns may cause dysphagia and pain. If

---

Table 10-15
Guide to Selected Procedures and Diagnostic Tests in Pediatric Gastroenterology

Test or Procedure	General Explanation/Purpose	Equipment Used	Patient Preparation
Radiologic			
Barium swallow	Fluoroscopic x-ray examination of esophagus by a radiologist; diagnostic of structural abnormalities, motor disorders, and mucosal integrity	X-ray machine including fluoroscopic screen	None needed
Upper GI	Fluoroscopic x-ray examination of esophagus, stomach, and duodenum by a radiologist; diagnostic of structural abnormalities, motor disorders, gastroesophageal reflux, ulcerative disease, delayed gastric emptying	X-ray machine including fluoroscopic screen	Newborn-2 yr: skip last feeding before examination ≥2 yr: skip meal before examination; if scheduled in afternoon, give clear liquid breakfast that day
Upper GI with small bowel follow-through	Fluoroscopic x-ray examination by a radiologist with follow-up spot films of esophagus, stomach, duodenum, and small intestines; allows diagnosis of small bowel abnormalities, including inflammatory bowel disease and rapid GI transit time	X-ray machine including fluoroscopic screen	Same as upper GI

Modified from Hazinski MF: *Nursing care of the critically ill child,* ed 2, St Louis, 1992, Mosby.

long-term therapy is anticipated, placement of a gastrostomy tube or a central venous catheter for parenteral nutrition is indicated. Antibiotics are usually prescribed to prevent secondary infection, and corticosteroids may be administered for 7 to 10 days to reduce inflammation.

If pharyngeal edema is severe, the child may develop evidence of upper airway obstruction and respiratory distress. If these signs develop, elective intubation is performed to ensure that a patent airway is maintained.

Esophagoscopy may be performed to determine the extent of the esophageal damage. Stric-

tures may be dilated with repeated procedures over several months.

Common Diagnostic Tests

For quick reference, Table 10-15 lists the most common GI diagnostic studies and provides information regarding the purpose, equipment, patient preparation, procedure, length, and postprocedure care for each.

Procedure Involved	Approximate Duration	Postprocedure Care
Patient given small amount of liquid barium by mouth, and x-ray films are taken	5-15 min	Routine postfeeding positioning of infants Nurse must ensure fecal elimination of barium
Patient given strawberry-flavored liquid barium by mouth or tube, and x-ray films are taken	15-45 min (depends on gastric emptying time)	Same as barium swallow
Same as upper GI with added spot films at 15-min and hourly intervals until barium reaches large bowel	30 min-several hours (depends on length of time until barium reaches large bowel)	Same as barium swallow

Continued

Table 10-15—cont'd
Guide to Selected Procedures and Diagnostic Tests in Pediatric Gastroenterology

Test or Procedure	General Explanation/Purpose	Equipment Used	Patient Preparation
Radiologic—cont'd			
Barium enema (BE)	Fluoroscopic x-ray examination of large intestine by a radiologist; diagnostic of structural abnormalities and mucosal integrity	X-ray machine including fluoroscopic screen	Beyond newborn period Liquids only on day of examination Cathartic may be ordered evening before examination (individualized to patient)
Air-contrast barium enema	Same as BE; thought to be more diagnostic of mucosal integrity, especially presence of inflammation or polyps	X-ray machine including fluoroscopic screen	Same as BE; however, an empty large bowel is essential for effective examination
Endoscopy			
Flexible upper endoscopy (esophagoscopy, gastroscopy)	Direct visualization of interior upper GI tract (esophagus, stomach, duodenum) for purpose of diagnosing mucosal injury, lesions, structural abnormalities, or source of upper GI bleeding	Pediatric fibroptic endoscope (approximately 30 Fr in diameter, tubing is made of flexible rubber; a light source is attached to scope)	With general anesthesia, follow regular preoperative routine; if intravenous sedation used: NPO 8 hr preceding procedure or gastric content is removed by NG tube before endoscopy Heparin lock or IV in place Oral suction at bedside Consent form required
Flexible sigmoidoscopy or colonoscopy	Direct visualization of interior large bowel for purpose of diagnosing mucosal injury or colonic lesions or source of lower GI bleeding; can be advanced further than a rigid proctosigmoidoscope	Pediatric fiberoptic endoscope (approximately 30 Fr in diameter, tubing is made of flexible rubber)	Determined by suspected abnormality; usually, either oral cathartic and clear liquid diet 24-48 hr before procedure or enema the night before procedure Consent form required
Rigid sigmoidoscopy	Direct visualization of lower bowel lining (rectum and sigmoid) for purpose of diagnosing mucosal injury, polyp, or source of lower GI bleeding	Hollow metal cylindric scope with tapered end (size used varies with age and size of child)	Depends on suspected abnormality; usually, either oral cathartic or enema the evening before procedure

Modified from Hazinski MF: *Nursing care of the critically ill child*, ed 2, St Louis, 1992, Mosby.

Procedure Involved	Approximate Duration	Postprocedure Care
Lubricated plastic enema tip placed in rectum; barium instilled into rectum while radiologist visualizes procedure on fluroscopic screen	15-60 min; varies with each patient and suspected abnormality	Observe for passage of barium, abdominal distension, or bleeding If no passage of barium in 24 hr, cathartic administration is recommended If procedure performed in presence of intussusception or volvulus, monitor for evidence of bowel perforation (see *Acute Abdomen*)
Same as BE except less barium is instilled and air is instilled by a radiologist via a hand bulb-pump similar to that on BP cuff	15-60 min; varies with each patient and suspected abnormality	Same as BE; patient may have gas pains and pass flatus because of air insufflation
Patient placed on left side; lubricated cated end of scope passed through mouth into esophagus by physician; bite block is placed around tube between patient's teeth to prevent damage to tube; oral suction of secretions prn Scope is advanced under direct visualization by physician	15-45 min depending on examination required and suspected abnormality	NPO for 1 hr Clear liquids after 1 hr; advance to preprocedure diet
Patient placed on left side with knees drawn to chest; following finger rectal examination by physician, lubricated end of scope is passed into rectum and scope is advanced under direct visualization by physician; air and water occasionally instilled through scope to ensure optimum visualization	15-120 min depending on examination and suspected abnormality	Resume diet as before Patient may have gas pains and pass flatus or small amount of blood
Patient placed in knee-chest position or on special proctosigmoidoscopy ta ble	5-30 min depending on abnormality suspected	May have small amount of bleeding per rectum after procedure

Continued

Table 10-15—cont'd
Guide to Selected Procedures and Diagnostic Tests in Pediatric Gastroenterology

Test or Procedure	General Explanation/Purpose	Equipment Used	Patient Preparation
Biopsy			
Percutaneous liver biopsy	To obtain liver specimen without laparotomy	Disposable soft tissue biopsy tray or sterilized biopsy tray per hospital regimen	IM, sedation IV or heparin lock in place PT and PTT results on chart Consent form required NOTE: If coagulopathy is present, blood component therapy may be required before or during biopsy biopsy to prevent hemorrhage
Nuclear Medicine			
Liver-spleen scan	Scanning technique used to determine liver and spleen size or presence of mass, abscess, or other abnormality in liver or spleen; radioactive substance used is taken up by a part of the liver cells and is then counted and imaged by scanner; *does not evaluate liver function*	Scanner and radioactive substance	IV or heparin lock in place; may have regular meals before test; sedation is ordered on prn basis
Liver excretion scans (DIS-IDA, PIP-IDA and rose bengal scans)	Scanning technique used to determine liver excretory function; radioactive substance used is taken up by liver cells directly and excreted in bile through biliary tree; lack of excretion or delayed excretion raises suspicion about extrahepatic biliary atresia	Scanner and radioactive substance	IV or heparin lock in place; may have regular meals before test; sedation is ordered on prn basis.
Meckel scan	Scanning technique used to identify presence of Meckel's diverticulum; radioactive substance administered is taken up by gastric mucosal parietal cells; if extragastric mucosa is present, it is usually detected by scan	Scanner and radioactive substance	IV or heparin lock in place; NPO 4 hr before scan

Modified from Hazinski MF: Nursing care of the critically ill child, ed 2, St Louis, 1992, Mosby.

Procedure Involved	Approximate Duration	Postprocedure Care

Patient supine with arms over head; local anesthesia given	5-10 min	Monitor for signs of blood loss
		Monitor VS, with BP q15min × 1 hr
		  q30min × 2 hr
		  q1h × 4 hr
		  q2h × 12 hr
		Do not remove pressure dressing on site for 24 hr
		Have patient lie on right side for 8 hr, providing additional pressure to puncture site
		Begin giving patient clear liquids when awake, and advance to preprocedure diet as tolerated
		Monitor Hct q4h × 3 hr; monitor for signs of hemorrhage

Radioactive substance is injected IV Patient lies flat on table Scanner is lowered close to patient's body, and scan is taken Patient must lie still	1 hr	Radioactive linen precautions per nuclear medicine protocol
Same as liver spleen scan; repeated scans are usually done at 1-hr intervals	Initial scan: 1 hr; return for 2-, 4-, and 24-hr scans as needed	Radioactive linen precautions per nuclear medicine protocol
Same as above scans	1 hr	Radioactive linen precautions per nuclear medicine protocol

Suggested Readings

Alter HJ et al: The incidence of transfusion-associated hepatitis G virus infection and its relation to liver disease, *N Engl J Med* 336:747-754, 1997.

Bortolotti F et al: Hepatitis G and C virus coinfection in children, *J Pediatr* 131:639-640, 1997.

Byrne TA, Nompleggi DJ, Wilmore DW: Advances in the management of patients with intestinal failure, *Transplant Proc* 28:2683-2690, 1996.

Cook DJ et al: Stress ulcer prophylaxis in critically ill patients: resolving discordant meta-analyses, *JAMA* 275:308-314, 1996.

Gecelter GR, Comer GM: Nutritional support during liver failure, *Crit Care Clin* 11:675-683, 1995.

Heymann MB et al: Transjugular intrahepatic portosystemic shunts (TIPS) in children, *J Pediatr* 131:914-919, 1997.

Levin DL, Morriss FC, editors: *Essentials of pediatric intensive care,* ed 2, New York, 1997, Churchill Livingstone and Quality Medical Publishing.

Mathew P et al: Antioxidants in hereditary pancreatitis, *Am J Gastroenterol* 91:1558-1562, 1996.

National Institutes of Health, Office of the Director: NIH consensus statement: Management of hepatitis C, *NIH Concens Statement 1997, Mar 24-26* 15:1-41, 1997.

Neu J: Necrotizing enterocolitis: the search for a unifying pathogenic theory leading to prevention, *Pediatr Clin North Am* 43:409-432, 1996.

Price MR et al: Management of esophageal varices in children by endoscopic variceal ligation, *J Pediatr Surg* 31:1056-1059, 1996.

Schneider BL: Neonatal liver failure, *Curr Opin Pediatr* 8:495-501, 1996.

Splawski JB: Gastrointestinal bleeding. In Levin DL, Morriss FC, editors: *Essentials of pediatric intensive care,* ed 2, New York, 1997, Churchill Livingston and Quality Medical Publishers.

Sussman NL, Kelly JH: Extracorporeal liver support: cell-based therapy for the failing liver, *Am J Kidney Dis* 30:S66-S71, 1997.

Sussman NL, Lake JR: Treatment of hepatic failure—1996: current concepts and progress toward liver dialysis, *Am J Kidney Dis* 27:605-621, 1996.

Thornton PS, Berry GT, Stanley CA: Disorders of intermediary metabolism. In Holbrook PR, editor: *Textbook of pediatric critical care,* Philadelphia, 1992, WB Saunders.

Tryba M, Cook D: Current guidelines on stress ulcer prophylaxis, *Drugs* 54(4):581-596, 1997.

Wolff JA, Gilbert-Barness E, Barness LA: Disorders /diseases of inborn errors of metabolism that produce critical illness. In Fuhrman BP, Zimmerman JJ, editors: *Pediatric critical care,* ed 2, St Louis, 1997, Mosby.

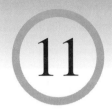

Hematologic and Oncologic Emergencies Requiring Critical Care

Pearls

- Severe anemia associated with a hemoglobin (Hgb) concentration <5 g/dl and a hematocrit (Hct) <15% is likely to produce congestive heart failure (CHF). Transfusion must be accomplished slowly (3 ml/kg/hr of packed red blood cells [PRBCs]).
- Complete bone marrow failure produces a fall in Hgb of approximately 0.8 g/dl/week; a more precipitous fall in Hgb is likely to be caused by bleeding or increased RBC destruction.
- The risk of spontaneous bleeding is increased if the platelet count is <20,000/mm^3, and intracranial hemorrhage is more likely once the platelet count is <5000/mm^3.
- Rule out intracranial hemorrhage in any child with severe thrombocytopenia and unilateral headache. If hemorrhage is suspected, stabilize first; obtain scans and radiographs later.
- Acute tumor lysis syndrome produces hypocalcemia, hyperkalemia, hyperuricemia, and hyperphosphatemia; disseminated intravascular coagulation (DIC) is also possible.
- An absolute neutrophil count [(percent polymorphonuclear neutrophils + percent bands) × white blood cell count] <500/mm^3 is associated with a significant risk of infection. Monitor these patients closely.
- Whenever blood products are administered, label the crossmatched specimen carefully and double-check patient and blood product identification (an extra time).

Additional Helpful Chapters

Chapter 2: Psychosocial Aspects of Pediatric Critical Care, entire chapter
Chapter 3: Analgesia, Sedation, and Neuromuscular Blockade in Pediatric Critical Care, entire chapter
Chapter 4: The Dying Child in the Intensive Care Unit, entire chapter
Chapter 5: Shock, Congestive Heart Failure, Sepsis
Chapter 6: Respiratory Failure, Airway Obstruction
Chapter 8: Increased Intracranial Pressure, Neurologic Assessment
Chapter 9: Fluid and Electrolyte Balance, Renal Failure
Chapter 10: Fluid and Electrolyte Balance

Essential Anatomy and Physiology

Blood Components

Blood transports oxygen and nutrients, buffers acid-base balance, and maintains hemostasis. It consists of a liquid phase (plasma), which contains clotting factors and serum (electrolytes, hormones, nutrients, etc.), and a formed phase, including red blood cells (RBCs), white blood cells (WBCs), and platelets. RBCs, WBCs, and platelets arise from multipotential stem cells in the bone marrow.

Red Blood Cells

RBCs are produced in the bone marrow, with a 120-day life span (shorter for transfused cells). Nuclei are normally extruded before the RBCs reach the peripheral circulation; thus the presence of nucleated RBCs in peripheral blood means that increased bone marrow activity is present. The *reticulocyte count* indicates the proportion of immature RBCs in the circulation:

- A high reticulocyte count indicates increased RBC production and possible increased destruction.
- A low reticulocyte count indicates that RBCs are not being produced.

The hemoglobin (Hgb) content of the peripheral circulation and the RBC count will reflect the oxygen-carrying capacity of the blood. Both can be directly measured; normal values vary with age.

The hematocrit (Hct), or packed cell volume (PCV) is the percentage of cells present in a volume of blood spun in a capillary tube. This result should be available immediately.

Polycythemia is an abnormally *high* Hgb or Hct. It is often a compensatory mechanism for chronic hypoxemia (e.g., in a child with cyanotic congenital heart disease) or alveolar hypoxia (e.g., in an infant born at high altitude). If the Hct approaches 60%, complications can result from increased blood viscosity (see Chapter 5, p. 196).

Anemia is an abnormally *low* Hgb or Hct, caused by a loss or decreased production of RBCs. Anemia may be asymptomatic if it develops gradually. Severe or acute anemia (e.g., caused by

trauma or hemolysis) often produces cardiovascular compromise.

Platelets

Platelets are important in hemostasis and in wound healing. Platelets are released into the peripheral circulation from megakaryocytes in the bone marrow, with a normal life span of 7 to 10 days.

White Blood Cells

The term *white blood cell (WBC),* or *leukocyte,* includes several different cell types. All WBCs defend the body from infection, but each has a different appearance and function. The WBC differential indicates the percent of the total WBC count contributed by each cell type. Analysis of the WBC differential can support or rule out the suspicion of bacterial infection or an inflammatory process (Table 11-1). WBCs are divided into two basic groups:

- *Granulocytes:* WBCs that contain granules in their cytoplasm (include neutrophils, eosinophils, and basophils)
- *Nongranular leukocytes:* WBCs that contain clear cytoplasm (include monocytes and lymphocytes)

Neutrophils provide the primary defense against bacterial infections. The neutrophil contains a multilobed nucleus, and it is referred to as a polymorphonuclear neutrophil (PMN, or "poly"). Neutrophils constitute approximately 40% of the total WBC count in children younger than 5 years of age, and approximately 60% to 70% of the WBCs in children older than 5 years of age. Neutrophils are subdivided in the report of the WBC differential according to the appearance of the nucleus. Segmented neutrophils, or "segs," are the mature form of neutrophils and constitute approximately 56% of the WBCs. Band neutrophils are the immature form of neutrophils and normally comprise only 3% of the WBCs.

During infection the bone marrow releases neutrophils in all stages of development, and the percentage of band forms is increased. This increase is referred to as a "left shift" (because the WBC differential was formerly reported horizontally on a sheet, with band forms on the left).

Table 11-1
Normal Differential and Function of White Blood Cells

Cell Type	Absolute No. (mm³)	Differential (%)	Function/Change
Total WBCs	5,000-10,000	100	↑With infection ↓With bone marrow suppression
Granulocytes			
Neutrophils	Newborn: (at birth) 2000-6000 12 hr-1 wk: 7000-14,000 1-4 wk: 1800-5400 6 mo: 1000-8500 1-5 yr: 1500-8000 >5 hr: 1800-7700	 32 30-42 50	↑With inflammation or infection ↓With bone marrow suppression
(Adult differential)	Adult: 3000-7000	60-70	
Segmented	2800-5600	56	↑Value = right shift
Bands	150-600	3-6	↑Value = left shift
Eosinophils	50-400	1-4	↑In allergy or parasitic infection
Basophils	25-100	0.5-1	Not affected by infection Involved in immediate hypersensitivity
Nongranulocytes			
Monocytes	100-800	2-8	↑With chronic infection, TB, malaria, some viruses
Lymphocytes	Infants: 2000-10,000 >6 hr: 1000-4000	60 30-40	↑In viral infection ↓In HIV disease
T cells	800-3200	80*	
B cells	1-600	10-15*	
NK	50-400	5-10*	

Modified from Tribett D: Immune system function: implications for critical care nursing practice, *Crit Care Nurs Clin North Am* 1:725-740, 1989; data from Dallman PR: White blood cells. In Rudolph AM, editor: *Pediatrics,* ed 19, Norwalk, Conn, 1991, Appleton & Lange.
*Percent of total lymphocyte count.

Leukemia is cancer of WBCs. Immature lymphoid or myeloid cells (blasts) fill the bone marrow and crowd out normal cells. When leukemia is present, leukemic cells may be found in the peripheral circulation, as well as in the marrow.

Clotting Cascade

Normal hemostasis is maintained by a complex balance of procoagulant and anticoagulant factors. These factors together provide rapid, localized control of bleeding at sites of injury, while preventing the clotting process in unaffected tissues. A simplified scheme of the coagulation process is shown in Figure 11-1.

The *partial thromboplastin time (PTT)* measures activity of the *intrinsic and common* pathways and thus can be used to screen for deficiencies of plasma coagulation. Since factors VII and XIII must be activated by tissue injury (the extrinsic pathway), they are *not* evaluated by PTT. A prolonged (abnormal) PTT can be caused by coagulation factor deficiencies, heparin administration, and disseminated intravascular coagulation (DIC).

The prothrombin time (PT) measures activity of the *extrinsic* pathway; thus it can screen for deficiencies of factor VII. A PT is useful to monitor warfarin (Coumadin) therapy and may be abnormal if DIC is present.

In normal clot formation, thrombin stimulates conversion of fibrinogen to fibrin, and fibrin monomers form clot latticework. The presence of *fibrin monomer* in the blood indicates activation of the clotting cascade and *clot formation.* Fibrin

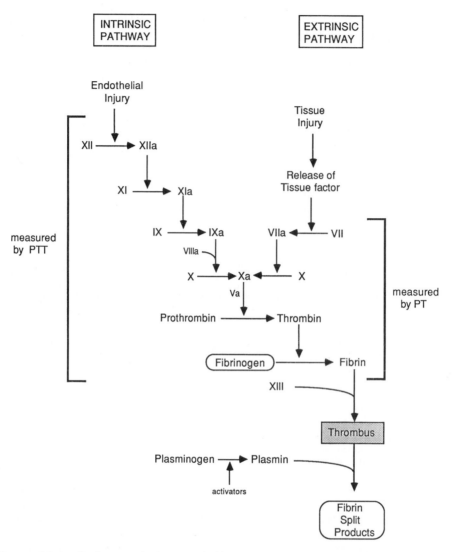

Figure 11-1 Clotting cascade. (From Hazinski MF: *Nursing care of the critically ill child,* ed 2, St Louis, 1992, Mosby.)

monomer can usually be detected by studies performed on the same blood sample as the PT and PTT.

Clot lysis begins whenever fibrin is formed to create a clot. *Fibrin split products* (FSPs) are released when factor XII activates the fibrinolytic system and fibrin is broken down. The presence and quantity of FSPs can be used to monitor the degree of activation of the fibrinolytic system. FSPs are quantified using a blood sample sent in a thrombin-containing tube. A rise in FSPs may be caused by normal clot breakdown after surgery, trauma, burns, DIC, or liver disease (FSPs are normally cleared by the liver).

Spleen

The spleen is a large, vascular organ located in the left upper quadrant of the abdomen behind the stomach and just beneath the left diaphragm. It removes aged and damaged RBCs, platelets, and encapsulated bacteria from the circulation. In addition, the spleen is a site of antibody production.

If the spleen is absent or nonfunctional, nuclear remnants within RBCs, called *Howell-Jolly bodies,* may be observed on a peripheral blood sample. The presence of Howell-Jolly bodies should raise the suspicion of asplenia or splenic dysfunction (functional asplenia).

Asplenia increases the risk for the development of infection from encapsulated organisms, such as *Haemophilus influenzae* or a pneumococcus *(Streptococcus pneumoniae),* which may produce overwhelming and fatal sepsis. Antibiotic prophylaxis with penicillin and pneumococcal vaccination are needed to decrease the risk of septicemia in patients with functional or true asplenia.

The spleen is normally palpable in infants and very young children. *Splenomegaly* is present if the spleen tip descends below the edge of the right costal margin in a child older than 6 months of age. *Hypersplenism* is increased splenic function usually associated with physical enlargement, with resultant entrapment and destruction of normal blood cells and consequent reduction in circulating blood cells.

Common Clinical Conditions

Acute Anemia

Etiology/Pathophysiology

Severe anemia reduces the oxygen content and oxygen-carrying capacity of the blood; thus cardiac output must increase to maintain oxygen delivery. If cardiac output *cannot* increase adequately, oxygen delivery will fall, and metabolic acidosis will develop. Causes of life-threatening anemia include acute blood loss, decreased RBC production, splenic sequestration, and hemolysis.

Acute blood loss produces equivalent loss of plasma and RBCs; thus Hgb and Hct may be normal until crystalloid solutions are administered. The crystalloid administration dilutes the remaining cells, and a fall in Hgb and Hct results.

Decreased RBC production can result from replacement of normal bone marrow by tumor or aplastic anemia (associated with hepatitis, administration of chloramphenicol or benzene, or an autoimmune process).

In *complete bone marrow failure,* Hgb falls by approximately 0.8 g/dl/week, producing chronic rather than acute anemia. If the Hgb falls more rapidly in the patient with bone marrow suppression, hemorrhage or increased RBC destruction is probably present.

Less common causes of decreased RBC formation include transient erythroblastopenia of childhood (TEC) and congenital RBC aplasia (Diamond-Blackfan syndrome).

Causes of acute RBC destruction (hemolysis) include intrinsic abnormalities of the RBC or altered antigen or antibody production (i.e., immune-mediated hemolytic anemia, which may be caused by infection or drugs). Antibodies may make crossmatching of the RBCs by standard Coombs testing impossible, so that *all units that are transfused will be labeled incompatible by the blood bank.*

Clinical Presentation

Signs of chronic anemia will differ from those of acute or severe anemia. When *chronic* anemia is present, cardiac output may increase commensurately, and intravascular volume is maintained through renal fluid retention. Decompensation will occur if cardiac output is compromised or oxygen requirements increase (e.g., fever).

Signs and symptoms of *acute* anemia include:

- Pallor, weakness, fatigue, and lethargy. A systolic flow murmur may be present.
- If Hct is < 9% or Hgb is <3 g/dl: development of high-output congestive heart failure (CHF), producing tachycardia (with gallop), pulmonary edema, and hepato-splenomegaly. NOTE: If the fall in Hct and Hgb is more acute, symptoms will likely develop earlier.
- If anemia is caused by hemorrhage: signs of shock, including signs of poor systemic perfusion, acidosis, altered level of consciousness.
- If anemia is caused by acute hemolysis: jaundice, splenomegaly.

Laboratory studies will reveal a fall in hematocrit. RBC hemolysis will produce elevated bilirubin and lactic dehydrogenase (LDH) levels. The reticulocyte count is decreased in disorders of RBC production and increased if RBC destruction is occurring (e.g., hemolytic process).

Management

If severe cardiorespiratory distress is present:

1. Administer oxygen.
2. Insert two large-bore venous catheters (or intraosseous needle, particularly for children younger than 6 years). Consider intraarterial monitoring if shock is present.
3. Obtain a complete blood count with reticulocyte count, and blood for type and crossmatch and venous pH. If possible, obtain and save a purple-top (EDTA) and green-top (heparin) tube for later determination of the cause of the anemia.
4. Begin RBC transfusion (see Care of the Patient During Transfusion Therapy, p. 569, and Box 11-4).
   a. *Chronic anemia:* Administer 3 ml/kg/ hr of PRBCs (this rate prevents hypervolemia and the development or worsening of CHF). Consider continuous diuretic therapy.
   b. *Severe CHF and anemia:* Partial exchange transfusion (remove anemic blood and replace with packed RBCs [PRBCs]).
   c. *Hemolytic anemia due to intrinsic RBC abnormalities:* RBC transfusions.
   d. *Immune-mediated hemolytic anemia:* May not respond to transfusions (antibodies may attack transfused, as well as native, RBCs). If transfusions are attempted, blood is crossmatched *in vivo*— blood is administered, and the patient is monitored closely for transfusion reaction (see Care of the Patient During Transfusion Therapy). Steroid therapy (prednisone, 2 to 10 mg/kg/day) or splenectomy may reduce RBC antibody destruction.

If cardiorespiratory distress is *not* present, transfusion can be accomplished on an elective basis. If chronic anemia is present, see step 4a.

Thrombocytopenia
Etiology/Pathophysiology

Thrombocytopenia is a decreased level of circulating platelets ($<150,000/mm^3$), which may result from decreased platelet production or increased platelet destruction. Common causes of thrombocytopenia are listed in Box 11-1. The etiology of thrombocytopenia must be determined to select the appropriate therapy.

Potential causes of *decreased platelet production* include bone marrow failure, bone marrow dysfunction, or temporary suppression of bone marrow. Increased platelet destruction may be immune-mediated. Immune-mediated platelet destruction occurs when antibodies bind to platelets, resulting in their removal by the spleen and liver. Platelet-specific antibody production may be triggered by viral infection, drugs (e.g., heparin), or breakdown in the body's ability to recognize its own antigens (e.g., systemic lupus erythematosus and other collagen vascular diseases).

Clinical Presentation

The thrombocytopenic patient must be monitored closely for evidence of bleeding:

- *Signs of external bleeding:* Petechiae, ecchymoses, epistaxis, or gingival oozing
- *Signs of internal bleeding:* Gross or microscopic hematuria, melena, guaiac-positive stools or emesis, a drop in PCV or Hct, and

---

Box 11-1

Causes of Thrombocytopenia

Decreased production: Bone marrow failure (aplastic anemia), bone marrow replacement, congenital amegakaryocytosis, bone marrow suppression

Increased destruction: Idiopathic thrombocytopenic purpura (ITP), disseminated intravascular coagulation (DIC), thrombotic thrombocytopenic purpura (TTP), collagen vascular diseases, hemolytic-uremic syndrome (HUS), isoimmune neonatal thrombocytopenia, hypersplenism, toxin (snakebite)

sudden cardiovascular changes consistent with hemorrhage (tachycardia, orthostatic hypotension, peripheral vasoconstriction)

Spontaneous bleeding may occur when the platelet count is <20,000. Spontaneous intracranial hemorrhage may occur when the platelet count is <5000.

Rule out intracranial hemorrhage in any child with critical thrombocytopenia who develops headache or a change in mental status. Other signs of intracranial hemorrhage include lateralizing neurologic signs, such as altered movement, strength, or sensation in extremities, or unilateral pupil dilation.

Management

For *severe thrombocytopenia* (platelet count <20,000), perform frequent neurologic examinations, particularly with any change in patient condition, to detect early signs of intracranial hemorrhage. Development of unilateral headache should be presumed to indicate intracranial hemorrhage until this complication has been ruled out. A bone marrow sample may be obtained before treatment of immune-mediated thrombocytopenia to establish the cause.

General Care   Monitor continuously for evidence of frank bleeding. Perform a guaiac test on any body fluid, but this test is routinely positive in thrombocytopenic patients.

Provide a soft mechanical diet and stool softeners. Do not administer rectal medications or evaluate rectal temperature. Avoid intramuscular injections and apply prolonged pressure over any venipuncture sites. Aspirin or other medications containing salicylates and any antiinflammatory agents that inhibit platelet function are contraindicated.

Treatment of Reduced Platelet Production   Care is largely supportive until the underlying cause resolves. Platelet transfusion will restore the platelet count only if the thrombocytopenia is due to decreased platelet production.

Treatment of Increased Platelet Destruction   Platelet transfusion is usually ineffective, since the transfused platelets will be destroyed by the underlying mechanism. When life-threatening bleeding is present, platelets will be administered. This may slow bleeding but usually will not result in an increase in the platelet count.

Severe *immune-mediated thrombocytopenia* may require drug administration to reduce the antibody-mediated platelet destruction:

- Corticosteroids: prednisone, 4 to 8 mg/kg/day
- Intravenous (IV) immunoglobulin: 0.5 to 1 g/kg of IgG
- High-dose methylprednisolone: 30 to 50 mg/kg/day for severe bleeding

The platelet count may rise over several hours or days, or effective platelet transfusion may be possible.

When immune-mediated thrombocytopenia produces intracranial or other life-threatening hemorrhage, emergent splenectomy is typically performed. Additional extreme measures include continuous infusion of platelets or administration of cytotoxic agents. The patient's blood may be filtered using an immunoglobulin G (IgG) absorbance column (absorbs the patient's IgG and may enable successful platelet transfusion).

Disseminated Intravascular Coagulation

Etiology/Pathophysiology

Disseminated intravascular coagulation (DIC) is a process of excessive coagulation that develops secondary to other diseases or disorders. DIC is most frequently associated with infection or shock but may complicate trauma (particularly head injury), malignancies, vascular abnormalities, poisoning, or hemolytic reactions (Box 11-2).

The patient with DIC demonstrates evidence of both excessive *clotting* (with a fall in fibrinogen, consumptive coagulopathy, and presence of fibrin monomer) and *clot breakdown* (with a resultant rise in levels of fibrin degradation products).

With low fibrin degradation product DIC, clot formation predominates and the risk of embolic vascular obstruction is high. Renal artery embolization will produce renal failure, and peripheral

Box 11-2

Causes of Disseminated Intravascular Coagulation

Infection: Gram-positive or gram-negative bacteria, viruses, rickettsiae (Rocky Mountain spotted fever)
Shock: Septic, hypovolemic, cardiogenic, anaphylactic
Trauma: Head injuries, crushing injuries, burns, surgery
Malignancies
Obstetrical problems: Placental abruption, retained dead fetus, amniotic fluid embolization
Vascular: Giant hemangiomas (Kasabach-Merritt syndrome)
Venomous snakebite
Transfusion reaction
Heat stroke

Table 11-2

Laboratory Findings Consistent With Disseminated Intravascular Coagulation

Laboratory Test	Normal Value	DIC
Platelet count	150,000-450,000/mm^3	<150,000
Partial thromboplastin time (PTT)	25-35 sec Patient/control ratio 1.0 Preterm newborn: 80-150 sec Term newborn: 65-84 sec Adult: 44-55 sec	Ratio >1.5
Prothrombin time (PT)	10-14 sec Patient/control ratio 1.0 Preterm newborn: 16-20 sec Term newborn: 13.5-16 sec Adult: 12-14 sec	Ratio >1.5
Fibrinogen	175-400	<175
Fibrin split products (qualitative)	<10	>10-40 or >40
Fibrin monomer	Negative	Positive (1+ to 4+)

From Hazinski MF: *Nursing care of the critically ill child,* ed 2, St Louis, 1992, Mosby.

extremity embolization will result in ischemia and necrosis of digits or extremities.

Clinical Presentation

Many PICU patients are at risk for the development of DIC, since they are hospitalized with conditions known to precipitate this disorder. The diagnosis should be suspected if new evidence of gastrointestinal bleeding or prolonged mucosal or skin oozing is observed.

Monitor the child closely for evidence of cerebrovascular accident or thrombotic manifestations, including pulmonary embolism, stroke, renal failure, or ischemia or gangrene of extremities. Report changes in level of consciousness, poor peripheral perfusion (particularly if localized), or decreased urine volume immediately.

Laboratory abnormalities consistent with DIC include thrombocytopenia, prolonged PT or PTT, decreased fibrinogen, elevated fibrin degradation products (fibrin split products), and anemia (Table 11-2). The presence of fibrin monomer is an early indication of DIC, indicating that fibrinogen is being broken down by thrombin and a clot is being formed.

Management

Once the diagnosis of DIC is made, the patient's clinical course and response to therapy must be closely monitored. *The primary goal in the management of DIC is treatment of the precipitating cause.*

Blood products may be administered to reverse existing coagulation abnormalities (e.g., platelets to treat thrombocytopenia, fresh frozen plasma to replace clotting factors, or cryoprecipitate to elevate fibrinogen levels). Heparin is not effective in the treatment of most forms of DIC. In fact, since heparin cofactor (antithrombin III [AT III]) concentration is low in DIC, heparin may be ineffective.

Box 11-3

Determination of Severity of Neutropenia

Absolute neutrophil count (ANC) = (Percent polys + Percent bands) $\times$ WBC count

ANC greater than 1000 = No increase in risk of infection
ANC of 500 to 1000 = Moderate risk of infection
ANC of less than 500 = Significant risk of infection
ANC of less than 300 = Profound risk of infection

From Hazinski MF: *Nursing care of the critically ill child,* ed 2, St Louis, 1992, Mosby.

The primary indication for heparin administration in DIC is *purpura fulminans* (i.e., DIC with necrosis of digits and thromboembolic phenomena). In this form of DIC, clot formation predominates, and the fibrin degradation products are only moderately elevated, suggesting that little clot breakdown is occurring. Plasma *must* be administered before heparin therapy, to restore levels of antithrombin III so that heparin will produce anticoagulation. Purified antithrombin III is now available and may be useful.

Neutropenia

Etiology/Pathophysiology

Neutropenia is a neutrophil count $<1500/mm^3$. Neutrophils provide the major defense against bacterial invasion; thus neutropenia is associated with increased risk of infection. Since the risk of infection is related to the severity of the neutropenia, the *absolute neutrophil count (ANC)* is calculated to monitor the infection risk (Box 11-3).

An ANC $<500/mm^3$ is associated with a significant risk of infection, and an ANC $<300/mm^3$ is associated with a profound risk of infection. If the neutropenia is immune mediated, the risk of infection may be lower at a given WBC count than it would be if the neutropenia resulted from failure to produce neutrophils.

Neutropenic patients most commonly become infected by organisms from their own stool or oral cavity. These opportunistic infections include *Staphylococcus epidermidis, Staphylococcus aureus, Klebsiella* organisms, *Escherichia coli,* and *Pseudomonas* organisms.

Clinical Presentation

Surveillance of neutropenic patients for sources of infection must be continuous, and presence of infection must always be suspected. Since the neutrophils participate in the inflammatory response, clinical signs of inflammation may not be observed when infection develops. Fever, nonspecific signs of distress, or characteristic skin lesions may be the only sign of infection in the neutropenic patient.

Blood cultures are frequently drawn to detect bacteremia, but they may be negative despite the presence of infection. Serial blood cultures are often ordered when the patient is severely neutropenic to increase the probability of bacterial capture. It is important that these cultures be obtained correctly despite the discomfort to the patient.

Management

Neutropenic patients must be thoroughly evaluated whenever infection is suspected. Evaluation and treatment are required when fever develops, and broad-spectrum antibiotics will be initiated immediately. Fungal infection should also be suspected and ruled out.

Administration of Colony-Stimulating Factors

Since severity and duration of neutropenia have

been directly linked with risk of infection, significant neutropenia may be treated with colony-stimulating factors (CSFs). CSFs are glycoproteins that stimulate the production of WBCs. Two forms of CSFs made by recombinant technology are now available: granulocyte CSF (G-CSF) and granulocyte-macrophage CSF (GM-CSF).

Administration of either G-CSF or GM-CSF leads to an increase in WBC number and function and reduces the incidence of infection and risk of sepsis in neutropenic patients. Administration guidelines include:

- G-CSF is approved for prophylactic use following chemotherapy, beginning 1 day after the last dose of chemotherapy. The most common adverse reaction is bone pain.
- GM-CSF is approved for use following bone marrow transplantation. Adverse reactions include sensitivity reactions, with fever, chills, lethargy, and erythematous lesions. GM-CSF may reactivate autoimmune diseases.
- Approximate dose is 5 to10 μg/kg/day over 1 hour intravenously or subcutaneously.
- Administration is usually discontinued when the neutrophil count is ≥5000 to 7000/mm^3.
- During CSF therapy, monitor complete blood counts with WBC differential and liver and kidney function twice a week. Blood sampling should be performed just before rather than just after CSF administration, since both types of CSFs cause a transient leukopenia before the increase in WBCs.

Reverse Isolation   Reverse isolation is *not* effective in preventing infection in neutropenic patients, since they are usually infected by their own indigenous organisms. *Good handwashing technique* must be practiced by hospital staff, the patient, and the family to prevent infection from other sources.

Suspected Infection   Obtain blood cultures and begin prophylactic *parenteral* antibiotics immediately. Administer doses on time. Since sepsis may be rapidly progressive in these patients, any delay in antibiotic therapy may be fatal.

Acute Tumor Lysis Syndrome
Etiology/Pathophysiology

Acute tumor lysis syndrome (ATLS) consists of several metabolic abnormalities that occur as a consequence of rapid tumor cell breakdown. ATLS is most likely to develop during initial administration of chemotherapeutic agents, in untreated patients with rapidly growing tumors (particularly Burkitt's lymphoma and T-cell leukemias and lymphomas), and in any patient with a bulky lymphoma or leukemia and a high WBC count.

The rapid destruction and lysis of tumor cells results in the release of their intracellular contents into the circulation, producing elevated levels of uric acid, potassium, and phosphate. Tissue thromboplastin is also released from myelogenous WBCs or tumor. ATLS is characterized by the following metabolic complications:

- Uric acid precipitates in the kidneys and urinary tract, producing renal obstruction and/or failure.
- Hyperkalemia can produce cardiac arrhythmias.
- Phosphate may precipitate with calcium in the kidney, resulting in ionized hypocalcemia and renal failure.
- Tissue thromboplastin release may precipitate DIC.

Clinical Presentation

ATLS is recognized by the electrolyte imbalances and organ failures it produces:

1. *Hyperuricemia and hyperphosphatemia* can cause urinary obstruction or renal failure. Uric acid precipitation is enhanced if the urine is acidic (pH <7). Suspect urinary obstruction or renal failure if urine output decreases. Hyperphosphatemia is usually asymptomatic, but symptoms do result from the hypocalcemia it produces.
2. *Hypocalcemia:*
   a. *Clinical signs:* Tingling, muscle cramping, lethargy, seizures, carpal-pedal spasm, or *positive Chvostek's sign* (contraction of facial muscles after tapping the facial nerve just anterior to the parotid gland).

b. *Electrocardiogram (ECG) changes:* Prolonged QT interval or bradycardia.
3. *Hyperkalemia:*
   a. *Clinical signs:* Weakness, tingling, and loss of sensation.
   b. *ECG changes:* Peaked T waves, increased PR interval, widening of the QRS complex, and arrhythmias.
4. *DIC:* Microscopic or gross bleeding, presence of fibrin monomer, and fibrin split products (see Disseminated Intravascular Coagulation).

Management

Prevention   The best treatment for ATLS is its prevention. This requires recognition of patients at risk and institution of therapy (including generous IV fluid administration) designed to minimize the complications of rapid cell breakdown. The initial chemotherapy dose may be reduced in patients with lymphoma to prevent rapid tumor breakdown.

Monitor renal function closely during initial chemotherapy. In high-risk patients, a urinary catheter is placed to enable continuous evaluation of urine output. Monitor urine pH and serum electrolytes and creatinine frequently. Mild renal dysfunction may respond to diuretic therapy; however, hemodialysis or peritoneal dialysis may be required if renal failure develops.

To prevent uric acid crystals and eliminate products of cell breakdown:

- If cardiac function is adequate, administer 1½ to 2 times maintenance fluid requirements (or 3000 ml/m^2 body surface area [BSA]/day).
- Alkalinize the urine (to pH of approximately 7) with IV sodium bicarbonate. Avoid excessive alkalinization (urine pH >8), which may precipitate calcium phosphate.
- Administer allopurinol (100 to 300 mg/day PO) to reduce uric acid production. Note that allopurinol administration may produce xanthine nephropathy and renal failure.

If urine output falls to <1 to 2 ml/kg/hr, assess the child's intravascular volume status. Insertion of a central venous pressure (CVP) monitoring catheter may be required:

- *CVP <2 to 5 mm Hg:* Additional fluid administration is probably required.
- *CVP >8 to 10 mm Hg:* Hypervolemia is present, and diuretic therapy is indicated.

Urgent Therapy   Urgent therapy is necessary for severe hyperkalemia or hypocalcemia. Hyperkalemia associated with arrhythmias requires urgent therapy:

1. Prevent potassium cardiac effects: administer calcium gluconate, 60 to 100 mg/kg IV or calcium chloride (20 to 25 mg/kg IV) (may repeat $\times$ 1).
2. Shift potassium from the vascular space (into cells):
   a. Administer sodium bicarbonate, 1 to 2 mEq/kg.
   b. Administer glucose (1 to 2 ml/kg of 25% dextrose) or glucose plus insulin (0.1 U/kg regular insulin).
3. Remove potassium from the body:
   a. *Gastrointestinal:* Administer sodium polystyrene resin (Kayexalate), 0.5 to 1 g/kg orally or as an enema (works over 4 to 6 hours).
   b. *Renal:* Administer furosemide, 1 mg/kg IV.
   c. *Total body:* Dialysis or exchange transfusion (see p. 469).

Monitor and maintain total (normal: 8.8 to 10.8 mg/dl) and ionized (normal: 4.5 to 5.6 mg/dl) serum calcium levels. Provide early correction of hypocalcemia, particularly if serum alkalinization is planned to prevent renal uric acid crystals or treat hyperkalemia. Such alkalinization will further reduce serum ionized calcium.

Hypercalcemia

Etiology/Pathophysiology

Hypercalcemia is associated with some malignancies (lymphocytic leukemia, many lymphomas, soft tissue sarcomas) that secrete a parathormone-like substance that stimulates bone reabsorption and release of calcium. Serum calcium levels as high as 19 to 20 mg/dl (normal 8.8 to 10.8 mg/dl) may result.

Significant hypercalcemia (total serum calcium ≥15 mg/dl) may produce renal and cardiovascular complications. The effects of the hypercalcemia will be exacerbated in the presence of acidosis or hypoalbuminemia, which increases serum ionized calcium.

Clinical Presentation

Classic signs and symptoms of hypercalcemia (the child with moderate hypercalcemia may be asymptomatic) include:

- Renal stones, osteoporosis, and neuromuscular pain or tingling
- Polyuria, polydipsia, and low urine specific gravity (renal concentrating ability is compromised)

Hypertension, which is common in adults, is rare in children.

Signs of severe/life-threatening hypercalcemia include:

- Lethargy or a change in mental status
- Decreased myocardial function or arrhythmias

Management

Monitor the serum calcium level closely in any child presenting with a lymphocytic leukemia, lymphoma, or soft tissue sarcoma, and report high or rising calcium level to a physician without delay.

During any therapy designed to reduce the serum calcium, the patient's ionized and total calcium levels must be monitored closely to prevent profound hypocalcemia.

Fluid administration replaces fluid losses and promotes urinary excretion of calcium. Steroid administration promotes calcium excretion, and calcitonin promotes calcium deposition in bone (Table 11-3). Antineoplastic therapy or chelation may also be required.

Hyperleukocytosis

Etiology/Pathophysiology

Hyperleukocytosis is a markedly high WBC count ($>300,000/mm^3$), which may be observed in children with leukemia, including those with acute nonlymphocytic leukemia (ANLL), such as acute myelogenous leukemia (AML), or those with acute lymphocytic leukemia (ALL). Patients with ANLL are at higher risk of complications from hyperleukocytosis than patients with ALL, because the myeloid blasts are more adherent than the lymphoid blasts.

Central nervous system (CNS) complications of hyperleukocytosis include intracranial hemorrhage (particularly likely when coagulopathy is present in patients with ANLL) or cerebral thromboembolus (e.g., infarction). Pulmonary complications may be directly related to this high WBC count. Sequestration of blast cells in

---

Table 11-3
Treatment of Hypercalcemia

Mild Hypercalcemia (<15 g/dl)	Severe Hypercalcemia (>15 g/dl)
Treat cause	Eliminate calcium intake; evaluate digitalis dose
Monitor cardiovascular function closely	Monitor cardiovascular function closely
Normal saline administration (bolus until urine output >1-2 ml/kg/hr)	Normal saline bolus (10 ml/kg) plus forosemide (1 mg/kg); may repeat
Increase phosphate intake	IV phosphate: 0.5-1 mmol/kg over 12 hr
Eliminate all sources of calcium intake	Calcitonin: 3-6 U/kg IV every 24 hr
Evaluate digitalis dose (hypercalcemia may perpetuate digitalis-related arrhythmias)	Consider chelation with EDTA (edetate disodium): 15-50 mg/kg over 4 hr
	Mithramycin (antineoplastic agent)
	Prednisone: 1-2 mg/kg/day in 4 IV doses or hydrocortisone: 1 mg/kg every 6hr

the lungs may produce intrapulmonary shunting and pulmonary infiltrates on chest x-ray examination.

Clinical Presentation

Frequent assessment of neurologic and pulmonary function is required to detect early evidence of cerebrovascular accident or pulmonary sequestration.

Evaluate level of consciousness, responsiveness, ability to follow commands, spontaneous movement, voluntary and antigravity muscle strength, and pupil size and response to light several times each day and hourly (or more frequently) when changes are noted. Unilateral headache in the child with hyperleukocytosis should be presumed to be caused by an intracranial hemorrhage or thromboembolism until these complications have been ruled out.

A computed tomography (CT) scan or magnetic resonance imaging (MRI) can confirm the development of cerebral thromboembolism or hemorrhage. However, these *diagnostic studies should be performed only if the child is stable.*

Clinical signs of pulmonary sequestration include tachypnea, increased respiratory effort, and hypoxemia despite oxygen therapy. Pulse oximetry should be used to detect hypoxemia.

Management

Prevention Preventive strategies include prophylactic CNS radiation, exchange transfusion, and leukapheresis before initiation of chemotherapy. CNS radiation may prevent cerebrovascular invasion and leukemic cell proliferation.

Fluid Therapy *Generous fluid administration is indicated for virtually every hospitalized child with leukemia* to reduce blood viscosity in the face of a high WBC count and prevent hyperuricemia. Initial treatment for hyperleukocytosis is fluid administration, titrated until diuresis is observed and maintained (urine output >1 to 2 ml/kg/hr).

Avoid or promptly treat dehydration, since it further increases blood viscosity. Metabolic abnormalities (e.g., high uric acid) should be corrected. Avoid transfusions unless the Hgb is dangerously low. Exchange transfusion and leukapheresis may be performed to lower the WBC count.

Graft-vs.-Host Disease

Etiology/Pathophysiology

Graft-vs.-host disease (GVHD) occurs when immunocompetent WBCs, specifically T cells, are transfused into a recipient, where they proliferate and attack recipient tissues. Typically, the recipient is immunocompromised and is incapable of destroying the foreign T cells. However, GVHD has been reported following directed blood transfusion in immunocompetent patients. GVHD is most commonly reported following bone marrow transplantation (particularly allogeneic bone marrow) or following blood transfusion to immunocompromised patients.

Clinical Presentation

Acute GVHD is most likely to develop within several days to 2 months after bone marrow transplantation and within 6 to 10 days after blood transfusion. *Chronic* GVHD develops 40+ days after bone marrow transplantation.

GVHD damages epithelial cells of target organs and also produces severe immunosuppression. Note that the kidney is often spared. Clinical signs of GVHO include:

- *Skin:* Maculopapular rash (particularly on the palms, soles, and ears)—may progress to bullae and desquamation
- *Gastrointestinal system:* Diarrhea (may contain blood), anorexia, nausea, abdominal pain, and ileus
- *Liver:* Coagulopathies, hyperbilirubinemia, and elevation in liver enzymes (alkaline phosphatase and aminotransferase)
- *Immune system:* Persistent immunodeficiency (after bone marrow transplantation) or bone marrow aplasia (after transfusion)

Management

Prevention Elimination of T cells from transplanted bone marrow may prevent GVHD but increases the likelihood of graft failure. More commonly, allogeneic bone marrow recipients are treated prophylactically with cyclosporine and possibly with methotrexate or corticosteroids. Isolation of bone marrow recipients in negative-flow rooms does reduce the incidence of GVHD in patients with underlying aplastic anemia by preventing activation of the recipient's macrophages; it is of questionable benefit in patients receiving bone marrow transplantation for leukemia.

Irradiation of blood products (≥2500 rad) prevents transfusion-related GVHD. It should be considered whenever transfusions are provided to very young infants, immunocompromised patients, bone marrow transplant recipients, or patients with bone marrow failure. Irradiation should also be performed on all granulocyte transfusions and transfusions from close family members or directed donors.

Therapy   Treatment of GVHD requires early detection and support of failing organ systems (e.g., treatment of coagulopathies) and immunosuppression. Corticosteroids and antithymocyte globulin or IV gamma globulin are administered. Experimental therapies that hold promise include anticytokines (to modulate the inflammatory response) and immunotoxins.

Spinal Cord Compression

Etiology/Pathophysiology

Growth of tumors in or near the spinal cord may result in spinal cord compression, with resulting pain, sensory deficits, and loss of motor function.

Clinical Presentation

Clinical signs and symptoms result from compression or direct invasion of the spinal cord and peripheral nerves and include:

- *Complaints:* Weakness, back pain, sensory deficits, or tenderness over the affected area of the spine
- *Motor deficits:* Reduced muscle tone and movement
- *Sensory deficits:* Loss of recognition of pain or touch at a sensory level
- *Loss of bowel and bladder function:* Inability to void, urinary retention, or incontinence

MRI and CT scanning provide the most rapid and least invasive imaging.

Management

If cord compression produces neurologic dysfunction, urgent surgical intervention is required to maintain or regain function. Unfortunately, permanent neurologic deficits often develop despite aggressive management.

If a compressive tumor has been identified, high-dose corticosteroids (dexamethasone, 1 to 2 mg/kg) are administered to decrease edema around the tumor. Emergent radiotherapy or chemotherapy may reduce sensitive tumors, and laminectomy or other surgical debulking procedures may relieve symptoms.

Obstructive Mediastinal Mass

Etiology/Pathophysiology

Tumors involving the mediastinum may grow rapidly, producing critical airway obstruction or superior vena caval (SVC) syndrome. The growth of the mass is often so rapid that the child develops symptoms of airway obstruction between the time of admission to the hospital and initiation of therapy.

Lymphomas most commonly involve the mediastinum. Other mediastinal tumors include T-cell acute lymphoblastic leukemia, Hodgkin's disease, neuroblastoma, and Ewing's sarcoma.

SVC obstruction can result from compression by lymphoma or tumor. It may also result from thrombus formation around long-dwelling central venous or implantable catheters or following cardiovascular surgery or SVC septic thrombus.

Clinical Presentation

Signs of respiratory distress in the child with a mediastinal mass usually indicate tracheal or bronchial compression and airway obstruction. These signs may develop rapidly and include stridor, dyspnea, wheezing, and increased respiratory effort. The diagnosis of airway obstruction is based on *clinical evaluation of respiratory effort and air movement,* since hypoxemia or hypercarbia will only develop if the child is exhausted and respiratory arrest is imminent.

SVC syndrome is suspected if the patient develops edema limited to the face, neck, and upper body. The upper extremities are less frequently involved. SVC obstruction can also produce cerebral edema with resultant headaches, visual disturbances, and neurologic abnormalities.

Management

Intubation and mechanical ventilatory support are required. Tracheal intubation may not relieve lower airway obstruction, but the use of positive pressure ventilation may ensure sufficient air exchange until the obstruction is relieved. Selective endotracheal intubation of one bronchus may be necessary.

An obstructive mediastinal mass must be removed or eliminated through urgent radiotherapy, chemotherapy, or surgical debulking, although the risks of anesthesia and biopsy are significant. The tumor is biopsied to enable treatment with appropriate chemotherapy, radiation therapy, or both.

These tumors are often very sensitive to radiation therapy and may shrink within days in response to radiation. However, radiation may also produce airway edema; thus temporary *worsening* of airway obstruction should be anticipated approximately 6 to 12 hours after radiation therapy, and respiratory support should be provided.

SVC thrombotic occlusion may be prevented with excellent care of central venous catheters. Pericatheter thrombi may be dissolved with urokinase infusion (5000- to 10,000-U bolus or 200 U/kg/hr) directly into the clotted central line or through a peripheral vein or a catheter positioned just above the obstruction. Surgical thrombectomy may be necessary.

Care of the Patient During Transfusion Therapy

A list of the standard blood components available for transfusion, together with their routine indications and doses, is provided in Table 11-4.

Red Blood Cell Transfusion

Purpose

The purpose of RBC transfusion is correction of hemorrhage or anemia and improvement in blood oxygen-carrying capacity and oxygen delivery (e.g., in the patient with respiratory failure).

Table 11-4
Transfusion Therapy

Blood Product	Indications for Use	Dose
Whole blood or packed RBCs	Exchange transfusion Acute blood loss	5-10 cc/kg
	Anemia	5-20 cc/kg
Fresh frozen plasma	Disseminated intravascular coagulation (DIC) Hemophilia B (factor IX deficiency) Other factor deficiencies (V,XI,XIII) Coumadin overdose	10-15 cc/kg
Random-donor platelets (RDP)	Thrombocytopenia DIC	1-8 U (see text)
Single-donor platelets (pheresed platelets)	Patient refractory to RDP	
Cryoprecipitate	Hypofibrinogenemia Von Willebrand's disease Mild hemophilia	1 bag/5 kg
Factor VIII concentrate	Hemophilia A	10-50 U/kg
WBCs	Life-threatening infection in neutropenic patients	
Irradiated blood products	Patient at risk for graft-vs.-host disease	

From Hazinski MF: *Nursing care of the critically ill child,* ed 2, St Louis, 1992, Mosby.

Types of Red Blood Cell Transfusions

Whole-Blood Transfusion   Whole blood is reserved for exchange transfusions, severe hemorrhage with depletion of coagulation factors, or when other products are unavailable. Fresh (unrefrigerated) blood from directed donators may be administered to provide RBCs and clotting factors after cardiopulmonary bypass.

Packed Red Blood Cell Transfusion   *Transfusion of 10 ml/kg of PRBCs should raise the Hct by 10 percentage points* (e.g., from 15% to 25%) and Hgb by 3 g/dl (e.g., from 5 to 8 g/dl). A more precise estimate of the volume required to achieve a desired Hct may be provided by the formula in Box 11-4.

If chronic compensated anemia or CHF is present, PRBC transfusion is provided at a rate of 3 ml/kg/hr to improve oxygen transport without a rapid increase in intravascular volume. When chronic anemia is present, the blood volume is normal; therefore transfusion may produce hypervolemia or worsen CHF. If severe CHF is present, a partial exchange transfusion (PRBCs replace patient blood) may be performed. This raises the Hct without changing the blood volume.

Procedure and Nursing Responsibilities

Appropriate (universal) blood and body fluid precautions must be followed.

Crossmatching   Obtain a sample of the patient's blood for typing and crossmatching with the proposed donor unit of blood. *Identify and label the sample carefully.*

Crossmatching may be waived with a physician's order if massive hemorrhage and shock are present (e.g., trauma); O-negative blood is then administered. Crossmatching is impossible when the child has immune-mediated hemolytic anemia; thus the physician must authorize administration of blood labeled "noncompatible" by the blood bank.

Checking of Blood   Two members of the health care team must verify the blood type, patient's name and hospital number, blood product and volume, donor and unit number, and expiration date of the blood product on both the transfusion request form and the blood product unit itself. The patient identification bracelet must be checked to confirm the patient's identity before blood administration. *Most severe (hemolytic) transfusion reactions are due to clerical error* and are therefore avoidable with careful verification procedures.

Transfusion   The administration rate is determined by the acuity of the blood requirement and the patient's cardiovascular function. Deliver blood as a bolus when hemorrhage is present, but transfuse over several hours if anemia is present (particularly if it is associated with CHF).

Warm blood to room temperature before administration in children and use a blood warmer (water bath heated to 37.5° to 40.5° C) to warm blood before administration to infants and young children. No other method of blood warming is recommended.

Box 11-4

Estimation of Appropriate Packed Red Blood Cell Transfusion Volume

$$\text{Volume of PRBC transfusion (in ml)} = \frac{\text{Estimated patient CBV} \times \text{Desired change in Hct}}{\text{Hct of transfused PRBCs}}$$

Patient circulating blood volume (CBV) is estimated as follows:
   Neonates at 85 ml/kg
   Infants and children at 75 ml/kg
Hematocrit (Hct) of transfused packed red blood cells (PRBCs) is approximately 65% to 70%.

From Hazinski MF: *Nursing care of the critically ill child,* ed 2, St Louis, 1992, Mosby.

Cold Antibodies Cold antibodies frequently develop following mycoplasma or certain viruses. If cold-activated antibodies are present in the patient's blood, transfusion of cold (i.e., less than body temperature) whole blood will result in binding of the antibodies to the transfused blood. As this transfused blood warms to body temperature in the patient, lysis of the transfused RBCs will occur, and the patient's Hct and Hgb will fail to rise. In fact, the presence of cold antibodies should be suspected as a cause of failure to respond to transfusion.

When cold antibodies are present, the transfused blood must be carefully warmed in a water bath before administration and must be kept warm *until it enters the patient.* The tubing between the water bath and the patient should also be warmed (in a water bath), so that the transfused blood is not allowed to cool before it enters the patient.

Platelet Transfusion

Purpose

Platelet transfusions are administered to thrombocytopenic patients who are at high risk for bleeding.

Types of Platelet Transfusions

- *Random-donor platelets:* Platelet fraction from a single unit of blood. In the absence of increased platelet destruction, *a single unit of random-donor platelets should increase the platelet count by approximately 10,000/mm³/m² BSA* (or 0.1 U/kg should raise the platelet count by 30,000 to 50,000/mm³).
- *Single-donor platelets:* Platelet pheresis from a single-donor, equivalent to 5 to 8 U of random-donor platelets. These platelets are used to minimize antibody development in patients who are anticipated to require multiple platelet transfusions.

The half-life of administered platelets is approximately 4 days but can be shorter in patients with infection, fever, or DIC.

Procedure and Nursing Responsibilities

Administer platelets intravenously over 20 to 40 minutes through a 170-μm filter that removes platelet aggregates. Agitate the platelet bag and Buretrol gently every 10 to 15 minutes during the transfusion. If the platelets settle out, they will activate in the bag and become nonfunctional. Obtain a 1-hour posttransfusion platelet count to determine the patient's response. Hemolytic reactions due to ABO incompatibility do not occur with platelet transfusions, but fever, chills, or rash may develop (treat with an antihistamine).

Frequent platelet transfusions can cause sensitization to foreign antigens found on the surfaces of random-donor platelets and rapid destruction of transfused platelets by the patient's antibodies. Sensitized patients may still benefit from single-donor platelets, which bear fewer foreign antigens. Ultimately, the patient may require platelets obtained by plasmapheresis from family members.

If frequent platelet administration is anticipated, transfusions should be limited to minimize the development of sensitivity. Indications include clinical evidence of bleeding, platelet count <50,000 before a surgical procedure, or profound thrombocytopenia (platelet count <10,000 to 20,000) with significant risk of bleeding.

Transfusion Reaction

Potential complications of transfusion therapy include mild to severe transfusion reaction and evidence of hypervolemia (Box 11-5).

Mild Transfusion Reaction

Mild transfusion reactions include fever, urticaria, rash, pruritus, and, occasionally, bronchospasm. These reactions are managed by administration of antipyretics, antihistamines (diphenhydramine, 1 to 2 mg/kg IV), or corticosteroids; interruption of transfusion is not required.

Severe Transfusion Reaction

Severe transfusion reactions usually result from blood type incompatibility; therefore proper identification of blood products is essential. A hemolytic reaction can be severe or fatal.

Clinical Presentation Clinical signs and symptoms include fever, chills, back (splenic) pain, hemoglobinuria, jaundice, DIC, hypotension, and renal failure.

Box 11-5

Recognition and Management of Transfusion Reaction

Mild Reaction

Febrile: Fever, chills
Allergic: Urticaria, itching, wheezing
Intervention: Administer antipyretics, antihistamines, corticosteroids.

Severe (Hemolytic) Reactions

Symptoms: Fever, chills, back pain
Hemolysis: Hemoglobinuria, renal failure, jaundice, disseminated intravascular coagulation, hypotension, shock
Interventions: Notify physician. *Stop transfusion immediately.* Administer generous amounts of intravenous fluids and diuretics. Monitor patient closely and support as needed.

Modified from Hazinski MF: *Nursing care of the critically ill child,* ed 2, St Louis, 1992, Mosby.

Management Stop transfusion immediately and send the unit back to the blood bank for recrossmatching. Administer crystalloids (20 ml/kg bolus) and osmotic diuretics (e.g., mannitol 0.25 to 1 g/kg) to avert renal tubular necrosis. Titrate fluid and diuretic therapy to maintain effective systemic perfusion and a urine volume ≥1 to 2 ml/kg/hr for 24 hours.

Hypervolemia

Clinical Presentation Clinical signs and symptoms include tachycardia, a gallop rhythm, worsening hepatosplenomegaly, and peripheral and pulmonary edema.

Management Diuretic therapy is required. Hypervolemia may be prevented by diuretic administration immediately before or following the transfusion.

Evaluation of Response

Check the Hgb and Hct. The Hgb should increase by approximately 3 g/dl, and the Hct should rise approximately 10 percentage points with the infusion of 10 ml/kg of PRBCs. An inadequate

Hgb/Hct rise may be caused by shortened RBC survival (e.g., cold antibodies or hemolytic reaction) or ongoing blood loss.

White Blood Cell Transfusion

WBC or granulocyte transfusions are occasionally provided for neutropenic patients with documented bacterial infection or sepsis who fail to respond to antibiotic therapy. However, the efficacy of this therapy is questionable.

Exchange Transfusion

Purpose

An exchange transfusion involves removal of the patient's blood with simultaneous administration of (replacement by) fresh blood or PRBCs. Exchange transfusion may be performed to remove an undesirable factor from the patient's blood (e.g., hyperbilirubinemia) or to avoid hypervolemia and heart failure in the severely anemic patient who requires transfusion.

Procedure and Nursing Responsibilities

Blood products are warmed using a water bath heated to 37.5° to 40.5° C. Exchange transfusion is accomplished through simultaneous withdrawal and infusion of blood (via two venous catheters or a venous and an arterial catheter). A volume of 4 to 5 ml of the patient's blood is slowly removed and transferred to a waste bag, and an equivalent volume of transfusion blood is then slowly administered. This cycle is repeated until the desired volume has been exchanged.

Blood volumes administered and removed are carefully recorded. The patient's systemic perfusion, temperature, vital signs, and electrolyte balance must be closely monitored. Alterations in blood pressure, heart rate, or cardiac rhythm should be investigated immediately.

Potential Complications

Hyperkalemia may result from potassium released from transfused blood cells. Hypocalcemia may develop when ionized calcium bonds to the phosphate present in citrate-phosphate-dextran–preserved blood; thus calcium administration is usually required. Other potential complications of exchange transfusion include acidosis, hypomagnesemia, hypoglycemia, and DIC (secondary to depletion of coagulation factors), or GVHD (see Graft-vs.-Host Disease under Common Clinical Conditions).

Specific Diseases

Sickle Cell Anemia

Etiology/Pathophysiology

Sickle cell anemia (SCA) is an inherited hematologic disorder that results in an abnormal Hgb protein (HbS) that polymerizes on desaturation. This alters the RBC membrane, causing it to assume the characteristic sickled shape.

The sickled RBCs can occlude small blood vessels, producing ischemia, infarction, pain, and organ dysfunction—the so-called vasoocclusive crises of SCA. A vasoocclusive crisis may involve the CNS, bone, the lungs, or other visceral organs.

The deformed RBCs are rapidly hemolyzed; thus chronic, compensated anemia develops. RBC production and the reticulocyte count will be increased.

Clinical Presentation of Sickle Cell Anemia Crisis

Hypoxemia, dehydration, or infection may contribute to the development of a vasoocclusive crisis. Clinical signs and symptoms of crisis include:

- *CNS crisis* (cerebrovascular accident [CVA], or stroke): Severe unilateral headache, motor deficits, change in responsiveness, signs of increased intracranial pressure (ICP), or seizures. Diagnostic studies, such as cerebral angiography or CT scanning can confirm the development of the CVA, but they are performed *only after therapy is initiated.*
- *Bone crisis:* Severe localized pain, and possible erythema, warmth, and tenderness.
- *Pulmonary crisis:* Chest pain and respiratory distress, including tachypnea and dyspnea. This can progress rapidly to respiratory failure. Pulmonary crisis or acute chest syndrome can be one of the most life-threatening

emergencies in sickle cell disease. The chest x-ray film may resemble that of a patient with pulmonary edema. However, the pathophysiology is pulmonary vasoocclusion, and, unlike pulmonary edema, the treatment is hydration and exchange transfusion. *Do not administer diuretics*—diuretic therapy will increase sickling and result in pulmonary infarctions.
- *Abdominal crisis:* Pain, abdominal tenderness, rigidity, and guarding.
- *Splenic sequestration crisis:* RBC trapping causes sudden anemia, hypotension, and shock. A massively enlarged spleen can be readily palpated. Chronic occlusion of splenic vessels leads to splenic infarction and subsequent loss of function at an early age; thus splenic sequestration is typically observed only in young children with SCA.
- *Aplastic crisis:* Transient suppression of bone marrow function with an acute decrease in RBC production produces symptomatic anemia and CHF. The reticulocyte count will be low.

Management of Sickle Cell Anemia Crisis

Maintenance of adequate hydration and oxygenation, and avoidance or prompt treatment of infection or hypothermia may prevent many SCA vasoocclusive crises. Parenteral fluids are administered at 1½ to 2 times the typical maintenance rate. Preoperatively, RBC transfusions are provided to reduce the HbS to <30% of the total Hgb.

Cerebrovascular Accident *If focal (unilateral) neurologic signs develop in the child with SCA, the presumption of a CVA should be made, and immediate transfusion is provided* to reduce the concentration of sickled RBCs. Partial exchange transfusion is then performed until the HbS level is <30% of the total Hgb. Diagnostic studies are performed only when the patient is stable.

Once one CVA has occurred, transfusions are provided on a regular basis (approximately every 3 weeks) to maintain the HbS level at <30% to prevent additional CVAs. Lifelong prophylactic transfusions may be required, and CVAs may be observed despite this therapy.

Pain Crisis Management of vasoocclusive pain crisis is largely supportive, but infection must be ruled out. Maintain hydration and provide analgesia (see Chapter 3) until the crisis resolves. Oxygen therapy is not beneficial.

Pulmonary Crisis Pulmonary infarction is treated with parenteral fluids, analgesics, and antibiotics. Oxygen therapy may improve arterial oxygen saturation and provide symptomatic relief. RBC transfusions are indicated to improve oxygen delivery and to avert further sickling. Emergency exchange transfusion may be required if evidence of pulmonary decompensation develops. *Do not administer diuretics;* hydration rather than diuresis is required.

Splenic Sequestration Crisis Management consists of immediate PRBC transfusion to restore intravascular volume and RBC mass. Splenectomy may ultimately be required.

Aplastic Crisis Symptomatic anemia is treated with RBC transfusions until marrow function returns. Partial exchange transfusion may be required if anemia with CHF develops.

Hemophilia

Etiology/Pathophysiology

Factor VIII deficiency, or hemophilia A, is an X-linked disorder causing a defective factor VIII protein with little or no clotting activity. Many hemophiliacs have also developed inhibitor to administered factor VIII; thus massive doses of factor VIII or activated concentrate products may be required to treat bleeding episodes. Factor IX deficiency (hemophilia B) is a less common X-linked disorder, caused by a defective factor IX gene and protein.

The lack of significant factor VIII activity prevents formation of a normal clot at bleeding sites. Persistent bleeding or severe hematoma formation may follow minor trauma, and recurrent hemarthroses (manifested by swollen, painful joints) are common.

Patients with severe hemophilia (less than 1% clotting activity) may suffer spontaneous or severe bleeding following trauma or surgery. Intracranial hemorrhages rarely occur spontaneously; most are associated with trauma.

Clinical Presentation

Persistent oozing at venipuncture sites or wounds is the most obvious sign of inadequate hemostasis in a hemophiliac patient. Subtle signs of bleeding include swelling or discoloration of soft tissues and joints.

Management

Management of bleeding requires administration of factor VIII. Severity of bleeding complications will be determined by the duration and magnitude of the bleeding; thus the initial dose of factor VIII cannot be delayed, and subsequent doses must be administered *on time*. Appropriate blood and body fluid (universal) precautions must be observed.

Minor Trauma A single bolus of factor concentrate should increase factor VIII activity to 20% to 40% of normal, providing adequate hemostasis.

Major Trauma or Surgery Frequent boluses or continuous infusion of factor VIII concentrate must be provided until the concentration of factor VIII reaches normal levels. A bolus of 1 U/kg will raise the clotting factor by 2%; thus a total infusion of 50 U/kg should raise the clotting factor to approximately normal levels (100% correction). The PTT should then be normal unless insufficient factor VIII was provided or inhibitors are present.

When major surgery is performed, factor VIII levels must be monitored. The PTT alone will not provide adequate information, since it can be normal once the factor VIII is >30% of normal in most laboratories. This factor VIII level will not protect the patient from serious bleeding.

Additional doses of factor VIII are provided every 8 hours for 24 hours, then approximately every 12 hours thereafter. Monitor PTT and factor VIII levels

Inhibitors will result in lack of response to standard doses of factor concentrates, and massive doses or activated concentrate products may be required

Joint Bleeding Wrap the joint with elastic bandage and consider application of ice. Casting may help preserve joint function.

General Care Avoid intramuscular injections and deep (femoral or subclavian) venipunctures. Only superficial (antecubital or external jugular) venipunctures can be safely performed, so that any bleeding will be readily detected and controlled by external pressure. Apply prolonged direct pressure (5 minutes or longer) following each venipuncture. Administration of aspirin and any other platelet inhibitors is contraindicated.

Acquired Immunodeficiency Syndrome

Etiology/Pathophysiology

Acquired immunodeficiency syndrome (AIDS) is a fatal disorder caused by human immunodeficiency virus (HIV), which is acquired through direct exposure to blood or other body fluids of infected patients, or by direct maternal-fetal transmission. HIV selectively destroys T lymphocytes (T4 or T-helper cells), producing loss of essential immune function. This increases the patient's risk of opportunistic infections and certain malignancies.

Not all persons who acquire HIV infection immediately develop AIDS. However, a person infected with HIV who has not developed AIDS can still transmit the virus to others through sexual contact, exposure to blood products, or maternal-fetal transmission.

Clinical Presentation

There are no signs or symptoms specific to infection with HIV. However, children with AIDS can develop recurrent bacterial infections, failure to thrive, opportunistic infections (including *Pneumocystis carinii* or other atypical pneumonias), chronic diarrhea, or chronic oral candidiasis. Critical care is generally required for treatment of sepsis or respiratory failure associated with pneumonia.

Management

There is presently no curative therapy for patients with AIDS. Zidovudine (AZT, Retrovir) may prolong survival of some AIDS patients by reducing opportunistic infections. Thus treatment consists primarily of supportive care and management of infections and other complications as they arise.

Hemolytic-Uremic Syndrome

Etiology/Pathophysiology

Hemolytic-uremic syndrome (HUS) is a group of disorders characterized by microangiopathic hemolytic anemia, thrombocytopenia, and uremia, which may progress to overt renal failure. Although a specific etiologic agent has not been isolated for all cases, *Escherichia. coli* infection is known to play a role in the development of one of the subgroups of HUS (prototypic HUS). Pathologic findings of HUS in the glomerular endothelium and small arteries resemble thrombotic thrombocytopenic purpura (TTP), which is part of the differential diagnosis. HUS is the most common cause of acute renal failure in children.

Clinical Presentation HUS is typically preceded by a history of diarrhea or upper respiratory tract infection. In fact, nondiarrheal forms of HUS have a worse prognosis than the diarrheal forms. Findings may include nonimmune hemolytic anemia, thrombocytopenia, hypertension, edema, and oliguria or anuria (see p. 483).

Management The management of anemia and thrombocytopenia in the child with HUS are discussed earlier in the chapter. The reader is referred to Chapter 9 for the management of renal failure secondary to HUS (see p. 472).

Common Diagnostic Tests

Bone Marrow Aspiration and Biopsy

A bone marrow aspiration or biopsy is performed to obtain bone marrow for diagnostic studies.

Procedure

The procedure is explained to the patient, and analgesics and sedatives are administered (see Chapter 3).

A bone marrow aspiration or biopsy is usually performed at the posterior iliac crest. The area is cleansed with a povidone-iodine solution, and a local anesthetic is injected into the overlying skin and subcutaneous tissue. Sterile technique must be maintained throughout the procedure.

The actual biopsy is performed by insertion of a Jamshedi needle with a trocar through the skin and through the periosteum and bony cortex, into the bone marrow cavity. Once the needle is in the marrow, the trocar is removed. If a bone marrow aspiration is performed, bone marrow is withdrawn using a sterile syringe (this may be painful). If a biopsy is performed, a marrow particle is removed from the Jamshedi needle barrel after the needle is withdrawn.

The skin puncture site is covered with a bandage. The site should be monitored for evidence of hematoma formation or other bleeding. If bleeding is observed, a pressure dressing is applied to the site.

Lumbar Puncture

A lumbar puncture (LP), or spinal tap, is performed to obtain cerebrospinal fluid (CSF) for diagnostic studies. Relative contraindications to performance of an LP include bleeding disorders and increased ICP. Therefore a CT scan of the head should be obtained before an LP to rule out increased ICP for any patient at risk for increased ICP.

Procedure

An LP is performed with the patient recumbent and on the side, or in a sitting position. The shoulders should be bent forward in order to flex the back and expose the intervertebral spaces.

Following sterile preparation and anesthesia of the overlying skin, a spinal needle with trocar in place is inserted through the skin and into the intervertebral space in the midline, between the third and fourth, or fourth and fifth, lumbar vertebrae. The needle is inserted through the dura and into the subarachnoid space. The trocar is removed, and the CSF opening pressure is measured (if appropriate) with a manometer. CSF is then allowed to flow from the needle into the appropriate specimen tubes. CSF closing pressure is measured (if appropriate) just before the needle's removal. Following removal of the needle, a bandage is applied to the skin puncture site to prevent bleeding.

Sterile technique must be maintained throughout the procedure. Following the procedure, the patient should be monitored for bleeding or a CSF leak at the procedure site. Some patients may develop headache following an LP; this may be averted by requiring the patient to remain in the supine position for several hours following the procedure.

Suggested Readings

Ablin AR: Supportive care of immunocompromised pediatric patients, *Curr Opin Pediatr* 6:52-57, 1994.

Allegretta GJ, Weisman SJ, Altman AJ: Oncologic emergencies, *Pediatr Clin North Am* 32:601, 1985.

Armitage JP: Bone marrow transplantation, *N Engl J Med* 330:827-838, 1994.

Consensus Conference: Platelet transfusion therapy, *JAMA* 257:1777, 1987.

Consensus Conference: Perioperative red blood cell transfusion, *JAMA* 260:2700, 1988.

Ferrara JLM, Deeg HJ: Graft-versus-host disease, *N Engl J Med* 324:667-674, 1991.

Ford R, Ballard B: Acute complications after bone marrow transplantation, *Semin Oncol Nurs* 4:15-23, 1988.

Goldmann D, Larson E: Hand-washing and nosocomial infections, *N Engl J Med* 327:120-122, 1992.

Kramer AB, Rubin P, Keller JW: Oncologic emergencies. In Rubin P, editor: *Clinical oncology: a multidisciplinary approach for physicians and students,* ed 7, Philadelphia, 1993, WB Saunders.

Lieschke GJ, Burgess AW: Granulocyte colony-stimulating factor and granulocyte-macrophage colony-stimulating factor, part I, *N Engl J Med* 327:28-35, 1992.

Lieschke GJ, Burgess AW: Granulocyte colony-stimulating factor and granulocyte-macrophage colony-stimulating factor. II: Therapeutic applications, *N Engl J Med* 327:99-106, 1992.

Mentzer WC, Matthay K: Hematology and oncology—editorial overview, *Curr Opin Pediatr* 6:43-45, 1994.

Rowe JM: AIDS. In Rubin P, editor: *Clinical oncology: a multidisciplinary approach for physicians and students,* ed 7, Philadelphia, 1993, WB Saunders.

Schwartz CL et al: Pediatric solid tumors. In Rubin P, editor: *Clinical oncology: a multidisciplinary approach for physicians and students,* ed 7, Philadelphia, 1993, WB Saunders.

Stewart CL, Tina LU: Hemolytic uremic syndrome, *Pediatr Rev* 14:218-225, 1993.

Tribett D: Immune system function: implications for critical care nursing practice, *Crit Care Nurs Clin North Am* 1:725-740, 1989.

Weitman SD, Sinick NJ, Kamen BA: "Above all do no harm": horizons in pediatric oncology, *Curr Opin Pediatr* 6:219-223, 1994.

12 Pediatric Trauma

Epidemiology of Pediatric Trauma

Frequency of Injuries

Injuries kill more children than all other diseases combined. Annually in children and adolescents, trauma is responsible for approximately 22,000 to 25,000 deaths, 600,000 hospitalizations, and 16 million emergency department (ED) visits, at an acute cost of more than $7.5 billion. In general, for every childhood injury death, 45 hospitalizations and 1300 ED visits occur.

Causes of Injuries

Young children in the United States are often injured in and around the home; thus injury prevention must target those responsible for the daily care of children. The most frequent causes of pediatric trauma are motor vehicle trauma, submersion, firearm injuries, fire, falls, and homicide, including child abuse.

Infants and children explore the environment. They have little concept of those activities that may be harmful to them, and they are unaware of their limitations. The child's balance and fine and gross motor skills are incompletely developed, contributing to falls, near-drowning, and "dart out" pedestrian injuries.

Traumatic injuries in the child can be categorized as either inflicted or unintentional:

- *Inflicted* injuries may be intentional (e.g., child abuse), or they may occur as a result of *neglect,* or failure to meet the community's minimal standards of care for children.
- *Unintentional* injuries caused by burns, submersion, and motor vehicles are often preventable.

Mechanisms of Pediatric Injury

Children are not "small adults," and their injuries are often quite different from what an adult might sustain under the same conditions. The child's small structure and physiologic immaturity play important roles in the physical consequences of injury. The following section describes those physical characteristics of children that influence the mechanism and significance of injury.

Types of Childhood Injury

The most common causes of severe childhood injury are motor vehicle crashes, falls, near-drowning, and firearms. In motor vehicle crashes and falls, *blunt injury* is the most common type of injury sustained. Anoxic injury is associated with submersion, and firearm injuries produce penetrating injuries. Approximately 80% of thoracic and abdominal injuries are blunt, and 20% are penetrating injuries.

Size

The small size of the child influences the degree and type of injury caused by traumatic forces. Forces impacting the thorax or abdomen of an adult

may not cause serious injury because they are dissipated over a large area. In a child those same forces may cause significant injury because they are concentrated over a smaller area.

The *location* of the impact is also influenced by the size of the child. An adult hit by the bumper of a car typically sustains lower extremity injuries. When an automobile strikes a child, lower extremity injuries may occur, but head, abdominal, and thoracic injuries are likely because these are the areas of the child's body most often struck by the car.

Any child with a history of pedestrian, bicycle, or motor vehicle occupant–related injury should be evaluated for internal abdominal and thoracic injuries, as well as head and spinal cord injuries and extremity fractures. The proper use of seat belts, child restraint devices, and bicycle helmets reduces the likelihood of such injuries but does not eliminate them.

Head and Skull

The child's head is relatively large in relation to body size. In addition, the child's neck and shoulder muscles are relatively weak and provide little head support. In acceleration-deceleration injuries such as those resulting from falls or motor vehicle crashes, the unrestrained child will likely fly "head first," resulting in head injury and possible spinal cord injury.

The child's skull is not as rigid as that of the adult, and it offers little protection for the child's brain. Although skull sutures can expand to accommodate a gradual increase in intracranial volume, such expansion cannot prevent a rise in intracranial pressure (ICP) associated with an acute rise in intracranial volume.

The brain of the young child has incomplete myelinization, and it has a higher water content than the brain of the adult. These factors make the child's brain more homogeneous than the adult's brain. As a result, blunt head injuries during childhood often result in gliding contusions, diffuse head injury, and diffuse brain swelling. Subdural, epidural, and intracranial bleeding following head injury are much less common in children than in adults.

Children with head injury demonstrate lower mortality than adults with similar head injury, particularly when outcomes following presentation with specific Glasgow Coma Scale (GCS) scores are compared. The reason for this lower pediatric mortality is debatable. It may be explained by a difference in the clinical signs of injury or by a difference in brain development and capacity for healing. Coma with fixed and dilated pupils on presentation often indicates severe brain stem injury or alcohol intoxication in adults, but it may be produced by less severe forms of diffuse head injury in children. Children with head injury do appear to have greater capacity for healing than do adults. The dendritic arborization in the child's central nervous system is incomplete; this may mean that the child is capable of compensating for injured areas of the brain through development of new intracranial fiber tracts.

Spinal Cord

Spinal cord injury is relatively uncommon in children because the child's spine is elastic and the vertebrae are less likely to fracture under minor stress. The elasticity of the spine is caused by relatively lax paraspinal ligaments; incomplete development of the neck, paraspinous, and paracervical muscles; incomplete ossification of the wedge-shaped vertebrae; and shallow orientation of the facet joints (so that the vertebrae may easily slip out of alignment).

Although the laxity of the spine can exert a protective effect during minor stress, major forces may result in subluxation and spinal cord injury without vertebral fracture. Very young children are likely to sustain subluxation injuries alone, whereas older children are more likely to sustain vertebral fractures or fractures with subluxation.

The upper cervical spine is particularly weak in infants and toddlers. The relatively large size of the pediatric head coupled with the relative instability of the cervical vertebrae can contribute to subluxation injuries during acceleration-deceleration trauma. During childhood the greatest vertebral joint mobility with the greatest angular displacement changes from the region of C1 to C2 during infancy to the region of C5 to C6 by school age (Box 12-1).

Many children with spinal cord injury do not demonstrate evidence of vertebral fracture or other radiographic abnormalities on routine (anteroposterior and lateral) spine radiographs. These children have spinal cord injury without radiographic

> ### Box 12-1
>
> ## Most Common Sites of Pediatric Cervical Spine Injury by Age
>
> *All children:* Injuries at the occiput-C2 level represent a significant portion of spinal injuries. Complete injury produces immediate respiratory arrest and is often fatal.
>
> *Infants and toddlers:* Sublaxation injuries are most commonly observed between the first and second (C1-C2) or the second and third (C2-C3) cervical vertebrae. Complete injury produces immediate respiratory arrest and is often fatal.
>
> *Children 3-8:* Sublaxation injuries are most likely to occur at the C3-C5 level. complete injury produces quadriplegia and loss of spontaneous breathing (respiratory arrest).
>
> *Children 9-15:* Fracture or fracture/sublaxation injuries are most likely to occur at C4-C6. Complete injury produces quadriplegia. Spontaneous respirations may persist with injuries lower than C5.

abnormality (SCIWORA), and one third of these patients develop permanent neurologic injury. Thorough assessment of movement and sensation in all extremities should be performed on admission and at frequent intervals throughout the child's hospitalization.

Spinal cord injuries in trauma victims may also be produced by lap belts or violent shaking. Lap belts may produce flexion-distraction fractures (Chance fractures) of the lumbar spine. The "shaken baby" syndrome can produce spinal cord hematoma or contusion.

Skeleton

The child's bones are incompletely calcified and are cartilaginous and compliant; thus they are less likely to fracture on impact than are the more ossified bones of the adult. For these reasons the absence of a fracture does not rule out serious injury.

The presence of rib fractures suggests that *major* thoracic trauma has occurred and that injury to underlying organs should be suspected. Upper rib fractures are most commonly associated with pulmonary and major vessel injuries, whereas lower rib fractures are typically associated with liver, spleen, lung, and kidney injury.

Abdomen

The thin abdominal wall and the protuberant abdomen of the infant and toddler mean that vital organs are close to impacting forces. As a result, minor forces may produce significant multiple-organ abdominal injuries. The kidneys, liver, and spleen are particularly vulnerable.

Blunt trauma is responsible for the majority of abdominal injuries observed in infants and children. However, penetrating trauma (e.g., from firearm injury) is increasing in frequency and is associated with higher mortality.

Abdominal injuries to motor vehicle occupants may result from lap belt trauma. Lap belts typically produce ecchymoses and bruising over the abdomen, and jejunal or small bowel transection or perforation is possible. Flexion-distraction fractures of the lumbar spine may be associated with the abdominal injuries.

Developmental Physiology Affecting Trauma Management

Children have smaller airways, a smaller blood volume, and a larger body surface area than adults. These factors increase the child's risk of development of cardiorespiratory distress and hypothermia when trauma occurs. For further information regarding the anatomic and physiologic differences between children and adults, see Chapter 1.

Prehospital Evaluation and Trauma Scoring Systems

Field Management of the Pediatric Trauma Victim

Priorities of Care

Children who die within the first minutes and hours after injury generally succumb to airway compromise or respiratory arrest, undetected or inadequately treated hemorrhagic shock, or devastating neurologic injury. Hypoxia, the final common pathway to death, is generally caused by one of these conditions.

Prehospital care providers should be able to accurately detect life-threatening conditions, resuscitate and support vital functions, and transport the patient to an appropriate facility. This prehospital (field) component of trauma care is critical and may have a major impact on patient outcome.

A *primary survey,* the first component of field care, is designed to detect and treat immediate threats to life and establish priorities of care. This survey includes assessment of airway, breathing, and circulation while the cervical spine is immobilized (Box 12-2). For further information regarding cardiopulmonary resuscitation (CPR), see p. 160, and Shock, p. 130.

Once immediate threats to life have been identified and treated, the first responder begins a *secondary survey* (head-to-toe assessment) to identify other injuries. This secondary survey will enable classification of trauma as major or minor and determine the number of organs injured.

Field Triage

Field care requires determination of the severity of injury with appropriate triage. Triage identifies those victims who require priority care through evaluation of:

- Airway, breathing, and circulation
- Location of injuries and general condition of the victim
- Mechanism and associated risks of hidden injuries
- Medical or physiologic factors that may increase the likelihood of life-threatening events

Each of these factors influences the selection of the mode of transportation and the destination facility. The field team must evaluate the hospital resources available and consider transport time and distance.

Injury Scoring Systems

Injury scoring systems enable quantification of injury severity. They provide objective criteria to determine the need to transfer the trauma victim to

Box 12-2

Priorities During Field Stabilization of the Pediatric Trauma Victim

A—Airway/cervical spine stabilization
    Position the patient.
    Clear the airway of debris.
B—Breathing/thoracorespiratory stabilization
    Bag-valve-mask (BMV) ventilation
    Oral intubation
    Decompress pneumothorax or hemothorax.
C—Circulation/control of external hemorrhage and shock
    Chest compressions, if needed
    Pressure dressings
    Establish venous access.
      Intraosseous, peripheral
      Begin volume resuscitation (if needed).
D—Disability/neurologic compromise
    Assess: Mental status
             Muscle tone
             Pupils
             Fontanelle (infants)
             Posturing
    If there are signs of increased intracranial pressure:
      Limit fluids (if the patient is *not* in hypovolemic shock).
      Elevate the head of the stretcher.
      Ensure adequate oxygenation, ventilation.
E—Exposure/hidden injuries
    Keep child warm.
    Fractures
    Lacerations
    Contusions

Forceful restraint of the child may exacerbate an existing problem. The benefit vs. risk of restraining a combative, agitated child must be weighed by the field team. There is inherent risk both in fighting to restrain struggling children and in allowing them to be transported in the parent's lap. This is a difficult decision for the prehospital care provider as well as the emergency department team to make.

From Hazinski MF: *Nursing care of the critically ill child,* ed 2, St Louis, 1992, Mosby.

Box 12-3

Injury Scoring Systems

Trauma Score (TS): Designed for scoring injury severity *in the field,* using the Glasgow Coma Scale (GCS), systolic blood pressure, capillary refill, respiratory rate, and respiratory effort. Each category is scored and then totaled.

Revised Trauma Score (RTS): Includes only the GCS, the systolic blood pressure, and the respiratory rate. Parameters are assigned coded values, which are then multiplied by assigned weights.

TRISS methodology formula: Combines the Revised Trauma Score, the Injury Severity Score (ISS), and the patient's age. The GCS score weighs most heavily in this formula.

Abbreviated Injury Scale (AIS): Rates anatomic injuries on a scale from 1 (minor) to 6 (fatal). The ISS uses AIS grades for injury but is designed to express the cumulative effect of injury to several body systems.

a pediatric trauma center. These scoring systems are described briefly in Box 12-3. The Modified Injury Severity Score (TRISS) is the most widely used score in trauma systems, the Pediatric Trauma Score (PTS) is the most widely used general scoring system for children, and the GCS score is the most widely used neurologic scoring system.

The *PTS* was developed to quantify the severity of injuries in children rather than adults. This system evaluates the patient's size, airway stability, systolic blood pressure, and mental status, and determines the presence of wounds or skeletal injuries (Table 12-1). Large size and optimal status yield a +2 for a parameter, whereas extremely small size and systemic dysfunction yield a −1 for the parameter. Potential scores range from −6 to +12. Children with a PTS <8 have the highest potential for preventable mortality or morbidity and should be transported to a tertiary care facility, such as a pediatric trauma center. Although this will result in the triage of some children with moderate injuries, conservative triage is appropriate.

The *GCS* was designed to enable rapid and reproducible evaluation of the neurologic status over time so that changes in the patient's condition can

Table 12-1
Pediatric Trauma Triage Criteria

Those injured persons with anatomic and physiologic characteristics of a person 15 years of age or younger that present with one or more of the following criteria:

(1) A *pediatric trauma score* of eight (8) or less* noted at any time during the prehospital care phase:

Component	+2	+1	−1
Size†	Orange or green; >20 kg (44+ lbs)	Yellow, white, or blue: 10-20 kg (22-43 lbs).	Red or purple; <10 kg (<22 lbs): **MOD**
Airway‡	Normal	Adjunct (e.g., O_2 mask, or cannula)	Assisted or intubated (oral/nasal airway, BVM, ETT, EOA, CRIC): **MAJ**
Consciousness	Awake	Amnesia or any reliable history of lost consciousness: **MOD**	Altered mental status (drowsy/lethargic/unresponsive) or paralysis or suspected spinal cord injury: **MAJ**
Circulation	Good peripheral pulses/perfusion; SBP > 90 mm Hg	Carotid/femoral pulses palpable; SBP 90-50 mm Hg: **MOD**	Weak or no palpable pulses: SBP <50- mm Hg: **MAJ**
Fracture	None seen or suspected	Single closed fracture anywhere	Any open long bone fracture or multiple fracture sites: **MAJ**
Cutaneous	No visible injury	Contusion, or abrasion, or laceration <3 in.	Amputation/tissue loss§ or 2°/3° burns to >10% TBSA or laceration >3 in. or any penetrating injury to head, neck, or torso: **MAJ**

MAJ = Major: any one (1): transport to trauma center
MOD = Moderate: any two (2): transport to trauma center
ALL OTHERS = Follow local protocols

Modified from Tepas JJ et al: The pediatric trauma score as a predictor of injury severity in the injured child, *J Pediatr Surg* 22:14-18, 1987.
*The color-coded system identified below the table may be used in place of calculating the Pediatric Trauma Score and the "less than eight" requirement.
†Colors correspond to color zones on length-weight based (Broselow) resuscitation tapes (see inside back cover).
‡Airway evaluation is designed to reflect the intervention required for effective care.
§Degloving injuries, major flap avulsions (> 3 in.) or amputations proximal to the wrist or ankle.

be easily recognized. Although the GCS was not designed as a triage or prognostic tool, it is used in many trauma scoring systems. The GCS characterizes the patient's eye opening and best motor and verbal responses. The lowest score is 3—one point earned for failure of response in each category, indicating that the child is flaccid, with no response to any stimulus. The highest score is 15 (eye opening—4, motor response—6, and verbal response—5).

When the child is unconscious, the key section of the GCS is the evaluation of the motor response (spontaneous movement, or movement or posturing in response to a painful stimulus). The GCS score should be determined by the *best* response observed (see Disability: Neurologic Evaluation under Initial Stabilization of the Pediatric Trauma Victim). A variety of pediatric modifications of the GCS have been developed, but only the Adelaide Coma Scale has been validated in children (Simpson et al.,

<table>
<tr><td colspan="1">

Box 12-4

Prognostic Indicators Following Submersion

Poor Prognostic Indicators

Absence of perfusing cardiac rhythm on arrival in the emergency department (ED)

Asystole on arrival in the ED

Glasgow Coma Scale (GCS) score of <4 with unresponsive pupils within the first 12-24 hr of intensive care unit (ICU) admission

Submersion duration >10 min or cardiopulmonary resuscitation (CPR) duration >25 min if victim was submerged in non-icy water (>5° C)

Good Prognostic Indicators

Submersion duration <5 min

Prompt bystander basic life support (BLS) at the scene

Prompt advanced life support (ALS; including intubation)

Total CPR duration <10 min

Sinus tachycardia, reactive pupils at the scene

Neurologic responsiveness in the ED

Data from Bratton SL et al: Serial, neurologic examinations after near-drowning and outcome, *Arch Pediatr Adolesc Med* 148:167–170, 1994; Kyriacou DN et al: Effect of immediate resuscitation on children with submersion injury, *Pediatrics* 94:137-142, 1994; Quan L, Kinder D: Pediatric submersions; prehospital predictors of outcome, *Pediatrics* 90:909-913, 1992.

</td></tr>
</table>

1991). The most important part of any scoring system is consistency in its application by each member of the health care team so that identification of trends in the patient's condition will be possible.

Prognostic Indicators Following Submersion

Predictors of outcome following pediatric submersion have been described in several studies (Box 12-4). Reported *poor prognostic signs,* associated with death or severe neurologic impairment in children submerged in *non-icy* (>5° C) waters include a long submersion time and absence of a perfusing rhythm on arrival in the ED. Increased survival among pediatric submersion victims has been

linked with a brief submersion duration, prompt bystander basic life support (BLS) at the scene, and sinus tachycardia and reactive pupils at the scene.

Although very small children may tolerate extended periods of submersion (>10 minutes) without neurologic sequelae, such intact survival is uncommon. It has only been documented in isolated reports involving *very* small children (<5 years of age) submerged in *icy* (<5° C) water.

Core *hypothermia* may develop in pediatric submersion victims whether or not they have been submerged in cold water. Such hypothermia may represent a *secondary* effect of inadequate perfusion, hypoxic brain injury, and heat loss during resuscitation, rather than initial cooling during the submersion itself. Protective hypothermia is unlikely to develop before hypoxic injury occurs unless the submersion occurs in *icy* water. Attempts should be made to restore normothermia before determining that CPR efforts are futile, but it may be impossible to restore or maintain normothermia if severe anoxic brain insult or cardiorespiratory arrest has contributed to a secondary fall in body temperature.

Initial Stabilization of the Pediatric Trauma Victim

Team Approach to Management

Optimal trauma care requires organization of resources and personnel; each member of the trauma team must have designated responsibilities. Team composition may vary from institution to institution based on the number and skill level of personnel, but intervention priorities remain the same (Table 12-2).

Emergency Department Stabilization and Transfer

The amount of care provided in the ED will be determined by the child's clinical status and the transport time required to reach the definitive treatment center. If the child can be transported to the pediatric intensive care unit (PICU) or operating room in the same hospital, a short ED stay is indicated. However, if the PICU is located in a separate hos-

Table 12-2
Responsibilities of the Pediatric Trauma Team*

Physician Team Leader	Trauma Team Members (MD, RN, EMT-P, PA)		
	Airway Maintenance	Assessment of Cardiovascular Status	Secondary Assessment
Assign team responsibilities	Open, maintain airway	Place on cardiac monitor	Evaluate head and neck trauma
Evaluate effectiveness of interventions	Immobilize cervical spine	Obtain vital signs	Stabilize cervical spine (C-collar, back board)
Reassign priorities as indicated	Assess ventilatory status	Assess capillary refill, color, proximal and distal pulses	Evaluate neurologic status; modified Glasgow Coma Scale
Determine need for specialty consultations	Clear airway of debris	Apply pneumatic anti-shock garments (PASGs) if indicated	Evaluate chest and heart
Evaluate for early or delayed life-threatening injuries	Suction oropharynx	Obtain vascular access	Perform needle thoracentesis for pneumothoraces
Perform needed critical procedures (central line placement, chest tube placement, pericardiocentesis)	Finger sweep visible debris	Peripheral	Evaluate abdomen
Determine need for secondary transport	Administer oxygen	Intraosseous	Insert nasogastric tube for gastric distension (no history of head trauma)
Maintain communication with child's family	Perform bag-valve-mask (BVM) ventilation and intubate when indicate	Femoral vein	Insert orogastric tube if head trauma is present
	Continuously assess ventilatory status	Obtain blood for hemocrit and hemoglobin, and type and crossmatch	Evaluate genitals and pelvis
	Hyperventilate when head trauma is suspected	Administer 20 ml/kg lactated Ringer's solution or normal saline boluses, as required, to treat shock	Observe for urinary tract trauma (i.e., blood in urethral meatus, scrotal hematoma); if present, consult urology (do not insert Foley)
		Administer blood when available	Evaluate pelvis for pain and deformity
			Observe for extremity trauma
			Assess distal perfusion
			Splint or evaluate previous splinting as required

Modified from Hazinski MF: *Nursing care of the critically ill child*, ed 2, St Louis, 1992, Mosby.
*Each trauma team member should be assigned specific responsibilities before the patient's arrival. Small emergency departments may consist of no more than 2 or 3 members; however, additional team members may be required depending on injury severity. Support service personnel (laboratory, x-ray, pharmacy, respiratory therapy), the appropriate medical consultants (e.g., surgeons, anesthesiologist, neurologist), and the operating room staff should be alerted.

pital, evaluation in the ED should be more thorough to detect any major occult injuries, and more time may be taken to stabilize the child (e.g., intubation, volume resuscitation) and establish reliable vascular access. Indications to consider transfer of the child to a pediatric trauma center have been developed by the American Pediatric Surgical Association (Box 12-5).

Primary Survey and Initial Resuscitation

Overview

The initial stabilization of the pediatric trauma victim is performed in the field and then, as needed, in the ED. By the time the child arrives in the PICU, the airway should be secure, intravascular access should be established, and a perfusing cardiac rhythm should be present. However, the primary and secondary assessments are repeated in the PICU; if major trauma is present and the child is extremely unstable, resuscitation may still be required (see p. 160).

The *primary survey* takes only a few minutes and focuses on assessment/detection and stabilization of life-threatening problems. Airway, breathing, circulation, and neurologic function are quickly assessed; any critical problems identified are treated immediately (Box 12-6). Initial resuscitation priorities include:

- *Airway:* Evaluate and maintain the airway while the cervical spine is immobilized.
- *Breathing:* Evaluate effectiveness of breathing; support oxygenation and ventilation.
- *Circulation:* Evaluate circulation and control hemorrhage. Begin shock/volume resuscitation.
- *Disability (neurologic function):* Evaluate level of consciousness and responsiveness, pupil size and response to light, and GCS score.

The airway and ventilation are supported as the cervical spine is stabilized. Circulation is assessed through *palpation of central and peripheral pulses.* This enables simultaneous evaluation of heart rate, quality of peripheral pulses, and skin temperature and capillary refill (consider ambient temperature).

Box 12-5

Possible Indications for Transfer of the Pediatric Trauma Victim to a Level I Trauma Center or a Pediatric Intensive Care Unit

History of injury

Patient thrown from a moving vehicle
Falls from >15 feet
Extrication time >20 min
Passenger cabin invaded >12 inches
Death of another passenger
Accident in a hostile environment (heat, cold water, etc.)

Anatomic Diagnoses

Combined system injury
Penetrating injury of the groin or neck
Three or more long bone fractures
Fractures of the axial skeleton
Amputation (other than digits)
Persistent hypotension
Severe head trauma
Maxillofacial or upper airway injury
Central nervous system injury with prolonged loss of consciousness, posturing, or paralysis
Spinal cord injury with neurologic deficit
Unstable chest injury
Blunt or penetrating trauma to the chest or abdomen
Burns, flame or inhalation

System Considerations

Necessary service or specialist not available
No beds available
Need for pediatric intensive care unit care
Multiple casualties
Family request
Paramedic judgment
Severity scores: Trauma Score 12 or less; or
                   Revised Trauma Score 11 or less; or
                   Pediatric Trauma Score 8 or less

From Harris BH et al: American Pediatric Surgical Association principles of pediatric trauma care, *J Pediatr Surg* 27:424, 1992.

Box 12-6

Primary Survey and Initial Resuscitation
of the Pediatric Trauma Victim

1. *Airway:* Open airway with jaw thrust while cervical spine is immobilized (if patient is not already intubated).
2. Suction airway if needed.
3. Evaluate airway patency and ventilation.
4. *Breathing:* Administer 100% oxygen:
   a. Via nonrebreathing mask or
   b. Bag-valve-mask (BVM) ventilation
   c. *If respiratory distress or depressed level of consciousness (LOC)* is observed, ventilate with 100% oxygen using BVM.
5. *If respiratory distress or depressed LOC:*
   a. Intubate (rapid sequence intubation if patient is conscious—see Box 12-8, p. 591).
   b. Ensure that airway is maintained if patient is not intubated.
   c. Monitor ventilation (rate, chest expansion, breath sounds).
6. Identify/treat tension or open pneumothorax or hemothorax if it prevents ventilation.
7. *Circulation:* Evaluate perfusion (including heart rate, pulses):
   a. If pulseless arrest is present, begin chest compression, cardiopulmonary resuscitation (CPR). Asystole in the victim of blunt trauma is an ominous finding.
   b. Bradycardia is often caused by hypoxia—ensure adequate airway, oxygenation, and ventilation; typically signals impending arrest—be prepared.
   c. Tachycardia is more appropriate than normocardia or bradycardia in the trauma patient.
   d. Ventricular arrhythmias or heart block may indicate presence of myocardial contusions, underlying congenital heart disease.
8. Determine presence of *shock*. Signs include:
   a. Heart rate that is rapid or inappropriately low
   b. Weak peripheral pulses
   c. Mottled color, pallor, or cyanosis (including gray color)
   d. Cold temperature (consider ambient temperature)
   e. Altered LOC (unusual irritability or lethargy) (A decreased response to painful stimulation is abnormal and often indicates compromise in cardiorespiratory status or head injury—evaluate further.)
   f. Hypotension (will be present with frank hypovolemic shock [>25% of circulating blood volume] but may not be present early in shock)
9. Identify/control major hemorrhage:
   a. Rule out/treat life-threatening thoracic injuries (tension pneumothorax, hemothorax).
   b. Consider need for urgent operative management of vascular injuries.
   c. Estimate circulating blood volume (CBV) and consider blood loss as a percent of CBV:
   (1) 80 ml/kg in infants
   (2) 75 ml/kg in children
   d. Identify/control external hemorrhage with pressure.
   e. Identify other potential hemorrhage sites: chest, abdomen, or retroperitoneal space.
10. Establish intravenous access—insert two large-bore catheters. Consider intraosseous route for children <6-7 years of age (particularly ≤3 years of age). Obtain blood sample for type and cross-match (and other laboratory work if possible—see step 17).
11. *If systemic perfusion is inadequate:* Administer 20 ml/kg isotonic fluid (normal saline or lactated Ringer's solution). Repeat if needed.
12. *Disability:* Evaluate neurologic status, immobilize neck with rigid collar, immobilize thoracic spine, and identify and begin to treat disability (increased intracranial pressure, status epilepticus)
13. Evaluate response to fluid bolus and determine need for additional fluid/blood boluses, or notification of pediatric surgeon (see Figure 12-6). Carefully regulate fluid administration—fluid boluses should be administered to restore systemic perfusion (avoid fluid overload).
14. *Exposure:* Maintain child's body temperature with warming lights or blankets. If hypothermia is present, warm intravenous fluids or blood before administration.

Box 12-6

Primary Survey and Initial Resuscitation of the Pediatric Trauma Victim—cont'd

15. Insert nasogastric tube if not accomplished with step 5. (If severe craniofacial trauma or maxillofacial or basilar skull fracture is present, insert orogastric tube to decompress stomach.)
16. Remove clothing and begin secondary survey.
17. Obtain additional blood specimens (for arterial blood gas analysis, complete blood count with differential and platelets, serum electrolytes, amylase, blood urea nitrogen, creatinine, glucose, prothrombin time, and partial thromboplastin time).

18. Evaluate and dress open wounds.
19. Obtain essential diagnostic studies (chest radiograph, head or neck computed tomography [CT] scan.)
20. Insert appropriate vascular monitoring catheters (including an arterial line); may be delayed until arrival in the pediatric intensive care unit (PICU).
21. Insert urinary catheter. *(Do not insert catheter if evidence of pelvic fracture, urethral injuries, or blood in the meatus is present.)*

The blood pressure is evaluated by the end of the primary survey.

If the ED or PICU is well organized, the primary survey is accomplished during the first 20 minutes of care (Box 12-6). Note that the primary survey is performed simultaneously with resuscitation.

Airway and Cervical Spine Immobilization

Open the Airway and Immobilize the Cervical Spine The first priority of management is to establish a patent airway while immobilizing the cervical spine. A patent airway must be maintained, particularly if the child is unconscious, because the child's tongue can fall into and obstruct the posterior pharynx.

A chin lift or jaw thrust is used to open the airway to avoid manipulation of the head until cervical spine injury has been completely ruled out. The patient's jaw can be lifted without compromising cervical spine immobilization (Figure 12-1).

When the child is placed supine (particularly on a firm surface such as a table or spine board), the prominent occiput of the child's head may produce neck flexion and airway obstruction. Use of pediatric spine boards with head wells will facilitate maintenance of a neutral position of the head and neck. If such a board is unavailable, the torso of the child should be elevated with a blanket folded to elevate the torso 2 cm (½ to 1 inch) so that the neck remains in neutral position.

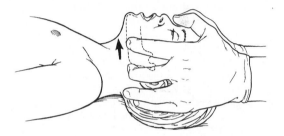

Figure 12-1 Proper method of simultaneous cervical spine stabilization during airway opening of the child with multiple injuries. (From Chameides L, Hazinski MF, editors: *The textbook of pediatric advanced life support,* Dallas, 1997, American Heart Association.)

Suction the Airway If large obstructing matter, such as blood, mucus, loose teeth, or vomitus is observed in the mouth or pharynx, clear it with a finger sweep (gloves should be worn). A rigid suction device or large suction catheter can then be used.

Airway, Breathing, and Oxygenation

Evaluation of Airway Patency and Ventilation
Ongoing assessment of airway patency and ventilation is mandatory if the child is breathing spontaneously. Continuously evaluate respiratory rate, effort, and effectiveness (air movement).

Signs of airway obstruction include changes in responsiveness, alteration in respiratory rate and depth, increased work of breathing, wheezing or

Box 12-7

Indications for Intubation in the Injured Child

Signs of Airway Obstruction

Stridor
Wheezing
Increased respiratory effort (particularly supra-
    sternal or supraclavicular retractions)
Nasal flaring
Weak cry
Tachypnea
Late signs:
    Hypoxemia or hypercarbia
    Decreased air movement
    Bradycardia
    Slowing of respiratory rate

Signs of Respiratory Failure and Need for Mechanical Ventilation

Severe respiratory distress (including grunting,
    retractions)
Hypoxemia despite oxygen therapy
Hypercarbia (particularly if rising rapidly)
Acidosis
Rising alveolar-arterial oxygen difference (A-a Do_2)
    or Oxygenation Index (OI) (see p. 305)
Late signs:
    Decreased air movement
    Apnea or gasping
    Bradycardia

Indications for Intubation

Respiratory arrest, apnea
Significant respiratory distress
Hypoventilation
Hypoxemia despite oxygen therapy
Respiratory acidosis
Signs of airway obstruction; stridor, increased
    work of breathing, suprasternal, supraclavic-
    ular retraction
Injuries associated with potential airway ob-
    struction (e.g., inhalation injuries, crushing
    facial or neck injuries)
Head injury or signs of increased intracranial
    pressure
Thoracic injury (rib fractures, pulmonary contu-
    sion, flail chest, penetrating injuries)
Anticipation of need for mechanical ventilatory
    support.

Modified from Hazinski MF: *Nursing care of the
critically ill child,* ed 2, St Louis, 1992, Mosby.

stridor, or prolonged inspiration or expiration (Box 12-7). Note that *hypoxemia may be only a late sign of airway obstruction* in the child who is breathing spontaneously; thus intubation should be accomplished before it develops.

Administration of Oxygen *If the child has a patent airway and effective spontaneous ventilation,* administer 100% oxygen via a nonrebreathing mask. If the frightened or irritable child refuses oxygen therapy, "blow-by" oxygen may be used but will result in unpredictable supplementary oxygen delivery.

If the child has ineffective spontaneous ventilation, provide ventilation with 100% oxygen through a bag-valve-mask (BVM). Signs of ineffective ventilation include apnea, gasping, increased respiratory effort, or cyanosis despite oxygen therapy.

If the child is unconscious or has a head injury, be prepared to provide BVM ventilation at the first sign of respiratory insufficiency. Maintain a $Paco_2$ of 32 to 34 mm Hg to prevent excessive cerebral blood flow and ICP but avoid extreme hyperventilation, which may create cerebral ischemia. The rate and tidal volume of ventilation should be approximately normal for size and age, although additional support may be required if shock or respiratory failure is present.

Respiratory rates delivered by BVM for the trauma victim include:

- *Infants:* Approximately 40 breaths/min
- *Preschoolers:* Approximately 30 breaths/min
- *School-age children:* Approximately 20 to 24 breaths/min

In most situations the proper use of a BVM device will support effective ventilation and oxygenation. If BVM ventilation does not produce visible chest expansion and adequate breath sounds, tension pneumothorax and hemothorax should be ruled out—these are the most likely causes of failure of ventilatory support in the trauma victim. Tracheal obstruction or direct injury to the lung or pleural space may cause persistent hypoxemia despite BVM ventilation with oxygen. Occasionally a needle cricothyrotomy is required to establish adequate oxygenation in the patient with upper airway obstruction, although this technique will not enable effective ventilation (carbon dioxide elimination).

The pulse oximeter is a useful adjunct to clinical assessment and enables continuous evaluation of patient oxygenation and response to therapy. Monitoring of end-tidal carbon dioxide is also useful. Although end-tidal carbon dioxide monitoring can be accomplished through a nasal cannula, it is most accurate via an endotracheal tube.

Airways Temporary use of artificial airways may facilitate spontaneous ventilation or BVM ventilation until intubation can be accomplished.

Both oropharyngeal and nasopharyngeal airways can help to maintain upper airway patency. *Oral* airways are reserved for *unconscious* children with spontaneous respirations—they *should not be used in the conscious child,* because insertion may stimulate gagging and vomiting. The airway must be sized appropriately because airways that are too small can push the tongue back into the oropharynx, and those that are too long can obstruct the trachea. The length of the airway should equal the distance between the mouth and the angle of the mandible.

To insert the oral airway, pull the tongue forward or use a tongue depressor to compress the tongue. The airway should be oriented to the proper position outside of the mouth and then inserted gently over the tongue. If a tongue depressor is not available, the airway can be inverted and used to depress the tongue and then rotated into proper position as it reaches the back of the oropharynx. However, this inversion method may produce trauma to the teeth and soft tissues in the oropharynx (see pp. 308-309).

Nasopharyngeal airways are soft rubber or plastic tubes that are inserted through the nose into the posterior pharynx. They can be inserted in the conscious patient, even if the gag reflex is intact. The nasopharyngeal airway should be slightly smaller than the diameter of the nares. The length of the airway should equal the distance from the nares to the tragus of the ear.

Intubation *If the child's ability to maintain a patent airway is in doubt, intubation should be performed by skilled personnel.* Intubation may be needed to establish a patent airway or to prevent an-ticipated airway compromise following inhalation injuries, facial burns, or severe trauma to the face and neck. When airway obstruction develops, elective intubation should be performed *before* signs of severe respiratory distress or hypoxia develop. Indications for intubation are listed in Box 12-7.

Preparation Appropriate sizes of intubation equipment can be estimated using formulas, tables, or a length-based reference system such as the Broselow Resuscitation Tape (Broselow Medical Technologies, Hickory, North Carolina); these aids should be readily available in the ED and PICU (Table 12-3). Cuffed tubes are not typically used in children less than 8 years of age because normal subglottic narrowing provides a snug fit when a tube of proper size is used. If a cuffed tube is inserted, the cuff is usually left deflated in younger children.

The child with respiratory distress tends to gulp air, and prolonged BVM ventilation may force air into the stomach, causing gastric distension. This complication may be prevented by application of pressure over the cricoid cartilage during ventilation (the Sellick maneuver). Before intubation, a *nasogastric tube* is often inserted to decompress the stomach (see p. 606).

Pharmacologic paralysis or sedation is not necessary during intubation of the comatose child. However, if the child is conscious, rapid sequence induction (RSI) anesthesia may be used to facilitate intubation (Box 12-8). RSI is preferred if it is suspected that the stomach is full, since it eliminates the possibility of gagging and regurgitation. Another neuromuscular blocker may be substituted for succinylcholine during RSI if head or eye injuries are present, because succinylcholine probably increases cerebral blood flow and intracranial and intraocular pressures.

Tube Placement *Oral* intubation is generally preferred over nasotracheal intubation, to minimize upper airway trauma. Emergent *nasotracheal* intubation is reserved for the child with severe craniofacial trauma, and it should only be performed by personnel experienced in the technique. Blind nasotracheal intubation in the presence of maxillary sinus fractures may result in intubation of the sinuses or cranium. If nasotracheal intubation is desirable to facilitate long-term ventilatory management, reintubation can be accomplished electively when the patient is stable.

Table 12-3
Selection of Proper Pediatric Resuscitation Equipment

Color on Broselow Pediatric Resus Tape	Infant (3-7 kg) RED	Small Child (8-11 kg) PURPLE	Child (12-14 kg) YELLOW	Child (14-17 kg) WHITE	Child (18-22 kg) BLUE	Young Adult (24-30 kg) ORANGE	Young Adult (32-34 kg +) GREEN
Bag-valve device	Infant	Child	Child	Child	Child	Child/adult	Adult
O₂ mask	Newborn	Pediatric	Pediatric	Pediatric	Pediatric	Adult	Adult
Oral airway	Infant/small child	Small child	Child	Child	Child/small adult	Child/small adult	Medium adult
Laryngoscope blade	0-1 straight	1 straight	2 straight or curved	2 straight or curved	2 straight or curved	2-3 straight or curved	3 straight or curved
ET tubes	Premie 2.5 mm uncuffed Term 3.0 mm uncuffed Infant 3.5 mm uncuffed	4.0 mm uncuffed	4.5 mm uncuffed	5.0 mm uncuffed	5.5 mm uncuffed	6.0 mm cuffed	6.5 mm cuffed
ET tube length (cm at lip)	10-10.5 cm	11-12 cm	12.5-13.5 cm	14-15 cm	15.5-16.5 cm	17-18 cm	18.5-19.5 cm
Stylet	6 Fr.	6 Fr.	6 Fr.	6 Fr.	14 Fr.	14 Fr.	14 Fr.
Suction	8 Fr.	8 Fr.	8-10 Fr.	10 Fr.	10 Fr.	10 Fr.	12 Fr.
BP cuff	Newborn-infant	Infant-child	Child	Child	Child	Child-adult	Adult
IV: Catheter	22-24 G	20-24 G	18-22 G	18-22 G	18-20 G	18-20 G	16-20 G
Butterfly	23-25 G	23-25 G	21-23 G	21-23 G	21-23 G	21-22 G	18-21 G
NG tube	5-8 Fr.	8-10 Fr.	10 Fr.	10-12 Fr.	12-14 Fr.	14-18 Fr.	18 Fr.
Urinary catheter	5-8 Fr.	8-10 Fr.	10 Fr.	10-12 Fr.	10-12 Fr.	12 Fr.	12 Fr.
Chest tube	10-12 Fr.	16-20 Fr.	20-24 Fr.	20-24 Fr.	24-32 Fr.	28-32 Fr.	32-40 Fr.

From Hazinski MF: *Nursing care of the critically ill child*, ed 2, St Louis, 1992, Mosby; modified from *Broselow Pediatric Resuscitation Tape*, Hickory, NC, Broselow Medical Technologies.

Box 12-8

Rapid and Modified Rapid
Sequence Induction

I. Rapid Sequence Induction

Rapid sequence induction is designed to induce loss of consciousness and muscle relaxation so control of the airway and intubation can be accomplished within seconds. This requires preoxygenation of the patient, assembly of all drugs and equipment at hand, and establishment of cardiorespiratory monitoring. The following steps occur sequentially:

1. Establish cardiorespiratory monitoring (ECG, pulse oximetry, noninvasive blood pressure monitoring)
2. Preoxygenate with 100% oxygen.
3. Atropine: 0.02 mg/kg (minimum: 0.1 mg) may be administered to prevent bradycardia (especially for children <7 years). Alternative: glycopyrrolate (Rubinul, 0.01-0.02 mg/kg).
4. Provide cricoid pressure and administer 100% oxygen by "blow by" technique.

The following drugs (Nos. 5 and 6) are administered in rapid sequence by intravenous push:

5. Thiopental: 3-5 mg/kg IV (unless patient hypotensive or in status asthmaticus) Alternatives: Midazolam: 0.1 mg/kg IV (Maximum dose: 5 mg) plus fentanyl
6. Succinylcholine: 1-2 mg/kg IV
   Pancuronium 0.01 mg/kg IV may be administered to reduce fasciculations (for children >12 years)
   Alternative: Vecuronium: 0.15-0.2 mg/kg IV (effects will last up to 60 minutes) or rocuronium (0.6-1.5 mg/kg, very rapid onset)
7. Intubate and maintain cricoid pressure while tube placement is verified.
8. Release cricoid pressure.
9. Tape endotracheal tube in place and reverify placement (including chest radiograph).

NOTE: The preceding sequence should not be used if head injury and increased ICP are present. Patients with increased ICP should be hyperventilated, and succinylcholine use is controversial because it will increase cerebral blood flow and ICP. Medical contraindications to the use of succinylcholine are provided in Box 3-2, p. 64.

II. Modified Rapid Sequence Induction

This procedure is recommended if head injury and increased ICP are present.

1. Establish cardiorespiratory monitoring (ECG, pulse oximetry, noninvasive blood pressure).
2. Preoxygenate with 100% oxygen.
3. Atropine (see dose in No. 3 at left)
4. Lidocaine: 1.5 mg/kg IV if severe head injury present (wait 2 minutes before administering succinylcholine–see No. 8, below).
5. Apply cricoid pressure while continuing to deliver 100% oxygen.
6. Thiopental: 3-5 mg/kg IV (unless patient hypotensive or in status asthmaticus) Alternatives: Midazolam: 0.1 mg/kg IV (Maximum dose: 5 mg) plus fentanyl.
7. Hyperventilate and continue to hyperventilate.
8. Succinylcholine: 2 mg/kg IV
   Alternative: Vecuronium: 0.2 mg/kg IV (effects will last up to 60 minutes)
9. Intubate when full muscle relaxation achieved.
10. Check tube placement with auscultation while maintaining cricoid pressure.
11. Release cricoid pressure.
12. Tape tube and reverify proper position (including chest radiograph).

Sources:

1. Pediatric Emergency Medicine Committee of the American College of Emergency Physicians, Gerardi MJ et al: Rapid-sequence intubation of the pediatric patient, *Ann Emerg Med* 28:55-74, 1996
2. Deshpande JK, Tobias JD, editors: *The pediatric pain handbook,* St Louis, 1996, Mosby.
3. Fitzmaurice LS: Approach to multiple trauma. In Barkin RM, editor: *Pediatric emergency medicine: concepts and clinical practice,* St Louis, 1992, Mosby.

Intubation of the child with multisystem trauma requires several people. The cervical spine must be immobilized by one person while a second person performs the intubation. That second person monitors the child's color during the attempt. A third person monitors the heart rate and hemoglobin saturation during the intubation attempt and gathers and provides equipment (Figure 12-2). The bedside cardiac monitor should be adjusted to provide an audible QRS tone during the intubation attempt, so that everyone at the bedside is aware of the heart rate at all times. If the heart rate falls or color or oxygenation deteriorates during an intubation attempt, the attempt should be interrupted to provide oxygenation and ventilation with BVM until the child's condition improves. For further information regarding intubation, see p. 310.

Evaluation of Tube Placement   If endotracheal intubation is successful and the tube is placed in proper position, bilateral chest expansion should be apparent during positive pressure ventilation, and bilateral breath sounds should be equal and adequate. Most important, the child's clinical status should improve. Breath sounds must be carefully evaluated, because sounds from one area of the lung may be transmitted through the thin chest wall to an area over atelectasis or a pneumothorax. One lung should be used as a control to compare sounds heard over the other lung, and chest expansion

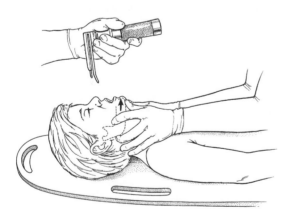

Figure 12-2   Simultaneous cervical spine stabilization and intubation. (From Chameides L, Hazinski MF, editors: *The textbook of pediatric advanced life support,* Dallas, 1997, American Heart Association.)

should be observed from the head or foot of the bed. Unilateral lung pathology (including pneumothorax, hemothorax, pleural effusion, or atelectasis) may produce a unilateral compromise in chest expansion and a unilateral change in *pitch* in breath sounds, rather than a decrease in *intensity* of breath sounds. Auscultate under the axilla and over the back to ensure that breath sounds are adequate bilaterally.

Causes of Acute Deterioration in Intubated Patients   If acute deterioration is observed following intubation and stabilization, the following should be ruled out (remember the mnemonic *DOPE*):

- *D:* Displacement of the endotracheal tube
- *O:* Obstruction of the tube
- *P:* Pneumothorax (tension)
- *E:* Equipment failure

Cricothyrotomy and Tracheostomy   When positioning of the head and jaw and BMV ventilation have not relieved airway obstruction, and intubation cannot be accomplished, injury to the larynx or trachea is likely to be present. Needle cricothyrotomy, although rarely necessary in the child, should be considered to enable oxygen delivery, and operative intervention may ultimately be required. Needle cricothyrotomy can be very difficult because the child has a relatively short neck, landmarks are not easily identified, and the needle is difficult to secure once it is inserted. Needle cricothyrotomy provides only a temporary route for delivery of oxygen; even large-bore catheters will provide oxygenation but inadequate ventilation. Prolonged hypoventilation through the small needle airway will eventually result in hypercarbia.

Emergency tracheostomy is *rarely* indicated in the child and should be reserved for times when both intubation and needle cricothyrotomy fail to produce adequate oxygenation. It is a difficult procedure in children, is associated with a high complication rate, and should only be performed by experienced physicians.

Crushing Airway Obstruction   Rare causes of airway obstruction include "clothesline" injuries with penetrating or crushing trauma to the larynx or trachea. When airway manipulation causes air hunger and ventilation is inadequate despite all methods of support (including BVM ventilation, intubation) operative intervention is indicated. Airway obstruction may also develop as a result of tracheobronchial tract edema associated with chemical or thermal burns. Treatment is supportive, and intubation will be required until the edema resolves.

Chest Injuries That Prevent Oxygenation and Ventilation

Note that some thoracic injuries are life threatening and may prevent establishment of effective oxygenation and ventilation. A *tension pneumothorax, open pneumothorax,* or *massive hemothorax* must be treated promptly. A flail chest may also interfere with initial oxygenation and spontaneous ventilation but will respond to positive pressure ventilation (see Flail Chest under Secondary Survey, Chest). These complications should be recognized on the basis of *clinical* rather than radiographic findings, and treatment should be initiated before a radiograph is taken.

Tension Pneumothorax   A tension pneumothorax develops from progressive air entry into the pleural space with an associated elevation of intrapleural pressure and collapse of the lung on the involved side. The pediatric mediastinum is extremely mobile; thus the *mediastinum shifts away from the affected side,* producing tracheal deviation and a shift in the cardiac point of maximal impulse (PMI) away from the pneumothorax, decreased breath sounds, and neck vein distension. When the lung on the involved side collapses, severe hypoxemia results and pulmonary vascular resistance increases dramatically (see Figure 7-11, *B*). Decreased cardiac output and oxygen delivery constitute immediate threats to life.

A tension pneumothorax is treated by immediate rapid needle or thoracostomy decompression, typically before a chest x-ray film is obtained (see Pneumothorax under Secondary Survey, Chest). Immediate improvement in the patient's condition with evidence of air evacuation confirms the diagnosis.

To perform needle decompression, a large-bore (14-, 18- or 20-gauge) over-the-needle catheter is inserted into the second intercostal space over the top of the third rib, at the midclavicular line of the affected side, or at the fourth or fifth intercostal space in the anterior axillary line. Successful needle decompression will result in a gush of air from the chest.

Occasionally the catheter is joined to a length of intravenous (IV) tubing before insertion in the chest. The distal 2 cm of the tubing can be submerged in a small bottle of sterile water, creating an underwater seal that prevents entry of room air into the chest during spontaneous inspiration. After the pneumothorax is decompressed by needle aspiration, a chest tube is inserted.

Venting of the pneumothorax can also be accomplished using a needle joined to a one-way flutter valve. The flutter valve enables evacuation of air from the chest but will not allow air entry into the chest.

A chest tube should be inserted as soon as feasible. The largest chest tube possible should be inserted (see Table 12-3). A local anesthetic should be provided, and the skin prepared with a povidone-iodine scrub. Gloves should be worn during the procedure.

The tube is inserted through a small stab wound made in the skin and subcutaneous tissue along the long axis of the rib, in the fourth, fifth, or sixth intercostal space at the anterior axillary line. The stab wound is made approximately one to two ribs below the desired insertion point for the chest tube, to reduce the risk of air leak after the tube is removed.

Before the tube is inserted, a hemostat is placed on the tube several centimeters from the tip (but beyond all drainage holes of the tube) to prevent excessive advancement of the tube into the chest. Using blunt dissection with finger and hemostat, the tube is inserted above the rib and threaded subcutaneously to the third or second intercostal space. At this point, it is advanced into the pleural space, directed posteriorly and apically (Figure 12-3). Once the tube is positioned appropriately, it is joined to a drainage device with underwater seal, and the hemostat is unclamped.

Sucking Chest Wounds   Sucking chest wounds result from penetrating trauma and produce an open pneumothorax that allows air to move into and out of the pleural space. This injury must be

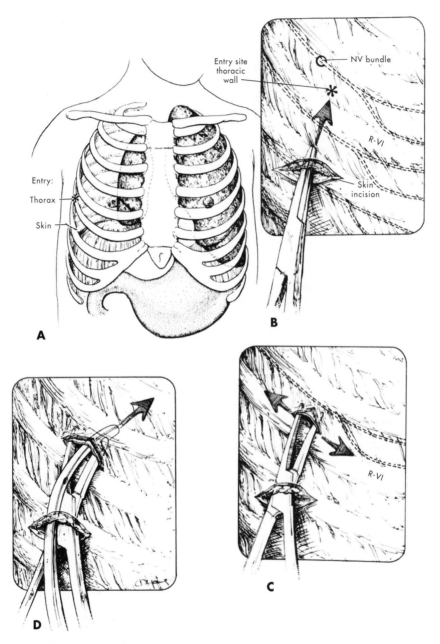

Figure 12-3 Chest tube insertion. Before chest tube insertion, the skin incision area is cleansed with povidone-iodine solution, and sterile gloves are worn. The skin incision site and the intercostal space are infiltrated with lidocaine (Xylocaine). **A,** Right pneumothorax is present. Skin incision will be made approximately one to two ribs below the entry into the thorax. **B,** Stab wound or small incision is made in the skin, and a hemostat is used to dissect to the desired entry site into the thorax. **C,** The hemostat enters the pleural space, and the arms are opened. **D,** The chest tube is inserted adjacent to the hemostat and into the thorax. (From Fleisher GR, Ludwig S: *Textbook of pediatric emergency medicine,* ed 3, Baltimore, 1993, Williams & Wilkins, p 1292.)

treated immediately with an occlusive dressing. If the child is intubated and receiving positive pressure ventilation, the chest wound should be sealed during inspiration to minimize the risk of a tension pneumothorax. Continuous observation is required to identify the possible development of a tension pneumothorax.

Hemothorax A hemothorax is the accumulation of blood in the pleural cavity; this may produce hypovolemic shock, as well as a compromise in ventilation. The severity of symptoms produced by the hemothorax will be determined by the extent and rapidity of blood loss and by the presence of associated injuries (i.e., lung or great vessel tears).

If the child is asymptomatic, the most effective immediate therapy is placement of an IV catheter to replace ongoing blood loss. An arterial blood gas measurement will indicate the degree of respiratory compromise produced. A chest tube is inserted to evacuate the hemothorax after initial volume replacement is accomplished.

Significant thoracic hemorrhage is associated with signs of poor systemic perfusion, as well as respiratory compromise. In this situation extremely rapid evacuation of blood from the pleural space can aggravate hypovolemia and lead to cardiac arrest. For this reason, it is extremely important to delay a chest tube placement until *after* initiation of volume resuscitation. If ongoing hemorrhage is apparent from the volume of chest tube drainage, rupture of a large vessel has probably occurred and an urgent exploratory thoracotomy is required.

Circulation

Evaluation and Support of Perfusion Evaluation and support of circulatory status requires (1) assessment of central pulses and determination of the need for cardiac compression and (2) evaluation and support of heart rate, systemic perfusion, and oxygenation.

Pulses Palpation of a central pulse enables determination of the need for CPR, as well as evaluation of the heart rate. If no pulse is palpable in a large central artery (the carotid or femoral artery) in an apneic, unconscious patient, pulseless cardiac arrest (asystole, ventricular fibrillation, pulseless ventricular tachycardia, or electromechanical dissociation) is present and CPR, including chest compressions,

is required. *The outcome of prehospital pulseless cardiac arrest in pediatric victims of blunt trauma is poor;* in the unlikely event that a perfusing cardiac rhythm is restored, severe hypoxic neurologic insult is likely to be present, and death may occur in the PICU. If pulseless arrest develops in the ED or PICU, immediate correction of causative factors (e.g., tension pneumothorax) must be accomplished to maximize the child's chance or survival.

Cardiopulmonary Resuscitation Basic components of resuscitation for pulseless arrest include (see also p. 160):

1. Asystole: Secure the airway and ventilate with 100% oxygen. Perform cardiac compressions and achieve IV or intraosseous (IO) access. Administer *epinephrine** every 3 to 5 minutes:
   a. Epinephrine, first IV/IO dose ("conventional dose"): 0.01 mg/kg (0.1 ml/kg of 1:10,000 concentration)
   b. Epinephrine, all endotracheal (ET) doses ("high dose"): 0.1 mg/kg (0.1 ml/kg of 1:1000 concentration)
   c. Epinephrine, second and subsequent IV/IO doses ("high dose"): 0.1 mg/kg (0.1 ml/kg of 1:1000 concentration)
2. *Electromechanical dissociation* (narrow QRS complex, no pulse): Manage as for asystole. Identify and *treat reversible causes:*
   a. Severe hypoxemia
   b. Severe acidosis
   c. Severe hypovolemia
   d. Tension pneumothorax
   e. Cardiac tamponade
   f. Profound hypothermia
   g. Severe electrolyte imbalances (e.g., hyperkalemia)
   h. Drug overdose
3. Ventricular fibrillation/pulseless ventricular tachycardia:
   a. Defibrillate up to three times (if needed) in rapid succession (2 J/kg, 4 J/kg, 4 J/kg).

---

*All epinephrine doses are 0.1 ml/kg. "Conventional dose" = 0.1 ml/kg of 1:10,000 (0.01 mg/kg). "High dose" = 0.1 ml/kg of 1:1000 (0.1 mg/kg).

b. Continue CPR, secure the airway, ventilate with 100% oxygen, and establish IV/IO access.

c. If ventricular fibrillation/ventricular tachycardia (VF/VT) persists, administer first dose of epinephrine—defibrillate 30 to 60 seconds after drug is administered.

    (1) IV/IO: 0.01 mg/kg (0.1 ml/kg of 1:10,000 concentration)

    (2) ET: 0.1 mg/kg (0.1 ml/kg of 1:1000 concentration)

d. If VF/VT persists, administer lidocaine, 1 mg/kg—defibrillate in 30 to 60 seconds.

e. If VF/VT persists, administer second dose of epinephrine, 0.1 mg/kg ET or IV/IO (0.1 ml/kg of 1:1000 concentration); repeat every 3 to 5 minutes—defibrillate 30 to 60 seconds after each dose.

f. If VF/VT persists, alternate epinephrine, 0.1 mg/kg, with lidocaine, 1 mg/kg—defibrillate 30 to 60 seconds after each dose.

g. If VF/VT persists, consider bretylium, 5 mg/kg (may be doubled and repeated)—defibrillate 30 to 60 seconds after each dose.

Heart Rate and Rhythm ECG monitoring is performed during evaluation and stabilization, so that the child's heart rate response to therapy can be continuously monitored. Systemic perfusion should also be constantly assessed. Pulse oximetry is a useful adjunct to enable continuous evaluation of oxygenation.

Evaluate the heart rate in light of the clinical condition. Cardiac output is almost linearly related to heart rate during early childhood, and stroke volume is relatively small. As a result, if the heart rate falls, it is likely that cardiac output will decrease commensurately.

Tachycardia *should* be observed in the frightened or injured child. In fact, *a normal heart rate may be inadequate in the seriously injured child.* Although tachycardia is often present following trauma, the heart rate should decrease toward normal levels if resuscitation is adequate; persistent tachycardia may indicate unrecognized hemorrhage (e.g., abdominal hemorrhage) or cardiopulmonary complications; therefore these should be ruled out.

Excessively high heart rates such as those produced by supraventricular tachycardia can result in a compromise in stroke volume and myocardial perfusion. A ventricular rate exceeding 180 to 200 beats/min may be caused by a supraventricular arrhythmia, requiring treatment.

Bradycardia is the most common terminal arrhythmia observed in children, and it is usually caused by hypoxia. If bradycardia is observed, assess airway patency and effectiveness of oxygenation and ventilation. If bradycardia develops during resuscitation of the intubated patient, rule out tube displacement, obstruction, pneumothorax, and equipment failure ("DOPE"). Note that chest compressions should be provided if, despite oxygenation and ventilation, the heart rate is <60 beats/min and is associated with poor systemic perfusion.

Heart block and malignant ventricular arrhythmias are relatively uncommon in pediatric trauma patients unless myocardial contusion, underlying congenital heart disease, drug toxicity, or profound hypoxia is present. Ventricular fibrillation in the near-drowning victim is often a poor prognostic sign.

Arterial Pressure *Accurate* blood pressure measurements require use of an appropriately sized cuff or an intraarterial catheter joined to a properly *zeroed and leveled* fluid-filled monitoring system. Cuff blood pressure measurements obtained with a sphygmomanometer may *underestimate* the intraarterial pressure in the unstable patient, since Korotkoff sounds may be difficult to hear. *Automated noninvasive oscillometric blood pressure monitors may fail to accurately reflect a rapidly falling or very low blood pressure.*

If the child demonstrates cardiovascular compromise, invasive intraarterial monitoring should be established as quickly as possible, since it provides access for serum and arterial blood gas sampling and enables continuous evaluation of the child's response to therapy. Typically, intraarterial monitoring is established in the PICU.

Shock A common cause of cardiovascular compromise in the trauma victim is shock secondary to hemorrhage. Signs of shock may be subtle in the child and include:

- Inappropriate heart rate, including extreme tachycardia or bradycardia, or normocardia in a child who is in pain, crying, poorly perfused, or unconscious

- Weak peripheral pulses
- Mottled skin; cool, pale extremities; prolonged capillary refill despite warm ambient temperature
- Inappropriate level of consciousness, such as unusual irritability, lethargy, or decreased response to a painful stimulus (e.g., placement of an IV catheter)
- Hypotension *(Shock may be present with a normal, low, or high blood pressure.)*

Hypotension beyond 1 year of age
  = Systolic BP <70 mm Hg + (2 × Age in years)

NOTE: Hypotension is not likely to be observed in the pediatric trauma victim unless/until approximately 25% of circulating blood volume is lost acutely.

Hemorrhage Identify external bleeding sites and control bleeding with application of pressure (wear gloves). Life-threatening thoracic injuries, particularly those that may interfere with ventilation and resuscitation, must be identified and treated. Such injuries include tension pneumothorax and hemothorax (see discussions of these conditions under Chest Injuries That Prevent Oxygenation and Ventilation).

The child's circulating blood volume should be calculated on admission (80 ml/kg for infants and 75 ml/kg for children), and all blood loss should be considered as a percentage of the child's circulating blood volume.

When the child hemorrhages, the blood pressure may not immediately change because systemic vascular resistance increases proportionately. This ability to compensate for blood loss with reflex vasoconstriction means that signs of hemorrhage may be insidious in the child, and vital signs alone may not identify "evolving shock." Ideally, signs of hemorrhage are detected and treated before evidence of decompensated shock (hypotension) develops. These signs include:

- Tachycardia
- Alteration in responsiveness
- Peripheral vasoconstriction (despite warm ambient temperature)
- Thready (weak) pulses, diminished pulse pressure

- Hypotension (a late and ominous sign of cardiovascular compromise and an indicator of decompensated shock)

Clinical findings may be used to classify the severity of the hemorrhage and to estimate the volume of blood loss (Table 12-4). As a rule of thumb, if hypotension is caused by hemorrhage, significant blood loss has occurred.

A discrepancy between the peripheral systemic oxygen saturation and the arterial oxygen saturation may indicate the need for further volume resuscitation. If the peripheral systemic oxygen saturation (obtained by pulse oximetry) is <80% of the arterial oxygen saturation, hypovolemia may be present, and additional volume resuscitation should be considered.

IV or IO access must be achieved, and blood loss must be replaced quickly. In addition, ongoing blood loss should be detected and stopped. External pressure is applied to accessible bleeding sites, and surgical exploration may be required.

Pericardial Tamponade Pericardial tamponade is the accumulation of blood in the pericardial sac, which compromises ventricular diastolic expansion and filling, producing a decrease in cardiac output. Tamponade is a relatively uncommon complication of trauma in children, but it should be suspected in any child with chest trauma associated with signs of shock unresponsive to establishment of effective oxygenation and ventilation, and volume administration. Classic signs of tamponade may be difficult to appreciate in the child in shock, but they may include:

- Persistent hypotension or other signs of shock despite fluid resuscitation
- Distension of neck veins, possible hepatomegaly
- Muffled heart sounds
- Pulsus paradoxus (a fall in arterial blood pressure of 8 to 10 mm Hg or more during spontaneous inspiration)

These signs may be particularly difficult to detect in the tachypneic infant or unconscious child in shock. An anterior hemopericardium can be confirmed by echocardiography, although a presumptive diagnosis is often made.

Treatment of tamponade requires pericardiocentesis or thoracotomy, and pericardial decom-

Table 12-4
Classification of Hemorrhagic Shock in Pediatric Trauma Patients Based on Systemic Signs

System	Class I: Very Mild Hemorrhage (<15% Blood Volume Loss)	Class II: Mild Hemorrhage (15%-25% Blood Volume Loss)	Class III: Moderate Hemorrhage (26%-40% Blood Volume Loss)	Class IV: Severe Hemorrhage (>40% Blood Volume Loss)
Cardiovascular	Heart rate normal or mildly increased Normal pulses	Tachycardia Peripheral pulses may be diminished	Significant tachycardia Thready peripheral pulses	Severe tachycardia Thready central pulses
	Normal BP Normal pH	Normal BP Normal pH	Hypotension Metabolic acidosis	Significant hypotension Significant acidosis
Respiratory	Rate normal	Tachypnea	Moderate tachypnea	Severe tachypnea
CNS	Slightly anxious	Irritable, confused Combative	Irritability or lethargy Diminished pain response	Lethargy Coma
Skin	Warm, pink	Cool extremities, mottling	Cool extremities, mottling or pallor	Cold extremities, pallor or cyanosis
	Capillary refill brisk	Delayed capillary refill	Prolonged capillary refill	Very prolonged capillary refill
Kidneys	Normal urine output	Oliguria, increased specific gravity	Oliguria, increased BUN	Anuria

Modified from Hazinski MF: *Nursing care of the critically ill child*, ed 2, St Louis, 1992, Mosby; American College of Surgeons: *Advanced trauma life support course*, Chicago, 1989, American College of Surgeons; and Fleisher GR, Ludwig S: *Textbook of pediatric emergency medicine*, ed 2, Baltimore, 1988, Williams & Wilkins.

pression. In addition, blood loss must be replaced. Emergency pericardiocentesis is accomplished with an 18-gauge metal spinal needle joined to a syringe by a three-way stopcock. Simultaneous electrocardiogram (ECG) monitoring or echocardiography should be performed to guide the depth of needle insertion (Figure 12-4). If ECG monitoring will be used, an alligator clip electrode is attached to the base of the needle and also to an ECG recorder. The needle is inserted in the left subxyphoid area and advanced toward the left scapula, with constant aspiration applied. When atypical ventricular (QRS) depolarizations are detected through the alligator clip electrode, the needle is in contact with the heart and should be withdrawn slightly. Alternatively, echocardiography may be used to guide needle insertion.

Ongoing pericardial hemorrhage requires insertion of a pericardial drain or catheter. Definitive treatment of a hemopericardium requires a thoracotomy, which is accomplished in the operating room if possible. Occasionally, emergent thoracotomy is performed in the ED or ICU.

Ongoing Hemorrhage Potential sources of severe ongoing hemorrhage include intrathoracic bleeding (including cardiac tamponade) or abdominal bleeding caused by injury of a solid organ or major vessel. Pelvic fracture may produce retroperitoneal hemorrhage, and a femoral shaft fracture can produce significant undetected blood loss into the thigh. Finally, head injury, cervical spinal cord injury (and spinal shock), and cerebral herniation should be ruled out if decompensated shock remains refractory to volume administration and thoracoabdominal hemorrhage is not present.

Medical Antishock Trousers A controversial adjunct to fluid therapy in the treatment of pediatric traumatic shock is the use of medical antishock trousers (MAST). Although MAST may increase blood pressure in children, the rise in blood pressure seems to result primarily from an increase in systemic vascular resistance. MAST have not been shown to improve survival in pediatric trauma victims with profound hypotension and may actually worsen the outcome in children with mild or moderate hypotension. Potential complications of MAST include lower extremity compartment syndromes and limb ischemia.

MAST may be helpful in stabilizing unstable pelvic fractures and halting or slowing pelvic bleeding. If MAST are used for this purpose, they should be inflated to a minimal pressure of 40 to 50 mm Hg. The abdominal section should not be inflated, since it may compress abdominal contents against the diaphragm, compromising ventilation.

If MAST are used, the child's blood pressure should be assessed as each section is inflated and deflated. Deflation should be performed *slowly,* with medical supervision. If the child's systolic blood pressure falls by ≥5 mm Hg, halt deflation and administer a fluid bolus before resuming inflation. Lactic acidosis may develop as lactic acid is mobilized from the extremities.

Intravenous Access and Volume Resuscitation

Intravenous Access Treatment of hypovolemia requires verification of adequate oxygenation and ventilation, and immediate establishment of venous access. Two short, large-bore peripheral catheters should be placed. If a small-bore catheter is in place, it should be used while attempts are made to insert a second, larger catheter. Upper extremity access is desirable in the presence of lower extremity injury. When an IV catheter is inserted, obtain necessary blood samples for laboratory analysis, including a complete blood count, electrolytes, and blood for type and crossmatch (see Diagnostic Studies and Catheter Insertion).

It is often difficult to establish IV access in the young child (less than 6 years of age), particularly if hypovolemia and poor systemic perfusion are present; therefore attempts to obtain a peripheral line during resuscitation should be limited (maximum time: 90 seconds or three attempts) before IO infusion is attempted.

Use of IO needles provides an acceptable emergent alternative to peripheral venous cannulation in children younger than 6 years of age, and particularly in children younger than 3 years of age. These needles provide access to the marrow cavity of a long bone in an uninjured extremity and are safe, effective, and require less time than venous cutdown. They can be inserted in the anterior tibia 1 to 3 cm below the tibial tuberosity or in the inferior third of the femur, 3 cm above the external condyle, anterior to the midline (Figure 12-5).

Central venous cannulation is not required during initial trauma resuscitation. Insertion requires particu-

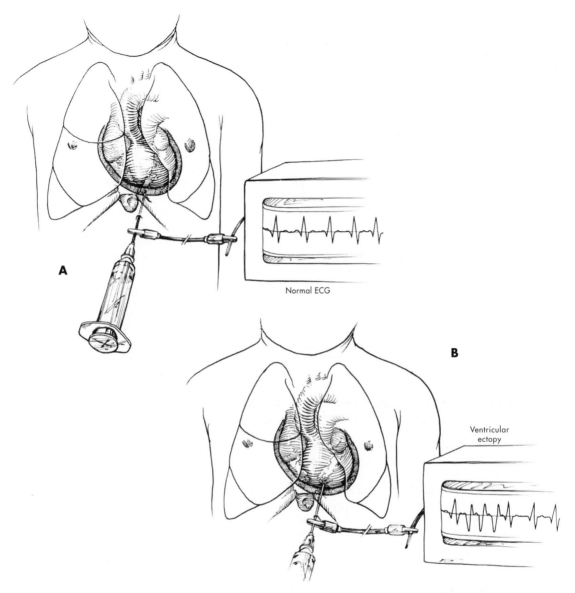

Normal ECG

Ventricular ectopy

Figure 12-4 Pericardiocentesis. The child is positioned upright at a 30- to 45-degree angle. Appropriate analgesia is provided. The xiphoid area is cleansed with a povidone-iodine solution, and sterile gloves are worn. The area (including the subcutaneous tissue and muscle layer) is infiltrated with lidocaine (Xylocaine), and a small skin incision is made just below the xiphoid. **A,** The pericardiocentesis needle (or a spinal needle) is joined to a stopcock or directly to a syringe. The V lead of the electrocardiogram is joined to the needle using a sterile alligator clip. The needle is inserted while held perpendicular to the skin. Once the skin is penetrated, the needle is inserted at a 60- to 70-degree angle from horizontal and advanced cephalad and to the left of the spine. The ECG is monitored during insertion. **B,** If the needle enters the pericardium, aspiration of fluid is possible. If the needle is inserted too far and penetrates the myocardium, ventricular ectopy or ST segment changes consistent with ventricular injury (depression or elevation of the ST segment—the segment is displaced in a direction opposite the orientation of the QRS complex) will be seen. These ECG changes indicate that the needle should be withdrawn, and the ECG pattern should return to normal. Alternatively, echocardiography may guide this procedure. (From Fleisher GR, Ludwig S: *Textbook of pediatric emergency medicine,* ed 3, Baltimore, 1993, Williams & Wilkins, p 1296.)

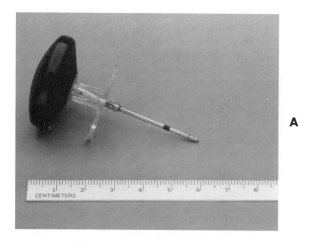

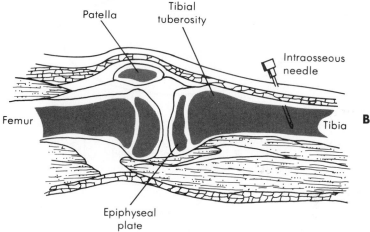

Figure 12-5   Intraosseous needle and insertion. **A,** One of the commercially available intraosseous needles. (Photo courtesy Cook, Inc.) **B,** The intraosseous needle is inserted in the medial aspect of the tibia, one finger-breath below the tibial tuberosity. When the periosteum is pierced, an immediate reduction in resistance is perceived. (From Barkin RM, Rosen P: *Emergency pediatrics,* ed 3, St Louis, 1990, Mosby.)

lar expertise and may produce complications such as pneumothorax or bleeding. If a central venous catheter is inserted, a short catheter should be used to minimize resistance to fluid infusion. In trauma centers with personnel experienced in central line insertion, jugular venous or subclavian line insertion may be accomplished rapidly with negligible morbidity.

Volume Resuscitation   Fluid resuscitation begins with a 20 ml/kg bolus of isotonic crystalloid solu-

tion, specifically normal saline or lactated Ringer's solution. Both isotonic crystalloids and blood are usually provided during intravascular volume resuscitation of the trauma victim, typically in a 3:1 crystalloid-blood ratio (Figure 12-6).

During volume resuscitation following hemorrhage, approximately three times as much fluid must be administered as the estimated volume lost, because administered isotonic crystalloids are distributed throughout the extracellular space; thus

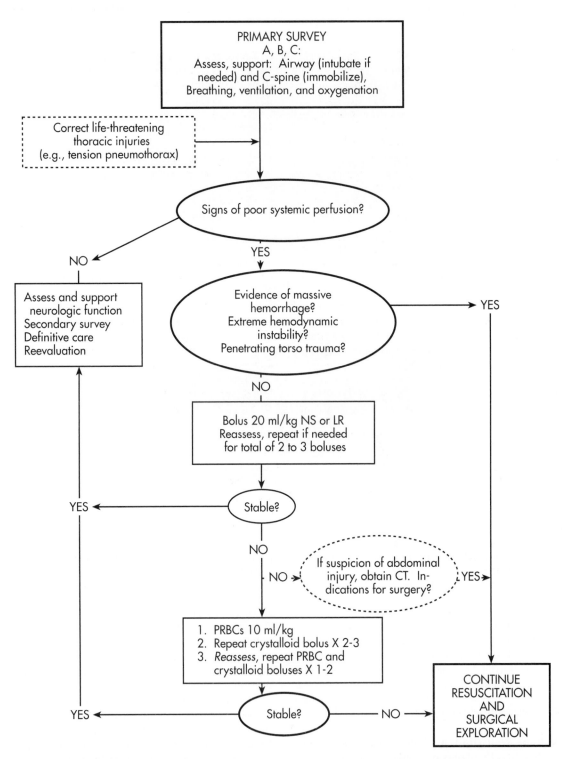

Figure 12-6 Fluid resuscitation and initial hemodynamic stabilization of the pediatric trauma victim.

only approximately one fourth will remain in the vascular space, with the remainder moving to the interstitial space. In the presence of shock, burns, or trauma, vascular permeability may be increased, resulting in an even greater loss of administered isotonic fluid from the vascular space.

A "three-to-one" rule is used to determine the ratio of crystalloid to blood administration in the pediatric trauma victim. This means that one bolus of blood (10 ml/kg of packed red blood cells or 20 ml/kg of whole blood) is typically administered for every two or three boluses of isotonic crystalloid (40 to 60 ml/kg of normal saline or lactated Ringer's solution) provided. The child often receives the first one to two boluses of crystalloid during pre-hospital stabilization and transport. Therefore the first blood bolus may be administered if signs of shock persist following an additional bolus of crystalloid in the ED.

Hypotonic fluid should *not* be used for rapid volume resuscitation in the trauma victim, because little hypotonic fluid remains in the vascular space. Most hypotonic fluid will move to the intracellular and interstitial spaces.

Blood administration is required for resuscitation of severely injured patients, and packed red blood cells (10 ml/kg) are typically used. Blood is a colloid; thus it will remain in the vascular space longer than crystalloids, exerting an osmotic effect. As a result, blood may enable more rapid restoration of the intravascular volume than would occur with crystalloid resuscitation alone.

Ideal blood therapy consists of type-specific packed red blood cells (10 ml/kg).Unmatched, type O, Rh-negative packed red blood cells (10 ml/kg) can be administered until type-specific blood is available.

Assessment of Response   If the child fails to respond to two to three boluses of blood plus the interspersed boluses of crystalloid, and external bleeding is controlled, urgent surgical intervention may be required (see Figure 12-6 and Abdomen under Secondary Survey).

Disability: Neurologic Evaluation and Stabilization

Rapid neurologic evaluation is an essential component of the primary survey. The initial neurologic examination consists of assessment of pupil size

and response to light, evaluation of mental status (using the GCS or the modified GCS), identification and treatment of status epilepticus, and (in the infant) palpation of the fontanelle. If head trauma has occurred, the scalp should be palpated to detect lacerations, edema, and fractures.

Pupil Size and Responsiveness   Pupil dilation with decreased response to light may indicate inadequate oxygenation or perfusion, or increased ICP. Both hypoxia and increased ICP are treated with ventilation with 100% oxygen. Systemic perfusion is supported as necessary.

Effective cerebral resuscitation in the pediatric trauma victim requires adequate shock resuscitation; cerebral perfusion will not be optimal in the presence of shock. Therefore shock resuscitation must be provided until effective systemic perfusion is achieved. Oxygenation and ventilation must also be supported effectively.

Children can lose a significant percentage of their blood volume from head wounds, and any external bleeding should be controlled with pressure. Following initial resuscitative efforts and treatment of any external bleeding, persistent shock is unlikely to result from head trauma unless increased ICP, brain death, or spinal shock has developed.

Level of Consciousness   The child's level of consciousness and responsiveness will provide a valuable indication of the degree of distress present. If the child is appropriately frightened and crying for the parents, the child is presumed to be relatively alert and oriented. However, irritability may be an early sign of cardiorespiratory or neurologic deterioration. Alternatively, if the child fails to respond to the parents and is unresponsive to painful stimuli, urgent evaluation and support is needed, since cardiorespiratory or neurologic compromise is probably present.

Two evaluation scales may be used to rapidly characterize the child's neurologic function. The child's responsiveness may be described in general terms or quantified using the GCS (see also p. 390).

Glasgow Coma Scale   The GCS characterizes the patient's eye opening and best motor and verbal responses (Table 12-5). The lowest possible GCS score is 3 (the child is flaccid, with no response to any stimulus). The highest possible GCS score is 15 (sponta-

Table 12-5
Glasgow Coma Scale and Modified Pediatric Glasgow Coma Scale Scores

	Child	Infant	Score
Eye opening	Spontaneous	Spontaneous	4
	To verbal stimuli	To verbal stimuli	3
	To pain only	To pain only	2
	No response	No response	1
Verbal response	Oriented, appropriate	Coos and babbles	5
	Confused	Irritable cries	4
	Inappropriate words	Cries to pain	3
	Incomprehensible words or nonspecific sounds	Moans to pain	2
	No response	No response	1
Motor response	Obeys commands	Moves spontaneously and purposefully	6
	Localizes painful stimulus	Withdraws to touch	5
	Withdraws in response to pain	Withdraws in response to pain	4
	Flexion in response to pain	Decorticate posturing (abnormal flexion) in response to pain	3
	Extension in response to pain	Decerebrate posturing (abnormal extension) in response to pain	2
	No response	No response	1

Adelaide Normal Aggregate Score

0-6 mo:	9	2-5 yr:	13
6-12 mo:	11	>5 yr:	14
1-2 yr:	12		

Modified from Hazinski MF: *Nursing care of the critically ill child,* ed 2, St Louis, 1992, Mosby; Davis RF et al: Head and spinal cord injury. In Rogers MC, editor: *Textbook of pediatric intensive care, Brain insults in infants and children,* New York, 1985, Grune & Stratton; Morray JP et al: Coma scale for use in brain-injured children, *Crit Care Med* 12:1018, 1984; and Simpson DA et al: Head injuries in infants and young children: the value of a pediatric coma scale; review of the literature and report on a study, *Child's Nerv Sys* 7:183-190, 1991.

neous eye opening, follows commands, and speaks coherently). *When the child is unconscious, the GCS score will be determined by the motor response* (spontaneous movement, or movement or posturing in response to a painful stimulus). The GCS score should be determined by the *best* response observed.

When a painful stimulus is applied to evaluate *localization* of painful stimulus in the obtunded or comatose patient, the stimulus should be applied to the *trunk above the nipple line* or to the neck or head. *Withdrawal* from a painful stimulus should be documented by application of the stimulus to the medial aspect of each extremity; withdrawal is indicated by abduction of each extremity.

Signs of Increased Intracranial Pressure Signs of increased ICP include deterioration in level of

consciousness, pupil dilation (unilateral or bilateral), lack of response to a central painful stimulus, and (in infants) a firm anterior fontanelle (Box 12-9). *Late* signs of increased ICP (often associated with brain stem herniation) include hypertension, bradycardia, and apnea.

Increased ICP during the first 24 to 48 hours following closed head injury is thought to result from *maldistribution* of cerebral blood flow. Some areas of the brain will receive inadequate blood flow whereas others will receive excessive blood flow. Hypoxemia and hypotension can contribute to the development of cerebral ischemia; thus these conditions must be avoided or promptly treated. Initial management of increased ICP requires control of cerebral blood flow through support of oxygenation, ventilation, and adequate blood pressure and systemic perfusion.

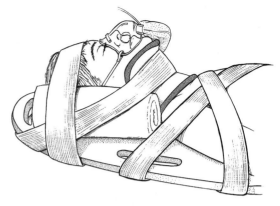

Figure 12-7 Proper method of cervical spine immobilization in the child with multiple injuries. (From Chameides L, Hazinski MF, editors: *The textbook of pediatric advanced life support,* Dallas, 1997, American Heart Association.)

If signs of increased ICP are present in the hemodynamically stable patient, furosemide (0.5 to 1 mg/kg) administration should be considered. Mannitol (0.25 to 1 g/kg) is generally avoided during initial resuscitation unless blood volume and perfusion are stable. (For further information see p. 394).

Seizures and Status Epilepticus Posttraumatic seizures occur in approximately 10% of all children with head injury, but in 35% of those with severe head injury. Seizures are treated (usually with diazepam, 0.25 mg/kg), because they increase cerebral oxygen demand. Factors that increase the risk of posttraumatic seizures include severe head injury, diffuse cerebral edema, acute subdural hematoma, and open, depressed skull fracture with parenchymal damage. Prophylactic anticonvulsant therapy should be considered in the presence of these risk factors.

Status epilepticus must be treated aggressively in the patient with increased ICP, because continuous seizures will increase cerebral metabolic oxygen consumption (see p. 406).

Cervical Spine Immobilization *Every trauma victim who has sustained blunt trauma to the head or upper body should be presumed to have a cervical spine injury,* and cervical spine immobilization must be maintained until definitive diagnostic studies can be performed.

Cervical spine immobilization requires that the torso, legs, and head be secured to a rigid spine board. A rigid cervical collar is an adjunct to this immobilization and can be placed before or after the patient is placed on the spine board (Figure 12-7). Ideally, the spine board contains a head well to prevent flexion of the child's neck from pressure on the occipital area of the skull. If there is no head well, folded sheets or pads should be placed on the torso section of the board before the child is placed on the board. The linens will elevate the torso approximately 2 cm (½ to 1 inch) and prevent neck flexion once the child is placed on the board.

The child's torso and legs are taped at three points (thighs, then pelvis, then shoulders) *before* the head is secured to the spine board. Rotation and lateral movement of the child's head is prevented through use of a cervical immobilization device (consisting of foam blocks and Velcro straps), or towel rolls or small pillows and tape. Particular care should be taken to eliminate any gaps between the child's head or body and the securing straps.

Any rigid collar used for cervical spine immobilization must fit correctly. An excessively large collar can produce hyperextension or permit flexion of the neck, whereas a collar that is too small can compromise the airway and enable neck flexion. If no collar of appropriate size is available, it would be better to leave the collar off than place one of inappropriate size. Foam collars should not be used because they provide *no* protection against head and neck movement.

Spinal cord injuries should be suspected following a fall or motor vehicle collision with evidence of acceleration-deceleration injuries (e.g., in the unrestrained passenger, the child with lap belt injuries, or the child struck by a vehicle). Spinal cord injuries should also be assumed to be present in near-drowning victims. In all of these victims, the spine should be immobilized, and the child should be log-rolled whenever turning is required until injury has been ruled out. For further information about treatment of spinal cord injuries, see Neck, Cervical Spine, and Face under Secondary Survey.

Diagnostic Studies and Catheter Insertion

Blood for Sampling Laboratory Analysis   Laboratory evaluation of the pediatric trauma victim typically includes arterial blood gases, a complete blood count with white blood cell differential and platelet count, serum electrolytes (including total and ionized calcium, glucose, and magnesium), serum amylase, blood urea nitrogen, creatinine, prothrombin time, and partial thromboplastin time. Additional laboratory studies (e.g., liver enzymes) may be ordered based on the location of the child's injury or based on evidence of organ injury or dysfunction.

Additional Diagnostic Studies   Diagnostic studies should only be obtained when the child is stable and systemic perfusion is adequate. A portable chest x-ray study is one of the first studies to be obtained. If head or cervical spine injury is present, a computed tomography (CT) scan is indicated. If abdominal hemorrhage is suspected, particularly in the unconscious child, a CT scan of the abdomen is required.

Nasogastric and Urinary Drainage Tubes   Gastric distension can have the following undesirable effects: it will increase the risk of vomiting and aspiration, it will compromise diaphragm movement, it may stimulate a vasovagal reflex and bradycardia, and it may mimic or mask symptoms of abdominal injury. Gastric distension is treated through insertion of a nasogastric tube.

Contraindications to nasogastric tube insertion include the presence of craniofacial trauma with a maxillofacial or basilar skull fracture. Blind advancement of the nasogastric tube in these patients may result in intracranial migration of the tube; therefore an orogastric tube should be inserted.

Insertion of a urinary catheter will enable continuous evaluation of urine output and should be considered when multisystem trauma or shock is present. Contraindications to urinary catheter insertion include pelvic fracture, urethral injuries, and blood observed at the urinary meatus. These conditions may be associated with urethral disruption.

Vascular Monitoring Catheters   Vascular monitoring catheters are typically inserted in the PICU once resuscitation and diagnostic studies are completed.

Exposure: Temperature Control and Preparation for Secondary Survey

In the ED the child's clothes should be removed to facilitate a complete inspection for injuries (the secondary survey—see the following section). If there is any question that the child's injuries were inflicted or if firearm injuries are present, the child's clothing should be saved in a sealed bag.

Infants and young children can rapidly become hypothermic when they are undressed. Cold stress can increase oxygen requirements and contribute to the development of hypoxia. For this reason, warm blankets or a radiant warming device should be used for all young pediatric trauma victims. IV fluids and blood products should be warmed (using approved blood warmers) before administration to hypothermic or very small children.

Throughout initial resuscitation and stabilization, monitor the skin and core body temperature closely. If hypothermia is present, the child's body temperature should be increased slowly (approximately 1° C/hr). If profound hypothermia is present, controlled rewarming may be accomplished with peritoneal lavage or extracorporeal membrane oxygenation.

Secondary Survey

General Description

The secondary survey begins as soon as all aspects of the primary survey and resuscitation are complete. The first goal of the secondary survey is to assess the patient's response to the initial resuscitative effort. The second goal is to perform a head-to-toe assessment, including a systematic examination to detect hidden injuries or further deterioration in organ or system function (Box 12-10).

Evaluation of Patient Response

Response to Cardiorespiratory Support

The child's airway, breathing, and circulation should be evaluated and reevaluated virtually constantly during initial stabilization. In addition, be alert for acute deterioration that may occur in the intubated patient, caused by tube displacement, tube obstruction, pneumothorax, and equipment failure.

Response to Fluid Bolus

If the blood pressure, capillary refill, and quality of peripheral pulses remain poor and the heart rate continues to be rapid despite administration of two or three fluid boluses (crystalloid plus blood), massive initial hemorrhage or a continuing source

---

Box 12-10

Overview of Secondary Survey: Head-to-Toe Assessment

1. **Head and Neurologic Status**
   Look for: Signs of increased intracranial pressure (ICP), head abrasions, contusions of the scalp, bruises, skull fractures, raccoon eyes
   Evaluate: Pupil size and response to light, Glasgow Coma Scale (GCS) score, computed tomography (CT) scan, skull films

2. **Neck, Cervical Spine, and Face**
   Verify: Cervical spine immobilization until injury has been ruled out
   Look for: Abrasions, facial bone fractures, broken teeth, cerebrospinal fluid drainage from the ear, tracheal deviation, jugular venous distension, cervical spine deformity or reported pain (do not insert nasogastric tube if severe facial fractures are present)

3. **Chest***
   Look for: Evidence of inadequate ventilation, shifting of cardiac point of maximal impulse (PMI), contusions, wounds, poor perfusion
   Auscultate lungs for evidence of: Decreased or altered breath sounds indicative of hemothorax, pneumothorax, or lung collapse; crackles or wheezes
   Auscultate heart sounds for: Murmurs, bruits, muffled heart tones

   Palpate ribs and sternum for: Crepitance, pain, fractures

4. **Abdomen***
   Look for: Abrasions, contusions, distensions (ensure that stomach has been decompressed by gastric tube)
   Auscultate for: Bowel sounds (all quadrants)
   Palpate for: Tenderness, size of liver, spleen
   Measure: Abdominal girth (mark measurement point on child's abdomen with pen)

5. **Pelvis and Genitalia**
   Look for: Abrasions, contusions, or lacerations; scrotal or labial hematomas; blood in the urinary meatus (if present, do not insert urinary catheter); rectal bleeding
   Palpate pelvis for: Crepitance, pain, instability (if pelvic fracture is suspected, do not insert urinary catheter)

6. **Musculoskeletal System and Extremities**
   Look for: Abrasions, contusions, lacerations, deformities, swelling
   Palpate for: Pain, crepitance, pulses

*Repeat examinations over time.

of blood loss must be suspected. Ongoing crystalloid and blood administration are then required, a pediatric trauma surgeon should be consulted, further diagnostic studies (e.g., CT of abdomen) are undertaken, and urgent surgical intervention may be needed.

Adequate shock resuscitation is required for the trauma patient with hemorrhage, but excessive fluid administration should be avoided. Once systemic perfusion is successfully restored, reduce fluid administration to a "keep open" rate and determine maintenance fluid requirements. In general, the child with head injury and multisystem trauma will receive less than the calculated "maintenance" requirements *after intravascular volume and systemic perfusion are restored,* since posttraumatic stress response can contribute to free water retention.

All fluids administered to the child should be administered via a syringe or volume-controlled infusion pump so that the total fluid administration rate may be accurately tallied. All fluid administration systems should be checked on an hourly basis so that any kinks or leaks in the tubing are immediately detected. The nurse must constantly be aware of the child's current fluid balance.

Additional Evaluation

Hemodynamic support should be established before extensive diagnostic studies (such *as chest radiographs or CT scans) are performed.* The radiology department is *not* the optimal location for initiation of resuscitation.

Head and Neurologic Status

The most common head injury in children is closed head injury, which may not produce visible signs of injury. Closed head trauma should be suspected in the unconscious trauma victim and should be assumed to be present if signs of increased ICP are observed.

Neurologic Evaluation

Following primary resuscitative measures (including intubation and establishment of oxygenation and adequate ventilation), ongoing evaluation of the patient's mental status is required with the use of a standardized scoring system (such as the GCS).

Causes of Acute Deterioration   Epidural hematomas or acute posttraumatic hydrocephalus may cause abrupt deterioration in the child's neurologic condition hours or days after head trauma. The child with an epidural hematoma classically suffers a relatively minor head injury with brief loss of consciousness. Approximately 25% of victims demonstrate a lucid interval, followed by clinical deterioration that may be heralded by headache and hemiparesis. Increased ICP produces pupil dilation and a decreased level of consciousness and may ultimately produce apnea and bradycardia. An emergent CT scan followed by immediate surgical decompression is required.

Children who have intraventricular blood noted on a CT scan following head injury are at risk for the development of acute posttraumatic obstructive hydrocephalus, because the blood can obstruct cerebrospinal fluid (CSF) flow through the narrow aqueduct of Sylvius. Such hydrocephalus may cause a sudden rise in ICP associated with pupil dilation and clinical deterioration. Urgent treatment includes ventriculostomy with CSF drainage and possible later insertion of a ventriculoperitoneal shunt.

Deterioration days or weeks after head injury may be associated with obstructive or communicating hydrocephalus or with meningitis. Obstructive hydrocephalus may develop in the child with posttraumatic intraventricular blood noted on the CT scan. The blood may obstruct the aqueduct of Sylvius, producing CSF accumulation. Communicating hydrocephalus may result from impaired absorption of CSF in patients with subarachnoid hemorrhage (SAH). Meningitis is an additional cause of late deterioration following head injury, particularly if penetrating head trauma was present or ICP monitoring was required.

Ongoing Assessment   A CT scan will help determine the extent and severity of the head injury and the need for surgical intervention, and it may indicate potential causes of further clinical deterioration. Skull radiographs may also be obtained.

Additional assessments that will contribute to neurologic evaluation include:

- Vital signs (note that increased ICP may produce bradycardia, hypertension, and apnea, but these "classic" signs typically appear late in the clinical course). Watch for any change associated with poor perfusion or neurologic deterioration.
- Pupil size and response to light.
- Cranial nerve function (Table 12-6) and spontaneous breathing pattern. Note presence or absence of cough, gag during suctioning (report absence immediately).
- Ability to follow commands. Ask child to hold up two fingers, wiggle the toes, or stick out his or her tongue. Document and report any deterioration in the child's condition immediately.

Management   Management of increased ICP requires identification and treatment of the cause, and prevention of secondary insults. Cerebral blood flow is maldistributed; thus systemic perfusion should be optimized and hypoxemia and hypotension avoided to prevent development of cerebral ischemia. Support oxygenation and ventilation, since both hypoxemia and hypercarbia can increase cerebral blood flow, as well as intracranial volume and pressure. Treat seizures and fever, since these factors can increase cerebral oxygen demand. If blood pressure and perfusion are adequate and oxygenation and ventilation are optimized, and ICP remains high, diuresis with furosemide (Lasix) or mannitol may be needed. Finally, barbiturates may be used if all other methods to control ICP have been tried (see p. 388).

Indicators of Poor Prognosis   The most consistent indicators of a poor prognosis following closed head injury in children are listed in Box 12-11. If a devastating neurologic injury is present and brain death has occurred or is imminent, the question of vascular organ donation should be raised with the family, and the local federally funded organ procurement agency should be contacted. The few contraindications to vascular organ donation include continued hemodynamic instability despite aggressive therapy, active infection, or failure of the organ.

External Examination of the Head

Palpate the head to identify fractures or wounds. Examine the nose and ears for blood or CSF

Table 12-6
Relationship Between Anatomic Site of Injury, Cranial Nerve Involvement, and Abnormal Clinical Posture and Respiratory Patterns

Anatomic Part	Cranial Nerve Exit	Posture	Respiratory Pattern
Cerebrum Cortex Subcortical structure Diencephalon	I (Olfactory) II (Optic)	Decorticate	Cheyne-Stokes
Midbrain	III (Oculomotor) IV (Trochlear)	Decerebrate	Hyperventilation
Pons	V (Trigeminal) VI (Abducent) VII (Facial) VIII Vestibulocochlear)	±Flaccid	Apneustic Cluster ventilation
Medulla	IX (Glossopharyngeal) X (Vagus) XI (Accessory) XII (Hypoglossal)	Flaccid	Ataxic Apneic

From Silverman BK, editor: *Advanced pediatric life support,* 1989, Elk Grove Village, Ill, American Academy of Pediatrics.

Box 12-11

Poor Prognostic Indicators Following Head Injury in Children

Cardiovascular collapse
  Pulseless cardiac arrest
  Profound hypotension (systolic blood pressure ≤50 mm Hg)
  Persistent hemodynamic stability despite resuscitation
Coma with absent pain response
Fixed and dilated pupils despite adequate oxygenation, ventilation, and systemic perfusion
Massive head injury associated with coagulopathy
Presence of diabetes insipidus on admission

drainage (indicative of a maxillofacial fracture or basilar skull fracture with a dural tear). Test any clear fluid draining from the nose or ears for the presence of glucose; this may indicate a CSF leak. Management of a CSF leak requires:

- Careful observation for signs of meningitis (may develop late)
- Consideration of possible surgical closure of the leak
- Consideration of possible prophylactic antibiotic therapy (This is controversial.)

An ocular examination must be performed to identify papilledema or lateralizing extraocular muscle paresis.

Neck, Cervical Spine, and Face

Spine

Assessment Spine immobilization should be maintained until spinal cord injury is ruled out. Examination to rule out injury should be performed after the child is stable and includes:

- Assessment of spontaneous movement of extremities and movement in response to pain

(a painful stimulus should be applied to the trunk, above the nipple line). The motor portion of the GCS can be used to score this assessment.
- Documentation of strength, muscle tone, and sensation in all extremities (test antigravity muscles). Spinal cord injuries and associated motor and sensory deficits are presented in Table 12-7 (see also Table 8-13, p. 432).
- If spinal trauma is suspected and hypotension persists in the absence of hypovolemia or pericardial tamponade, spinal shock should be considered. Spinal shock causes vasodilation due to spinal cord injury.
- If the child is awake and oriented, the presence of neck, head, or back pain or tenderness is highly suggestive of spinal injury. If clinical examination findings, the mechanism of injury, or associated injuries suggest the likelihood of a spinal injury, spinal films are indicated, and the spine is immobilized.
- The cervical spine of the unconscious child cannot usually be "cleared" on the basis of anteroposterior and lateral radiographs alone. A complete cervical spine series includes anteroposterior and lateral cervical spine radiographs, as well as oblique and odontoid views, on all patients. The head should be in neutral position, and the arms should be placed at the sides of the body with the hands pointing toward the feet. Dynamic flexion and extension films may also be obtained once fracture and subluxation have been ruled out.
- A CT scan provides definitive evidence of cervical spine subluxation or vertebral fracture in the unstable or unconscious patient; this scan is often obtained to evaluate head injury and includes "cuts" through the upper cervical spine. Magnetic resonance imaging (MRI) is helpful, but not practical during initial stabilization.

Management Steroid administration is now administered during the first 23 hours after a spinal cord injury to prevent or minimize secondary edema and inflammation. Methylprednisolone (bolus of 30 mg/kg plus continuous infusion of 5.4 mg/kg/hr for 23 hours) is prescribed.

Table 12-7
Correlation of Motor and Sensory Deficit with Levels of Spinal Cord Injury

Level of Lesion	Motor Function Lost	Sensation Lost at and Below	Reflex
C2	Breathing	Occiput	
C3	Spontaneous breathing and	Thyroid cartilage	
C4	trapezius function	Suprasternal notch	
C5	Shoulder flexion and abduction	Infraclavicular with or without lateral arm sparing	Biceps brachialis*
C6		Infraclavicular with or without lateral arm, forearm sparing	Brachioradialis*
C7	Elbow and wrist extension	Infraclavicular with sparing as above to middle finger	Triceps*
C8	Small muscles of hand (lumbricales and interossei)	Infraclavicular with sparing as above to little finger	
T1		Infraclavicular with upper extremity sparing to axilla	
T4		Nipple line	
T7	Intercostal and abdominal musculature	Inferior costal margin	Upper abdominal†
T10		Umbilicus	
T12			Lower abdominal†
L1	Hip flexion	Groin	
L2		Anteromedial thigh	
L3	Hip adduction and knee extension	Medial knee	Knee/patellar*
L4	Hip abduction and knee extension	Anterior knee and medial calf	
L5	Foot and great toe dorsiflexion	Lateral dorsum foot and lateral sole foot	
S1	Foot and great toe plantar flexion	Lateral dorsum foot and lateral sole foot	Ankle/Achilles tendon*
S2			
S3	Perianal and rectal sphincter tone	Perianal and rectal sensation	
S4			

From Barkin R, Rosen P: *Emergency pediatrics: a guide to ambulatory care,* ed 4, St Louis, 1994, Mosby.
*Deep tendon.
†Superficial.

Urgent surgical intervention for spinal cord injury is indicated if progressive neurologic dysfunction (e.g., ascending paralysis or sensory loss) is observed. If a cervical spine injury is unstable or if subluxation is present, immobilization is necessary through use of Gardner-Wells tongs or halo traction. If the vertebral bodies are not aligned, weight is added to the traction device and repeated radiographic evaluations are performed until the vertebrae are realigned and reduced (Figure 12-8). Spinal fusion is then accomplished after 10 days to 2 weeks.

Face

Examine the face for evidence of abrasions, fractures, or broken teeth. Examine the neck for evidence of tracheal deviation or jugular venous distension (may indicate pneumothorax or pericardial tamponade).

Chest

Blunt thoracic trauma is often associated with parenchymal injury (e.g., pulmonary contusion) in the absence of rib fractures in children. During the

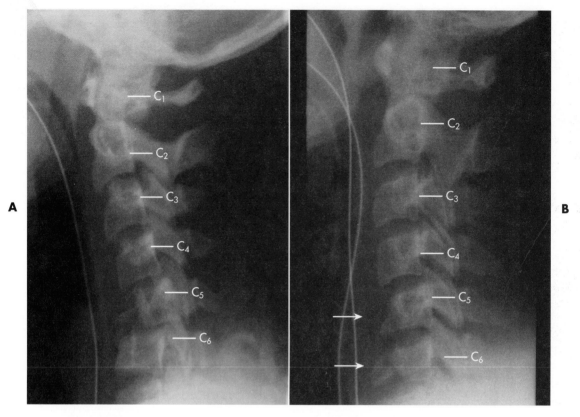

Figure 12-8   Unstable cervical spine injury and effects of cervical spine traction. The patient in these films is a 13-year-old who suffered a three-column (teardrop) (burst suppression) fracture of the fifth and sixth cervical vertebrae. The child was found floating unconscious in a home swimming pool. Because a diving injury was not suspected, his head and neck were not immobilized by lay rescuers at the scene. Proper immobilization was provided by EMS personnel on their arrival and during transport. **A,** Initial lateral cervical spine radiograph showing teardrop fracture of C5 with retrolisthesis of C5 on C6 and kyphotic angulation. **B,** Lateral radiograph of the cervical spine following application of halo traction (10 pounds), showing restoration of cervical alignment. Contiguous teardrop fractures of the fifth and sixth cervical vertebrae are now apparent.

primary survey, life-threatening injuries (hemothorax or tension pneumothorax or cardiac tamponade) are detected and treated. Chest inspection and palpation should detect external injury. Careful auscultation should localize any alteration in the intensity or pitch of breath sounds or the presence of pulmonary edema. The chest must be reexamined if at any time during the secondary survey any of the following are observed: tachypnea with or without respiratory distress, continuous hemodynamic in-

stability, chest pain or tenderness, hypoxemia, hemoptysis, crepitus, or abnormal breath sounds. These signs may be caused by thoracic injury. Comparison of clinical findings of the most common critical thoracic injuries are presented in Table 12-8.

Common thoracic injuries that may be detected during the secondary survey include pulmonary contusion, pneumothorax, hemothorax, cardiac contusion, flail chest, rib fractures, and diaphragm rupture. Chest x-ray studies, including anteroposte-

Table 12-8
Differential Diagnosis of Life-Threatening Cardiothoracic Injury

	Tension Pneumothorax	Massive Hemothorax	Cardiac Tamponade
Breath sounds	Ipsilaterally decreased	Ipsilaterally decreased	Normal
Percussion note	Hyperresonant	Dull	Normal
Tracheal location	Contralaterally shifted	Midline	Midline
Neck veins	Distended	Flat	Distended
Heart tones	Normal	Normal	Muffled

From Cooper A, Foltin GL: Thoracic trauma. In Barkin RM et al, editors: *Pediatric emergency medicine: concepts and clinical practice*, ed 2, St Louis, 1997, Mosby.

rior and lateral upright films and computerized tomography (CT) scanning, should be performed on any child with injury to the chest or torso.

Pulmonary Contusion

Clinical Presentation A pulmonary contusion is a lung parenchymal injury that may cause alveolar hemorrhage and pulmonary edema. It produces impaired gas exchange and may produce acute respiratory distress syndrome (ARDS) and respiratory failure after blunt chest trauma. A pulmonary contusion will produce localized opacification of the lung and increased density on a CT scan.

Management Treatment requires positive pressure ventilation with oxygen support and positive end-expiratory pressure (PEEP) if signs of respiratory failure are observed. Diuretic therapy will also be provided if intravascular volume status is acceptable. For further information regarding ARDS, see p. 332.

Pneumothorax

Clinical Presentation Pneumothorax is the most common complication of blunt thoracic injury in children. Clinical signs include dyspnea, chest pain, severe respiratory distress, hypoxemia, asymmetric chest wall movement, and decreased breath sounds or altered pitch of breath sounds on the involved side (this may be difficult to appreciate in the small child).

Management Aspiration of the air may be accomplished with a needle and syringe. However, chest tube insertion will be required for evacuation of a significant pneumothorax.

Hemothorax

Clinical Presentation If massive hemorrhage indicates major vascular injury, immediate surgical exploration is required. After the child has been stabilized, upright and lateral decubitus films will enable quantification of the fluid accumulation.

Management Insertion of a chest tube may be the only treatment required. Urgent surgical exploration is indicated for massive hemorrhage (>10 to 15 ml/kg of blood or 25% of estimated circulating blood volume), ongoing hemorrhage (>2 to 4 ml/kg/hr), uncontrolled air leak, continuing hemodynamic instability, or penetrating trauma present below the intermammary line. A thoracotomy may be performed in the ED if penetrating trauma produces cardiopulmonary arrest.

Rib Fractures

Clinical Presentation Rib fractures are relatively uncommon in children. When they are present, they often result from application of severe forces; therefore significant underlying organ injury (e.g., liver, spleen, lung) must be suspected.

Management No treatment is required unless flail chest develops (see Flail Chest), although assessment for other injuries is necessary.

Flail Chest

Clinical Presentation When multiple rib fractures are present (three or more ribs fractured at two points), flail chest can occur. Paradoxical chest wall movement, hypotension, and respiratory distress indicate the need for immediate positive pressure ventilatory support. A posterior flail chest is very poorly tolerated in the child. Such thoracic injury may remain undetected until the child has been resuscitated and careful examination is performed.

Management Management is with positive pressure ventilation.

Cardiac Contusion

Clinical Presentation Cardiac contusion may be present in any child with a history of blunt thoracic trauma. However, the criteria for diagnosis have not been standardized, and this complication is rarely symptomatic in children. Potential signs of cardiac contusion include ST segment depression or elevation (ischemia) on a 12-lead ECG, elevation in cardiac isoenzymes, chest pain, and potential arrhythmias or compromise in myocardial function.

Management Close monitoring and support of cardiovascular function and systemic perfusion are required. Cardiac contusion in children does not commonly produce congestive heart failure or shock (see pp. 118 and 130).

Diaphragm Rupture

Clinical Presentation Rupture of the diaphragm (usually on the left side) is a relatively uncommon complication of pediatric blunt chest trauma. It will produce significant respiratory distress if the trauma victim is breathing spontaneously, but it may be impossible to detect once positive pressure ventilation is instituted. During spontaneous inspiration, the diaphragm is drawn up into the ipsilateral chest; this compromises ventilation of that lung. Thus increased respiratory effort, atelectasis, and fatigue develop. Occasionally, herniation of abdominal contents will be apparent on a chest radiograph.

Management Controlled positive-pressure ventilation will prevent the development of atelectasis and respiratory failure. Surgical repair (through an abdominal or thoracic approach) is required.

Abdomen

Hemorrhage from thoracoabdominal injuries is second only to head trauma as the leading cause of death in pediatric trauma victims. Most abdominal trauma is *blunt*. Although *penetrating* abdominal injuries are less common, they are associated with significant morbidity and mortality. In the alert child, signs of abdominal hemorrhage may be subtle; in the unconscious child, signs of hemorrhage may be impossible to detect.

The pediatric patient with a history of blunt trauma must be monitored continuously, and the nurse must be able to recognize subtle signs of pain and developing shock. If patient deterioration is observed, surgical intervention is usually required on an emergent basis. Surgical exploration is also required following penetrating injury to the thorax below the intermammary line and anterior to the midaxillary line to rule out bowel perforation. Appropriate resuscitation equipment should always be readily available (see p. 160).

Signs of Abdominal Hemorrhage

Clinical Presentation Clinical signs of abdominal hemorrhage can include abdominal pain, tenderness, or distension; bruising or discoloration of the abdomen; and respiratory distress in the absence of rib fracture or other chest injury. Abdominal ecchymosis and bruising may indicate abdominal injuries caused by lap belts (Box 12-12). Signs of abdominal hemorrhage are very difficult to detect in the comatose patient or one with spinal cord injury and loss of abdominal sensation. In these patients, evaluation and diagnostic studies should include a flat-plate radiograph of the abdomen. Presence of free air in the peritoneal cavity indicates a hollow viscous rupture. A CT scan (see Diagnostic Studies) is also indicated.

A careful *rectal examination* is performed to rule out the presence of blood within the rectum, to assess sphincter tone, and to ensure that there has been no disruption of the lower urinary tract. Absence of sphincter tone may indicate spinal cord injury.

Diagnostic Studies Diagnostic *peritoneal lavage* is *not* routinely performed in the assessment of children with blunt abdominal trauma, because it is not organ or injury specific and because it fails to detect retroperitoneal hemorrhage. This technique tends to be reserved for patients in whom other diagnostic modalities are unavailable or the clinical examina-

> # Box 12-12
> ## Physical Findings Suggestive of Abdominal or Genitourinary Injury
>
> ### Clinical Signs of Abdominal Injury
>
> Rapid, shallow breathing
> Abdominal tenderness
> Flank or abdominal mass, contusion, or wound
> Increasing abdominal girth
> Blood in the urethral meatus, hematuria
> Inability to void
> Genital swelling or discoloration
> Referred shoulder pain with upper abdominal palpation:
>   Right shoulder pain—hepatic injury
>   Left shoulder pain—splenic injury
>
> ### Signs Suggestive of Hepatic Injury
>
> Abdominal pain and tenderness
> Referred right shoulder pain
> Elevation in serum transaminases (aspartate transaminose [AST] >450 IU/L and alanine transaminase [ALT] >250 IU/L)
>
> ### Signs Suggestive of Splenic Injury
>
> Signs of hemorrhage (tachycardia, possible hypotension)
> Abdominal pain or tenderness, Kehr's sign (referred pain to the left shoulder during compression of the left upper quadrant)
> Leukocytosis
> Rise in serum amylase
>
> ### Signs Suggestive of Renal Injury
>
> Hematuria, presence of threadlike clots in the urethra
> Abdominal or flank pain
> Flank hematoma
>
> ### Signs Suggestive of Urethral Injury
>
> Blood in the urinary meatus
> Consider the possibility with a pelvic fracture
>
> ### Injuries Frequently Associated With Abdominal Injury
>
> Fractured lower ribs
> Penetrating trauma to the lower chest
> Pelvic fracture
> Multisystem trauma sustained during a motor-vehicle accident
>
> ### Laboratory Results
>
> Elevated serum transaminases (hepatic injury)
> Elevated serum amylase (pancreatic, small bowel injury)
> Leukocytosis (may be nonspecific sign of stress or splenic trauma)
>
> From Hazinski MF: *Nursing care of the critically ill child*, ed 2, St Louis, 1992, Mosby.

tion is equivocal (including comatose or paralyzed patients), and it may be used when bowel rupture is suspected. Peritoneal lavage should only be performed by physicians skilled in the technique.

A double-contrast CT scan is the diagnostic study of choice when hepatic, splenic, or renal injury is suspected. This scan allows visualization of organs in the peritoneal cavity and the retroperitoneal space. Abdominal ultrasound and radionuclide scanning may also be performed to document solid organ and retroperitoneal injury but will not provide the anatomic detail apparent with the CT scan.

Nonoperative Management of Abdominal Trauma

Conservative management of hepatic, splenic, or renal contusions or lacerations includes supportive care and close observation in a PICU. Typically, bleeding produced from such lacerations has ceased by the time the child arrives at the hospital, and these organs will often heal themselves. If rapid deterioration is observed, surgical intervention is required on an urgent basis.

Surgical Intervention

Indications for urgent surgical intervention (Box 12-13) are based predominantly on the patient's physio-

---

Box 12-13

Indications for Emergency Surgery for Abdominal and Genitourinary Injury

Hemodynamic instability despite administration of >40 ml/kg of blood (or transfusion requirements equivalent to 50% of estimated blood volume)

Decompensated shock on admission

Evidence of ongoing bleeding (falling hematocrit)

Penetrating trauma anterior to midaxillary line and below intermammary line

Evidence of peritonitis

Evidence of devastating organ injury by computed tomography (CT) scan (e.g., shattered organ or associated vascular injuries) using the American College of Surgery Committee on Trauma Solid Organ Injury Scale

Radiologic evidence of pneumoperitoneum (including intraperitoneal or retroperitoneal gas), intraperitoneal bladder rupture, renovascular pedicle injury

Peritoneal lavage findings:
  >100,000 red blood cells/mm^3
  Bile, bacteria, stool
  >500 white blood cells/mm^3

Modified from Foltin GL, Cooper A: Abdominal injury. In Barkin RM et al, editors: *Pediatric emergency medicine: concepts and clinical practice,* ed 2, St Louis, 1997, Mosby.

---

logic status and include hemodynamic instability despite administration of >40 ml/kg of blood (or equivalent to 50% of estimated blood volume), evidence of ongoing bleeding (falling hematocrit), penetrating trauma, or evidence of devastating organ injury on a CT scan (e.g., shattered organ or associated vascular injuries). Typically, the injured organ is repaired rather than removed. Removal of the injured spleen or kidney is usually required only for shatter or avulsion injuries or if the organ is separated from its vascular supply. Attempts are made to salvage remnants of splenic tissue whenever possible.

Late Complications

Three late complications of abdominal trauma include (1) ongoing hemorrhage, (2) sepsis due to peritoneal contamination, and (3) organ dysfunction (early or late).

Hepatic Trauma

Clinical Presentation   The liver is the organ most likely to be injured with blunt abdominal trauma. Signs of hepatic trauma include abdominal pain and tenderness, and referred *right* shoulder pain. Severe lacerations associated with hemorrhage may produce hemorrhagic shock. Most significant hepatic injury will result in elevation of the serum transaminases (aspartate transaminase [AST] >450 IU/L and alanine transaminase [ALT] >250 IU/L).

Management   Minor hepatic lacerations are managed nonoperatively. Surgical intervention is likely to be required for lesions producing hemodynamic instability despite administration of >40 ml/kg of blood or for large, stellate lacerations and subcapsular hematomas that have eroded through Glisson's capsule.

Splenic Trauma

Clinical Presentation   Signs of splenic trauma include evidence of hemorrhage, abdominal tenderness, Kehr's sign (referred pain to the left shoulder during compression of the left upper quadrant), leukocytosis, and a rise in serum amylase.

Management   Most splenic injuries can be managed nonoperatively. Indications for urgent surgical intervention include hemodynamic instability despite significant (>40 ml/kg) transfusion requirements. If surgery is required, attempts are made to salvage at least 50% of the splenic tissue or transplant some splenic tissue into the omentum (autotransplantation) to maintain protection against sepsis from encapsulated organisms. If splenic removal is necessary, the child will require vaccination against *Streptococcus pneumoniae.* Also, the lifetime risk of overwhelming infection from encapsulated organisms (e.g., *Haemophilus influenzae*) is significant following splenectomy.

Genitourinary Trauma

Genitourinary trauma is common in children because the kidneys are relatively unprotected. This form of trauma is seldom life threatening, and most renal injuries can be managed nonoperatively.

Box 12-14

Indications for Radiographic Evaluation Following Genitourinary Trauma

Indications for Intravenous Pyelogram (or Limited-View IVP) in Evaluation of Genitourinary Injury

Genitourinary injury alone suspected

Flank pain, hematoma, or ecchymosis

Penetrating trauma of the abdomen

Suspected ureteral injury

Patient too unstable to undergo computed tomography (CT) scan for evaluation

Microscopic hematuria >20 red blood cells per high-powered field

Gross hematuria

Indications for Abdominal CT Scan

Stable patient

Gross hematuria

Microscopic hematuria >20 red blood cells per high-powered field in patient with multiple injuries

Mechanism suggesting intraabdominal or renal injury

IVP result equivocal for injury or indicative of severe injury

Modified from Gausche M: Genitourinary trauma. In Barkin RM et al, editors: *Pediatric emergency medicine: concepts and clinical practice*, ed 2, St Louis, 1997, Mosby.

Renal Injury

Clinical Presentation Hematuria, abdominal pain, and flank hematomas are all signs of renal injury. The presence of threadlike clots in the urethra is a pathognomonic finding associated with major renal injury. Although the amount of hematuria does not correlate with the severity of renal trauma, >20 red blood cells visualized per high-powered field indicates the need for radiologic renal evaluation (Box 12-14).

Urinary catheter insertion is a routine procedure during resuscitative management for most patients. Contraindications to catheter insertion in the trauma victim include frank blood in the urinary meatus, gross hematuria, perineal hematoma or injury, or severe pelvic fracture, because these conditions may be associated with urethral disruption. In the presence of any of these findings, a urology consultation should be obtained. In the stable trauma victim with no evidence of pelvic or urethral injuries, it is advisable to wait for spontaneously voided urine before inserting a urinary catheter.

Severe renal injury with separation of the kidney from the urethra will not be associated with hematuria; these patients will demonstrate evidence of extravasation of urine, which will be detected by a CT scan or intravenous pyelogram (IVP).

Management Many renal injuries can be managed nonoperatively. Indications for surgery include hemodynamic instability (despite administration of >40 ml/kg of blood), presence of associated injuries requiring surgical intervention, and severe renal injury (e.g., renal pedicle injury or expanding hematoma).

Pelvis and Genitalia

Pelvic Fracture

When a pelvic fracture is suspected, the integrity of other structures within the pelvis (including the urethra, bladder, and pelvic vessels) must be ensured. If the pelvic vessels are disrupted, rapid blood loss can occur. Blood replacement is required, and stabilization with the use of MAST should be considered.

Genitalia

Testicular Injury Testicular injury requires ultrasonography and urology consultation. Surgery is occasionally required.

Female Perineal Trauma Vaginal trauma may result from blunt abdominal trauma or from straddle injuries. Most perineal trauma will result from sexual abuse and requires skilled evaluation and thorough documentation (see Sexual Abuse under Child Abuse).

Musculoskeletal System and Extremities

Extremities should be observed for tenderness, deformity, swelling, pallor, coolness, and decreased peripheral pulses. Long bone fractures and pelvic fractures can produce significant blood loss. Fractures should be splinted.

Compartment Syndrome

Clinical Presentation Compartment syndrome may complicate any skeletomuscular injury, particularly injury to the lower leg and the forearm. Compartment syndrome occurs when external forces (such as pneumatic antishock garments or a tight bandage) compress an area of muscle or when bleeding or edema increases pressure within the muscle compartment. The high pressure in the compartment compromises vascular supply to the muscle and tissue and can cause ischemia and nerve damage. Signs of compartment syndrome include the "six *P*s": pain (which worsens with movement), pallor, pulselessness, paresthesia (altered sensation), puffiness (edema), and paralysis

Intracompartmental pressures may be measured using a needle joined to a fluid-filled monitoring system (with a transducer). Pressures equaling or exceeding 30 to 60 mm Hg require treatment, since compression of muscle and nerves can compromise perfusion.

Management Treatment of compartment syndrome requires surgical release of the restriction surrounding the muscle. A fasciotomy is performed, and the area is left open (but covered with a sterile dressing).

Skin

Wounds

During initial stabilization of the trauma victim, pressure dressings are placed on sites of external bleeding, and hemorrhagic shock is treated with fluid boluses. Once the primary survey and stabilization have been accomplished, the patient should be undressed and examined carefully for the presence of contusions or burns.

Tetanus prophylaxis may be required. Clean, minor wounds do not require prophylaxis unless the patient has not received tetanus toxoid in more than 3 years or the history is unknown (Table 12-9).

Burns

If burns are present, they should be evaluated for depth and extent (Box 12-15). More details regard-

Table 12-9
Guidelines for Tetanus Prophylaxis in Routine Wound Management From the Centers for Disease Control, 1985

History of Adsorbed Tetanus Toxoid (Doses)	Clean Minor Wounds		All Other Wounds*	
	Td†	TIG	Td†	TIG
Unknown or < three	Yes	No	Yes	Yes
≥three‡	No§	No	No‖	No

From Centers for Disease Control and Prevention: *MMWR* 39(3):37-41, 1990.
*Such as, but not limited to, wounds contaminated with dirt, feces, soil, saliva, etc.; puncture wounds; avulsions; and wounds resulting from missiles, crushing, burns, and frostbite.
†For children under 7 yr old: DPT (DT, if pertussis vaccine is contraindicated) is preferred to tetanus toxoid alone. For persons 7 yr old and older, Td is preferred to tetanus toxoid alone.
‡If only three doses of *fluid* toxoid have been received, a fourth dose of toxoid, preferably an adsorbed toxoid, should be given.
§Yes, if more than 10 yr since last dose.
‖Yes, if more than 5 yr since last dose. (More frequent boosters are not needed and can accentuate side effects.)

Box 12-15

Classification of Burn Severity

Minor Burns
Partial-thickness injuries of <15% body surface area (BSA)
Full-thickness burns <2% BSA*

Moderate Burns
Partial-thickness injuries of 25% BSA
Full-thickness burns <10% BSA

Major Burns
Partial-thickness injuries of >25% BSA
Full-thickness burns >10% BSA
Combined partial- and full-thickness burns of the hands, face, genitalia, or feet

*Full-thickness burns of the face, hands, genitalia, or feet <2% may require more extensive treatment.

---

ing assessment and treatment of the patient with burns is presented in Chapter 13.

Reliable venous access must be established, since fluid resuscitation is required for all major burns. Analgesics are required to alleviate pain (see

Chapter 3). Children with significant burns will lose body heat rapidly, and the use of a radiant warmer should be considered.

The majority of fire-related deaths are secondary to smoke inhalation, and for this reason the most common cause of death during the first hour after burn injury is respiratory failure. A history of closed space confinement should lead to further patient evaluation for the presence of carbon monoxide poisoning. Inhalation injuries should be anticipated in the presence of: singed eyebrows and nose hair, dark sputum, carbon deposits and inflammatory changes in the mouth, cyanosis and dyspnea, and altered level of consciousness.

Initial treatment of smoke inhalation includes oxygen administration and close observation for deteriorating respiratory status. Carbon monoxide (CO) levels should be assessed, and hyperbaric oxygen may be considered for severe carbon monoxide poisoning. *Pulse oximetry will not reliably detect hypoxemia resulting from carbon monoxide poisoning,* since the oximeter does not recognize carboxyhemoglobin.

Medical History of the Trauma Patient

The trauma victim's past medical history is obtained from the patient (as age appropriate) and the parent(s) and friends. Information to be recorded includes allergies, past illnesses, current medications, events leading up to the trauma, the mechanism of injury, the child's status at the scene, the location and degree of pain, the child's last meal, and changes in the child's status during initial stabilization and transport.

Child Abuse

Definition and Epidemiology

Definition

The term *child abuse* applies to any maltreatment of a child, including infliction of physical injuries, sexual exploitation, infliction of emotional pain, or neglect of the child. Child abuse is usually a pattern of maladjusted behavior rather than a random, isolated act of violence.

Epidemiology

The three components of the child abuse syndrome include the maladjusted adult, the vulnerable child, and the presence of situational stressors.

Failure to Thrive Maternal deprivation in an abusive pattern during infancy can result in failure to thrive. This syndrome occurs when the primary caretaker fails to provide for the infant's basic needs. A vicious cycle is created by the primary caretaker that begins with the caretaker's feelings of inadequacy; as the child is neglected and becomes sickly, the child's condition reinforces the caretaker's feelings of inadequacy, and further neglect occurs.

Munchausen Syndrome by Proxy Munchausen syndrome by proxy (MBP) is a form of child abuse in which a parent fabricates or induces illnesses in the child and then seeks medical care for the child. The child is subjected to illnesses by the parent and to needless hospitalizations and diagnostic studies. Gastrointestinal illnesses, bleeding, seizures, and cyanosis are the most common presenting complaints. Some children have been suffocated, and illnesses induced by the parent may be fatal. MBP is an extremely difficult problem to confirm or rule out. However, if MBP is suspected, the parent must be closely watched during all visits to the bedside, to protect the child.

Sexual Abuse Sexual abuse is a symptom of seriously disturbed family relationships, almost invariably associated with both physical and emotional neglect or abuse of the child. The sexually abusive adult typically was sexually abused as a child and has subconsciously justified this form of behavior. Family relationships are usually complex, and silent complicity by at least one parent is usually present.

History of Injuries Suggesting Abuse

Health care workers must be vigilant in attempting to detect evidence of abuse and are obligated to report suspected abuse to the local child protective agency. Explanations for traumatic injuries that should be questioned include the following: unknown injury, implausible sequence of events, self-inflicted injury, and sibling-inflicted injury.

Any injury followed by a delay in seeking medical care is suspicious. Finally, any time a child or a spouse names an adult as the cause of the injuries, such accusations should be considered seriously.

Characteristics of Injuries Suggestive of Abuse

Implausible Injuries

Implausible injuries are those that are inconsistent with the history. For example, if a child allegedly sustained multiple bruises when falling down the stairs, all of the bruises should be the same color and at the same stage of healing. Bruises caused by such falls are usually located over bony prominences (e.g., the tibia) and are rarely present over soft tissues (e.g., inside the thighs). The presence of a skull fracture, rib fractures, or multiple bruises is inconsistent with a simple fall.

Suspicious bruises are located on the buttocks, on the insides of the child's legs, over the cheeks or flanks, near the upper lip or inside the mouth, and around the neck. Any bruises or lacerations near the genitals should be carefully examined and investigated. Bilateral black eyes, retinal hemorrhages, detached retinas, and traumatic cataracts are usually inflicted.

Marks of Injury

The marks of injury can be characteristic of the method of injury. Human hand marks can often be identified, and bite marks may be used to confirm the identity of the abuser. Characteristic marks of belt buckles, hair brushes, curling irons, or radiators may be identifiable.

Inflicted burns may be splash burns, hot water immersion burns, or branding. Inflicted splash burns may be difficult to distinguish from unintentional burns. Hot water immersion burns usually have circumscribed borders; burns on the hands and feet will resemble the areas covered by gloves or socks. If the buttocks are dunked in the water, a characteristic V-shaped burn will be associated with the water level on the back and thighs. Irregular margins consistent with splashing or movement by the child will be notably absent, indicating that the child was intentionally held in the water.

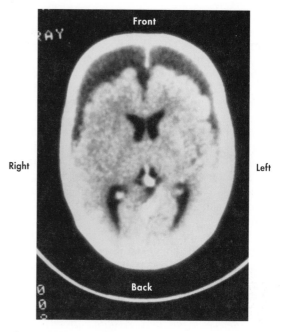

Figure 12-9 Subdural hematomas caused by child abuse. Bilateral significant subdural hematomas are apparent on computerized axial tomography scan as the darkened areas in the front of both sides of the brain. (Photograph courtesy Scott McKercher.)

Branding burns will usually reflect the shape of the hot object.

Subdural Hematomas and Shaken Baby Syndrome

Subdural hematomas are among the most common results of inflicted head injury in children (Figure 12-9). Many are associated with a skull fracture, and some may be associated with retinal hemorrhage (the shaken baby syndrome). Scalp bruises and traumatic alopecia may also be observed.

The shaken baby syndrome refers to a constellation of clinical findings that are observed in infants with little or no evidence of external cranial trauma. The injuries result from vigorous shaking or shaking plus impact (e.g., the child is shaken and struck or is shaken while being held against a mattress in bed). Signs of this syndrome include retinal hemorrhages and subdural hemorrhage/hematoma documented by CSF examination and a CT scan (MRI is helpful when the infant is stable). Additional injuries may include brain stem and spinal cord hematoma, subdural hematoma or contusion, or unexplained diffuse cerebral edema with or without hypoxic-ischemic insult.

Responsibilities of the Health Care Team

The first priority in care of the abused child is provision of necessary resuscitation, and restoration and support of cardiopulmonary and neurologic function. In addition, the child must be protected from further abuse and must receive compassionate emotional support. As soon as feasible, injuries observed should be carefully recorded. If possible, color photographs of the child's injuries should be made with a ruler visible to indicate sizes.

Suspected abuse must be reported to the local child protective services agency. The child protective services agency will usually arrange for temporary custody of the child to be awarded to the hospital or to the state. The child's appointed custodian will then be the person to provide permission for any elective surgery or procedures. The state child protective services agency will investigate the child's condition, as well as the condition of the home and family, to determine if the child should be temporarily removed from the home.

If a child abuse team is present in the hospital, they should be consulted about proper recording of injuries and documentation of parental statements. This team is also experienced in the examination of abused children and will frequently identify additional injuries that may be related to abuse.

The parents should also be informed about the contact with the child protective services agency. Unless or until custody of the child is removed from the parents, the parents should continue to be informed of the child's condition and progress. If the child is legally removed from the parents' custody, the agent of the court will provide a written document from the court specifying the contact the parents are allowed to have with the child.

As soon as possible after stabilization of the child, the child's injuries should be described in the chart. The location, size, and color of bruises and lacerations must be described and drawn on a human figure drawing. The age of the bruises can be estimated according to the color of the bruise

Table 12-10 Dating of Bruises by Color	
Color	**Age**
Reddish blue or purple	Immediate or <24 hr
Dark blue to purple	1-5 days
Green	5-7 days
Yellow	7-10 days
Brown	10-14 days or longer
Resolution	2-4 wk

From Hazinski MF: *Nursing care of the critically ill child,* ed 2, St Louis, 1992, Mosby; and Wilson EF: Estimation of the age of cutaneous contusion in child abuse, *Pediatrics* 60:750, 1977.

(Table 12-10), although the accuracy of this dating has been recently called into question. If possible, color photographs signed and dated by the nurse should be attached to the chart. Thorough notes and photographs will provide incontrovertible documentation of the child's condition (Figure 12-10) and will assist the nurse's recollection if testimony in court is required at a later time.

A "child abuse" long bone series of x-ray films will ultimately be obtained to detect evidence of healed fractures. These radiographs should be copied, and a summary of the radiologist's report must be part of the hospital record.

When abuse is suspected, every explanation of the injuries stated by the parents or primary caretakers should be quoted verbatim in the hospital record. Conflicting statements should be quoted and noted.

Throughout the child's hospitalization, the child will require sensitive support and care. It may be difficult for the child to trust unfamiliar adults, and the child will frequently feel responsible for angering the abusive adult. The child's guilt and feelings of rejection are likely to be compounded if parents are forbidden to visit (as the result of a court order). Psychologists and child abuse experts and therapists should participate in the child's care whenever possible.

Sexual Abuse

Epidemiologic Factors

Pediatric sexual abuse requires the association of four preconditions: an adult with a motivation for sexual abuse of children, absence of internal in-

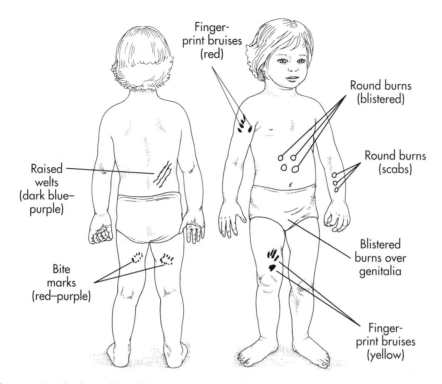

Finger-
print bruises
(red)

Round burns
(blistered)

Round burns
(scabs)

Raised
welts
(dark blue–
purple)

Blistered
burns over
genitalia

Bite
marks
(red–purple)

Finger-
print bruises
(yellow)

Figure 12-10   Recording of bruises on a human figure drawing. The Eland human figure drawing is used here with notations to indicate size, location, and color of bruising resulting from intentional trauma. The date and time are recorded on the figure, and the figure becomes part of the child's hospital record. The bruises are in various stages of healing, some of identifiable shapes. The injuries include burns, as well as bruises over soft tissue areas. These findings are inconsistent with the explanation that the child fell down the stairs. (Outlines from Stevens B: Nursing management of pain in children. In Foster RL, Hunsberger MM, Anderson JJT, editors: *Family-centered nursing care of children,* Philadelphia, 1989, WB Saunders.)

hibitors in the adult's life, absence of external inhibitors, and breakdown of the child's resistance.

History Suggestive of Possible Sexual Abuse

When sexual abuse begins, the child often demonstrates a noticeable change in behavior, including a change in school performance, development of temper tantrums, withdrawal, depression, and guilt. The child may no longer associate with friends, may associate with new friends, or may run away. The child may make comments of a sexual nature.

Physical Signs Suggestive of Sexual Abuse

The development of venereal disease or diagnosis of pregnancy indicates that sexual abuse has oc-

curred. Other infections such as chlamydia and herpes are suggestive but not pathognomonic of sexual abuse. The female victim may develop repeated urinary tract infections, evidence of urethral irritation, enuresis, and encopresis.

If sexual abuse is suspected, the child and parents should be separated and interviewed individually. The examination of the perineal area should be performed only by a clinician experienced in these examinations, and only after witnessed interviews have been conducted and the child has had an opportunity to become more comfortable with the health care team.

Physical examination of the child should be accomplished using established hospital protocols (approved by the local law enforcement agencies and the coroner) with appropriate witnesses (Box 12-16). A "rape kit" is typically used to collect clothing, scrapings of dried blood or semen, and any materials from under the fingernails. *All clothing, whether visibly stained or not, should be saved for forensic examination.* It is likely that the results of this examination will be used in courtroom proceedings; therefore all specimens should be handled and labeled carefully. Either a nurse or a police officer should witness the physical examination of the child.

Examination of the sexually abused child may not yield any concrete evidence of sexual abuse. However, the child's body should also be examined thoroughly for evidence of trauma and tenderness. A bone scan is also performed to detect other evidence of physical abuse.

A Wood's lamp should be used during the inspection, since it will aid in the detection of semen

---

Box 12-16

Suggested Examination When Sexual Abuse Is Suspected

Careful, Complete Physical Examination

Document sites of bleeding, bruising, and any ligature or teeth marks.

Note child's general appearance (including state of cleanliness) and manner.

Examination of genitalia should be performed only by experienced member of child abuse team. Child requires adequate explanation, preparation, and possible sedation prior to examination. Speculum examination of prepubescent females is often not required.

Thorough documentation and description of physical findings, including color, location, and size of any bruises or marks, and location of any blood or fluids.

Examination using a Wood's lamp will cause fluorescence of semen, so may allow identification of presence of semen on skin or clothing.

Save All Clothing in Sealed Bag

Obtain Photographs of Any Wounds or Injuries

Laboratory Studies

Pharyngeal, rectal, and vaginal swabs to culture for gonorrhea. Urethral cultures may be obtained from male victims. Plate on Thayer-Martin medium.

Vaginal culture for chlamydia.

Cultures may be obtained from suspicious lesions, for identification of additional sexually transmitted diseases, including herpes, genital warts, trichomonas, or HIV.

Pubescent females should be screened for possible pregnancy.

Forensic Examination

Specimens and examination should be obtained to comply with recommendations of local coroner or medical examiner. Therefore the local forensic medical authority should be consulted prior to the examination. A kit is often provided with written instructions regarding the obtaining and preservation of specimens, and these instructions should be followed precisely. Specimens required usually include the following:

Swab pharynx, vagina, and rectum, and plate for gonorrheal culture.

Swab pharynx, vagina, and rectum, and smear on slides to check for presence of motile sperm.

Swab vagina, pharynx, and rectum for acid phosphatase determination (elevation in acid phosphatase is consistent with presence of semen). This specimen will be air dried.

Vaginal specimens may be obtained by vaginal lavage with normal saline. If sperm are detected, additional specimens may be obtained to detect the presence of blood group antigens. This also requires that a salivary sample be obtained from the victim (to separate antigens secreted by the victim from those potentially secreted by the perpetrator).

Photograph the victim completely.

Use Wood's light to detect presence of semen.

From Hazinski MF: *Nursing care of the critically ill child,* ed 2, St Louis, 1992, Mosby.

and pubic hairs on the child's body or clothing. Collect any dried blood or semen or pubic hair found, and submit it for laboratory analysis. Bucchal scrapings should be collected and tested for semen and cultured for evidence of venereal infection. Any specimens obtained should be tested for acid phosphatase (present in semen), and ABO testing will be performed on any semen collected.

Signs consistent with rectal penetration include tenderness, lacerations, and scarring of the anus, and a decrease in rectal sphincter tone. Rectal tenderness and blood may also be present. Rectal swabs should be collected and tested for semen or acid phosphatase.

Vaginal examination may confirm the presence of hymenal tears or thickening, and the presence of a vaginal opening of greater than 4 mm in a prepubescent girl is strongly suggestive of sexual abuse. Labial adhesions and neovascularization of scarred areas may be seen following a variety of injuries but may also occur as a result of vaginal sexual abuse. The use of a colposcope, a combination magnifier and camera, enables detailed examination of the perineal area; it also provides a green light to assist in the examination of perineal vascularity.

Interviewing the Child

It is extremely important that victims of possible sexual abuse be questioned by *only those members of the health care team specifically trained in and skilled in such an interview.* The child may be asked to draw pictures or to reenact the assault using anatomically correct dolls.

Any statements made by the child outside of the formal interview should be recorded in the chart. The child requires compassionate support, and it is important that caregivers avoid creating the impression that discussion of the abusive event is wrong.

Discharge Preparation

The child cannot be returned to the home until that home environment will be safe for the child. The child requires ongoing psychologic therapy, and such therapy should be provided for the family.

Post–Intensive Care Unit Care of the Pediatric Trauma Patient

Comprehensive care of the pediatric trauma patient should ideally include a transfer agreement between the acute care center and rehabilitation facilities so that the child is automatically transferred to a known rehabilitation facility as soon as it is appropriate. This frequently does not occur, however, because admission to rehabilitation facilities is likely to require demonstration of the family's ability to pay for the costs of care.

Obviously, patient care must assume the highest priority while the child requires critical care interventions. However, preparation for discharge should begin while the child is in the ICU.

Conditions Requiring Rehabilitation

To effectively coordinate the discharge of a pediatric trauma patient, the child's rehabilitative needs and potential for recovery must be established. Most children who require inpatient rehabilitative care have sustained severe head injuries and may show signs of recovery for years after the injury. Additional effects of the head injury may also become apparent at a later date.

Potential sequelae of head injuries include learning disabilities, attention deficits, and disinhibition. The child's family and teachers should be aware of these possible sequelae to ensure that appropriate therapy is provided.

Rehabilitation services may also be necessary for children with musculoskeletal deficits, those requiring medications, and those requiring skilled care as a result of the injury. The specific level of rehabilitative services needed can only be determined after careful evaluation of the child, the family and their support systems, and the home environment.

Selection of a Facility

The Delta scoring system (Table 12-11) can be used to help formulate the child's problem list. Once a problem list is drafted, the child's specific rehabilitative needs can be determined.

The pediatric trauma discharge coordinator must be familiar with the specialties of each reha-

Table 12-11
Delta Scoring System for Evaluation of Outcome Following Pediatric Injury

Function, Central Nervous System (CNS)
  −1 Attention deficit, nightmares, fixation, and distraction despite otherwise normal function
  −2 Reading, speaking learning deficit
  −3 Objective CNS deficit: obtundation, paresis, seizures, etc.

Function, Musculoskeletal (M/S)
  −1 Temporary deficit—e.g., cast, bandage
  −2 Long-term defect—e.g., loss of muscle group, scarring dysfunction, limb
  −3 Permanent disability—e.g., limb loss, wheelchair, walker dependent

Lifestyle, Medication (Rx)
  −1 Finite, short-term drug dose—e.g., antibiotics
  −2 Lifelong prn medication—e.g., antibiotics for asplenia, seizure, meds
  −3 Lifelong, ongoing medication

Lifestyle, Care (Care)
  −1 Temporary finite help from cast, dressing, etc.
  −2 Special education, care
  −3 Custodial care

	Discharge	3 Months	6 Months	12 Months
Function (CNS) (MS)	_____ _____	_____ _____	_____ _____	_____ _____
Lifestyle (Rx) (Care)	_____ _____	_____ _____	_____ _____	_____ _____
Total	_____	_____	_____	_____

From Tepas JJ: Problems in the management of multiple trauma. In Luten RC, editor: *Problems in pediatric emergency medicine,* New York, 1988, Churchill Livingstone.

bilitation facility in the trauma referral region. Many rehabilitation facilities will transport members of the trauma team and potential patients and families to their centers.

The location of the rehabilitation facility must also be considered. The development of pediatric trauma centers with large referral populations has fostered the growth of pediatric rehabilitation facilities. This allows for more specialized care but often also means that the centers are remote from the family's home. The health care providers must weigh the relative benefits offered by a facility against the consequences of separation from or disruption to the family.

Needs Assessment

Once a rehabilitation facility has been selected by the pediatric trauma team and the family, an evaluator from that center is invited by the hospital and family to visit with the patient to determine the child's rehabilitation needs. Parents are usually required to sign a consent form to give the evaluator access to the patient's chart. It is important to compare the problem list the evaluator formulates with the one drafted by those already involved in the patient's care to ensure that the evaluator's facility offers all of the services the child will need.

Funding

Rehabilitation facilities usually operate on a for-profit basis. As such, they require identification of a funding source before the patient is accepted. At present, the issue of an appropriate method of payment for rehabilitation services continues to be debated on a national level. There are a number of potential funding sources that should be explored for any child who would benefit from rehabilitative services.

If the child has any insurance, the admitting office at the prospective rehabilitation facility will contact the insurance company to discuss the child's coverage. If the child has insufficient or no insurance benefits, other potential funding sources are possible, including state funds as distributed through the state Medicaid offices, as well as those funneled through the state's division of the Department of Health and Human Services. Various service organizations such as the Elks and the Shriners sponsor children who fall within their guidelines. Families may also receive financial assistance from church groups or with the assistance of the local media.

Transition From the Pediatric Intensive Care Unit

Relatively few pediatric trauma patients require inpatient treatment at a rehabilitation center. Most pediatric trauma victims are discharged to their home and require minimal follow-up (usually a return outpatient visit or two). Some children require home health nurses, physical or occupational therapy, or outpatient services provided by either the acute care facility or the rehabilitation facility. These children should spend some time in a non-ICU setting before discharge.

The transition from the PICU to a general unit ("the floor") may be frightening to the patient, family, and floor nurses. PICU nurses can help to make the transition to the floor more relaxed for

everyone involved. The family and child require time to adapt to noncontinuous care.

Before transfer of a complex trauma patient to the floor, the floor nurses responsible for the patient's care should participate in joint PICU-floor rounds. In addition, if staffing permits it, the floor nurses should spend a shift or two with the patient while the child is still in the PICU. This gradual introduction of the child and family to the floor nurses will make the transition from the ICU to the floor much less frightening for the family and the nursing staff.

It is very important that everything possible be done to make the transition out of the PICU as smooth as possible. If possible, transfer the child with complex care needs early in the week (*not* on

---

Table 12-12

Sample Supply List in Preparation for Discharge of Trauma Patient to Rehabilitation Facility

Pediatric ostomy supplies	Pediatrics pouches
	4×4 Duoderm wafers
	Stomahesive paste (optional)
Tracheostomy supplies	Tracheostomy tubes
	Same size as child uses, ties in place
	One size smaller than child uses
	Tracheostomy ties
	Blunt scissors
	Bulb suction
	Suction catheters
	Suction machine and tubing
	Ambu bag and tubing
	Oxygen source
	Hydrogen peroxide
	Respiratory saline
Central venous line supplies	Betadine wipes
	Alcohol wipes
	Examination gloves
	Luer-Lok male adapters
	Dressing change kits
	Heparin flush kits
	Normal saline kits
Wet-to-dry dressing supplies	Normal saline
	Gauze dressings
	Tape
	Duoderm (optional)

From Hazinski MF: *Nursing care of the critically ill child,* ed 2, St Louis, 1992, Mosby.

Friday afternoon!) and in the morning. It may be more difficult to accomplish this if the child is being sent to a rehabilitation facility or home. Be sure that all supplies and instructions go with the child. Sample checklists of supplies for patients with an ostomy, a tracheostomy, a central venous line, or wet-to-dry dressing changes are provided in Table 12-12.

The transition will be facilitated if the child and family visit the new unit or facility and if the staff members of the facility that will be involved in the child's care go to the PICU to meet the child and family and to be given any particular instructions before the time of discharge. The more comfortable the new staff is with the child's care, the more comfortable the family and child will be with the transition.

Long-Term Follow-Up

All effects of a head injury may not be apparent during hospitalization; in fact, many deficits related to a child's injury may only be detected once the child resumes activities of daily living. It is important that injured children receive regular follow-up examinations and evaluations.

Suggested Readings

American Academy of Pediatrics, Committee on Child Abuse and Neglect: Shaken baby syndrome: inflicted cerebral trauma, *Pediatrics* 92:872-875, 1993.

American College of Emergency Physicians: *Pediatric basic trauma life support,* Oakbrook, Ill, 1995, The College.

American College of Surgeons: Pediatric trauma. In *Advanced trauma life support for doctors,* ed 6, Chicago, 1997, The College.

Baker SP et al: *Injury to children and teenagers: state-by-state mortality facts,* Johns Hopkins Center for Injury Research and Policy, Vienna, Va, 1996, The National Maternal and Child Health Bureau.*

Barkin RM et al, editors: *Pediatric emergency medicine: concepts and clinical practice,* ed 2, St Louis, 1997, Mosby.

Bracken MB et al: A randomized controlled trial of methylprednisolone or naloxone in the treatment of acute spinal cord injury: results of the second national acute spinal cord injury study, *N Engl J Med* 322:1405-1414, 1990.

Bratton SL et al: Serial, neurologic examinations after near-drowning and outcome, *Arch Pediatr Adolesc Med* 148:167-170, 1994.

Centers for Disease Control and Prevention: Airbag-associated fatal injuries to infants and children riding in front passenger seats—United States, *MMWR* 44:845-847, 1995.

Chameides L, Hazinski MF, editors: *Textbook of pediatric advanced life support,* ed 3, Dallas, 1997, American Heart Association.

Champion HR et al: Trauma score, *Crit Care Med* 9:672, 1981.

Chestnut RM, Prough DS: Critical care of severe head injury, *New Horizons* 3:365-593, 1995.*

Cooper A, Foltin GL: Thoracic trauma. In Barkin RM et al, editors: *Pediatric emergency medicine: concepts and clinical practice,* ed 2, St Louis, 1997, Mosby.*

Crone KR, Lee KS, Kelly DL: Correlation of admission fibrin degradation products with outcome and respiratory failure in patients with head injury, *Neurosurgery* 21:532, 1987.

Cywes S et al: Blunt liver trauma in children, *Injury* 22:310-315, 1991.

Enos WF, Conrath TB, Byer JC: Forensic evaluation of the sexually abused child, *Pediatrics* 78:385, 1986.

Foltin GL, Cooper A: Abdominal trauma. In Barkin RM et al, editors: *Pediatric emergency medicine: concepts and clinical practice,* ed 2, St Louis, 1997, Mosby.*

Gausche M: Genitourinary trauma. In Barkin RM et al, editors: *Pediatric emergency medicine: concepts and clinical practice,* ed 2, St Louis, 1997, Mosby.*

Hamilton MG, Myles ST: Pediatric spinal injury: review of 174 hospital admissions, *J Neurosurg* 77:700-704, 1992.

Hazinski MF et al: Pediatric injury prevention, *Ann Emerg Med* 22:456-467, 1993.*

Hazinski MF et al: Outcome of cardiovascular collapse in pediatric victims of blunt trauma, *Ann Emerg Med* 23:1229-1235, 1994.

Hennes HM et al: Elevated liver transaminase levels in children with blunt abdominal trauma: a predictor of liver injury, *Pediatrics* 86:87, 1990.

Hertzenberg JE et al: Emergency transport and positioning of young children who have an injury of the cervical spine; the standard backboard may be hazardous, *J Bone Joint Surg Am* 71:15-22, 1989.

Huerta C, Griffith R, Joyce SM: Cervical spine stabilization in pediatric patients: evaluation of current techniques, *Ann Emerg Med* 16:1121, 1987.

Kyriacou DN et al: Effect of immediate resuscitation on children with submersion injury, *Pediatrics* 94:137-142, 1994.

Lacey SR et al: Munchausen syndrome by proxy: patterns of presentation to pediatric surgeons, *J Pediatr Surg* 28:827-832, 1993.

Luten RC et al: Length-based endotracheal tube and emergency equipment selection in pediatrics, *Ann Emerg Med* 21:900-904, 1992.

Meadow R: Munchausen syndrome by proxy, *Arch Dis Child* 57:92-98, 1982.

Medina FA: Neck and spinal cord trauma. In Barkin RM et al, editors: *Pediatric emergency medicine: concepts and clinical practice,* ed 2, St Louis, 1997, Mosby.*

Moore EE et al: Organ injury scaling: spleen, liver, and kidney, *Surg Clin North Am* 75:294-302, 1995.*

Nypaver M, Treloar D: Neutral cervical spine positioning in children, *Ann Emerg Med* 23:208-211, 1994.

---

*Excellent overeiw.

Proehl JA: Compartment syndrome, *J Emerg Nurs* 14:283, 1988.

Quan L, Kinder D: Pediatric submersions: prehospital predictors of outcome, *Pediatrics* 90:909-913, 1992.

Schoenfeld PS, Baker MD: Management of cardiopulmonary and trauma resuscitation in the pediatric emergency department, *Pediatrics* 91:726-729, 1993.

Simpson DA et al: Head injuries in infants and young children: the value of the paediatric coma scale; review of literature and report on a study, *Childs Nerv Syst* 7:183-190, 1991.

Smith JS, Wengrovitz MS, DeLong BS: Prospective validation of criteria, including age, for safe, nonsurgical management of the ruptured spleen, *J Trauma* 33:363-369, 1992.

Stafford PW, Harmon CV: Thoracic trauma in children, *Curr Opin Pediatr* 5:325-332, 1993.

Steele B: Psychodynamic factors in child abuse. In Helfer RE, Kempe RS, editors: *The battered child,* ed 4, Chicago, 1987, University of Chicago Press.

Tepas JJ et al: The Pediatric Trauma Score as a predictor of injury severity in the injured child, *J Pediatr Surg* 22:14-18, 1987.

Tepas JJ: Blunt abdominal trauma in children, *Curr Opin Pediatr* 5:317-324, 1993.

Wilson EF: Estimation of the age of cutaneous contusion in child abuse, *Pediatrics* 60: 750, 1977.

Resources for Patients and Families

American Paralysis Association
500 Morris Avenue
Springfield, NJ 07081
(800) 225-0292
Newsletter and hot line for information about spinal injury research.

Kriegsman KH, Zaslow EL, D'Zmura-Rechsteiner J: *Taking charge: teenagers talk about life and physical disabilities,* Bethesda, Md, 1992, Woodbine House. Excellent, honest discussion about communication, relationships, dating, sexuality, and family life for adolescents.

Maddox S: *Spinal network 3: the total wheelchair book:* Malibu, Calif, In press, Miramar Communications. Excellent reference, including anatomy and physiology, activities of daily living, rights and legal/financial information, and state-by-state resources. (Phone: 800-543-4116; address: PO Box 8987, Malibu, CA 90265-8987.)

National Spinal Cord Injury Association (NSCIA)
8300 Colesville Rd, Suite 551
Silver Springs, MD 20910
800-962-9629
Provides excellent printed material, chapter network in most states, and information about rehabilitation programs.

New Mobility Magazine
800-543-4116

13 Care of the Child With Burns

Joshua Pietsch, John Pietsch

Pearls

- Intentional injury (child abuse) should be considered and ruled out as a cause of burns and scalds in children.
- Burns are painful; therefore analgesia should be provided and should be supplemented as needed before burn care.
- "Adult" burn formulas should not be used to calculate the burn surface area and fluid resuscitation requirements for children.
- Children with large burns should be cared for in units with nurses and physicians who have pediatric expertise. Strong consideration should be given to transfer of a child to a pediatric intensive care unit (PICU) when large burns or complicating factors, such as smoke inhalation, are present.

Additional Helpful Chapters

Chapter 3: Analgesia, Sedation, and Neuromuscular Blockade
Chapter 4: Care of the Dying Child and Family
Chapter 5: Cardiovascular Disorders, Particularly Hypovolemic and Septic Shock and Cardiopulmonary Resuscitation
Chapter 6: Pulmonary Disorders: Respiratory Failure, Inhalation Injuries, and Acute Respiratory Distress Syndrome

Introduction

Fires and burns are the leading cause of accidental death in the home in children ages 1 to 14 years in the United States. Scald burns are most common in infants and toddlers, whereas flame burns and smoke inhalation are more often seen in older children. Unfortunately, approximately 15% of burns in children are due to child abuse or neglect.

The vast majority of childhood burns occur in the home, and most burns are preventable. Simple measures such as placing smoke detectors in every home, keeping hot liquids out of the reach of children, using back burners on stoves, and reducing the hot water temperature from 150° to 120° F can be very effective in reducing injuries and deaths resulting from fires and scalds.

Anatomy and Physiology of a Burn

Burn Severity and Classification

The severity of thermal injury and the fluid resuscitation required are determined by the depth of the burn and the surface area involved. The burn depth can be estimated based on the clinical appearance of the wound and is characterized as a superficial, partial-thickness, full-thickness, or fourth-degree burn (Table 13-1).

The burn size can be estimated using a variety of formulas. The "rule of nines" and the Lund and Browder chart (Figure 13-1) are probably used most frequently. The "rule of nines" does enable rapid, preliminary assessment of the burn size, but

Table 13-1
Characteristics of Burn Injury

Depth	Appearance	Healing Time	Scarring	Examples
Superficial (First-degree burn)	Erythema; mild edema and pain; blanches with pressure	3-7 days	No	Sunburn; flash burn
Partial thickness (Second-degree burn)	Pink to red; moist; moderate edema; extremely painful; vesicles	14-21 days	Variable	Scalds; flames; brief contact with hot objects
Full thickness (Third-degree burn)	Waxy white to black; dry; leathery; thrombosed vessels; edema; painless	Requires grafting	Yes	Flames; scalds; prolonged contact with hot objects; electrical; chemicals
Fourth-degree burn	Dry; leathery; black; painless; possibly exposed bones, tendons, or muscles	Requires grafting, flaps, or amputation	Yes	Prolonged contact with flame, electrical

Modified from Hazinski MF: *Nursing care of the critically ill child,* ed 2, St Louis, 1992, Mosby.

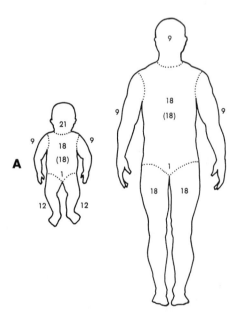

Lund and Browder Chart

Burned Area	1	1-4	5-9	10-14	15	Adult
			Total Body Surface			
Head	19 %	17 %	13 %	11 %	9 %	7 %
Neck	2	2	2	2	2	2
Anterior trunk	13	13	13	13	13	13
Posterior trunk	13	13	13	13	13	13
Right buttock	2.5	2.5	2.5	2.5	2.5	2.5
Left buttock	2.5	2.5	2.5	2.5	2.5	2.5
Genitalia	1	1	1	1	1	1
R.U. arm	4	4	4	4	4	4
L.U. arm	4	4	4	4	4	4
R.L. arm	3	3	3	3	3	3
L.L. arm	3	3	3	3	3	3
Right hand	2.5	2.5	2.5	2.5	2.5	2.5
Left hand	2.5	2.5	2.5	2.5	2.5	2.5
Right thigh	5.5	6.5	8	8.5	9	9.5
Left thigh	5.5	6.5	8	8.5	9	9.5
Right leg	5	5	5.5	6	6.5	7
Left leg	5	5	5.5	6	6.5	7
Right foot	3.5	3.5	3.5	3.5	3.5	3.5
Left foot	3.5	3.5	3.5	3.5	3.5	3.5

Figure 13-1 Lund and Browder method of estimating burn extent. **A,** Estimation of body surface area (BSA) in the infant and adult. **B,** Lund and Browder chart for estimation of BSA involved in burns during childhood. This chart should be used to accurately estimate the extent of burns in children of all ages. (**A** from Dressler DP, Hozid JL, Nathan P: *Thermal injury,* St Louis, 1988, Mosby; **B** from Emergency Nurses Association: *Trauma nursing core course (provider) manual,* ed 2, Chicago, 1988, The Association.

Table 13-2
Criteria for Classification of Burns in Pediatric Patients

	Minor	Moderate	Critical
Partial thickness	<10% TBSA	10%-15% TBSA	>15% TBSA
Full thickness	<2% TBSA	2%-10% TBSA	>10% TBSA
Age	Children older than 2 years of age	Children younger than 2 years with otherwise minor injury	Children <10 years of age with otherwise moderate injury
Involvement of face, ears, hands, feet, and perineum	No	Small areas	Large areas
Electrical	No	Small areas	Yes
Chemical	No	Small areas	Yes
Inhalation	No	Suspected	Significant
Treatment location	Outpatient	Burn unit or general hospital	Designated pediatric burn unit or PICU

From Hazinski MF: *Nursing care of the critically ill child,* ed 2, St Louis, 1992, Mosby.

it is somewhat imprecise. The Lund and Browder chart provides a more precise estimation of the burn size in relation to the body surface area (BSA).

Burns are also classified as minor, moderate, or critical in children, with consideration given not only to the burn depth and size, but also to complicating factors, such as involvement of the hands and face and presence of inhalation injuries (Table 13-2). Triage of children to a pediatric intensive care unit (PICU) or designated pediatric burn unit is required for critical burns.

Fluid Resuscitation

Thermal injury results in the loss of fluid both through the burn wound and into the adjacent tissue (third space loss). Injury to the skin also results in heat loss, which can be extremely problematic in small children.

Fluid resuscitation is critically important in children with burns to replace fluid losses and to prevent organ damage from dehydration. Intravenous (IV) access should be obtained in any child with a burn greater than 15% of the total body surface area (TBSA), and a urinary catheter should be placed in children with burns greater than 20% of the TBSA.

The fluid administration rate should be adjusted based on the child's clinical response; these clinical

responses are summarized in Table 13-3. Urine output is commonly used to monitor adequacy of fluid resuscitation, and fluid administration can be adjusted based on hourly urine output. Adequate pediatric urine output is approximately 1 ml/kg/hr, or 30 ml/m^2 BSA/day.

A variety of formulas can be used to calculate fluid resuscitation and administration rates (Table 13-4); pediatric-specific formulas (Carvajal, 1988) should be used because resuscitation formulas designed for adults can be inaccurate when applied to the infant or small child.

A balanced salt solution is provided to replace fluid loss, based on the burn size and the patient's weight or BSA. The BSA can be determined by plotting the patient's height and weight on a standard surface area nomogram (see inside back cover).

The first 12 to 36 hours after a burn are characterized by a fluid shift from the intravascular to the interstitial space ("third spacing") as a result of increased capillary permeability. The IV fluids provided to replace fluid lost to "third spacing" during the first 24 hours are generally administered in two increments: half of the calculated fluid replacement volume is administered during the first 8 hours of therapy, and the second half is provided during the next 16 hours. As noted above, a balanced salt solution is used, although some pediatric formulas use a colloid solution during the initial 24 hours of

Table 13-3
Clinical Responses to Fluid Resuscitation in Children With Burns

Parameter	Desirable Response	Potential Hypovolemia	Potential Hypervolemia
Urine output	1 ml/kg/hr	<1 ml/kg/hr	>2 ml/kg/hr
Specific gravity	1.010-1.025	>1.025	<1.010
Blood pressure	Normal for age	Hypotension	Hypertension
Pulse	Normal for age	Tachycardia	Normal or tachycardia
Level of consciousness	Alert	Lethargy	Alert or lethargy
Hematocrit	34%-45%	48%-55%	25%-30%
Blood urea nitrogen	5-20 mg/dl	>25 mg/dl	<5 mg/dl
Serum sodium	136-148 mEq/L	>150 mEq/L	<130 mEq/L
Peripheral circulation	Normal	Vasoconstriction—diminished pulses	Bounding pulses

Table 13-4
Burn Fluid Resuscitation Formulas

Type	Formula	Solution
Brooke	2 ml/kg/% burn + 2000 ml/24 hr	¼ colloid and ¾ crystalloid
Parkland	3 ml/kg/% burn/24 hr	Lactated Ringer's (LR)
Carvajal	5000 ml/m^2 burn + 2000 ml/m^2/24 hr	5% Dextrose and lactated Ringer's with 12.5 g albumin/liter

therapy. There is evidence that the addition of colloid results in a more rapid resuscitation with less total fluid administration and less edema formation.

Injured capillaries generally heal approximately 24 to 36 hours after a burn; thus intravascular fluid loss typically ceases at this time. After the initial 24 hours of therapy, most fluid loss results from evaporative losses, which are largely electrolyte free. Fluid also begins to shift from the interstitial space back into the vascular space, where it is eliminated by the kidneys. Therefore the composition and rate of fluid administration are modified after the first 24 to 48 hours of therapy to provide less sodium and less total fluid intake.

The child's weight should be measured daily. Children with large burns will gain weight as a result of fluid administration. The maximum weight gain will be observed 2 to 3 days following the burn. The weight gradually decreases, however, as the child eliminates this fluid during the diuretic phase. Preinjury weight is typically reached approximately 2 weeks after the burn.

Common Clinical Conditions: Complications of Burns

Potential Organ System Failure Associated With Burns

Myocardial Dysfunction

Cardiac output falls after a burn as a result of decreased intravascular volume and also as a result of myocardial dysfunction. This decrease in cardiac function has been linked to the presence of a circulating myocardial depressant factor, which has been implicated in a fall in cardiac output by as much as 30% following a large burn. A catecholamine (stress)–induced increase in systemic and pulmonary vascular resistance may contribute to the fall in cardiac output. Cardiac output may remain depressed for 18 to 36 hours after a burn, but it generally returns to preburn levels even before intravascular volume has been completely restored.

Treatment of inadequate cardiac output requires support of maximal oxygen delivery. This requires support of oxygenation (oxyhemoglobin saturation), ventilation, hemoglobin concentration, heart rate, cardiac preload, cardiac contractility, and appropriate vascular tone (see Shock, p. 130).

Pulmonary Dysfunction

Respiratory failure may result from inhalation of smoke or toxic fumes (see Inhalation Injury), airway edema or obstruction, or increased pulmonary capillary permeability with resultant pulmonary edema. Carbon monoxide is produced in almost every fire and particularly in fires in closed spaces. Carbon monoxide may produce death or significant tissue or organ ischemia.

Gastrointestinal Dysfunction

Gastrointestinal perfusion is often compromised after a burn, particularly if cardiac output falls. Decreased gastrointestinal perfusion, in turn, will compromise gastrointestinal motility and can also contribute to increased gastrointestinal permeability and translocation of gram-negative bacteria or endotoxin from the gastrointestinal lumen into the lymphatics or circulation. Gastrointestinal perfusion, motility, and permeability should return to normal if cardiac output is maintained and early enteral feedings are instituted.

Metabolic Changes

The burn patient is in a hypermetabolic state with high oxygen consumption and caloric requirements. The metabolic rate peaks at double or more the normal value approximately 4 to 12 days after a burn. Increased muscle protein catabolism will occur to provide amino acids for gluconeogenesis and fuel sources for local tissue needs. Insufficient protein administration and nutrition will result in marked catabolism and a delay in healing.

Immune Dysfunction

A thermal injury destroys the protective barrier of the skin, creating an open wound. In addition, the burn activates the inflammatory response, including activation of the complement system and other mediators, which compromises immune function. Burn toxin, a high-molecular-weight protein, is thought to contribute to postburn immunosuppression. Immune-enhancing enteral feedings containing glutamine, arginine, and omega-3 fatty acids may ameliorate this immune dysfunction.

Box 13-1

Clinical Signs of Possible Inhalation Injury

Burns to the head and neck region (closed space)
Tachypnea (bradypnea a late sign)
Nasal flaring
Retractions
Drooling
Sputum containing soot
Singed nasal hairs
Wheezing
Hypoxemia
Altered mental status

Inhalation Injury

Respiratory compromise associated with thermal injury is almost always due to the inhalation of toxic products that cause airway edema and respiratory distress. Direct airway burns are very rare and are usually caused by exposure to steam. Flame burns that occur in a closed space are likely to be associated with inhalation injury.

Signs and symptoms of smoke inhalation are listed in Box 13-1. The definitive diagnosis of inhalation injury is made via flexible fiberoptic bronchoscopy.

Treatment of all patients with suspected inhalation injury begins with the administration of supplemental oxygen at the scene of the injury. Monitoring with pulse oximetry is mandatory in these children. Carbon monoxide (CO) poisoning should be suspected in all children with burns who have been exposed to smoke from burning wood or furniture. The relationship between plasma carboxyhemoglobin (COHgb) levels and clinical signs are summarized in Table 13-5.

Pulse oximetry is *not* useful in determining the degree of carbon monoxide exposure in these children, because the pulse oximeter does not detect carboxyhemoglobin (COHgb). As a result, the pulse oximeter will only reflect the oxygen saturation of *normal* hemoglobin. If the patient has a 40% COHgb level, the pulse oximeter may still reflect 97% saturation because the normal hemoglobin is 97% saturated; this patient probably actually has a 58.2% oxyhemoglobin saturation, indicating 97% saturation of the 60% of the patient's hemoglobin

Table 13-5
Relationship Between Blood Carboxyhemoglobin
Levels and Symptoms

CoHgb Level	Symptoms
<10%	None
10%-20%	Mild headache, dyspnea, visual changes, confusion
20%-40%	Dizziness, shortness of breath, nausea and vomiting, irritability, weakness, ringing in the ears, hypotension, tachycardia
40%-60%	Hallucinations, confusion, coma, cardio-pulmonary instability, dysrrhythmias
>60%	Usually fatal

From Hazinski MF: *Nursing care of the critically ill child,* ed 2, St Louis, 1992, Mosby.

Table 13-6
Clinical Stages of Inhalation Injury

Stage	Onset	Characteristics
Ventilatory insufficiency	0-8 hr	Bronchospasm and alveolar damage
Pulmonary edema	8-48 hr	Edema of upper or lower airways and pulmonary interstitial edema, hypoxemia and decreased lung compliance
Bronchopneumonia	72 hr and later	Bronchorrhea, pneumonia, decrease in ciliary and mucosal activity

From Hazinski MF: *Nursing care of the critically ill child,* ed 2, St Louis, 1992, Mosby.

that is *not* bound to carbon monoxide. To determine true hemoglobin saturation, the patient's arterial blood sample should be sent for measurement of hemoglobin saturation by co-oximeter. The binding of carbon monoxide to hemoglobin is strong but reversible with oxygen administration.

Hyperbaric oxygen can be used for treatment of extreme cases of carbon monoxide poisoning. Although hyperbaric oxygen will enable more rapid reduction of carbon monoxide/COHgb levels than oxygen delivered at barometric pressure, it is not clear if this therapy affects the neurologic outcome following carbon monoxide poisoning.

Children with severe smoke inhalation or airway compromise require intubation and mechanical ventilation. These treatments should be instituted electively *before* arterial desaturation occurs and the patient deteriorates. Succinylcholine is probably contraindicated for rapid sequence induction intubation of burn patients, particularly beyond the first day after a burn, because it may produce potassium release from muscles and severe hyperkalemia.

If severe facial burns are present, it will be impossible to secure the endotracheal tube with tape; therefore it will be necessary to use twill tape or a commercially available system to secure the endotracheal tube around the child's neck. This system must be checked frequently to prevent loosening of the ties and spontaneous extubation. IV sedation and/or paralysis (with analysis) may be necessary to prevent tube dislodgment (see Chapter 3).

Inhalation injury adds substantially to the morbidity and mortality of burn injury. The clinical stages of this injury and causes of respiratory deterioration are listed in Table 13-6. For further information regarding respiratory failure, see Chapter 6.

Burn Care

Burn care should begin after adequate airway management, oxygenation, ventilation, and fluid resuscitation have been accomplished. The objectives of burn care include:

- To eliminate nonviable tissue
- To reduce or eliminate bacterial colonization
- To preserve distal extremity perfusion and chest wall motion

Burn Care on Arrival in the Emergency Department and Pediatric Intensive Care Unit

Initial burn care in the emergency department (ED) should focus on airway management, initiation of fluid resuscitation, and restoration of perfusion of distal extremities. Full-thickness or circumferential

Table 13-7
Topical Antimicrobial Agents for Treatment of Burns

Agent	Duration	Side Effects	Comments
Silver sulfadiazine	q12h	Rare	Painless on application; resistance may develop on large burns
Mafenide acetate	q12h	Metabolic acidosis	Very effective on deep burns, especially ears; painful
Silver acetate	q12h	Leaching of electrolytes	Poor penetration of burn; dressings must be kept wet
Antibiotic ointment (gentamicin, Neosporin, bacitracin)	q8h	Rare	May result in antiobiotic resistance

burns may restrict chest wall motion or perfusion of distal extremities. In these circumstances escharotomies are indicated to relieve the tourniquet effect of the burn wound. Burns should be dressed with clean, dry dressings in the ED. Definitive burn wound care can begin once the child has been transferred to the burn unit or PICU.

Initial and Daily Burn Debridement, Cleansing, and Dressing

Analgesia must be adequate throughout the child's hospitalization, but it is particularly important during burn care. Bolus supplementation of continuous infusion analgesics should be provided before the burn care, and adequate time should be allowed for the drugs to take effect before beginning the care (see Pain Management and Chapter 3). Whether continuous or intermittent analgesia is provided, additional analgesia should be administered before burn care, with sufficient time allowed to ensure that analgesia is adequate during burn care.

Gowns, head coverings, masks, and sterile gloves should be used during initial debridement and burn care. Subsequent wound care should be performed using aseptic technique. Heat loss during dressing changes is common in infants and small children; therefore use of radiant warming devices is required to prevent hypothermia.

All loose and necrotic tissue should be debrided using either forceps and scissors or a washcloth. Broken blisters should also be debrided. Intact blisters may be left in place. Following debridement, the burn areas should be cleansed

gently with a washcloth and antibacterial soap. The areas are then rinsed with water or normal saline solution.

A topical antimicrobial agent (Table 13-7) is applied to the burn areas after debridement and cleansing. Silver sulfadiazine is the most common topical agent used for burn care in the United States. The areas are then covered with sterile dry gauze dressings and wrapped with a sterile bandage. Burns to the face or ears are covered with a nonadherent dressing or left uncovered using an antibiotic ointment (for superficial burns). Burns to the fingers and toes are individually dressed.

Following initial burn care, burns are debrided, cleansed, and dressed twice a day. Burns to the face usually require dressing changes three times a day.

At the time of initial burn assessment and subsequent dressing changes, the burns should be evaluated for extent, depth, color, and appearance, as well as the condition of the surrounding skin. Determination of the depth of scald burns in children may require as long as 5 days, and decisions regarding suitability for excision and grafting are made based on the appearance of the burn wound.

Pain Management

All children with burn injuries will experience pain. Although full-thickness burns are insensate, all other burns, as well as tissue surrounding even full-thickness burns, can be extremely painful.

The awake and alert child may be able to verbalize pain and discomfort. However, in the preverbal, disoriented, or intubated child, pain assessment is more difficult. The nurse should assess for non-verbal signs of discomfort, including tachycardia, facial expressions of discomfort, pupil dilation, hypertension, diaphoresis, and irritability.

IV and oral narcotics are frequently used in pain management for the pediatric patient with burns. The use of patient-controlled analgesia (PCA) pumps in older children is beneficial. Psychotropic drugs such as midazolam may be added at the time of dressing changes, to relieve anxiety and induce amnesia. If the child is breathing spontaneously when narcotics or muscle relaxants are administered, respiratory rate and effort must be closely monitored. Pulse oximetry will enable detection of hypoxemia but will not signal the development of hypercarbia. For further information regarding pain management, see Chapter 3.

Infection

Following a burn injury, the child is at risk for infection from a variety of sources, including the burn wound and the lungs. Infection is the leading cause of death from burns in children. Clinical signs of a burn wound infection are listed in Box 13-2. Systemic signs of infection in the child with burns are listed in Box 13-3. For further information regarding the pathophysiology, clinical presentation, and management of septic shock, see Shock, p. 137).

Proper burn wound care, as described in previous paragraphs, is an essential element in burn infection prevention. Effective topical antimicrobial agents have also helped to reduce the incidence of burn wound sepsis. Systemic antibiotics are not administered prophylactically to children with fresh burn wounds, because they do not reduce the incidence of infection and they will contribute to the development of resistant organisms. Systemic antibiotics are reserved for the treatment of documented infection.

The single most important factor in the prevention of cross-contamination between patients is proper handwashing. In addition, early and aggressive nutritional therapy has been shown to reduce infectious complications in burned children.

Nutrition

Adequate nutritional management of the child with burns is crucial to recovery. The body's response to a burn injury is one of hypermetabolism, leading to increases in caloric requirements of as much as twice normal predicted values. If these requirements are not met, deterioration of body mass, delayed wound healing, and increased risk of infection occur.

A variety of formulas can be used to estimate caloric requirements in children. Hildreth and Carvajal (1982) recommend 1800 Cal/m^2 BSA/day to provide maintenance calories *plus* 2200

Box 13-2
Signs of Possible Burn Wound Infection

Conversion of partial-thickness to full-thickness injury
Hemorrhagic discoloration or ulceration of healthy skin at the burn margins
Erythematous, nodular lesions in unburned skin and vesicular lesions in healed skin
Edema of healthy skin surrounding the burn wound
Excessive burn wound drainage, odor
Pale, boggy, dry, or crusted granulation tissue
Sloughing of grafts and wound blisters after closure

Box 13-3
Potential Systemic Signs of Sepsis in the Child With Burns

Altered level of consciousness (irritability or lethargy)
Changes in vital signs (tachycardia, tachypnea, persistent fever, hypotension)
Increased fluid requirements
Oliguria
Gastrointestinal dysfunction (diarrhea, vomiting, abdominal distention, paralytic ileus)
Fever (>40° C) or hypothermia in presence of other symptoms
Hyperglycemia

Cal/m^{2}BSA/day to provide for calories to heal the burn ("burn" calories).

Although some nutritional intake can be provided parenterally, parenteral nutrition is not the ideal method of feeding for a variety of reasons and is associated with a higher complication rate than use of the gut for feeding. Enteral nutrition should be initiated as soon as possible following the burn, ideally within 24 hours of the burn. Use of the gut for nutrition decreases translocation of gram-negative bacteria and endotoxin from the gut and reduces the risk of infection.

Oral feedings will provide adequate nutrition in children with burns covering less than 15% of the TBSA. In children with larger burns, tube feedings are usually necessary to meet nutritional goals. Transpyloric feeding is preferred in the neurologically depressed patient, since the risk of vomiting and aspiration is reduced. Tube feedings should be started with a slow infusion rate (1 to 2 ml/kg/hr) and increased as tolerated every 4 to 8 hours until the target number of calories is provided. The head of the child's bed should be elevated, and gastric residual volume should be checked every 4 hours. Infusion pumps should be used to ensure a consistent volume and feeding rate. Continuous feeding is better tolerated than bolus feedings.

The ideal composition of enteral nutrition for children with burns has not been determined. There is evidence that enteral formulas containing specific proteins (glutamine and arginine), fats (omega-3 fatty acids), and other components (zinc and vitamins A and C) may be particularly beneficial.

Late Complications of Burns

Joint contractures and hypertrophic scars may develop following burn injury. Contractures will impair movement of extremities and are much easier to prevent than to treat. This prevention must begin during the acute phase of burn care, through neutral positioning of joints and use of passive range-of-motion exercises.

The child's neck should be kept in neutral position or slightly extended. If burns involve the anterior side of the neck, the use of standard pillows should be avoided. Doughnut pillows may be used in place of standard pillows to keep the neck extended and prevent flexion of the neck at the area of the burn.

When burns involve the upper extremities, these extremities should be splinted in neutral position. Deep axillary burns are likely to heal with contractures; therefore the arms should be splinted and positioned at a 90-degree angle from the child's body.

When burns involve the lower extremities, these extremities also should be splinted in neutral position. The foot should be positioned at a 90-degree angle from the leg, avoiding flexion or foot-drop. The knees should be extended, and the hips should not be flexed.

Active and passive range-of-motion exercises are crucial to maintenance of proper joint function. Although the rehabilitative process may be interrupted by grafting procedures, physical therapy should resume as soon as the graft is stabilized.

Hypertrophic scars (keloids) may occur with any partial-thickness or full-thickness burn. These scars can be very disfiguring and contribute to joint contractures. Preventive measures include excision and grafting of deep burns and the use of pressure garments on both the donor sites and grafted and ungrafted burns for approximately 1 year after the injury.

Suggested Readings

Ashburn MA: Burn pain: the management of procedure-related pain, *J Burn Care Rehab* 16:365-371, 1995.

Baxter CR, Shires GT: Physiological response to crystalloid resuscitation of severe burns, *Ann NY Acad Sci* 150:874-893, 1968.

Carvajal JF: Resuscitation of the burned child. In Carvajal HF, Parks DH, editors: *Burns in children: pediatric burn management,* Chicago, 1988, Year Book Medical Publishers.

Cortiella J, Marvin JA: Management of the pediatric burn patient, *Nurs Clin North Am* 32:311-329, 1997.

Crawley T: Childhood injury: significance and prevention strategies, *J Pediatr Nurs* 11:225-232, 1996.

Dietch EA: Nutritional support of the burn patient, *Crit Care Clin* 11:735-750, 1995.

Gordon M, Goodwin CW: Burn management: initial assessment, management, and stabilization, *Nurs Clin North Am* 32:237-249, 1997.

Hildreth M, Carvajal HF: Caloric requirements in burned children: a simple formula to estimate daily caloric requirements, *J Burn Care Rehabil* 3:78-86, 1982.

Pruitt BA Jr: Fluid and electrolyte replacement in the burned patient, *Surg Clin North Am* 58:1291-1312, 1978.

Pruitt BA Jr et al: Burn wound infections: current status, *World J Surg* 22:135-145, 1998.

Walker AR: Emergency department management of house fire burns and carbon monoxide poisoning in children, *Curr Opin Pediatr* 8:239-242, 1996.

Index

Selection of Proper Pediatric Resuscitation Equipment

Color on Broselow Pediatric Resus Tape	Infant (3-7 kg) RED	Small Child (8-11 kg) PURPLE	Child (12-14 kg) YELLOW	Child (14-17 kg) WHITE	Child (18-22 kg) BLUE	Young Adult (24-30 kg) ORANGE	Young Adult (32-34 kg +) GREEN
Bag-valve device	Infant	Child	Child	Child	Child	Child/adult	Adult
O₂ mask	Newborn	Pediatric	Pediatric	Pediatric	Pediatric	Adult	Adult
Oral airway	Infant/small child	Small child	Child	Child	Child/small adult	Child/small adult	Medium adult
Laryngoscope blade	0-1 straight	1 straight	2 straight or curved	2 straight or curved	2 straight or curved	2-3 straight or curved	3 straight or curved
ET tubes	Premie 2.5 mm uncuffed Term 3.0 mm uncuffed Infant 3.5 mm uncuffed	4.0 mm uncuffed	4.5 mm uncuffed	5.0 mm uncuffed	5.5 mm uncuffed	6.0 mm cuffed	6.5 mm cuffed
ET tube length (cm at lip)	10-10.5 cm	11-12 cm	12.5-13.5 cm	14-15 cm	15.5-16.5 cm	17-18 cm	18.5-19.5 cm
Stylet	6 Fr.	6 Fr.	6 Fr.	6 Fr.	14 Fr.	14 Fr.	14 Fr.
Suction	8 Fr.	8 Fr.	8-10 Fr.	10 Fr.	10 Fr.	10 Fr.	12 Fr.
BP cuff	Newborn-infant	Infant-child	Child	Child	Child	Child-adult	Adult
IV: Catheter	22-24 G	20-24 G	18-22 G	18-22 G	18-20 G	18-20 G	16-20 G
Butterfly	23-25 G	23-25 G	21-23 G	21-23 G	21-23 G	21-22 G	18-21 G
NG tube	5-8 Fr.	8-10 Fr.	10 Fr.	10-12 Fr.	12-14 Fr.	14-18 Fr.	18 Fr.
Urinary catheter	5-8 Fr.	8-10 Fr.	10 Fr.	10-12 Fr.	10-12 Fr.	12 Fr.	12 Fr.
Chest tube	10-12 Fr.	16-20 Fr.	20-24 Fr.	20-24 Fr.	24-32 Fr.	28-32 Fr.	32-40 Fr.

From Hazinski MF: *Nursing care of the critically ill child*, ed 2, St Louis, 1992, Mosby; modified from *Broselow Pediatric Resusciation Tape*, Hickory, NC, Broselow Medical Technologies.